An Introduction to
Children
with
Language Disorders

Second Edition

Vicki A. Reed

The University of Sydney
Sydney, Australia

Merrill, an imprint of
Macmillan College Publishing Company
New York

Maxwell Macmillan Canada
Toronto

Maxwell Macmillan International
New York   Oxford   Singapore   Sydney

Cover art: Student artwork by Danielle Coble of Indian Mound
  Elementary School, Marion, Ohio
Editor: Ann Castel Davis
Production Editor: Jonathan Lawrence
Art Coordinator: Lorraine Woost
Photo Editor: Anne Vega
Text Designer: Rebecca Bobb
Cover Designer: Cathleen Norz
Production Buyer: Pamela D. Bennett
Illustrations: Steve Botts

This book was set in Garamond by Compset, Inc., and was
printed and bound by Book Press, Inc., a Quebecor America
Book Group Company. The cover was printed by Lehigh Press,
Inc.

Macmillan College Publishing Company
866 Third Avenue
New York, NY 10022

Macmillan College Publishing Company is part of the
Maxwell Communication Group of Companies.

Maxwell Macmillan Canada, Inc.
1200 Eglinton Avenue East, Suite 200
Don Mills, Ontario M3C 3N1

Library of Congress Cataloging-in-Publication Data

Reed, Vicki.
    An introduction to children with language disorders /
  Vicki A. Reed.—2nd ed.
       p.   cm.
    Includes bibliographical references and index.
    ISBN 0-02-399150-X
    1. Language disorders in children.   I. Title.
  RJ496.L35R44   1994
  618.92′855—dc20   93-2404
                                                         CIP

Printing: 6 7 8 9   Year: 8

Photo credits: pp. 3, 36, 61, 95, 139, 153, 230, 251, 442 by Todd
Yarrington/Macmillan; p. 26 by Don Franklin; pp. 34, 54, 63, 105,
117, 211, 274, 277, 290, 318, 352 by Anne Vega/Macmillan; pp.
109, 169, 257, 401, 456 by Barbara Schwartz/Macmillan; p. 192
by Linda Peterson/Macmillan; pp. 308, 385 by Larry Hamill/
Macmillan; p. 364 by Paul Conklin; pp. 377, 435 by Tom Watson/
Macmillan; p. 415 by Dan Floss/Macmillan.

To Monnie and Meeanne
and the children who managed to generate
such creative names for one amazing woman

Preface

Language is the most powerful, fascinating skill that humans possess. It affects educational achievements, human relationships, and entire life-styles. Without language, we never would have known the great ideas of the world. Language has been a catalytic factor in starting and stopping wars. Yet, despite its power, most of us rarely think about our abilities with language. We take our skills with it very much for granted until these skills are lost to us or until our proficiencies with language are disrupted.

When we look at what is involved in language learning, we see a complex interaction among cognitive, physiological, linguistic, psychological, and sociological factors. Although language is an extremely complex phenomenon, most children seem to learn it easily. But, for those children who do not, the impact on their lives can be profoundly debilitating. A language disorder in a child can alter the child's relationships with caregivers, undermine academic success, disturb interpersonal relationships, limit vocational possibilities, and generally isolate the child from the mainstream of society.

This book is about children who do not acquire language normally. It is an introductory text primarily for students who are learning about children's language disorders to help children with language problems. Individuals presently working with such children will also find the book a valuable resource.

In this second edition we continue to take the position that neither the traditional etiological approach nor the noncategorical approach to children's language disorders is, by itself, sufficient to describe the complex problems presented by these children. However, we believe each approach has something to contribute to our understanding of children with language disorders. Because the book is about children with language disorders, this edition has retained an organization that does not lump the children and their language behaviors together. And, as with the first edition, we believe our discussions of the children and their language go far beyond the usual discussions organized around the etiological approach, including information normally not found in books organized around the noncategorical approach.

The book continues to be divided into three parts. Part One consists of three chapters that review normal aspects of language. Part Two begins with a chapter providing an overview of children's language disorders. This chapter is followed by nine chapters that focus on language performances often encountered with different populations of children. As with the first edition, each chapter provides an overview, followed by a discussion of issues related to and descriptions of the language performance of these children and a section on intervention implications. Part Three addresses general principles and practices related to assessment and intervention for children with language disorders.

In revising the book, we have updated the information presented. Chapters on language and children with mental retardation, learning disabilities, autism, and hearing impairments continue to be found in this edition. The chapters addressing the language of bilingual-bicultural children and language-disordered adolescents remain, too. But we also did some rearranging and adding. We added a chapter on youngsters with specific language impairments and one on children with acquired language disorders. We combined formerly separate chapters on language and gifted children and language and children with physi-

v

cal disabilities into one chapter, "Language and Other Special Populations of Children." In this chapter we then included a section on language related to children with visual impairments, a frequently neglected topic in discussions of children's language disorders. In fact, in the first edition, we believed that we had addressed topics not often encountered in books on children with language disorders, such as children with physical handicaps, gifted children, and adolescents with language disorders. In this second edition, we retained these unique features and added others.

Help with writing this text came from many quarters. Our reviewers—Joyce E. Bernstein, Alabama A&M University; Judy Flanagin, University of South Dakota; Jennifer Ryan Hsu, William Paterson College; Karyn Bobkoff Katz, University of Akron; and Peter B. Smith, Jr., Northern Michigan University—offered suggestions and comments that helped to improve this edition. Some people were exceptionally good at helping the author and contributors maintain sanity and at providing a reminder that other things existed besides the book. But especially to Mariana, Susan, and Tony, we are grateful, even if we did not always appear so. Gaye Gurney also played a key role. Armed with quiet competence and gentle assertiveness, she managed to "keep the wolves at bay" long enough for the project to reach completion. Thank you to all of you.

Vicki A. Reed

Contents

11

Language-Disordered Adolescents   318

12

Children with Acquired Language Disorders   364

Steven H. Long

13

Language and Other Special Populations of Children   385

Steven H. Long

Part One

Aspects of Normal Language

· Chapter 1 ·

An Introduction to Language

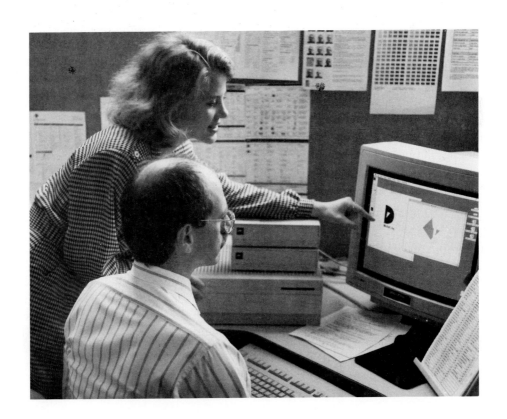

OBJECTIVES

Upon completion of this chapter, the reader should be able to:

► Define language and speech and understand the difference between them.

► Understand the phonological, semantic, syntactic, morphological, and pragmatic components of oral language.

► Describe various communication modes.

► Define metalinguistics.

► Discuss how oral language relates to reading and writing, literacy, and education.

As a species, humans survive by cooperating. In one of the near-classic books on language, Hayakawa (1964) wrote, "Cooperation within a species (and sometimes with other species) is essential to the survival of most living creatures" (p. 10). This cooperative behavior is facilitated by communication because it provides a way of sharing what is happening to or within one organism with another. As humans, we have the capacity to acquire and use a complex communication system of symbolic processes called language. Language is a powerful and effective communication system. In fact, language allows us to draw on the information of others in order to increase our own knowledge, thereby making it unnecessary for us to experience personally all that we know. Classroom lectures and textbooks are common examples of the ways humans share their experiences and increase their knowledge through language. Language is also one of the ways through which we establish our social identities, and how we use language influences, in part, how we are evaluated as individuals in our society (Burroughs & Tomblin, 1990; Gumperz & Cook-Gumperz, 1982; Hudson, 1980).

Our concern here is with this system of symbolic processes called language and the ways in which children use or do not use it. Before we talk about children's language disorders, we first examine normal aspects of language. In this chapter, we discuss the differences between speech and language, the components of language systems, the relationship between understanding and using language, and the relationship between language and education.

LANGUAGE AND SPEECH DEFINED

The terms *language* and *speech* are not synonymous, although they are related to each other. **Language** is a *code* in which we make specific symbols stand for something else. Bloom (1988) defines language as "a code whereby ideas about the world are represented through a conventional system of arbitrary signals for communication" (p. 2). According to this definition, coded symbols refer to real things, concepts, or ideas. The things that the symbols represent are the **referents**. Hayakawa (1964) has analogized that a linguistic symbol is to the referent as a map is to the territory it represents. Furthermore, the symbols chosen for the code are *arbitrary*. As Hayakawa (1964) points out, there is *"no necessary connection between the symbol and that which is symbolized. . . .* Symbols and things symbolized are independent of each other; nevertheless, we all have a way of feeling as if, and sometimes acting as if, these were necessary connections" (p. 27). In our code system there is no reason why an animal with four legs that is noted for tail wagging and barking is labeled a "dog." Such an animal could as easily be coded as a "sloot," and perhaps it is in a code system other than English. Although the symbols are arbitrary, the symbols and their appropriate referents must be mutually agreed on by the members of a community using the code if the code is to be meaningful. In this sense, language is a *convention* (Bloom, 1988).

In addition to being an arbitrary code, language is a system in which *rules* or regularities guide what coded symbols may be combined with other symbols and in what order, and what symbols can be used in what situations. These rules or regularities are predictable and can be used to identify what are and are not acceptable uses of language. For example, in the English language, the word order in the sentence "The ball is not red" is acceptable and considered correct, while the word order in the sentence "The ball not is red" violates accepted rules even though the words in the two sentences are identical. The number of rules that delimit a language is finite. Once these finite rules are learned, however, a person can then generate an infinite variety of meaningful messages by combining and recombining the symbols according to the agreed-on rules. The system of rules that results in the ability to produce an infinite number of expressions gives language its *creative* feature. By applying systematic rules, a language user can generate expressions never used or heard before, and another user of the same language can understand those expressions by employing the same rules.

Because a language consists of regularities or sets of rules, members of a language community (including children) must learn the rules and induce the regularities in order to use the language. Among the rules that must be learned are those that determine who can say what to whom and how. Language is, therefore, a *learned* behavior.

Speech, on the other hand, is the actual behavior of producing the code by making vocal sound patterns appropriate for the language (Hubbell, 1985). It involves the sensorimotor processes by which language users reproduce the coded symbols that are stored in their central nervous systems so that others can hear the symbols. Consequently, speech production requires the neurological control of physical movements to create sound patterns. These sound patterns are produced as a result of the coordinated, rapid muscular activities of the chest (which controls the lung action), the larynx (which houses the vocal folds), and the throat and mouth (in which movements of the tongue, lips, and palate occur). Speech includes such things as how rapidly or how rhythmically one talks, how well one makes specific sounds of the language (e.g., "s" or "th"), how one raises or lowers the pitch for intonation or inflection, and how pleasing or dis-

pleasing the quality of one's voice is. *Language is the code; speech is the sensorimotor production of that code.*

As we indicated, language and speech are closely related even though they are not the same. The two sentences "The dog is black and white" and "Is the dog black and white?" consist of the same sounds. However, the order of the sounds, and therefore the words, in the two sentences is different, as is the resultant meaning of the two sentences. By producing the sounds in a different order, the word order in the sentences is changed, which then alters the meaning. Furthermore, in the sentences "I want it to *fit*" and "I want it to *sit*," a child must only alter speech movements slightly to produce the difference between "f" and "s." Yet, the meaning of the two sentences is quite different based on the one sound variation.

It is possible for a child's code system (language) to be intact but for the child to have a problem speaking (speech). For example, a child who says "w" for "r" might say the words "reads" and "weeds" the same way, but from the context we can tell that the child knows that the words mean different things:

1. The boy "weads" the books.
2. The boy weeds the lawn.

It is also possible for a child's speech production to be intact but for the child's language system to be deficient. As examples, a child who says "I want it no to go," "The gooses are flying," or "I don't want for you to sick" with well-pronounced sounds in a highly fluent manner is demonstrating problems with language, not speech.

COMPONENTS OF LANGUAGE

Spoken languages are made up of components. Some authors call these *elements*; others call them *parameters*; still others call them *aspects*. Whatever they are labeled, the intent is to break language into its parts in order to discuss and describe it. There are five basic components of language: (1) phonology, (2) semantics, (3) syntax, (4) morphology, and (5) pragmatics. Each of these components is part of a system and is, therefore, governed by regularities and sets of rules that all speakers of a specific language must learn if they are to communicate effectively. Although we can discuss each of these components separately, they are all interrelated in language functioning, as we will see in later chapters.

Phonology

One aspect of **phonology** is concerned with the sounds that comprise a language and the rules that determine how the sounds are used. (This is sometimes referred to as **segmental** phonology.) When we look at these sounds, we see that some differentiate one word from another. That is, they distinguish meaning. For example, in the word pair "bin/pin," the main sound differences occur in the initial positions of the words. Although these words differ by only one speech sound, this sound difference results in two words, each with its own distinct meaning. This is an example of a **phoneme**. In a broad sense, a phoneme conveys differences in word meanings. However, we rarely produce each phoneme in exactly the same way every time we use it. To illustrate, the "l" in "light" is usually produced differently than the "l" in "cold," even though both words contain the phoneme "l." Hubbell (1985) defines a phoneme as "a set of speech sounds considered the same for the purpose of distinguishing between words. To put it the other way around, the differences between versions of a particular phoneme are ignored" (p. 25).

The exact number of phonemes in American English is difficult to determine because there are acceptable variations within the language. Some of these variations result from individual differences in pronunciation, while others result from dialectal differences. Most estimates of the number of phonemes suggest that there are 40 to 46 (Dale, 1976; Fairbanks, 1960; Owens, 1992).

One problem that becomes painfully clear as we watch children attempting to learn to read is the lack of consistency between the way an English sound is said and the way it is written. For example, the letter "c" is pronounced as a "k" sound in "cat" and as an "s" sound in "center," and the long vowel "a" is spelled "ay" in "bay," "a" in "fade," and "ea" in "break." Trying to use the usual alphabetic symbols to write English as it is said is very difficult. However, the International Phonetic Alphabet (IPA) is a system that has a correspondence between a written symbol and a sound. That is, a spoken sound is represented by one consistent printed symbol. In the IPA, for example, the symbol /s/ represents the "s" sound in "sun" and "cement," the symbol /ʤ/ represents the "j" sound in "jest," "sage," and "drudge," and the symbol /θ/ represents the "th" sound in "thumb" and "tooth." In using the IPA, a word in the language is transcribed on paper as a speaker produces it. Therefore, the speech of a child who uses the "th" sound instead of the "s" sound in words like "sun" and "cement" would be written as /θʌn/ and /θəmɛnt/. When utterances are noted in IPA, the transcription is placed between two slash marks as in /sʌn/ for "son." Occasionally in this book, some sounds and words will be indicated by IPA symbols in order to avoid possible confusion with other sounds. To help with the few instances in which these IPA symbols are used, the IPA with key words for pronunciation is shown in Appendix A.

Phonemes can be classified as either vowels or consonants. The production of *vowels* requires that the air from the lungs pass relatively unobstructed out of the mouth once the air vibrates the vocal folds. The various positions of the tongue and lips change the size and shape of the mouth and result in the production of specific vowels. In contrast to vowels, production of *consonants* requires that differing degrees of obstruction be placed in the path of the air flow from the lungs. The placement and movement of the lips and tongue are primarily responsible for the obstruction of the air flow. This obstruction can be complete, as for the /p/ or /g/ phonemes, or much less so, as for /w/ or /r/.

The way in which the air is obstructed for different consonants gives them specific characteristics, such as the complete obstruction for /p/ and /g/ that then classifies them as stop plosives or the less complete obstruction combined with a high-pitched (high-frequency) hiss of air for sounds like /s/ and "sh" /ʃ/. The latter sounds are classified as *fricatives,* the term coming from the word "friction." Still other sounds are produced by completely blocking the air and then creating friction noises. These sounds, like "ch" /tʃ/ and "j" /ʤ/, are called *affricates.* Unlike vowels, for which production always requires vocal-fold vibration, production of some consonants, such as /f/, requires no vocal-fold vibration. Conversely, production of other consonants, such as /v/, does necessitate vibration of the vocal folds. An additional characteristic of each consonant is created by the place in the mouth where the air flow is restricted. For some sounds, the air is obstructed by the lips, as for /p/ and /b/; for others the tongue tip is raised to the roof of the mouth, like /l/, /n/, and /t/; and for still others the back of the tongue is raised, such as /k/ and /g/. Finally, a few consonants, like /m/ and /n/, have air flowing into the nasal cavity, although for most English consonants the air is directed only into the mouth. When these characteristics are combined, each consonant can be described in terms of its unique combination of features.

Just as each language has a limited set of phonemes that comprises the sound system, each language has its own set of rules governing which phonemes can be combined with other phonemes in what order. In English, "ksunt" is not a word and never could be, even though all the individual sounds that make up the word are acceptable English phonemes. On the other hand, "skunt," which is also not an English word, potentially could be a word in the language. One of the phonological rules of English permits the /k/ phoneme to follow the /s/, but at the beginnings of words /s/ cannot follow /k/. However, it is permissible for both the /sk/ and /ks/ sequences to occur at the ends of words ("husk" and "books"). Children learning the phonological system of their language must learn not only to use the acceptable set of phonemes but also the rules for combining these phonemes sequentially into words.

Descriptions of children's uses of sounds in words are somtimes done in terms of the *phonological processes* they are demonstrating. For example, if a child regularly substitutes consonants produced in the front of the mouth (e.g., /t/, /d/) for those that are supposed to be produced in the back of the mouth (e.g., /k/, /g/), the child might be said to be using a fronting process. Similarly, if a child regularly omits one or more consonants when they occur together as **clusters**, as in "fea*st*," so the production sounds more like "feet" or /fis/, the child might be described as using a cluster reduction process.

The **prosodic features** of a language (also known as **suprasegmental** phonology) refer to the melodic and rhythmic aspects of the phonological system, including stress, juncture, and pitch (intonation), and they are superimposed on and used simultaneously with the sounds of the language. Just as the phonemes vary among languages, different languages have differing rules governing the use of prosodic features. *Stress* is the relative loudness with which certain syllables in words are produced. For example, in the word "sofa," the vowel in the first syllable is said more loudly than the vowel in the second syllable. However, in the word "adore," the first-syllable vowel is weaker than the second. The two word combinations "white house" and "White House" contain exactly the same sounds, but one of the distinctions in meaning between the house that is white and the president's residence is the stress pattern used. Additionally, when speakers refer to the house that is white, they produce a small catch or break between the adjective and noun. When referring to the president's house, no such catch occurs and the two words are blended together. Finally, *pitch,* or *intonation,* patterns are superimposed on sequences of sounds. The sentence "He said that word" could be said as a statement of fact, in which case the speaker's pitch would drop at the end. However, the same sentence could be expressed with surprise and amazement, in which case the speaker's pitch would rise at the end. In both examples, the sequence of phonemes remains the same, but a difference in meaning is signaled by the pitch variation. Typically, it is the combination of prosodic features that helps transmit the meaning of utterances creat d by sequences of speech sounds.

Semantics

Semantics deals with the referents for words and the meanings of utterances. At a basic level, semantics involves the vocabulary of a language, or the **lexicon**. Sequences of phonemes combine to form words. The words are then used to represent items, attributes, concepts, or experiences. As we know, many words can have multiple meanings, depending on the situations in which they are used. "Girdle" can refer to an item used to compact flesh or the process of encircling another item. "Square" can mean a geometric shape composed of four right angles and four equal sides, a person whose thinking and actions are somewhat out of date, or the action of creating a right angle. In identifying the meanings of words, we typically think of the dictionary meanings. These dictionary meanings are the **referential meanings** or denotative meanings of words. However, words may have connotative or emotionally associated meanings. These meanings can, in fact, be so strong as to produce physical responses to the word. To many, the word "snake" can create chills even though the denotative meaning of the word refers to one of several kinds of limbless reptiles.

A word and its referents can trigger associations with another word and its referents. In some instances, the associated words belong to the same category as the original word. For example, the word "cow" may trigger the thought of "pig," "horse," and "sheep." In other instances, the associated word or words may be the category for the original word—"animal" or "farm animal."

Words can be categorized and recategorized through the process of abstraction. In the process of categorizing words, we identify or abstract the similarities among the referents for the words and use the similar characteristics to form another category that is also labeled. Hayakawa (1964) used the example of Bessie the cow to demonstrate the categorization and abstraction of referents. One of the lowest levels of categorization of Bessie is that of "cow," some of the abstracted characteristics of which include animal, four legs, tail, milk giver, and "moo." This category of abstracted qualities ignores the individual differences among all the other cows that make up the group and focuses only on the similar characteristics. The similar characteristics or attributes form the category "cow." However, cows have characteristics similar to those of chickens, pigs, and horses. Those abstracted similar characteristics can be categorized and labeled as "livestock." The term "livestock" becomes a *superordinate* category for cows, chickens, and pigs. In turn, livestock is similar to all other salable farm items, and based on these attributes a new category of "assets" is abstracted. Livestock is now *subordinate* to the superordinate category of assets. The abstracted similar attributes of all possible assets allow the formation of a new category—"wealth."

The process of abstraction and categorization of referential attributes has taken us from Bessie the cow to wealth. Each time a new category was created, we increased our level of abstraction. Bessie is a tangible object that can be directly seen and touched. Bessie has relatively concrete referents. With each level of abstraction we moved further and further away from the **concrete,** or that which can be perceived by the senses. "Wealth" is an abstract concept. Its attributes cannot be perceived by the senses; therefore, its referents are said to be relatively **abstract.**

The use of superordinate and subordinate categories in the lexicon helps to bring order to our experiences. By categorizing and labeling our experiences, it is not necessary for us to treat each experience as a totally new one. Because we have finite memories, this skill is efficient and allows us to store cognitively more information than if it were not used. Unfortunately, we sometimes fail to acknowledge that categorization is based primarily on similarities, and our grouping of attributes may become inflexible when the differences in these attributes are forgotten. Nevertheless, children learning the semantic system of their language must acquire a categorization system somewhat consistent with that of others in the language community. Much of the educational system does, in fact, center on teaching children the categorization of attributes and how to move from superordinate categories to subordinate categories and vice versa. Teachers develop units of instruction—on colors, animals, and transportation, for example. How a transportation unit might be categorized is shown in Figure 1.1. Again, we have moved from concrete to abstract and vice versa through a system of superordinate and subordinate categories.

Not only does the semantic component of language deal with the lexicon, it also involves the meanings conveyed by the relations among words. This aspect of semantics is termed **relational meaning**. In fact, some words, such as "an" or "if," really take on meaning only as they are used with other words. Furthermore, when the individual meanings of words interrelate in a multiword statement, the statement

FIGURE 1.1 An Example of the Categorization of Attributes in a Transportation Unit.

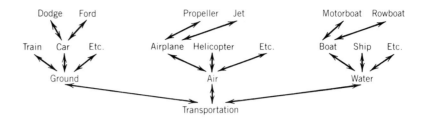

takes on a meaning that goes beyond the separate words. This meaning is the statement's **propositional meaning** and is partly derived from the logical relationships inherent in the sequence of words. In the sentences "The boy climbs the tree" and "The tree climbs the boy" the words are identical. The first sentence is plausible while the second is not, even though the individual words within the sentences retain their usual referents. The order in which the words are arranged imposes certain restrictions on the logical relationships among the words, and these restrictions are violated in the second sentence. Therefore, semantics is not independent of syntax, the rules affecting word order. Kempson (1977) writes:

> In all languages, words can be arranged to form sentences, and the meaning of those sentences is dependent on the meaning of the words it contains [*sic*]. But this is not a simple accumulation process. *Cats chase dogs* and *Dogs chase cats* do not mean the same, though the words in each sentence are identical. And sometimes word-order will change meaning, but sometimes not. *The opera house had never been closed before* and *Never before had the opera house been closed,* like *Cats chase dogs* and *Dogs chase cats,* contain identical words but in a different order, but unlike the latter, this pair do [*sic*] not differ in meaning. (p. 2)

Earlier, in discussing semantics, reference was made to the *multiple meanings* of many individual words. In situations where a word may have several different referents, we typically determine its meaning from the contexts in which it is used and its relationship to other words uttered. We can use the word "table" to illustrate the derivation of meaning by employing cues regarding the word's logical relationship to other words in a sentence. Although "table"

has several meanings, we can surmise from the sentence "The table was too small to fit six chairs around" that the referent for the word is a piece of furniture; from the sentence "As the rains continued the table continued to rise" that the referent is probably a water level; and from the sentence "The table contained numbers she had never seen before" that the referent for the word is an organized grouping of figures such as those of an accountant. However, using the word in some sentences may not aid in deriving the word's meaning. For example, the sentence "Read about the table" gives us no clue as to the meaning of "table." In these instances we must depend on previous utterances or the situation in which the sentence was expressed to determine the referent of "table." Verbal humor is frequently based on multiple meanings of words.

Two other aspects of semantics involve **figurative language** and **inferential meaning**. Figurative language goes beyond meaning that can be derived from literal interpretations of phrases. For example, "It's raining cats and dogs" is implausible if interpreted at its literal level. Metaphors, similes, proverbs, and idioms all involve figurative meanings. Inferential meaning refers to meaning that is derived not from what is explicitly stated, but from the logical relationships of statements. As an example, consider the following sequential statements:

> Sally went to the restaurant and ordered from the standard menu. She loved her tacos and refried beans.

The kind of restaurant is not explicitly stated. Yet, if we were asked the kind of restaurant Sally went to, we would be able to derive sufficient information through inferential meanings to increase the odds of making a correct, educated guess of a Mexican restaurant.

Syntax

All languages have systems of **syntax**, or sets of rules that govern how words are to be sequenced in utterances and how the words in an utterance are related. Phonemes combine to form words, and words combine to form **phrases** and sentences. In the same way that phonological rules govern what phonemes can be combined in what order, syntactic rules determine what words can be combined in what order to convey meaning.

A basic English syntactic rule is the subject + verb + object sequence, which places the actor first, followed by a description of the action, followed by the receiver of the action. Although the words in the sentences "The boy hits the girl" and "The girl hits the boy" are identical, reversal of the word order signals a different meaning. Word combinations typically convey more specific information than any of the individual words alone do. For example, a child who utters the word "milk" may be indicating that the item is present, may simply be labeling it, may wish to have more of the item, or may not want it at all. If the child uses the utterance "more milk," additional specificity is obtained, although the child may be indicating that a larger quantity is present or that an increase in the amount is requested. But when the child says, "I want more milk," the child's meaning is specific. If the child says, "More milk I want," the listener may be able to understand the child's wish, but the utterance violates the syntactic rules for the intended meaning. In most instances, however, precise sequencing of words using correct syntactic rules is essential if the exact intended meaning of an utterance is to be conveyed. The words in the sentences "When she was 10 years old she reported that a dog had bitten her" and "She reported that a dog had bitten her when she was 10 years old" are identical, but the meanings of the two sentences are different, depending on the location of the clause "when she was 10 years old."

Combining words provides a way of expressing an infinite number of ideas. Syntactic rules are, therefore, a basis of the creative aspects of language previously referred to. According to Chomsky (1972), once one has acquired these rules, "one is able, with greater or less facility, to produce such expressions on an appropriate occasion, despite their novelty and independently of detectable stimulus configurations, and to be understood by others who share this still mysterious ability" (p. 100). This view is fundamental to the linguistic theory called *generative transformational grammar* (Chomsky, 1957, 1965).

The theory is *generative* in that once syntactic rules are learned, numerous sentences or phrases can be generated and, thus, numerous ideas can be expressed. Table 1.1 shows a number of the multiple phrases and ideas that are possible with knowledge of a single syntactic rule—article + attributive + noun sequence. The theory is *transformational* in that, with a set of operational rules, sentences can be changed by adding, deleting, and/or rearranging the words to derive sentences of various types. To illustrate, the sentence "The girl is riding a horse" can, by rearranging the words, be transformed into the question "Is the girl riding a horse?" or, by adding the word "not" in the correct place, transformed into the negative "The girl is not riding a horse." In both transformations the meaning conveyed by the first sentence is altered. However, both transformed sentences are based on the structure of the original sentence "The girl is riding a horse."

In transformational grammar there is a distinction between surface structure and deep structure. **Deep structure** relates to meaning, or the meaningful base that underlies a string of words. It also involves the phrase structure rules required to convey the meaning. **Surface structure** is the string of words we produce. Perhaps the easiest example to differentiate the

TABLE 1.1   Use of a Syntactic Rule to Generate Multiple Phrases

Article	+	Attributive	+	Noun
The		Pretty		Dress
A		Big		Doll
An		Old		Apple
A		Round		Face
The		Tremendous		Crowd
An		Exhaustive		Experience

two structures is the active/passive sentence contrast. If our intended meaning is to convey that the specific piece of fruit (apple) was masticated and ingested (eat) by a specific individual (Simon), this would be our deep structure and we would know the phrase structure rules to produce it. We have at least two options at the surface structure—"Simon ate the apple" (active) and "The apple was eaten by Simon" (passive). Alternatively, we can sometimes generate two possible meanings with one surface structure—"Fighting men can be dangerous."

As previously stated, a basic English syntactic structure is the subject + verb + object sequence in sentences. This sentence structure is called, alternatively, the **kernel sentence**, *base structure,* or *phrase structure* (Lee, 1974), and is often defined as a simple, active, affirmative, declarative sentence. The kernel sentence and its accompanying subject + verb + object relationship is a fundamental structure underlying other sentence types. Lee (1974) stated that "throughout the transformational processes the base structure of actor-action-acted upon remains a kind of constant, an invariant under transformation" (p. 4). Table 1.2 demonstrates several transformations that can be made to the kernel sentence "The horse eats the hay."

There are numerous transformations of the kernel sentence structure, including several forms of the three already mentioned. For example, the following sentences are negative, but each requires the application of different operational rules to arrive at the transformed sentence:

The ball is not red.

The girl does not run.

The flower is not blooming.

TABLE 1.2   Various Transformations of the Kernel Sentence "The Horse Eats the Hay"

Transformation	Sentence
Negation	The horse does not eat the hay.
Question	Does the horse eat the hay?
Passive	The hay is eaten by the horse.

The same is true for question transformations. Furthermore, English has several types of question forms, some of which require the inclusion of a wh- word:

Is the ball red?

Does the girl run?

Is the flower blooming?

What color is the ball?

When is the girl running?

Why is the flower blooming?

What is this?

The negative and question transformations can sometimes be used together to derive sentences such as these:

Isn't the ball red?

Doesn't the girl run?

Isn't the flower blooming?

Why isn't the flower blooming?

And, in some instances, transformations may involve joining two kernel sentences or embedding one kernel sentence in another, as shown in Figures 1.2 and 1.3.

This discussion has not explained the operations required to make the transformations mentioned, nor have all possible forms of transformations been reviewed. Such a review is not essential in order to understand the basic concepts of how kernel sentences can be altered. However, once the rules for any specific transformation are acquired, the speaker can generate transformed sentences that have never been spoken or heard previously:

Does the robin sing a song?

Does the ball roll?

Does the child fly a kite?

Does a proton revolve around an atom's nucleus?

Unfortunately, Chomsky's generative transformational grammar permitted implausible sentences to be generated. It also did not account for the learnability of all the grammars of the world. That is, the theory was neither sufficiently restrictive nor flexible to ac-

FIGURE 1.2   Tree Diagrams Showing a Transformation That Joins Two Kernel Sentences.
S_1 = The horse eats the hay.
S_2 = The pig eats the corn.
S_3 = The horse eats the hay, but the pig eats the corn.

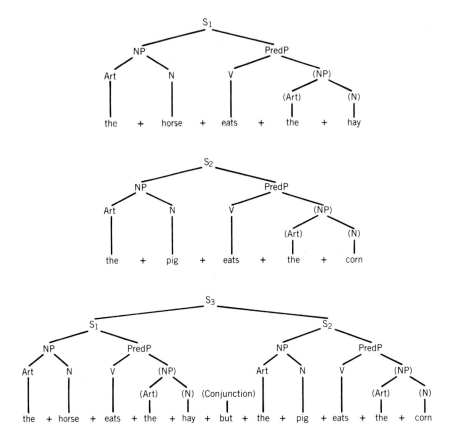

count for the limitations found in grammatical structure, as well as for the creativity and variability evidenced in generating novel utterances (Leonard & Loeb, 1988). Chomsky's (1981) later theory of grammar, *government-binding theory,* attempts to address these difficulties. Government-binding theory has roots in generative transformational grammar theory, and some of the concepts are similar. That is, it is still a grammatical theory that attempts to explain how humans represent syntactic knowledge mentally, it continues to employ concepts of deep and surface structure, and it maintains a focus on rules. We also see tree diagrams used to illustrate the rules. It is not, however, simply a revision of generative transformational grammar. Government-binding theory strives to include descriptions of the constraints in language patterns, guided, in part, by notions of *well-formedness.* Therefore, different rules and principles are employed. It

also emphasizes language learnability. A complete review of government-binding theory is beyond the scope of this chapter. It is sufficient to understand that, as in generative transformational grammar, rules govern how we manage to map meaning through systematic applications of grammatical rules.

Morphology

Morphology deals with the rules for deriving various word forms and the rules for using grammatical markers or inflections. These derived word forms include plurals, verb tenses, adverbs, and superlatives. For example, consider the number of forms for the words "drive" and "gentle":

drives (either the third person singular present tense verb or the plural form of motor paths)

FIGURE 1.3   Tree Diagrams Showing a Transformation That Embeds One Kernel Sentence in Another. S_1 = The girl sees the boy. S_2 = The girl is a student. S_3 = The girl who is a student sees the boy.

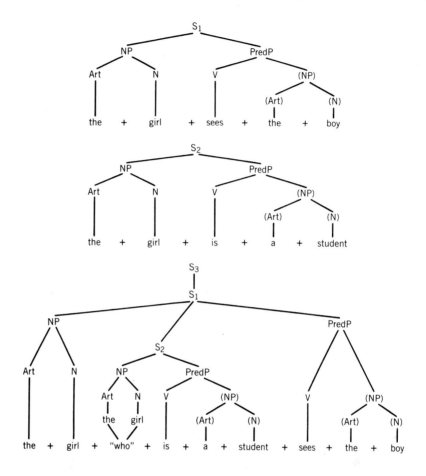

drove

driven

driving (either a verb form or an adjective)

gently

gentleness

gentleman

gentlemanly

ungentlemanly

Because morphology is concerned with sequences of phonemes, it is sometimes discussed as part of the phonological system. Sometimes it is considered part of the semantic system because of the meaning derived from the phoneme sequences, and sometimes it is classified as part of the syntactic system because of the interrelationships among varying word forms, their functions within sentences, and word order. Furthermore, morphology is sometimes considered as a separate component of language because of the unique rules affecting differing word forms.

In all instances, morphology is concerned with meaning, and the "smallest or most elementary meaningful units in a language" are called **morphemes** (O'Malley & Tikofsky, 1972, p. 7). In some instances, the smallest unit or form that conveys meaning is a word, such as "drive" in the previous example. Even though the word is composed of phonemes, none of them is meaningful by itself. The phonemes obtain meaning only when combined to form the word. Therefore, "drive" cannot be broken into smaller units and retain its meaning. "Drive" is a morpheme. In other instances, however, the smallest unit that conveys meaning is not a word. For example, "ing" when added to a verb denotes the progressive tense and its associated meaning. Therefore, when "ing" is added to the verb, it signals a meaning that is somewhat different from the meaning of "drive" alone. While "ing" is not a word, it is still a morpheme.

There are basically two classes of morphemes: roots and affixes. *Roots* are words that cannot be divided into any smaller units, while *affixes* are morphemes that are attached to roots in order to alter meaning. In the word "driving," the root is "drive" and the affix, in this case a suffix, is "ing." In the word "redo," the root is "do" and the affix, in this case a prefix, is "re." As we see in these two examples, sometimes the affix involves deriving a grammatical form and conveying grammatical information, such as "ing" on "drive." Other terms used for such affixes are *inflections, inflectional morphemes, grammatical markers,* and *grammatical inflections*. In other instances, the affix involves deriving an altered word meaning that conveys semantic information, such as the "re" on "do." A term used for these affixes is *derivational morphemes.*

Another classification of morphemes uses the terms **free morphemes** and **bound morphemes** to identify the two different kinds. A free morpheme is able to occur alone in the language. In the previous example, "drive" is a free morpheme because it can occur meaningfully by itself. However, "ing" is a bound morpheme because it cannot occur by itself and be meaningful; it derives its meaning only when attached to another morpheme. Therefore, its function is bound to that of another morpheme. There is a parallel between free morphemes and roots and between bound morphemes and affixes. "Drive" is both a root and a free morpheme, and "ing" is both an affix and a bound morpheme. However, "driving," which is capable of occurring alone, is not a single morpheme but a combination of two morphemes, a free morpheme (root) and a bound morpheme (affix). Words must, therefore, be viewed in terms of the smallest units of meaning they possess ("drive" + "ing") to determine the number and types of morphemes they contain. The word "ungentlemanly" contains two free morphemes ("gentle" and "man") and two bound morphemes ("un" and "ly").

Examples of common rules for attaching bound morphemes to free morphemes include the formation of plural nouns by adding "s" (pronounced as the /s/ sound) to the root noun ("cat" to "cats"), past tense verbs by adding "ed" (pronounced as a syllable "uhd") to the root verb ("bait" to "baited"), superlative adjectives by adding "est" to the root adjective ("short" to "shortest"), and reflexive pronouns by adding "self" to the objective pronoun ("him" to "himself"). However, such rules do not explain the formation of plural nouns for which the "z" sound is used ("home" to "homes"), for which a syllable with "z" (pronounced as "uhz") is used ("house" to "houses"), or for which the entire word changes ("man" to "men"). The examples do not explain past-tense verbs pronounced with a "t" or "d" at the end ("kick" to "kicked" or "comb" to "combed"), superlative adjectives that use a different word ("good" to "best"), or reflexive pronouns that use "selves" ("them" to "themselves"). The concept of allomorphs is needed to explain such variations. An **allomorph** is a variation of a morpheme that does not alter the meaning of the original morpheme. Table 1.3 lists several examples of allomorphs that are used to indicate noun plurals, verb tenses, and verb person and number.

In some cases, the use of allomorphs is determined by specific rules; for example, to form a noun plural when the root ends with a voiceless consonant, like "p," add "s" to the root, except when the voiceless consonant is a fricative or an affricative, like "sh" or "ch," in which case "uhz" is added to the root. However, in English many of the allomorphs to be used are irregular. That is, there are no specific rules governing their application. Why do we pluralize "child" by using "children," and why do we use "was" as a past tense of "be"? Because no rules can be used for the irregularities, they must simply be memorized. Children, in the process of learning the morphology of their language, often overgeneralize the morphological rules and use the rules in place of the irregular allomorphs ("comed" instead of "came," "deers" instead of "deer," and "gooder" instead of "better"). Even adults may have difficulty with some of the irregular allomorphs.

Context and/or syntax are often the only ways to determine the meaning of some irregular allomorphs or to know whether or not an allomorph has been

TABLE 1.3   Examples of Allomorphs for Noun Plurals, Verb Tenses, and Verb Person and Number

Noun Plurals

book	books	("s")
robe	robes	("z")
twitch	twitches	("uhz")
leaf	leaves	

Verb Tenses

kick	kicked	("t")	kicked	("t")
comb	combed	("d")	combed	("d")
eat	ate		eaten	
ring	rang		rung	
do	did		done	
bait	baited	("uhd")	baited	("uhd")
tear	tore		torn	

Verb Person/Number

kick	kicks	("s")
comb	combs	("z")
eat	eats	("s")
ring	rings	("z")
do	does	
have	has	

used correctly. For example, "deer" does not change its form from singular to plural. If "deer" is the subject of a sentence, a verb may indicate whether the noun is singular or plural ("The deer is jumping" or "The deer are jumping"). However, the speaker may have a problem using correctly the "is" and "are" forms of the irregular verb "be," in which case the verb cue may not be reliable. Context then becomes the best cue. Syntax and/or context are also the ways to determine whether or not a speaker is correctly using the possessive form of the singular noun "foot" ("foot's") or incorrectly using a plural marker for the noun ("foots"), because both are pronounced the same way.

Pragmatics

Language is used for specific reasons, and without these there would be no purpose for language. That is, the use of language is aimed at achieving communicative or social functions (McLean & Snyder-McLean, 1978). This aspect of language is referred to as **pragmatics**, and, as Bates (1976) points out, pragmatics concerns the "rules governing the use of language in context" (p. 420). Because the area of pragmatics is concerned with the whys and, therefore, the hows of language use, some prefer to see pragmatics not as a component of language that is equal in status to the other components, such as syntax or semantics, but rather as the "super" component that drives, organizes, and encompasses the other components (Owens, 1992). As Owens (1992) explains, "it is only when the child desires a cookie that he employs the rules of syntax, morphology, phonology, and semantics in order to form his request" (p. 23).

Like the components of language we have discussed previously, the pragmatic aspect is rule governed. Certain ways of using language vary from context to context, and what is socially and culturally acceptable in one situation violates the appropriate rules in another. For example, we might say to a 4-year-old child, "Close the door," but a more appropriate request to an adult peer would be, "Can you close the door?" Wood (1982) writes that the pragmatic aspects of language include:

1. Conveying the intent of the message through appropriate verbal and nonverbal devices for communicative interaction (that is, by selecting content, form, and gestures that fit the context and the situation).
2. Developing language competencies for intrapersonal growth, creativity, and direction and organization of behavior. (p. 24)

Prutting (1982) even described pragmatics as social competence. Children, in the process of learning the form and content of language, must also learn how to vary these aspects to communicate effectively in a variety of situations.

There are a number of elements that make up pragmatics:

1. The various functions and acts that utterances serve.
2. The coherence of sequential statements.
3. The fluency with which messages are delivered.

4. The ability to take turns during dialogues and at the same time maintain topics of conversation.
5. The provision of adequate information for listeners to comprehend spoken messages without supplying redundant information.
6. The responsibility to repair communication breakdowns and request additional information when messages are not understood.
7. The appropriate use of nonverbal communicative cues.
8. The codes or styles of communicative behavior employed in different situations.

Skill in employing these elements, combined with the ability to use the phonological, semantic, syntactic, and morphological systems accurately, embodies what we refer to as *communicative competency* or proficiency.

Some confusion exists in the literature about two terms often used in discussions of pragmatics—*discourse* and *narrative*. For our purposes, **discourse** will be used to refer to the connected flow of language. This frequently relates to conversations and communicative interactions between people, but different kinds of discourse may also occur in speeches or soliloquies. **Narrative** will be used to refer to one form of discourse, that of telling a story. A narrative is a frequently used logical description of a sequence of events. We employ narratives in discourse when describing a movie we have seen or giving an account of what happened when we went shopping. Stories, as in children's fairy tales or novels, are another type of narrative.

One element of language use identified earlier concerns the functions for which language is employed. In some instances, language functions as a means of establishing a human relationship (Halliday, 1975). For example, if we wish to meet a person sitting next to us in an audience, we might ask what time the performance is expected to start even though we already know. The function of the utterance in this instance is not to acquire information, but rather to make contact. The same query, of course, could be made for the purpose of receiving information, and another important function of language is to acquire information (Halliday, 1975). For most adults, messages often serve more than one function at the same time (Chapman, 1978; Halliday, 1975), and adults usually vary their messages

appropriately between direct and indirect speech acts. That is, they use alternative forms of language to accomplish similar purposes, depending on the context and the person to whom they are addressing the messages. Previously, we indicated that an imperative (a direct speech act like "Close the door") is acceptable in some instances and a question (an indirect speech act like "Can you close the door?") is more appropriate in others. As we can see, the form (syntax, phonology, semantics, and morphology) of a message does not always correspond to the intents or functions of the message.

Fluency in the delivery of messages refers to the number of false starts, hesitations, fillers, and revisions that take place as speakers say their utterances. While these fluency disrupters occur in most people's speech, they interfere with communication if they are too frequent or long. Sometimes we use these fluency disruptors deliberately to help convey part of our message. For example, if we wish to appear thoughtful about what we are saying, we might introduce more hesitations and false starts into our utterances than if we said the same thing with total assurance. These aspects of message delivery in combination with some of the suprasegmental phonological features we discussed previously (e.g., stress, intonation) are known as **paralinguistic behaviors**. Nonverbal behaviors, such as facial expression, gestures, and eye contact, are also important aspects of communicative competency. These behaviors can add and supplement meaning, counter the meaning of the oral message (e.g., sarcasm), or in some cases substitute for the oral message.

Effective language use requires that sequential utterances be related to each other. This aspect of pragmatics, termed **cohesion**, refers to the organization and order of utterances in a whole message so that the individual ideas of each utterance build logically on the previous ones. The following is part of an example, provided by Wiig and Semel (1984), in which cohesion problems are illustrated in the sequential utterances of a boy producing a narrative, in this case an explanation of the plot of a television show:

So he was scared to tell John-boy that he stoled his poem, but he didn't really. He just got an idea from John-boy's poem. And then John-boy was trying to figure out what who shot this man he knows. And then the man stole the chickens and then that night he bring 'em back. (p. 288)

The adequate inclusion of temporal words and grammatical **inflections** indicating time references to help listeners orient themselves to the interrelationships of ideas and events, and the use of appropriate referent identification for pronouns, are parts of delivering coherent messages. Another important aspect of delivering coherent messages involves using not only coordinating conjunctions (e.g., "and," "so") but also subordinating conjunctions (e.g., "because," "if," "when") to produce complex sentences that contain more than one proposition. Adverbial conjuncts (e.g., "nevertheless," "however") are other devices that contribute to cohesion.

Being able to provide coherent messages also depends, in part, on determining what listeners already know about the topics under discussion. Shared knowledge between listener and speaker is not given emphasis or, in some cases, even reported. However, knowledge that only the speaker has must be stated in order for a listener to comprehend a message. This aspect of pragmatics is termed *presupposition* and refers to the provision of sufficient, but not too much, information for adequate listener comprehension. Appropriate use of presuppositions requires that a speaker gauge listeners' needs for specificity and frames of reference. We have all experienced irritation with speakers who waste valued communicative time reporting what is obviously known without proceeding to the key parts of a message. In contrast, we have attempted to engage in conversations in which we were unable to follow the speaker's sequence of ideas because adequate background information was not supplied.

In the latter situations, we would likely determine that a communication breakdown had occurred and attempt to repair it. We indicated previously that repairing communication breakdowns is one of the several elements of pragmatic language behaviors. The process of **conversational repair** is twofold. First, speakers are obligated to identify when listeners have not understood their messages and supply additional information or modifications of the ways in which previously given information was delivered. Second, listeners must signal their lack of understanding. These

signals may be verbal, such as the statements "I don't understand," "What did you say?" or "Would you repeat that, please?" Or listeners may use nonverbal cues, such as puzzled facial expressions, to indicate that they have not understood.

During a conversation, both the speaker and the listener take turns responding to each other's utterances. One part of this rule-governed behavior is that one does not interrupt or talk over the other. However, *turn taking* also involves acknowledging the previous utterances but without repeating unnecessary content and expanding the content of the conversation with appropriate additional information (Dore, Gearhart, & Newman, 1978). Such behavior facilitates topic maintenance. *Topic maintenance* requires that a person about to speak abide by the constraints of the topic created by a previous speaker and reply with responses appropriate to the topic. For example, an appropriate response and one that would continue the topic of the statement "I bought a new car" would be "What kind is it?" In contrast, the response "It's cold outside" would be startling and disconcerting to the previous speaker and would probably discontinue the first topic, if not the interaction. However, there are times when we wish to change a topic that has already been introduced. These are referred to as *topic shifts.* Topic shifting is acceptable if it is not done so frequently that our conversational partners begin to think we are uninterested in them and if it is done smoothly rather than abruptly.

In certain situations with certain people, specific rules dictate the way we are supposed to communicate. For example, it would be very inappropriate during an interdisciplinary educational staffing on a child to relate the results of testing, such as "Sally sure did ace the hearing test but bombed the IQ test." In contrast, it might be acceptable to say to a friend and colleague that "Tom aced the continuing ed. course he took." Joos (1976) describes five styles of communication: intimate, casual, consultative, formal, and frozen. In the previous examples, the people and the situation at the staffing probably dictated the use of the consultative or formal style rather than the casual and intimate styles that were used, and it would seem strange in the second situation to employ a formal or consultative style, such as "I believe I understand that Tom did exceptionally well in the academic course he completed at the university in order to renew his credential." Effective use of language involves determining in communicative situations which styles are appropriate and wording messages accordingly.

We indicated earlier that narratives are a frequently employed aspect of communication. Narratives have predictable structures, and their organization is rule governed. Several approaches have been used to examine the organization, structure, and rules of narratives. One approach looks at narrative level. Applebee (1978) proposed six levels of narratives; from least to most complex, these are heaps, sequences, primative temporal narratives, unfocused temporal chains, focused temporal or causal chains, and proper narratives. Another common approach to examining narratives is story grammar (Johnston, 1982; Stein & Glenn, 1979). Stein and Glenn (1979) propose seven elements of story grammar, which are listed in Table 1.4. A story consists of a setting (the first element listed in Table 1.4) and one or more episodes (Johnston, 1982). The remaining elements listed in Table 1.4 constitute episode structure. When a story contains more than one episode, these need to be interrelated

and can be linked causally, temporally, and/or additively. The more episodes used and the more they are interrelated, the more a narrative is considered to be complex.

COMPREHENSION AND PRODUCTION

In our discussion of the pragmatic aspects of language, we saw that language use often involves at least two people interacting in a communicative situation—the sender of a message and the receiver of a message, who typically take turns in the roles of sender and receiver. This communicative process is referred to as **dyadic communication** and is illustrated in Figure 1.4 (Skinner, 1985). A basic assumption is that for the communicative act to be complete, both the sender and the receiver use the same code and know the same rules of the language. The sender takes an idea, applies the appropriate language rules to put the idea into code, and then transmits the code through speech **production.** The listener hears the sound transmission, applies the same language rules to match the code with the one already neurologically stored, and then, one hopes, comprehends the message. In other words, the sender **encodes** the message and the receiver **decodes** the message. Terms often used synonymously with *encoding* are *expression* and *production,* while *reception, understanding, interpretation,* and **comprehension** are terms often considered synonymous with *decoding.*

As we can see, language has both a production and a comprehension aspect. As language users, we both talk and listen, both express and receive at different times. Therefore, we must be competent in both comprehension and production. We must be able to decode the phonological, morphological, semantic, pragmatic, and syntactic aspects of the language, as well as to encode them. It is generally agreed, however, that for adults in most situations, comprehension skills are greater than production abilities. For example, for most of us, our understanding vocabularies are superior to our expressive vocabularies (the words we use to convey our thoughts to others). There is also a general belief that this superiority of comprehension over production applies to children in their acquisition. This belief appears reasonable when one considers the superiority of receptive to expressive skills in

TABLE 1.4   Elements of Story Grammar

Element	Description
Setting statement(s)	Introduces character(s); describes usual states (locale, habits, situations, temporal context)
Initiating event(s)	Event(s) causing character to act; event(s) changing the usual status
Internal response(s)	Internal reaction(s) of character(s) to initiating event(s); establishes motivation
Internal plan(s)	Strategies developed to respond to the situation; plans to resolve the problem created by the initiating event
Attempt(s)	Action(s) taken to resolve the problem
Direct consequence(s)	Result(s) of action(s)
Reaction(s)	Responses of the character(s) to the consequences

Source: Based on Stein and Glenn (1979).

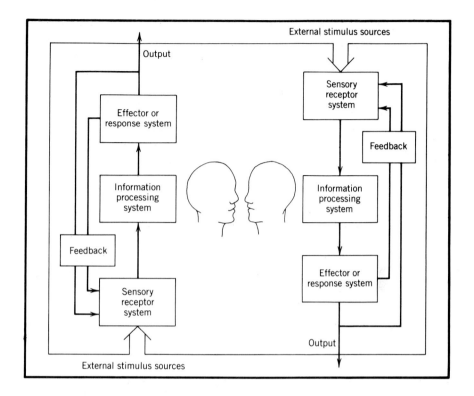

FIGURE 1.4 Dyadic Communication. (From *Speech, Language, and Hearing*, 2nd ed. [p. 11], ed. by P. Skinner and R. Shelton, 1985, Columbus, OH: Merrill. Copyright © 1985 by the authors. Reprinted by permission.)

adults and when one observes that very young children often appear to understand much more language than they produce. Ingram (1974) stated that "comprehension ahead of production is a linguistic universal of acquisition" (p. 313).

Early studies attempted to investigate the relationship between language comprehension and production. For example, Fraser, Bellugi, and Brown (1963) examined children's comprehension and production skills in a study designed to look at abilities in imitating, understanding, and expressing grammatical relationships. The results indicated that the children's abilities in imitating the language structures exceeded their skills in comprehending the structures. Furthermore, the children were better able to comprehend grammatical relationships than to produce them. Lovell and Dixon (1967) expanded and repeated the Fraser et al. (1963) study, and their results were similar to those of the earlier investigation. Imitation skills were superior to comprehension skills, which were, in turn, superior to production skills. However, others (Baird, 1972; Fernald, 1972) questioned the procedures used by Fraser et al. Three methodological questions concerned the differences in the odds for correct chance responses among the imitation, comprehension, and production tasks; the scoring systems employed; and the response patterns used by the children. Because of these questions regarding research design, some researchers doubted the results of the investigations. However, support for the belief that comprehension does, in fact, precede production and for the findings of Fraser et al. (1963) and Lovell and Dixon (1967) was found in an investigation by Monroe (1971). She examined children's receptive and expressive abilities for selected morphological endings, such as plural nouns and superlative adjectives, and found that the children's comprehension skills developed either before or simultaneously with their production skills.

Conflicting results were found in a study by de Villiers and de Villiers (1973). They investigated children's ability to comprehend word order (specifically, the sequences of subjects and objects in active and passive sentences) by having the children act out commands. The results indicated that the children were less successful in understanding the word order of subjects and objects in varying sentence types than in using correct word order. Chapman and Miller (1975) later found that children's receptive skills related to word order were poorer than their expressive skills. In studying receptive versus expressive skills for subject-verb agreement, Keeney and Wolfe (1972) found that production skills exceeded comprehension skills. Their results indicated that the children were better able to use correct subject-verb agreement than to understand it. Others have also challenged the belief that children's comprehension skills precede and exceed their production skills (e.g., Chapman, 1981; Nelson & Bonvillian, 1978).

The research on the acquisition of comprehension and production skills in children has yielded some conflicting results, as we can see. It appears that in some situations children's comprehension of language does precede their production, and in others, production abilities appear superior. Factors such as the definition of comprehension being used, the degree of comprehension being measured (e.g., depth and/or breadth of comprehension of the word "snake"), and the amount of contextual support attached to the comprehension tasks likely affect how we interpret the relationship between production and comprehension. It may be that the relationship between comprehension and production changes with age (Bloom & Lahey, 1978; Owens, 1992). It may also be that comprehension and production are related but distinct skills.

METALINGUISTICS

The prefix *meta* as it is used in *metalinguisitics* means something like "beyond" or "higher" or "transcending," not unlike its use in the word "metaphysics." As such, metalinguis*c*s refers to the ability to use language to think about and to analyze language. It involves talking about language, seeing it as an entity separate from its function as a way of communicating, and using language to judge the correctness of language and to correct it; it is an awareness of the components of language; it is seeing language as a tool and controlling how we use language. Rhyming words involves metalinguistic awareness. Frequently, monitor-

ing whether or not our messages are understood and consciously deciding how to clarify them involve metalinguistic skills. Writing and reading this chapter, especially the section on language components, reflect metalinguistic awareness.

Unless children actually acquire phonological, semantic, syntactic, morphological, and pragmatic skills, they may be limited in the extent to which they can spontaneously acquire metalinguistic skills related to these components of language. The better one is at using language, the better one is likely to be with metalinguistic skills. However, once this process starts, it appears that the relationship becomes reciprocal. That is, the better one is with metalinguistic skills, the greater are one's possibilities for further expanding language skills. The early processes of learning to read and write depend heavily on certain metalinguistic abilities, but as we become better readers and writers these abilities also appear to help us develop further our metalinguistic skills (e.g., Johnson, 1985; Menyuk, Chesnick, Leibergott, Korngold, D'Agostino, & Belanger, 1991; Snyder & Downey, 1991; Tunmer & Bowey, 1984; van Kleeck, 1990; van Kleeck & Schuele, 1987). Again, we see developmental reciprocality.

COMMUNICATION MODES

We have previously discussed comprehension and production. In that discussion, hearing was used as the input modality for comprehensio , and speaking was used as the output modality for production. These are the input-output **modalities** that comprise the auditory-oral system for language. The auditory-oral system is the most common way of using language and the one that most children acquire first. However, other combinations of input-output modalities that people may use include the visual-graphic (reading and writing) and the visual-gestural systems.

Auditory-Oral System: Hearing and Speech

The functional components of the auditory-oral system are hearing and speaking. Phylogenetically, humans heard and comprehended before they read, and they spoke before they acquired the ability to write. In some ways, the auditory-oral mode of language is more flexible than the visual-graphic mode. Vision is a unidirectional sense, whereas hearing is multidirectional. We can see in only one direction at a time, but we can hear sounds originating from many directions despite the positions of our heads. Furthermore, we can talk when our hands are busy, but we cannot write. Speaking needs no special instruments, whereas writing requires the use of a pencil, a pen, or (these days) a computer.

Children typically learn to use the auditory-oral system before they learn to use the visual-graphic system. That is, they can listen and speak before they know how to read and write. Developmentally, maturation of the physiological bases for audition and speech occurs before those used for reading and writing. Yet, developmental maturation is not the only reason for children's earlier proficiencies with the auditory-oral system. For most Western languages, writing evolved as a system of visual symbols used to represent auditory symbols. The auditory-oral system is generally the basis of the visual-graphic system.

Visual-Graphic System: Reading and Writing

In the visual-graphic system, reading is employed as the input mode and writing is used as the output mode. The functions of reading and writing are closely related to the auditory-oral system. In many respects, the visual-graphic system is a code for another code— the auditory-oral system. As a code, language symbolizes experiences and thoughts. This code can then be represented by a system of sounds combined to form words and sentences. However, these sounds (which are themselves a code) can be recoded and rerepresented as visual, rather than auditory, symbols. That is, reading and writing are codes for hearing and speaking, which themselves are codes for the actual experiences or ideas. In the process of learning the visual-graphic language system, children learn a new coding system based on a previously learned code system. In an early explanation, McGrady (1968) wrote that the relationship between the auditory-oral and visual-graphic systems "presumes a reciprocality among all language functions, but assumes the development is hierarchial. Hence, the developmental process re-

quires that later developing modalities are superimposed upon earlier developing systems. Consequently, reading and writing are most adequately developed if a functional base of oral comprehension and expression has been formed" (p. 200).

Given the complex reciprocal relationships between the auditory-oral and visual-graphic systems, it is no surprise that children who have problems with the auditory-oral system often have difficulties learning to read and write. Most professionals emphasize the importance of an adequate auditory-oral system in learning to read and the relationship between oral language skills and reading achievement. Wiig and Semel (1984) state, "Beginning reading depends upon accurate, deliberate, analytical decoding of letters and upon conscious translation of these letters into their auditory-vocal equivalents, which the child has already learned" (p. 33). This description is consistent with a theory of reading known as the *bottom-up theory*. A child learning to read must be able to segment printed words, decode letters in them, match them to some stored auditory model (phonetic and phonemic segmentation), and then retrieve a corresponding word (lexical retrieval). However, reading also involves using already known semantic-syntactic information, world knowledge, and narrative structure information to predict and organize what is being seen on the printed page. This is consistent with the *top-down theory* of reading, in which higher-order linguistic and cognitive skills play an important role in reading. Skills associated with both the bottom-up and top-down theories (phonological and syllabic segmentation, rapid lexical retrieval, semantic-syntactic abilities, narrative skills, general knowledge level) have been found to be factors in learning to read. It may be, however, that these different skills play more dominant roles in the process at different stages in learning to read and in different children at different times (e.g., Menyuk et al., 1991; Owens, 1992; Snyder & Downey, 1991). This perspective is consistent with the *parallel, or interactive, theory* of learning to read.

There are several analogies between the visual-graphic and auditory-oral systems. The auditory and visual modalities are the receptive aspects of the two systems, whereas the oral and graphic modalities are the expressive aspects. The auditory component is based on a set of sounds that combine to form spoken words; the visual component is based on a set of letters that combine to form written words. Just as oral production for speech is a sensorimotor process, the same is true for graphic production for writing. Reception for the auditory-oral system involves transduction (conversion of waves into neural impulses) and auditory **perception** and processing of sound waves. Similarly, reception for the visual-graphic system involves transduction and visual perception and processing of light waves. Rules govern the use of both systems.

Although there are a number of analogies between the auditory-oral and visual-graphic systems, there are also differences (Gillam & Johnston, 1992). One difference is the sequence in which the two systems are acquired. Furthermore, although rules govern both systems and although some rules are similar, there are also different rules. One obvious difference deals with punctuation. Another relates to spelling. These are not factors in the auditory-oral system. Another difference deals with the level of grammatical complexity. The semantic-syntactic level used in the auditory-oral system is generally less complex than that found in the visual-graphic system once one progresses beyond the early learning stages. Still another difference relates to the amount of context available. Reading and writing are more decontextualized modes of communication than listening and speaking. That is, fewer cues to decipher and impart meaning are available in reading and writing compared to listening and speaking. We cannot point or use facial expressions to communicate in reading and writing, although graphs, illustrations, and pictures are attempts to supplement written material. Additionally, speech consists of sounds that occur over time, and these are generally temporary and fleeting. Writing consists of marks in space that are relatively permanent and can be referred to repeatedly. As such, the visual-graphic mode has the potential to reduce demands on individuals' processing and cognitive systems. However, it is faster to speak than to write. Another difference is the fact that most children acquire the auditory-oral system without formalized instruction, whereas carefully planned instructional processes are typically offered in schools in order to teach most children to read and write. And, while use of the auditory-oral system can develop independently

of the visual-graphic system, proficiency with the visual-graphic system is exceedingly difficult to achieve without first acquiring at least some proficiency with the auditory-oral system. This point will be reiterated in later parts of this text.

Visual-Gestural Systems

The visual modality combined with gestures, body postures and movements, and/or facial grimaces can be used as communication modes. Here we discuss three visual-gestural communication systems: nonverbal communication, manual communication, and other forms of alternative/augmentative communication such as communication boards and electronic communication aids. Although this chapter has focused primarily on normal aspects of language, we include discussions of manual communication and other alternative/augmentative communication systems, systems sometimes used with children who have language and/or speech disorders, in order to illustrate the variety of visual-gestural communication systems.

Nonverbal Communication   In our discussion of pragmatics, we indicated that effective employment of nonverbal communication is one aspect of language use. In many respects, nonverbal communication can be considered a system itself. Hall (1959), in the title of his book on nonverbal communication, referred to it as the "silent language." Reception in nonverbal communication is accomplished primarily through the visual modality. Expression includes such things as facial grimaces, gestures, or combinations of these forms. The parameter of nonverbal communication that refers to body movement is called **kinesics**, or body language. A second parameter of nonverbal communication is **proxemics**, or the use of space and distance for expression. Consciously or unconsciously, we engage in nonverbal communication, sometimes to emphasize concurrent oral messages, sometimes to contradict simultaneous oral messages, and sometimes to substitute for oral messages. Our understanding and use of nonverbal cues can largely determine the quality and effectiveness of our interpersonal relationships. In fact, some suggest that nonverbal communication carries more than half of the social meaning in interpersonal communication situations.

Cultures differ in the uses of and meanings associated with specific elements of nonverbal communication. It is not unusual for travelers in a foreign country to find themselves in awkward situations because of their ignorance of the nonverbal communication system of the indigenous culture. In a country with multicultural groups, differences in nonverbal communication exist. In a culture, inaccurate or ineffective interpretation and use of nonverbal communication may lead to problems in establishing and maintaining social relationships with others. An awareness of nonverbal communication and the ways in which it influences relationships is important because some language-disordered children experience deficits in the ability to understand and express nonverbal cues correctly (e.g., Bryan, 1977, 1978; Kretschmer & Kretschmer, 1980; Wood, 1982). Wiig and Semel (1976) suggest that such difficulties can result in the development of poor self-images and self-concepts, potentially leading to even more impaired interpersonal relationships.

Manual Communication   One of the more familiar visual-gestural systems is manual communication, or sign language, sometimes used by people who are deaf or severely hearing impaired. Children with other speech and/or language problems also sometimes use manual communication. While there are many forms of manual communication (Moores, 1978), two forms use manual signs that correspond closely to or match exactly the sequence of morphemes in English syntax. These are **Seeing Essential English** (**SEE**) (Anthony, 1971) and **Signing Exact English** (**SEE**) (Gustason, Pfetzing, & Azwolkow, 1972). In other words, the two SEEs are basically the English language communicated through visual-gestural modalities.

American Sign Language (ASL) is also one of the common forms of manual communication. As with the two SEEs, reception takes place through the visual modality, and expression is in the form of gestures. However, research indicates that ASL is not simply English communicated through a system of gestures, but a different language from English. That is, the coding system and the rules for coding are different from those

of English. Bellugi and Klima (1972) write, "In its deepest and most interesting respects, sign [ASL] seems to be a language in its own right, with properties that are different from spoken language in general and English in particular" (p. 61). These same authors (1978) even suggest that ASL is often misunderstood:

1. American Sign Language is not a derivative or degenerate form of written or spoken English. It has a lexicon that does not correspond to English, but must be considered a different language. The grammatical principles governing the modification of meaning of signs are different, in form and content, from the grammatical processes in English and in spoken language in general.
2. American Sign Language is in no way limited to "concrete ideas." It is a full-fledged language with the possibility for expression at any level of abstraction. There is vocabulary dealing with religion, politics, ethics, history, and other realms of mental abstraction and fantasy. . . .
3. American Sign Language is not a universal form of pantomime. For example . . . it differs from British Sign, and, for all but the most rudimentary purposes, the two sign languages are mutually incomprehensible. (pp. 46–47)

Viewing ASL as a language raises several questions about the education of deaf or severely hearing-impaired children. Are we, in teaching reading and writing to children who already know ASL, attempting to teach them to use a visual-graphic system of a language (English) for which they have little background? Is this a second-language visual-graphic system for them? For those who are capable of acquiring some oral communicative skills, are these oral skills based on a different language than the one they may already know (ASL)? We do not yet know the answers to these questions.

Alternative/Augmentative Communication   In addition to manual communication, there are a number of alternative/augmentative systems that rely primarily on visual-gestural modes for communication. With professionals' increased understanding of and emphasis on communication, greater acceptance and use of alternative modes of communication for individuals with speech and/or language problems has occurred. In some cases, as we will see later in this text, alternative/augmentative systems have been used as methods of facilitating oral language learning in children with language disorders. Advances in computer technology and electronics in general have also facilitated the development of a wide variety of more sophisticated and efficient alternative/augmentative communication systems.

Communication Boards.   When functional speech is not present, one alternative system is a communication board. Symbols, which can be written words or sentences or other symbolic visual representations, are placed on a board. Through some type of motor response, the user indicates on the board which symbols convey the thoughts. Motor responses may consist of activating an electronic indicator or pointing; however, the output modality is, in some way, gestural. Input for the receivers of the messages is visual—the symbols indicated on the board. Input to the user of the board may be visual (the "listener" replies by pointing to symbols on the board), may be auditory (the "listener" replies by speaking), or may be both (the "listener" replies by pointing to symbols and talking simultaneously).

Words and sentences on communication boards are appropriate for individuals who have some reading ability. For those who do not, other more graphically representative symbols, such as pictures, may be used. One visual system that is sometimes used is the Bliss symbols system, or **Blissymbolics** (Bliss, 1965). The symbols in the system consist of pictographs (⌂ for house) and arbitrary symbols, which often indicate some grammatical function (? for a question or ⌐ for past tense) that are illustrated with black line drawings (Archer, 1977). Because of the iconic nature of many of the Bliss symbols, children may be able to code their environments and thoughts more easily than with the arbitrary symbols used for the code in the auditory-oral system. Frequently on communication boards, the words that the visual symbols represent are written below the symbols, permitting people not familiar with the system to understand the user's messages. In contrast to the auditory-oral or visual-graphic systems, there are far fewer elements in the system, which reduces the complexity of the learning

task. However, by varying positions, sizes, and number, a wide variety of ideas can be conveyed (Archer, 1977). Furthermore, certain symbols represent categories and, when slightly modified, represent items within the categories. For example, the category of transportation is symbolized by ⊗ (wheel), and when it is altered to ⊗̸ and ⊠, it becomes an airplane and a wheelchair, respectively. There are also symbols to indicate opposites, thereby allowing new concepts to be communicated (Symbol Communication Research Project, 1974). Since the original Bliss symbols were developed, some of the more abstract symbols have been enhanced by the addition of pink line drawings to the original black line drawings in order to give cues to the meanings (Blissymbolics Communication Institute, 1984). In a recent study of normal 3-year-old children, the enhanced symbols were more easily identified than the original standard symbols, suggesting that the enhancements helped the children attach more meaning to the symbols (Raghavendra & Fristoe, 1990). This may be an important factor when considering the use of Bliss symbols on communication boards for children.

Electronic Communication Aids.   Electronic communication aids are generally used with children whose motor skills are sufficiently impaired to hinder severely, if not preclude, the use of speech and/or writing for communication. The advent of computer-generated speech and miniature/micro electronic systems has increased the variety of alternative/augmentative systems available for these children. These systems typically require that the "speaker" make a movement or gesture that electronically activates some form of output (e.g., printed words, synthesized speech, lights on a board). Some systems are so sophisticated that only a minimal amount of movement is necessary to generate electronically a limited repertoire of synthesized speech.

At least two issues become apparent when considering possible systems. One is the language level and the other is the motor ability of the child. As we will see later in this text, language impairments are not uncommon in some physically handicapping conditions. Systems that require the user to generate letters or words and sentences, even if these are then converted electronically into synthesized speech, obviously require at least basic language functioning. Even pictures or symbols, such as the Bliss symbols just introduced, require some form of coding system. "Listener" familiarity with the symbolic nature of the system is also a consideration. When motor disabilities do not allow a child to point, as with a communication board, many different types of switches that activate an electronic system are available. These include the following (Silverman, 1980):

1. Push/touch switches, pads, or plates.
2. Wobble sticks or a mouse that move in any direction.
3. Squeeze bulbs that are activated by hand squeezes.
4. Position switches that are activated by changing body or body part position.
5. Foot trolleys that are activated by foot movement.
6. Pneumatic switches that are activated by blowing or sucking.
7. Sound-controlled switches that are activated, as the name implies, by sound.
8. Light-controlled switches activated by a beam of light.

For the more severely motorically disabled children, even **neuroassisted** modes are available. These can use brain wave activity, muscle action potentials, or eye movements to activate electronic communication devices. Unfortunately, however, none of these systems is as efficient and effective as either the auditory-oral or visual-graphic systems.

LANGUAGE, LITERACY, AND EDUCATION

Language and language-related skills comprise the majority of the curricula in the early grades, which emphasize learning to read and write and, later, improving reading and writing skills. In the upper grades, the language and language-related skills acquired earlier become the modes through which the content areas are learned. Students are asked to do independent reading in content areas and to write about what they have learned. Language is, therefore,

a fundamental aspect of literacy and the educational process.

When children enter school, often at the kindergarten level, they typically bring with them a solid base in the auditory-oral language system. This is not to say that their oral language system is wholly developed by age 5, but children beginning kindergarten have usually had 5 years of listening experiences and 4 years of talking experiences. They use fairly well-formed, complex sentences to express their ideas and needs and to ask questions. Six-year-old children have been estimated to have expressive vocabularies of about 2,600 (Owens, 1992) to 7,000 words (Zintz, 1970). They may understand between 20,000 and 24,000 words (Owens, 1992). This competence in the auditory-oral language system is a significant factor in learning to read and write. Loban's (1963, 1976) investigations of the language skills of school children demonstrated the importance of the auditory-oral language system in the acquisition of the visual-graphic system. In his studies, children whose listening and speaking skills were well developed had better reading and writing skills than those whose auditory-oral language systems were less advanced. Conversely, elementary school children described as "low-achieving" (but not receiving special education services or diagnosed as language disordered) have been found to have poorer language skills than their academically achieving peers (Hill & Haynes, 1992). Oral language development in the preschool years prepares the child for formalized education. It is also integrally related to literacy.

Emergent Literacy

Achieving literacy in Western societies is no longer seen as only acquiring the abilities to read and write, that is, having literacy skills (Miller, 1990). Rather, literacy is viewed as engaging in literate behaviors. These include reading spontaneously for pleasure and learning; writing to convey analyzed and synthesized thoughts and ideas; and listening and speaking to argue, discuss, and plan. Recent views of literacy have also discarded the notion that literacy begins when children go to school and learn to read and write. The acquisition of literacy is now seen to begin basically at

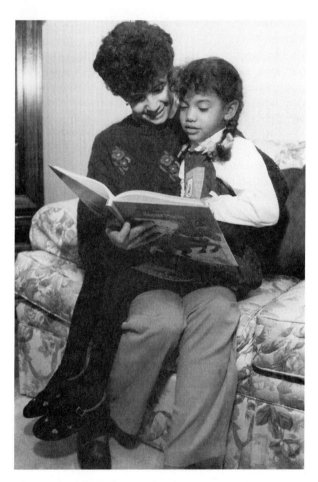

Literacy begins in the preschool years.

(crayons, pencils) and paper easily available to the child, with adults who are responsive to the child's attempts to read and write (Cochrane-Smith, 1984; Heath, 1983; Teale, 1978, 1980). In literacy-promoting homes, reading and writing have also been found to be integrated with and embedded in the daily family routine as regular activities of living (Heath, 1983; Teale, 1978, 1980). Another factor associated with emergent literacy is adult–child storybook reading. Storybook reading that is a social, interactive event, contains routinized dialogue cycles, and varies differentially to allow children to take more responsibility for the reading as their language skills grow has been found to enhance literacy development (Teale, 1987). Factors such these are seen as helping to prepare young children for the more formal learning activities they will experience during their elementary and secondary school years. These young children begin school knowing that print represents oral language and, therefore, that it is meaningful and serves a variety of functions (van Kleeck & Schuele, 1987). They may even know something about the visual-graphic symbols associated with printed material. Combined with metalinguistic skills, these developmental factors play important roles in children's learning the literacy skills (reading, writing, spelling) that allow them to engage in literate behaviors, that is, to become literate individuals.

School

The educational system is divided into the elementary and secondary school grades. The primary emphasis of the elementary grades is acquisition of basic learning skills (reading, writing, spelling, arithmetic abilities), although as children progress into the upper elementary grades, somewhat more importance is placed on using basic skills for content learning. In secondary school, emphasis shifts dramatically to acquiring content area information, with gradually increasing expectations for independent learning. At this level, basic skills are assumed to have been acquired.

The Elementary Grades

Kindergarten.   Kindergarten is often considered as a readiness grade to prepare children for the learning experiences to come in first grade. Because of the in-

birth, and toddlers and preschool children are considered to be in the process of becoming literate (Miller, 1990; van Kleeck, 1990; van Kleeck & Schuele, 1987). *Emergent literacy* is the term that has been applied to the development occurring during the preschool years in the child's early environments that lead to literacy. These are prereading and prewriting behaviors and skills that develop into conventional reading and writing abilities.

Several factors are associated with emerging literacy skills in children. One of these is the preschooler's home and family environments. Characteristics of home and family environments that have been found to promote literacy include having a variety of print materials in the environment and writing instruments fluence that listening and speaking skills have on reading and writing abilities, kindergarten learning activities frequently focus on further developing the children's oral language skills. Although kindergarten may emphasize the listening and speaking skills, most children are also introduced formally to reading and writing skills. Kindergartners may learn to recognize the printed words for the days of the week, their classmates' printed names, or the names of printed letters. Learning activities may involve having the children clearly formulate their thoughts and dictate them to the teacher, who writes them on the board. Such an activity emphasizes the relationship between the spoken and printed word and is an initial stage in the development of written composition skills. The children's early experiences with the sensorimotor processes of the visual-graphic language system typically include learning to write the letters of the alphabet and their names. The children may also be shown how to improve their drawings of circles and lines, the elements of writing. In some schools, limited formal instruction in reading and writing may be introduced in kindergarten. In other schools, formal instruction in reading and writing may not be introduced until first grade.

First Grade.   Formal reading and writing instruction typically begins in first grade. Children learn to use word recognition skills, acquire information from printed words, distinguish among beginning sounds of spoken words, and read for meaning. In writing, children learn to form both lower- and uppercase letters and print short words. Skill levels in writing, however, usually lag behind those in reading. Although the primary emphasis on language skills in first grade may shift from the auditory-oral system to the visual-graphic system, learning activities continue to involve listening and speaking skills. The children are encouraged to dictate letters and stories; because their writing skills are still limited, the teacher acts as a scribe. Such experiences further demonstrate to children the relationship between the spoken and written word and encourage them to learn to write the words they say.

Second Grade.   Second-grade curricula emphasize increased skill in listening, speaking, reading, and writing. Children may be asked to rhyme words, fol-

low sequences of orally presented directions, write short stories, increase their spelling vocabularies, and improve printed forms. In reading, the emphasis turns to independence. Students are expected to develop independent word recognition and reading comprehension skills; typically, the curriculum also encourages the children to spend time in independent reading. Learning activities move from concrete, hands-on experiences to abstract, language-related experiences. Wiig and Semel (1976) suggest that the "demands for auditory language processing, oral presentations, and verbal recall increase significantly in the second grade" (p. 6).

Third Grade.   Third grade is a transition grade. Increased attention is given to independent reading, with emphasis on reading more complex, longer stories. Instruction in cursive writing typically begins, although printed forms may continue to be used in situations where speed is expected. If we look at the demands of cursive writing, we see that we are asking children to recode previously learned printed symbols, which were themselves coded symbols for the auditory code. Children are asked to answer questions by writing sentences and to write increasingly complex paragraphs. Continued emphasis is placed on increasing spelling vocabularies. Children in third grade are also typically expected to proofread and correct their written work. Oral activities include participating effectively in group discussions and making presentations.

Fourth, Fifth, and Sixth Grades.   The curricular emphases in these grades continually shift from learning activities directed to building skills in the auditory-oral and visual-graphic language systems to using these language skills for acquiring content area information. Students gain information through class discussions and short teacher lectures and demonstrations (Bashir, 1989; Owens, 1992; Wiig & Semel, 1984). Students may even be given independent reading assignments and asked to write short reports about what they have read. They are expected to use their language skills to seek out information from resources. Without the necessary underlying basic skills in both the auditory-oral and visual-graphic systems, we can see how children may be at risk for failure.

The Secondary Grades   The shift from elementary to secondary education generally occurs somewhere around sixth or seventh grade. Lectures as the means of instruction become more common, and students are increasingly expected to be able to take written notes on the lecture content. Additionally, students may have different teachers for different subjects. This means that students need to adjust to varying lecture delivery styles (Bashir, 1989; Comkowycz, Ehren, & Hayes, 1987). Independence in all forms of learning is stressed, and teachers expect students to be able to seek out and organize information for themselves (Boyce & Larson, 1983). The emphasis is on learning content and on demonstrating what information has been acquired (Ehren & Lenz, 1989). There is a significant increase in the use of the written mode for demonstrating knowledge, and performance on written tests of content knowledge takes on greater importance (Comkowycz et al., 1987). Students are also expected to know the rules for classroom communication and to take on the "student role" when necessary (Bashir, 1989; Comkowycz et al., 1987).

Table 1.5 summarizes some of the changing language demands at different grade levels. Children's language skills evolve dramatically from kindergarten on. Although the development is a complex process, with listening, speaking, reading, and writing skills closely related to and interacting with one another, a large part of the early educational achievement in reading and writing depends heavily on the children's abilities with the auditory-oral language system. Later educational achievements depend on both the auditory-oral and visual-graphic language systems.

Whole Language

Increasing recognition of the relationship between oral language, reading and writing, and literacy in general and awareness of the importance of emergent literacy skills has led some to suggest that learning to

TABLE 1.5   *Changes in Language Demands at Different Grade Levels*

Starting in . . .	A child should be able to . . .
Kindergarten	Follow directions Answer questions and speak in small groups Produce short narratives
First grade	Learn decoding strategies necessary for reading
Third grade	Read text in order to acquire information
Fourth grade	Engage in dialogues with teachers and peers in order to clarify misunderstandings and facilitate learning Learn multiple word meanings Begin to make inferences and draw conclusions about information presented in print Understand text organization (e.g., titles, chapters)
Fifth-eighth grades	Read independently outside of class Adapt to class formats in which the lecture is a primary means of conveying information Learn to read and produce different written language forms (e.g., poems, essays, term papers) Adjust to language differences in various content areas (e.g., history, mathematics) Adapt to the lecture styles of different teachers Modify the communication style to suit different educational and social contexts (e.g., classroom, gym, peer social activities)

Source: Adapted from Bashir (1989), Owens (1992), Wiig and Semel (1984).

read and write should not be viewed as an activity that is taught only in a formal and fragmented sense when a child enters school or as anything separate from what children do in the whole process of learning to communicate and becoming literate (Goodman, 1986; King & Goodman, 1990; Norris, 1992; Norris & Damico, 1990; Schory, 1990). Rather, reading and writing and speaking and listening are all integrally intertwined, development in one area enhances development in the others, and children learn the various communication modes (reading/writing, speaking/listening) naturally as they interact in context-relevant situations in which meaning for some purpose is what is being made sense of. This approach to literacy has been termed *whole language.*

Whole language is a philosophy of literacy and education, as opposed to a teaching method or theory (Norris, 1990, 1992). Kamhi (1992), in summarizing the assumptions underlying the philosophy of whole language that Norris and Damico (1990) discussed, writes:

1. Language is closely linked with other semiotic and cognitive abilities and is influenced by such things as motivation, experience, learning, and anxiety.
2. All of the components of language are always present and interacting in any instance of language use.
3. Language is not learned by first acquiring the smallest component parts but by exposing the child simultaneously to all language components in a meaningful context.
4. Language learning is viewed as an active constructive process. (p. 58)

Accordingly, the strongest proponents of whole language suggest that children can learn to read and write as naturally as they learn to talk and listen, that is, without specific instruction that breaks language into artificial, smaller units. Rather than direct teaching of literacy skills or oral language, education encompass-

ing a whole language philosophy views teachers as facilitators, not instructors, and curriculum as an environment, not a set of learning objectives.

Although whole language may be inherently appealing (Kamhi, 1992), not all professionals agree with all of its principles, the ways in which the philosophy has been translated into practice, and/or its application to children with language disorders. One area of disagreement relates to equating oral language acquisition with written language acquisition (Altwerger, Edelsky, & Flores, 1987; Liberman & Liberman, 1990; Shapiro, 1992). This objection points to the evolutionary differences in how humans learned to speak and listen, and how they came to read and write, with the auditory-oral language system being the more "biologically" natural system. Another concern focuses on the whole language approach that discourages attention to language structures and the components of oral and printed language (Chaney, 1990; Kamhi, 1992; Shapiro, 1992). The basis for this concern relates to metalinguistic skills (language analysis skills), skills that have been associated with reading proficiency, and the need to employ at least some bottom-up analysis skills both in learning to read and in situations where proficient readers encounter unknown reading structues, such as unfamiliar printed words. A third objection relates to the assumption that what may be a "natural" learning approach or a "normal process" that works for young, normal children is an approach that will work for children with language disorders and/or learning problems (Olswang & Bain, 1991). Here the question is, if children are not developing normally, can we assume that providing the kinds of learning experiences that are normal or doing more of what is normal is what the children need to overcome their difficulties? Although there may be good aspects of the whole language approach, there may also be some bad aspects (Chaney, 1990; Kamhi, 1992).

SUMMARY

In this chapter we have seen that:

▶ Language consists of a system of phonological, semantic, morphological, syntactic, and pragmatic rules that are used to put ideas and thoughts into a

code in order to communicate them to others and to relate to others. Language is the code; speech is one of several sensorimotor processes that can be used to produce the code.

▶ Communication involves both comprehension and production, but the relationship between them is not fully agreed upon.

▶ Metalinguistics refers to the ability to treat language as an object and to analyze it; metalinguistic skills are important in learning to read and write.

▶ Communication can be accomplished through several modes: auditory-oral (hearing and speech), visual-graphic (reading and writing), and visual-gestural. Nonverbal communication and manual communication are two forms of the visual-gestural mode. Other visual-gestural modes are sometimes used in alternative/augmentative communication systems for individuals who are limited in their abilities to use speech and/or language.

▶ Auditory-oral language is integrally related to and permeates literacy and the educational process; literacy begins in the preschool years; and the language demands of the educational process increase with advancing grades. Whole language is a philosophical approach to literacy and education that recognizes the interrelationships among all aspects of language, although concerns about the use of whole language as an appropriate approach for children with language and/or learning problems have been raised.

If we are to understand the nature of children's language disorders and their impacts on children's lives, we must first understand the various aspects of language. We also need to recognize the role language plays in communication, literacy, and the educational process.

REFERENCES

Altwerger, B., Edelsky, C., & Flores, B. (1987). Whole language: What's new? *The Reading Teacher, 41,* 144–154.

Anthony, D. (1971). *Seeing essential English.* Anaheim, CA: Anaheim School District.

Applebee, A. (1978). *The child's concept of story.* Chicago: University of Chicago Press.

Archer, L. (1977). Blissymbolics—A nonverbal communication system. *Journal of Speech and Hearing Disorders, 42,* 568–579.

Baird, R. (1972). On the role of change in imitation, comprehension and production. Test results. *Journal of Verbal Learning and Verbal Behavior, 11,* 474–477.

Bashir, A. (1989). Language intervention and the curriculum. *Seminars in Speech and Language, 10,* 181–191.

Bates, E. (1976). Pragmatics and sociolinguistics in child language. In D. Morehead & A. Morehead (Eds.), *Normal and deficient child language.* Baltimore: University Park Press.

Bellugi, U., & Klima, E. (1972). The roots of language in the sign talk of the deaf. *Psychology Today, 6,* 60–64.

Bellugi, U., & Klima, E. (1978). Structural properties of American Sign Language. In L. Liben (Ed.), *Deaf children: Developmental perspective.* New York: Academic Press.

Bliss, C. (1965). *Semantography—Blissymbolics* (2nd ed.). Sydney, Australia: Semantography.

Blissymbolics Communication Institute. (1984). *Picture your Blissymbols.* Toronto: Author.

Bloom, L. (1988). What is language? In M. Lahey, *Language disorders and language development.* New York: Merrill/Macmillan.

Bloom, L., & Lahey, M. (1978). *Language development and language disorders.* New York: Macmillan.

Boyce, N., & Larson, V. Lord. (1983). *Adolescents' communication: Development and disorders.* Eau Claire, WI: Thinking Publications.

Bryan, T. (1977). Learning disabled children's comprehension of nonverbal communication. *Journal of Learning Disabilities, 10,* 36–41.

Bryan, T. (1978). Social relationships and verbal interactions of learning disabled children. *Journal of Learning Disabilities, 11,* 58–66.

Burroughs, E., & Tomblin, J. B. (1990). Speech and language correlates of adults' judgments of children. *Journal of Speech and Hearing Disorders, 55,* 485–494.

Chaney, C. (1990). Evaluating the whole language approach to language arts: The pros and cons. *Language, Speech, and Hearing Services in Schools, 21,* 244–249.

Chapman, R. (1978). Comprehension strategies in children. In J. Kavanagh & W. Stange (Eds.), *Speech and language in the laboratory, school, and clinic.* Cambridge, MA: MIT Press.

Chapman, R. (1981). Mother–child interaction in the second year of life: Its role in language development. In R. Schiefelbusch & D. Bricker (Eds.), *Early language: Acquisition and intervention.* Baltimore: University Park Press.

Chapman, R., & Miller, J. (1975). Word order in early two and three word utterances: Does production precede comprehension? *Journal of Speech and Hearing Research, 18,* 355–371.

Chomsky, N. (1957). *Syntactic structures.* The Hague: Mouton.

Chomsky, N. (1965). *Aspects of the theory of syntax.* Cambridge, MA: MIT Press.

Chomsky, N. (1972). *Language and mind.* New York: Harcourt Brace Jovanovich.

Chomsky, N. (1981). *Lectures on government and binding.* Dordrecht, Holland: Foris.

Cochrane-Smith, M. (1984). *The making of a reader.* Norwood, NJ: Ablex.

Comkowycz, S. M., Ehren, B. J., & Hayes, N. H. (1987). Meeting classroom needs of language disordered students in middle and junior high schools: A program model. *Journal of Childhood Communication Disorders, 11,* 199–208.

Dale, P. (1976). *Language development: Structure and function* (2nd ed.). New York: Holt, Rinehart and Winston.

de Villiers, J., & de Villiers, P. (1973). Development of the use of word order in comprehension. *Journal of Psycholinguistic Research, 2,* 331–341.

Dore, J., Gearhart, M., & Newman, D. (1978). The structure of nursery school conversation. In K. Nelson (Ed.), *Children's language* (Vol. 1). New York: Garden Press.

Ehren, B. J., & Lenz, B. K. (1989). Adolescents with language disorders: Special considerations in providing academically relevant language intervention. *Seminars in Speech and Language, 10,* 192–203.

Fairbanks, G. (1960). *Voice and articulation drill book.* New York: Harper & Row.

Fernald, C. (1972). Control of grammar in imitation, comprehension and production. Problems of replication. *Journal of Verbal Learning and Verbal Behavior, 11,* 606–613.

Fraser, C., Bellugi, U., & Brown, R. (1963). Control of grammar in imitation, comprehension, and production. *Journal of Verbal Learning and Verbal Behavior, 2,* 121–135.

Gillam, R., & Johnston, J. (1992). Spoken and written language relationships in language/learning-impaired and normally achieving school-age children. *Journal of Speech and Hearing Research, 35,* 1303–1315.

Goodman, K. (1986). *What's whole in whole language?* Portsmouth, NH: Heinemann.

Gumperz, J., & Cook-Gumperz, J. (1982). Introduction: Language and the communication of social identity. In J. Gumperz (Ed.), *Language and social identity* (pp. 1–21). Cambridge: Cambridge University Press.

Gustason, G., Pfetzing, D., & Azwolkow, E. (1972). *Signing exact English.* Rossmoor, CA: Modern Signs Press.

Hall, E. (1959). *The silent language.* New York: Fawcett.

Halliday, M. (1975). *Learning how to mean: Explorations in the development of language.* London: Edward Arnold.

Hayakawa, S. (1964). *Language in thought and action* (2nd ed.). New York: Harcourt, Brace & World.

Heath, S. (1983). *Ways with words: Language, life and work in communities and classrooms.* Cambridge: Cambridge University Press.

Hill, S., & Haynes, W. (1992). Language performance in low-achieving elementary school students. *Language, Speech, and Hearing Services in Schools, 23,* 169–175.

Hubbell, R. (1985). Language and linguistics. In P. Skinner & R. Shelton (Eds.), *Speech, language, and hearing: Normal processes and disorders* (2nd ed.). New York: Wiley.

Hudson, R. (1980). *Sociolinguistics.* Cambridge: Cambridge University Press.

Ingram, D. (1974). The relationship between comprehension and production. In R. Schiefelbusch & L. Lloyd (Eds.), *Language perspectives—Acquisition, retardation, and intervention.* Baltimore: University Park Press.

Johnson, D. (1985). Using reading and writing to improve oral language skills. *Topics in Language Disorders, 5,* 55–69.

Johnston, J. (1982). Narratives: A new look at communication problems in older language-disordered children. *Language, Speech, and Hearing Services in Schools, 13,* 144–155.

Joos, M. (1976). The style of the five clocks. In N. Johnson (Ed.), *Current topics in language: Introductory readings.* Cambridge, MA: Winthrop.

Kamhi, A. (1992). Three perspectives on language processing: Interactionism, modularity, and holism. In R. Chapman (Ed.), *Processes in language acquisition and disorders.* St. Louis, MO: Mosby Year Book.

Keeney, T., & Wolfe, J. (1972). The acquisition of agreement in English. *Journal of Verbal Learning and Verbal Behavior, 11,* 698–705.

Kempson, R. (1977). *Semantics theory.* Cambridge: Cambridge University Press.

King, D., & Goodman, K. (1990). Whole language: Cherishing learners and their language. *Language, Speech, and Hearing Services in Schools, 21,* 221–227.

Kretschmer, R., & Kretschmer, L. (1980). Pragmatics: Development in normal-hearing and hearing-impaired children. In J. Subtelny (Ed.), *Speech assessment and speech improvement for the hearing impaired.* Washington, DC: Alexander Graham Bell Association for the Deaf.

Lee, L. (1974). *Developmental sentence analysis.* Evanston, IL: Northwestern University Press.

Leonard, L., & Loeb, D. (1988). Government-binding theory and some of its applications: A tutorial. *Journal of Speech and Hearing Research, 31,* 515–524.

Liberman, I., & Liberman, A. (1990). Whole language vs. code emphasis: Underlying assumptions and their implications for reading instruction. *Annals of Dyslexia, 40,* 51–76.

Loban, W. (1963). *The language of elementary school children.* Urbana, IL: National Council of Teachers of English.

Loban, W. (1976). *Language development: Kindergarten through grade twelve.* Urbana, IL: National Council of Teachers of English.

Lovell, K., & Dixon, E. (1967). The growth of the control of grammar in imitation, comprehension, and production. *Journal of Child Psychology and Psychiatry, 8,* 31–39.

McGrady, H. (1968). Language pathology and learning disabilities. In H. Myklebust (Ed.), *Progress in learning disabilities* (Vol. I). New York: Grune & Stratton.

McLean, J., & Snyder-McLean, L. (1978). *A transactional approach to early language training.* Columbus, OH: Merrill.

Menyuk, P., Chesnick, M., Leibergott, J., Korngold, B., D'Agostino, R., & Belanger, A. (1991). Predicting reading problems in at-risk children. *Journal of Speech and Hearing Research, 34,* 893–903.

Miller, L. (1990). The roles of language and learning in the development of literacy. *Topics in Language Disorders, 10,* 1–24.

Monroe, N. (1971). *Concept learning in the acquisition of inflectional endings.* Unpublished doctoral dissertation, University of Kansas, Lawrence.

Moores, D. (1978). Current research and theory with the deaf: Educational implications. In L. Liben (Ed.), *Deaf children: Developmental perspectives.* New York: Academic Press.

Nelson, K., & Bonvillian, J. (1978). Early language development: Conceptual growth and related processes between two and 4½ years of age. In K. Nelson (Ed.), *Children's language* (Vol. 1). New York: Gardner Press.

Norris, J. (1990). Introduction. *Language, Speech, and Hearing Services in Schools, 21,* 205.

Norris, J. (1992). Some questions and answers about whole language. *American Journal of Speech-Language Pathology, 1,* 11–14.

Norris, J., & Damico, J. (1990). Whole language in theory and practice: Implications for language intervention. *Language, Speech, and Hearing Services in Schools, 21,* 212–220.

Olswang, L., & Bain, B. (1991). Intervention issues for toddlers with specific language impairments. *Topics in Language Disorders, 11,* 69–86.

O'Malley, M., & Tikofsky, R. (1972). The structure of language. In J. Irwin & M. Marge (Eds.), *Principles of childhood language disabilities.* Englewood Cliffs, NJ: Prentice-Hall.

Owens, R. (1992). *Language development: An introduction* (3rd ed.). New York: Merrill/Macmillan.

Prutting, C. (1982). Pragmatics as social competence. *Journal of Speech and Hearing Disorders, 47,* 123–134.

Raghavendra, P., & Fristoe, M. (1990). "A spinach with a *V* on it": What 3-year-olds see in standard and enhanced Blissymbols. *Journal of Speech and Hearing Disorders, 55,* 149–159.

Schory, M. (1990). Whole language and the speech-language pathologist. *Language, Speech, and Hearing Services in Schools, 21,* 206–211.

Shapiro, H. (1992). Debatable issues underlying whole-language philosophy: A speech-language pathologist's perspective. *Language, Speech, and Hearing Services in Schools, 23,* 308–311.

Silverman, F. (1980). *Communication for the speechless.* Englewood Cliffs, NJ: Prentice-Hall.

Skinner, P. (1985). Speech and hearing in communication. In P. Skinner & R. Shelton (Eds.), *Speech, language, and hearing: Normal processes and disorders* (2nd ed.). Columbus, OH: Merrill.

Snyder, L., & Downey, D. (1991). The language–reading relationship in normal and reading-disabled children. *Journal of Speech and Hearing Research, 34,* 129–140.

Stein, N., & Glenn, C. (1979). An analysis of story comprehension in elementary school children. In R. Freedle (Ed.), *New directions in discourse processing* (Vol. 2). Norwood, NJ: Ablex.

Symbol Communication Research Project. (1974). *Teaching guideline.* Toronto: Crippled Children's Centre.

Teale, W. (1978). Positive environments for learning to read: What studies of early readers tell us. *Language Arts, 55,* 922–945.

Teale, W. (1980). *Early reading: An annotated bibliography.* Newark, DE: International Reading Association.

Teale, W. (1987). Emergent literacy: Reading and writing development in early childhood. *National Reading Conference Yearbook, 36,* 45–74.

Tunmer, W., & Bowey, J. (1984). Metalinguistic awareness and reading acquisition. In W. Tunmer, C. Pratt, & M. Herriman (Eds.), *Metalinguistic awareness in children: Theory, research, and implications.* New York: Springer-Verlag.

van Kleeck, A. (1990). Emergent literacy: Learning about

print before learning to read. *Topics in Language Disorders, 10,* 25–45.

van Kleeck, A., & Schuele, C. M. (1987). Precursors to literacy: Normal development. *Topics in Language Disorders, 7,* 13–31.

Wiig, E., & Semel, E. (1976). *Language disabilities in children and adolescents.* New York: Merrill/Macmillan.

Wiig, E., & Semel, E. (1984). *Language assessment and intervention for the learning disabled* (2nd ed.). New York: Merrill/Macmillan.

Wood, M. (1982). *Language disorders in school-age children.* Englewood Cliffs, NJ: Prentice-Hall.

Zintz, M. (1970). *The reading process.* Dubuque, IA: William C. Brown.

Chapter 2

Bases of Language Functioning: An Overview

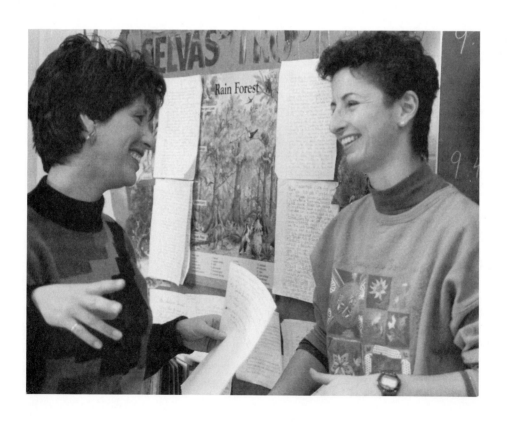

Upon completion of this chapter, the reader should be able to:

▶ Discuss several different views of the relationship between language and cognition.

▶ Define metacognition.

▶ Discuss the components of information processing, with special reference to auditory processing, its relationship to language and speech, and some of the controversial issues regarding this relationship.

▶ Summarize the physiological mechanisms that underlie speech and language functioning.

▶ Discuss the characteristics of a child's language learning environment that contribute to language acquisition.

Language is a complex linguistic, cognitive, physiological, psychological, and sociological phenomenon. All of these factors are involved in language functioning, but the ways in which they interact are not fully understood. In Chapter 1, we discussed the linguistic aspects of language. Here we introduce some of the cognitive, physiological, psychological, and sociological aspects of language. Volumes have been written on each of these topics. We cannot hope to cover them in depth in one chapter. Rather, this chapter provides an overview or, for some readers, a refresher.

LANGUAGE AND COGNITION

Few of us would disagree with the idea that language and cognition are related. However, there is no universal agreement concerning the nature of the relationship. Does cognitive development for specific mental processes precede the acquisition of language structures that incorporate the concepts involved in cognitive development? Does language influence cognition? Are the developments of language and cognition separate entities that become entwined at some point? If so, when? Finally, how do language and cognition influence each other? We have no definitive answers to these questions yet, although a number of theoretical positions regarding the relationship of language and cognition have been advanced. Several theories attempting to describe the relationship between language and cognition are discussed here.

Dependency of Language on Cognition

According to one view of the relationship between language and cognition, language use is a function of cognition and its acquisition is dependent on underlying cognitive processes: "Language and verbal behavior are first and foremost cognitive behaviors. Our verbal behavior is determined by what we know, by what we perceive and think in a given circumstance, and by the cognitive operations in production and comprehension" (Muma, 1978, p. 35). Proponents of this position strongly support the notion of cognitive precursors to language. That is, they believe that there are prerequisite cognitive abilities that children need to develop before learning various language skills, a viewpoint sometimes referred to as the *strong cognition hypothesis*.

Piaget is one of the best-known advocates of this position. He has described four stages in the cognitive development of children: (1) the sensorimotor stage from birth to about 2 years, (2) the preoperational stage from about 2 to 7 years, (3) the concrete operations stage from about 7 to 11 years, and (4) the formal operations stage from about 11 to 15 years (Table 2.1). (Interested readers are referred to Piaget [1957] or Flavell [1977] for more in-depth descriptions of Piaget's theory of cognitive development.) According to Piaget, children progress through each of these cognitive developmental stages in order, without skipping any of them, and each stage of development is the foundation for each succeeding stage. As children progress through the stages, they acquire the necessary

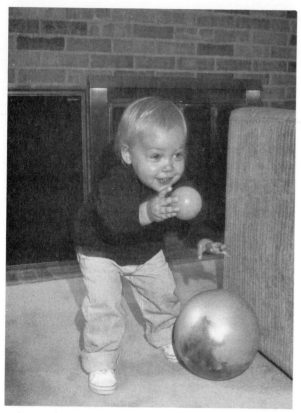

Cognition is important for language development, but the relationship between language and cognition is not well understood.

cognitive operations that lead to the development of succeedingly higher levels of language. Piaget, therefore, believes that thought precedes language. Language use is a reflection of underlying cognitive skills.

Sinclair-deZwart (1973), a coworker of Piaget's, agrees that cognitive development provides the basis for language acquisition. She suggests that children's cognitive developments during the sensorimotor period take place through their experiences with the environment and that this enables them to initiate language production toward the end of the sensorimotor period—18 to 24 months—typically when we see children using single words and some two-word combinations. She states:

Knowledge is acquired through the subject's action upon, and inter-action with, people and things. Action patterns become established, extended, combined with others, and differentiated under the influence of internal regulator mechanisms; later, they become interiorized (i.e., mentally representable) and organized into grouplike structures. Acting upon environment, rather than copying it or talking about it, is the source of knowledge. Language is only one way among others to represent knowledge. Representation in general does not appear until the end of sensorimotor period (around the age of 1½) when direct-acting-on-objects has become organized in a first grouplike structure. (p. 13)

Clark (1973) extended the discussion of thought as the basis for language to children's acquisition of spatial and temporal concepts. In discussing the relationship between children's learning of space and time concepts and their use of appropriate expressions for these concepts, he suggested that they first acquire a priori knowledge of the concepts and then apply the language.

A related view of language functioning as dependent on cognition is the *weak cognition hypothesis.* This position proposes that cognition accounts for many of a child's language abilities but not all of them. There remain some aspects of language that do not derive directly from cognition. Rice (1983) referred to this as a partial "mismatch" between language and cognition and presented, as examples, "language acquisition not rooted in parallel change in meanings, linguistic competence exceeding the supposed cognitive base, and language-specific difficulties with the expression of meanings" (p. 353).

Language and Cognition as Separate (But Sometimes Related) Entities

A differing point of view concerning language and cognition is that although language and cognition are related, cognitive activity without language and language without underlying cognitive bases are both possible. For example, a composer or a sculptor at work is not necessarily directed by language processes (Langacker, 1968). Langacker suggested that if cognitive processes were not possible without language, we would never encounter situations in which we know

TABLE 2.1   Characteristics of Piaget's Stages of Cognitive Development

Sensorimotor (0–2 years)	Preoperational (2–7 years)
Substage 1: 0–2 months Reflexive sensorimotor behavior Reflexive vocal/prelinguistic behavior	*Preconceptual: 2–4 years* Experiences difficulty with sub- and supraclassifications Uses transductive reasoning (inferences from one specific to another specific) Over- and underextends word meanings
Substage 2: 2–4 months Coordinated hand-mouth movements Coordinated eye-hand and auditory orienting movements Anticipatory gestures	*Intuitive: 4–7 years* Thought is guided by perceptions Deals with only one variable at a time Lacks conservation and reversibility Employs improved but still inadequate classification skills Egocentric Concreteness of thought
Substage 3: 4–8 months Begins to act motorically on objects Searches for objects Babbles and imitates sounds	**Concrete Operations (7–11/12 years)**
Substage 4: 8–12 months Begins to recognize own ability to cause objects to move Early stages of walking Searches for objects based on memory of last location Uses first word	Uses effective classification skills Acquires conservation and seriation skills Uses coordinated descriptions Employs logical causality Reasoning limited to concrete experiences Less egocentric
Substage 5: 12–18 months Experimentation with objects' functions and properties Imitates models' behaviors when models present Walks Evidence of object permanency	**Formal Operations (11/12–14/15 years)**
Substage 6: 18–24 months Represents objects internally Problem solving with thought Acquires basic cause-effect relations Uses memory for deferred imitations Uses words when referents not present	Uses hypothetical and propositional reasoning Demonstrates lack of egocentricity Employs adequate verbal reasoning and logical "If . . . then" statements Can deal with the abstract Uses deductive and inductive thought processes

the ideas we wish to convey but are unable to find the right words to express them. Whereas Langacker suggested that cognition without language is possible, Vygotsky (1962) proposed that language without appropriate underlying cognitive bases also occurs. He cited examples in which children correctly use conjunctions, such as "because," "but," and "if," before they fully understand the logical relationships expressed by the terms.

Vygotsky also suggested that the developments of language and thought stem from completely different roots. A child progresses independently through a "preintellectual" language period and a **prelinguistic** thought phase. Although these lines of development are separate for some time, the two developmental processes do eventually merge. The child's thought then becomes verbal and language rational. According to Vygotsky (1962), once the union of language and thought has occurred, language becomes the foundation of further cognitive development: "The speech [language] structures mastered by the child become the basic structures of his thinking.... The child's intellectual growth is contingent on his mastering the social means of thought, that is, language" (p. 51).

The *local homology model* offers a different point of view (Bates, Benigni, Bretherton, Camaioni, & Volterra, 1977, 1979). Some researchers have observed that certain cognitive and linguistic skills develop at the same time, but not necessarily in a predetermined order (Kelly & Dale, 1989; Thal, 1991). That is, a specific language ability sometimes emerges first, and in other instances a cognitive ability appears. This perspective suggests a correlative relationship between language and cognition for some skills at certain points in time. As an example, there is a strong correlation between the use of recognitory gestures and naming when very young children begin to use single words (Bates, Bretherton, Snyder, Shore, & Volterra, 1980). However, the correlation between cognitive and language skills may not be maintained over time. Language and cognition are seen as distinct functions that both derive from a common but separate source. Thal (1991) wrote that the homology model "predicts that at one time we will see a correlation between two behaviors (for example, a linguistic and a nonlinguistic skill), reflecting their common underlying source, but after a period of time they will grow apart" (p. 35). The local homology model appears to have been widely adopted among professionals and researchers in the child language area.

Language Mediation of Cognition

Although there may not be agreement on the exact nature of the early relationship between language and cognition, many suggest that, once acquired, language does mediate many of our cognitive processes. Although Piaget believed that in the earlier stages of a child's development thought precedes language use, he stressed the importance of language in the acquisition of conceptual thinking in the later stages of a child's development. Bruner (1964), a psychologist who views language as a powerful mediating force of cognition, has described the cognitive development of children as consisting of three sequential stages: the enactive stage in early infancy, the iconic stage from about 2 to 6 years, and the symbolic stage from about 6 years on. During the enactive and iconic stages, cognitive processing takes place either through motoric interaction with the environment or by perceptual or image representations. As children enter the symbolic stage of cognitive processing, they are able to internalize stimuli and experiences and represent them in the forms of categories. Bruner (1964) suggested that the use of language is the means by which symbolic processing occurs and views language as a tool for cognition during the symbolic stage. He wrote:

> In effect, language provides a means, not only for representing experience, but also for transforming it.... Once the child has succeeded in internalizing language as a cognitive instrument, it becomes possible for him to represent and systematically transform the regularities of experience with far greater flexibility and power than before. (p. 4)

Both Vygotsky (1962) and Luria (1961) have proposed that language mediates cognitive activity. They used their concepts of *inner speech* and language as a *second signal system* to explain. Vygotsky and Luria viewed inner speech as thought processes that take place in the forms of words. Once language and thought have merged (as previously discussed), thinking occurs in terms of language or word meanings. Vygotsky stated:

> The relation of thought to word is not a thing but a process, a continual movement back and forth from thought to word and from word to thought. In that process the relation of thought to word undergoes changes which themselves may be regarded as development in the functional sense. Thought is not merely expressed in words; it comes into existence through them. (p. 125)

Vygotsky's concept of inner speech led him to disagree with Piaget on the role of children's **egocentric** speech. Piaget described the egocentric speech of young children as speech that occurs with no intent to communicate with others, whether or not others are present, or with no attempt to consider the informational needs of others in communication. It is speech emanating from children who see themselves as the center of the universe, without communicative concern for others. According to Piaget, egocentric speech disappears as children develop, and socialized speech—speech specifically aimed at interpersonal communication—emerges. Vygotsky, however, proposed that the egocentric speech of children is a forerunner of inner speech. He viewed the function of egocentric speech as an overt act of thought, or putting thought into expressed words. According to Vygotsky, the acts of expressing cognitive processes in words are children's ways of guiding and regulating their actions and thoughts. He suggested that as children develop, they are able to turn the overt expressions of thought inward into language, which is used for the same purposes of regulating and guiding thoughts and actions but is not heard by others, that is, inner speech. In contrast to Piaget, Vygotsky described egocentric speech as evolving into inner speech rather than disappearing and being replaced by socialized speech.

The discussion of egocentric speech functioning to regulate and guide thought and action, and then evolving into inner speech for the same guiding and regulating purposes, leads us to Luria's view of language functioning as a second signal system. As children interact with the environment and with the verbalizations of adults, complex connections between perceived phenomena and words are formed (Luria & Yudovich, 1971). Initially, adult verbalizations in the presence of stimuli serve to guide children's behaviors, either to focus the children's attention on specific, essential features of stimuli or to modify and direct their actions in certain directions. That is, in the early developmental stages, the regulation (or direction) of children's cognitive activities and behaviors is externally controlled by the verbalizations of adults, which occur simultaneously with perceived phenomena. Because of the connections between these perceptions and others' verbalizations, children eventually begin to use the verbalizations internally to regulate their own behaviors. Luria and Yudovich (1971) explained:

> The child acquires a system of these verbal instructions and gradually begins to utilize them for the regulation of his own behavior. . . . He begins to act according to verbally elaborated influences by reproducing the verbal connections reinforced by earlier adult instructions, and

thereafter modifies them, isolating verbally the immediate and final aims of his behavior, indicating the means of achieving these aims to verbally formulated instructions. (pp. 24–25)

Through this process, children learn to use language to direct their own thoughts and actions. Language becomes a mediator of cognition and purposeful behavior. Pavlov's terminology is used to describe this process of language self-regulation. The *first signal system* is the cue provided by the actual event or perceived stimuli. The *second signal system* is the verbal mediation of the first signal system. For Luria, language is the basis of the development of higher mental processes because of the second signal function it plays in mediating experiences.

We have seen here several different views on the relationship between language and cognition. Rice (1983) was reassuring when she stated that confusion about the nature of the relationship between cognition and language is justified in light of the diversity of views and the array of empirical data. In summarizing the various positions, she stated:

> Accounts that emphasize the influence of cognition are centered on the earlier stages of acquisition, whereas explanations that emphasize linguistic influence or uniqueness concentrate on later stages. . . . An obvious conclusion is that the relationship between cognition and language may vary as a function of age, linguistic abilities in question, and the type of cognition involved. . . . If that is the case, then any attempt to characterize the relationship in global terms is misdirected. (p. 354)

Metacognition

In chapter 1 we introduced the concept of metalinguistics. Like metalinguistics, **metacognition** relates to the ability to stand back from what we know and the cognitive skills that we have and consciously analyze, control, plan, and organize them (Flavell, 1976; Wellman, 1985). As adults, we can think about our thinking and can decide what learning and cognitive strategies we might want to use in specific situations. We can even monitor our performances and may decide to employ different learning or cognitive strategies. For example, if we need to memorize a list, we might choose to use any of several types of *rehearsal strate-*

gies—saying the list over and over, writing the list over and over, or making up sayings (associations). If one strategy does not work, we may choose to abandon it for another or to use several strategies simultaneously. In other instances, we may ask ourselves: "What else do I know with which I can associate this new piece of information?" or "How can I organize this information so that it makes sense?" These are all metacognitive activities.

In order to engage in metacognitive activities, we need to *decenter,* that is, be less egocentric, to use a Piagetian term. Like metalinguistics, true metacognition in children is a later-developing skill, with some suggesting a shift to metacognitive abilities occurring sometime in the early elementary grades, from kindergarten to grade 2 (Wiig, 1989). If we review Table 2.1, we see that these grades/ages tend to correspond to about the time children enter Piaget's concrete operations stage. Another shift to higher-level, more refined metacognitive skills is generally seen at about grade 6 or at 11–12 years of age, about the time children enter Piaget's formal operations stage.

Not surprisingly, metacognitive skills are important in school success. Expectations for how children are to solve problems and approach learning increase as children progress through school. By senior high, students are expected to monitor and plan their own learning and to think and reason with adultlike abilities. We suspect some relationship between metacognitive and metalinguistic skills (e.g., van Kleeck, 1984; Wiig, 1989), but as with the relationship between cognition and language generally, the exact nature of the relationship is not clear. We do know, however, that many children with language disorders evidence problems with metacognitive tasks (e.g., Kamhi, 1987; Kamhi, Gentry, Mouer, & Gholson, 1990; Wiig, 1989).

INFORMATION PROCESSING

Another way to look at language is from an information processing point of view. Information processing focuses on the ways in which humans deal with incoming stimuli, that is, the steps in taking in stimuli and analyzing and retaining them for future use. A number of information processing models have been proposed. In comparing these models, however, it is not unusual to find that they include different component processes, label the processes differently, and use different definitions for what appear to be similar processes. No one information processing model has been universally adopted. However, some of the processes that have been included in many models are attention to stimuli, rate at which stimuli are dealt with, discrimination among stimuli, determining the sequence of the stimuli, and memory of the stimuli. We will discuss these processes here. And of these processes, those dealing with auditory processing, as opposed, for example, to visual processing, have received the greatest attention in the area of language. They will, therefore, receive more attention in the following discussion. Of course, adequate processing of stimuli requires that the system be sufficiently sensitive to the stimuli. For auditory functioning this requires adequate auditory sensitivity (hearing acuity). We will begin with a brief introduction to auditory sensitivity. We will then present an overview of several aspects of processing and conclude with a discussion of some of the controversy that surrounds the area of auditory processing.

Auditory Sensitivity

Hearing is the primary sensory modality through which oral language is acquired. The effects of reduced **auditory sensitivity**, or hearing loss, on oral language skills are dramatically illustrated in the language and speech difficulties experienced by deaf children. However, less severe hearing losses can also interfere with the acquisition of language and speech skills. Although there is no one-to-one relationship between the degree of hearing loss and the extent of language and speech impairment, generally the greater the loss, the more impaired the oral communication skills will be. There is also some evidence in the literature that even mild, intermittent hearing losses due to middle ear infections in children can adversely affect language and speech acquisition and, later, academic achievement. In reviewing the results of numerous investigations, Northern and Downs (1984) conclude that "investigators have pointed up the role of minimal auditory deficiencies in lowering school achievement or language skills" (p. 17). Although auditory sensitivity and **auditory perception** and processing are frequently discussed separately, they are not as distinct as these discussions might imply. For example, some auditory sensitivity problems result in distortions of incoming acoustic signals, as well as reduced sensitivity to the sounds themselves. Even though a speech signal may be heard, it may be decoded inaccurately because it is distorted. Van Tasell (1981) suggests that the "inability of the abnormal auditory system to preserve speech information constitutes the speech recognition impairment caused by hearing loss" (p. 14). Katz (1978) and Brandes and Ehinger (1981) even suggest that slight, fluctuating hearing losses, typical of middle ear infections, can lead to inadequate acquisition of auditory perceptual abilities, as well as language skills, especially when children experience these mild losses at early ages. Adequate auditory sensitivity is, therefore, a critical factor in normal language and speech development in children. In Chapter 9 the implications of disorders of auditory sensitivity are examined.

Some Processing Components

Attention   At any one time, the human organism is bombarded with many environmental stimuli in many sensory forms. Although multimodality stimuli are constantly present in the environment, we cannot consciously process all of them at the same time. We selectively choose which stimuli to pay attention to, and our selection is often based on our purposes and motivations at the time. Stimuli that are relevant to our immediate behavior are consciously brought to the foreground, and other, less relevant stimuli are ignored until such time as they become important.

The abilities to attend selectively to certain stimuli and ignore others, and to maintain attention long enough for the stimuli to be interpreted, are critical for active learning. Unless children can sort out the numerous stimuli by attending only to some, they attempt to deal with all. Few stimuli, if any, actually get processed. Processing information from stimuli takes time, and children must continue to attend to the selected stimuli until processing is completed. If children cannot maintain attention to specific stimuli without being distracted by other stimuli, only part of

the important stimuli is processed and the rest is missed. Conversely, children must be able to shift their attention when incoming stimuli indicate that changes are appropriate or when the reasons for attending change. Without being able to shift attention to new stimuli when the situation requires it, children continue to respond inappropriately to previous stimuli.

Both cognitive abilities and language skills can be negatively affected by problems with attention. Attention to stimuli in the environment is a necessary prerequisite for the acquisition of concepts that underlie language. The perceptual attributes of objects and activities to which a child attends provide the input needed to form classifications and categorizations that become the referents for words. Language-disordered children are often described as demonstrating difficulties with one or more of these aspects of attention, and the literature abounds with terms such as *distractibility, inattentiveness, short attention span,* and *perseveration.*

Selection of which stimuli to attend to depends largely on how salient the stimuli are. Stimuli that have more salient features are attended to more quickly, more frequently, and for longer periods than are stimuli with less salient aspects. *Saliency* can be determined not only by the relevance of the stimuli but also by the energy, or strength, of the composite features and the degree to which the stimuli change or differ from the background. Children tend to pay more attention to stimuli that are louder or brighter and that represent change, especially if the children themselves are the agents of the change. Objects and activities with these characteristics will most likely be the ones that form the early experiential bases for language.

Auditory attention is the ability to focus selectively on important aspects of speech signals and ignore other acoustic stimuli that, at any moment in time, are not relevant to the listener. The ability to attend to speech signals has been described as a critical factor in learning, and a number of authors have identified auditory inattentiveness as a characteristic of children with impaired language skills (Costello, 1977; Sanders, 1977; Wiig & Semel, 1976; Witkin, 1971). Without the ability to attend selectively to certain speech stimuli and ignore irrelevant acoustic signals, it is suggested that the listener experiences a sensory overload because all incoming sounds are treated as equally important and none gets decoded. It may also mean that important aspects of speech do not get sorted out for language acquisition.

Auditory attention is a developmental skill. Children improve in their ability to focus auditorily as they grow older (Hedrick, 1967; Maccoby, 1967; Maccoby & Konrad, 1966, 1967). It is unclear whether the developmental trend is a phenomenon of increasing skill in auditory processing itself or a function of improved language abilities that reduces the need to process much of the incoming stimuli. The relationship may be reciprocal. However, there is evidence that young infants (7 and 8 months old) attend more to the language of their environment than to other languages and more to speech that contains pauses at clause boundaries (syntactic boundaries) than to speech that has pauses in the middle of clauses (Hirsh-Pasek, Nelson, Jusczyk, Cassidy, Druss, & Kennedy, 1987; Mehler, Jusczyk, Lambertz, Halsted, Bertoncini, & Amiel-Tison, 1988). Infants as young as 4 weeks old have also been found to attend longer to facial (lip) movements that match the vowels being heard than to those that do not match the vowels being heard (Kuhl, 1990; Kuhl & Meltzoff, 1988). Apparently, infants' attending skills are intermodal in that they associate lip movements with the appropriate speech sounds. These findings suggest very early development taking place with regard to auditory attending behaviors.

Rate   Rate refers to the speed with which we can process bits of information. *Speed reading* became popular because its techniques purported to increase the rate at which adults could process print. The faster we can process information, the quicker we can move on to and attend to new stimuli.

Auditory rate refers to the ability to process acoustic stimuli presented at varying speeds. Speech consists of very rapid sequences of different sounds. The suggestion has been made that children with language-learning problems need to have speech stimuli presented at slower rates in order to process the incoming messages. The implications are, therefore, that there is a base rate at which children with normally developing language can process incoming speech signals and that children experiencing language-learning difficulties cannot decode speech quickly

enough to keep up with the flow of messages. In a review of the literature exploring children's performances on tasks in which the rates of stimuli presentation had been electronically altered (compressed or expanded), Lubert (1981) indicates that there is some evidence that language-impaired children have more difficulties than children with adequate oral communicative skills in perceiving separations and differences between speech sounds presented at *rapid* rates. She adds that a consistent finding in the literature suggests that language-impaired children demonstrate deficits in determining the sequence of rapidly presented speech sounds when their performances are compared to language-normal children. Lubert summarizes the research results as follows: "Language-disordered children are unable to adequately process rapidly incoming acoustic information, though they may be able to deal with slower auditory signals" (p. 6).

Like auditory attention, auditory rate has been found to be a developmental process. Tallal (1976) found that normal 8½-year-old children performed as well as adults on rapidly presented auditory stimuli but that 6½-year-old children could achieve at the same performance levels only when the incoming stimuli were given at slower rates. Further support showing a developmental trend for auditory rate skills has been demonstrated by Beasley, Maki, and Orchik (1976).

Discrimination   Discrimination involves recognizing differences among stimuli. Discrimination between objects and events is important in children's language. Not only must children recognize similarities in order to form semantic classes of objects, they must recognize differences. For example, not all balls are alike, yet they belong to the same class. Differences between balls allow children to form subordinate classifications, for example, footballs, basketballs, and baseballs. Sometimes differences in the characteristics of stimuli are so great that it is relatively easy to recognize them. In other instances, differences can be much less marked, making recognition of the differences more difficult. In reading, it is generally easier to recognize visually the differences between the letters "o" and "t." It is typically more difficult to recognize visually the differences between "b" and "d" or between "b" and "p."

Auditory discrimination is the act of identifying differences between sound stimuli. Witkin (1971) has stated that adequate "auditory discrimination is essential for the acquisition of language and for learning to read" (p. 42). Although auditory discrimination has been one of the most studied and discussed of the auditory operations, it is also one of the most confusing. The variety of tasks used to study auditory discrimination skills has created much of the confusion. Aram and Nation (1982) summarized these various tasks as consisting of metalinguistic, linguistic, and/or nonlinguistic operations. Knowledge of and skills with language can affect the results of studies that use tasks involving linguistically meaningful stimuli (Atchison & Canter, 1979; Locke, 1980a, 1980b). Furthermore, nonlinguistic sounds may be neurologically processed differently than linguistic stimuli, so the results of investigations that utilize nonlinguistic tasks cannot be generalized to auditory discrimination skills for linguistic material. Many tests designed to measure auditory discrimination skills in children have been developed. Most of these involve asking children to tell whether two sounds are the same or different (e.g., "s" and "th"), to identify one of several minimally paired words (words that differ only by one phoneme, such and "beet" and "sheet"), or to tell whether two minimally paired words said by an examiner are the same or different. The validity of such commercially available tests has been questioned (Locke, 1980a, 1980b; Rees, 1973).

Although the role of auditory discrimination in language acquisition and the methods of examining auditory discrimination abilities remain areas of debate and confusion, children with language disorders have sometimes been described as having poorer auditory discrimination skills than their normal-language peers (e.g., Elliott & Busse, 1987; Elliott, Hammer, & Scholl, 1989; Tallal & Piercy, 1974; Tallal, Stark, Kallman, & Mellits, 1981). There is also a suggestion, as with the previously discussed auditory operations, that children improve in their ability to discriminate auditory stimuli as they grow older (Elliott, 1986; Elliott, Busse, Partridge, Rupert, & DeGraaf, 1986; Weiner, 1967; Wepman, 1960). Other studies have found that infants,

some as young as 4 weeks of age, can discriminate auditorily between syllables differing only by one phoneme (Eimas, 1974; Moffitt, 1971; Morse, 1972; Trehub, 1973), 6-month-old infants can discriminate vowels and recognize them as the same or different when they are spoken by different speakers (Grieser & Kuhl, 1989), and 4-month-old infants can not only discriminate between vowels but can imitate vocally the main features of the vowels (Kuhl, 1990). Again we see remarkably early ability for auditory functioning.

Sequencing   Sequencing involves the ability to identify the order in which stimuli occur. Visual sequencing is an important part of reading and writing. **Auditory sequencing** skills, which involve the ability to identify the temporal order of acoustic stimuli, have been described as important for adequate language and speech acquisition and for analysis of meaning (Sanders, 1977; Witkin, 1971). The ability to determine the sequences of auditory stimuli also requires memory for the units and discrimination among the individual components of the signal. Studies of auditory sequencing skills have, therefore, frequently been contaminated by requiring the use of auditory processing tasks in addition to sequencing operations alone. In such instances, differentiating among the auditory operations that affected the results is difficult, if not impossible.

As we indicated earlier, children with normal language skills appear to be able to identify the temporal order of rapidly presented speech sound sequences better than children with language disorders. These differences in auditory sequencing abilities might be interpreted as the reasons for the differences in the children's language proficiencies. However, when the rate of presentation for auditory sequences has been reduced, language-impaired children have been able to improve in determining sequences accurately (McCroskey & Thompson, 1973; Peck, 1977; Tallal & Piercy, 1975). Therefore, the rate of auditory stimuli presentation for language-disordered children appears to affect the ability to determine the sequence. This is a variable that has not always been controlled in auditory sequencing investigations, making interpretation of results equivocal. Other investigations have incorporated matching motor sequential responses with auditory stimuli and/or matching a second type of representation with auditory sequences, such as ordering different colored blocks to correspond with different sequences of sounds. The reasons for children's failures or successes with these activities cannot be differentiated when such complex tasks are involved. The role that auditory sequencing skills play in language has not yet been isolated from the influences of other auditory, linguistic, or cognitive operations.

Memory   Memory is a critical aspect of language learning. If events and stimuli cannot be retained in memory, categorizing and abstracting processes necessary for language fail to occur. Hubbell (1981) writes:

> Memory is the cornerstone of our information-processing capacities. Memory is at the very heart of language learning and use. . . . In fact, one way to look at learning is in terms of getting information into permanent memory and out again at appropriate times. (p. 28)

Brown (1975) identified two types of memory—episodic and semantic. *Episodic memory* involves recall of entire units despite their meaningfulness. Remembering telephone numbers ascertained from a directory long enough to dial them is episodic memory. In contrast, *semantic memory* involves remembering reproductions of initial events. The mnemonic reconstructions of these events are not exact. Rather, only the critical elements or main points are recalled. Because only the major points are remembered, some points are forgotten, and much is integrated and associated with other representations in memory. As we might expect, semantic memory for events leads to categorization and classification.

Some remembering is purposeful, whereas other remembering is involuntary (Brown, 1975). In instances of intentional memory, rehearsal strategies and mnemonic devices are typically employed. Although voluntary memory usually involves mnemonic strategies, these strategies often impose associative or categorization activities on the information. As a result, the information is made meaningful. In contrast, unintentional memory is the result of "the involuntary product of our continuous interactions with a relatively meaningful environment" (Brown, 1975, p. 113). Hubbell (1981) suggests that in the process of learning, including learning language, children rarely demonstrate the intention to remember. However, the more meaningful an experience, the more likely the major points of the experience will be remembered. As we see, meaning may very well lead to more information being stored in memory. Memory for experiences leads to information storage that can be classified and associated, and that provides the foundation for remembering more information, since meaning is imposed on the events.

Auditory memory, or the ability to store speech stimuli mentally, is closely related to auditory sequencing, and certainly affects and is affected by discrimination abilities. Speech signals occur in series over time. In order for auditory stimuli to be differentiated, the speech signals must be remembered long enough to be compared. Furthermore, the ability to perceive a temporal sequence of sounds depends, in part, on being able to remember the stimuli. With the close relationship of auditory memory to auditory sequencing, as well as discrimination, most of the investigations in this area have incorporated tasks that require several forms of processing.

Concepts of short- and long-term auditory memory are presented in most discussions of auditory memory. *Short-term memory* is the relatively brief retention of auditory stimuli. This is similar to Brown's (1975) concept of episodic memory. However, there is a fairly severe limit on the number of auditory units that can be held in short-term memory. This limit has been estimated at between five and seven (some suggest nine) discrete units (Anderson, 1975; Sanders, 1977; Simon, 1974). Because such limits exist for short-term auditory memory, this aspect of processing cannot account for the larger amounts of auditory information we are able to remember in order to interpret them. By grouping the discrete units, or *chunking* the stimuli into related elements, we are able to retain a larger amount of information. However, the chunking process requires that the relationships among units be identified. This is similar to Brown's concept of semantic memory. This process also closely resembles classification and categorization activities, skills that are integrally related to language. Sanders (1977) states that a child who experiences deficits in the ability to chunk auditory stimuli

> soon faces an overload situation, since he lacks the patterns which would further reduce dependency upon individual components. Instead of being able to process a limited number of logical auditory language units, the child has to attempt to retain a long string of single sounds or words, a task beyond the capacity of his short term memory system. (p. 209)

The ability to retain and immediately repeat sequences of unrelated words, such as digits, increases with age. One might conclude that as children grow older, their auditory memory spans increase. However, this does not appear to be the case. Rather than true increases in auditory memory spans with age, more efficient abilities to impose structure on auditory stimuli seem to account for the longer sequences of information that can be stored as age increases. That is, organizational skills or strategies for remembering improve with maturation, but the absolute storage capacity itself does not likely increase. This perspective suggests that language and language-related skills, such as cognitive abilities and categorization and classification abilities, influence retention and recall of auditory stimuli. For example, in a study examining children's ability to imitate auditorily presented sequences of related words (sentences), Menyuk and Looney's findings (1972a, 1972b) indicated that the grammatical structure of sentences was more influential in affecting children's ability to remember and reproduce the utterances than the length of the sentences. Remedial activities aimed at improving children's auditory memory skills might, therefore, be better directed toward helping children organize incoming information rather than emphasizing repetition of increasingly longer sequences of items.

Long-term memory is the more permanent retention of acoustic signals. Although long-term auditory memory is an often-referred-to aspect of processing, its nature is even less well understood than that of other auditory operations. Most adult language users can recall the acoustic characteristics of a phoneme or word. There is a stored model that can be retrieved and against which incoming stimuli can be compared. Certainly, practice and repeated experiences would enhance these abilities. However, the process by which auditory stimuli are transferred to long-term memory storage is not precisely known, with Berry (1980) concluding that the neurophysiological "evidence on the difference between short-term memory and long-term storage is inconclusive" (p. 98). Meaningfulness and usefulness of incoming stimuli likely affect what information is retained on a long-term basis. Perhaps the more relevant the incoming stimuli are viewed, the greater the probability that the person will remember them for longer periods of time. However, this view suggests that auditory stimuli that are to be transferred to long-term memory must first be analyzed for meaningfulness. Once they are transferred to long-term memory, the question then becomes one of retrieving the memory for use on demand. Retrieval mechanisms are also not fully understood.

Controversy About Auditory Processing

Auditory processing and its relationship to normal and impaired language and speech are areas of considerable confusion and debate. Yet, having made this statement, we know that most humans are particularly good at processing speech- and language-related auditory information. Some suggest that the human nervous system is especially adapted for this task. We even know that infants, some within a month of birth, are attending to, discriminating, and recognizing certain aspects of auditory stimuli that are important for speech and language development. Such information suggests that very early in development the human organism is capable of critically analyzing auditory information. This ability may well provide a basis for language and speech learning. It would seem reasonable, therefore, to conclude that adequate perception and processing of auditory information is fundamental to normal oral language development. It would also follow logically that deficits in auditory processing could lead to impaired acquisition of oral language and later to other learning problems. And, in fact, professionals working with language-impaired children have often noted what appear to be problems in processing auditory stimuli. The children seem to pay little attention to auditory stimuli or appear not to recognize differences in sounds. We have alluded to some of these problems in the foregoing discussions. In light of these statements, one might wonder why the area is surrounded with controversy and debate. Part of the debate has centered on the direction and nature of the effect, with some suggesting that inadequate auditory processing skills negatively influence the acquisition of language and speech and with others proposing that deficient oral communication skills adversely affect auditory processing abilities. Embodied in the debate is the controversial diagnostic label termed *central auditory processing disorder* (CAPD).

In support of the viewpoint that poor auditory processing skills negatively affect language and speech acquisition, a number of studies examining the auditory skills of children with language and/or speech disorders or with learning problems in language-related areas have found that these children experience difficulties in one or more aspects of auditory processing (e.g., Eisenson, 1968; Elliott et al., 1989; Haggerty & Stamm, 1978; McReynolds, 1966; Rosenthal, 1970; Tallal & Piercy, 1974; Tallal et al., 1981; Weiner, 1969a, 1969b). The assumption is that adequate auditory processing abilities are prerequisite to normal language and speech learning, and inadequate functioning can lead to language and/or speech deficits. These observations and findings have led some to suggest the children have what are believed to be central auditory processing disorders stemming from neurological disruptions in the auditory pathways beyond the ear, that is, in the central nervous system. The children have adequate hearing sensitivity but problems sorting and integrating what they hear.

In contrast, others argue that the evidence indicating that auditory processing skills are basic to some language and/or speech problems is weak, if nonexistent, or that interpretation of findings as causal factors must be done cautiously (Leonard, 1982; Rees, 1973; Tomblin & Quinn, 1983). One frequently used task in these studies has been to have children make distinctions auditorily between /ba/ and /da/ presented rapidly. Leonard and his colleagues (Leonard, McGregor, & Allen, 1992) state that

> although the [ba]–[da] distinction is difficult for children with SLI [specific language impairment] in these studies,

substitutions of [b] for [d] or vice versa are very rare in the speech of these children. In addition, even normally developing children under the age of 4 years, 6 months cannot perform the simplest of the tasks used in this line of research—the target identification task—yet these children produce language that seemingly requires the perception of many of the same fine distinctions. (pp. 1076–1077)

For some, difficulties with auditory processing skills are viewed as possible results of deficits in oral communicative abilities. Normal language users auditorily process incoming speech signals in light of their linguistic knowledge, an ability that reduces dependency on each specific aspect of auditory signals. Pierce (1969), in describing how people understand spoken language, proposes that comprehension occurs "not because they hear the phonetic features or words distinctly, but because they have a general sense of what a conversation is about and are able to guess what has been said" (pp. 1049–1050). Linguistic knowledge provides the listener with predictive abilities about what the upcoming auditory signals in a sequence will be. Sanders (1977) writes that "prediction greatly enhances the rate of perception and consequently the rate at which spoken language can be perceived" (p. 8). This latter viewpoint places less emphasis on the importance of inadequate auditory processing skills as factors underlying disruptions in language and speech acquisition or at least questions the relationship between language learning and auditory processing.

An alternative perspective on these two possible relationships of auditory processing and language is that auditory processing and linguistic deficits are concomitants of each other, and the skills evidenced in both aspects of behavior are the result of some other factor (Lahey, 1988; Tallal & Piercy, 1978). In other words, some third capability leads to adequate acquisition of both auditory processing and oral communicative functioning, and disruption of this still unidentified third factor can lead to impaired language learning and auditory processing skills. It is also likely that the relationship between auditory processing and language changes as a child develops and as skills in both aspects are acquired and extended. Some evidence of this comes from research on children younger than 1 year of age. Werker (1989) reported that at about 6 months of age, infants from English-speaking homes can discriminate between phonemes used in other languages but not in English. At 8 to 10 months of age, infants have more difficulty making such discriminations, and by 12 months of age very few can make the discriminations for the foreign language. Children seem to start with a universal discrimination ability, but the language of the environment appears very early to affect what they can and cannot discriminate auditorily later on. The relationship between oral language and auditory processing is probably more complex than the viewpoints proposing that development of one ability results in development of the other or that an impairment of one causes impairment of the other.

The methods used to investigate auditory processing skills have also led to some of the controversy surrounding the role of these skills in language. Many of the studies have employed behavioral tests of auditory processing that use naturally spoken stimuli, semantic concepts such as same-different, and/or spoken responses on the part of the subjects (Aten & Davis, 1968; Flowers & Costello, 1963; McReynolds, 1966; Stark, Poppen, & May, 1967; Weiner, 1969a, 1969b). Critics of these studies have suggested that children may perform poorly because of the tasks involved rather than because of true deficits in auditory processing. Furthermore, the tests may not examine auditory processing at the appropriate neuropsychological processing levels or control for other acoustic factors such as the sound level of the input or background noise. In light of the concerns about the validity of these investigations, Lubert (1981) writes that examination of auditory processing function might better be accomplished in controlled conditions with "synthetically produced or synthetically altered stimuli, in tasks that do not require a verbal response" (p. 5). A number of studies have incorporated such technological modifications (Rosenthal, 1970; Tallal & Piercy, 1973a, 1973b, 1974). However, language-impaired children have been found to perform equally well or better on auditory tasks involving linguistic stimuli compared to tasks incorporating nonlinguistic tones (Thal & Barone, 1983). These results suggest that, in contrast to synthetically produced

auditory stimuli, naturally produced linguistic (meaningful) stimuli may ease the tasks involved in processing auditory stimuli. It is possible that artificially produced stimuli do not truly measure the skills used in language processing, whereas the use of linguistically meaningful stimuli confounds the measurement of auditory processing abilities with a measurement of language skills.

To address some of the concerns about other methods of examining auditory processing skills, testing for central auditory processing disorders is generally done with relatively sophisticated equipment in specially sound-treated environments in an attempt to control background noise and the level and timing of auditory stimuli. Conditions are similar to those used by audiologists to test hearing sensitivity. Some of the tasks children are asked to perform involve comprehending speech in conditions of controlled background noise (figure-ground), **dichotic** listening, and pitch-pattern sequencing (Chermak & Musiek, 1992; Keith, 1984). The concerns raised earlier regarding the nature of the auditory stimuli used in auditory processing tasks are relevant to these tasks as well. That is, these are not always tasks children encounter in daily life. Concern has also been raised about the need to standardized the stimuli being used (Noffsinger, 1992).

Additional confusion has resulted from a lack of agreement regarding the components of the holistic concept termed *auditory processing,* the components' labels and their definitions, and their relationships to each other (Chalfant & Scheffelin, 1969; Sanders, 1977; Weener, 1974; Wiig & Semel, 1976). This confusion is not unlike the problems associated with information processing models generally, as raised in the introduction to this topic. Although attempts have been made to delineate the individual components making up auditory processing, Sanders (1977) states that "each [component] is so intimately involved with all other aspects of processing that it is impossible to define any as truly autonomous" (p. 201).

Several years ago, Aram and Nation (1982) summarized the area of auditory processing in four statements. The statements continue to apply:

1. We only know what we know, which is not enough. (p. 108)

This statement is true for both auditory processing as a requisite for normal language development and deficient auditory perception as a possible cause of language and speech disorders.

> 2. All child language disorders do not stem from auditory processing disruptions. (p. 108)

Multiple factors influence language and speech acquisition or disrupt its development. The exact role that auditory processing plays is still unclear.

> 3. Children may fail auditory processing tasks because of the task rather than because of an auditory processing deficit. (p. 109)

Many of our research and testing instruments do not presently allow us to make discriminative statements about the relationship between language and speech skills and auditory processing abilities.

> 4. We must maintain alternative perspectives on the causal relationship of auditory processing disruptions and child language disorders. (p. 110)

We must view normal language and speech acquisition as a process affected by many interacting variables and requisite skills. Anyone attempting to understand children's acquisition of language and speech must be aware of the many parameters that may affect language learning; auditory processing is only one of those factors, although it may be an important one.

PHYSICAL MECHANISMS UNDERLYING SPOKEN LANGUAGE

In chapter 1, hearing and speaking were identified as the primary modalities used in spoken languages. Although other modalities, such as vision and gesture, may contribute to the total communicative process, our discussion here provides an overview of the major physical bases of auditory-oral language: the ear, the speech mechanism, and the nervous system.

The Ear

The ear is the sensory mechanism that receives sound waves and converts them sequentially into mechanical, hydraulic, and finally electrical/electrochemical energy (neural impulses). If the ear is not adequately sensitive to a variety of sound frequencies and intensities, auditory information needed to receive and understand the spoken code of others is prevented from being converted to neural impulses and reaching the brain.

The ear consists of three parts: the outer ear, the middle ear, and the inner ear—that is, the **peripheral hearing mechanism** (Figure 2.1). In the *outer ear,* the auricle and ear canal (external auditory meatus) collect sound waves and funnel them toward the middle ear, where the waves hit the eardrum (tympanic membrane) and make it vibrate. The movement of the eardrum, now mechanical energy, is transferred to three small bones of the *middle ear*—the malleus, incus, and stapes—which pass the movement to the inner ear. The major structure for hearing in the *inner ear* is the cochlea. The *cochlea* contains a membranous structure suspended in fluid. As the mechanical energy in the middle ear reaches the inner ear, the fluid is set in motion. Mechanical energy now becomes hydraulic energy. As the fluid moves, it impinges on the membranous structure—the *cochlear duct*—which also contains fluid, and the end organ of hearing, the *organ of Corti*. The movement of the membrane causes the fluid in the membrane to move, and the result is a rubbing or shearing action on parts of the organ of Corti. This rubbing converts the hydraulic energy to neural energy, which travels to the brain via cranial nerve VIII (the vestibulocochlear, or auditory, nerve).

The Speech Mechanism

The anatomical structures used to produce speech are actually parts of the respiratory and digestive systems (Figure 2.2). The exhaled air from the lungs provides the basic source of energy for speech. It is this air that is modified by the vocal folds in the larynx and/or the structures of the mouth to produce speech sounds.

The *larynx,* located in the front of the neck, houses the *vocal folds.* During production of approximately one-half of the English consonants, the vocal folds are basically inactive. These sounds are termed *voiceless consonants* because they require no vibration of the vocal folds. Air from the lungs passes unobstructed to-

FIGURE 2.1   The Ear. (From *Basic Anatomy and Physiology of Speech and Hearing: A Learning Guide,* 2nd ed. [p. 210], by Vicki Reed, 1982, Austin, TX: PRO-ED. Copyright 1982 by PRO-ED. Used with permission.)

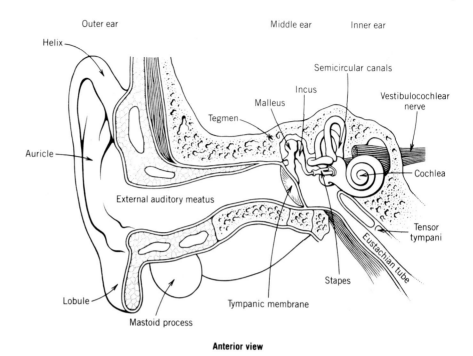

Anterior view

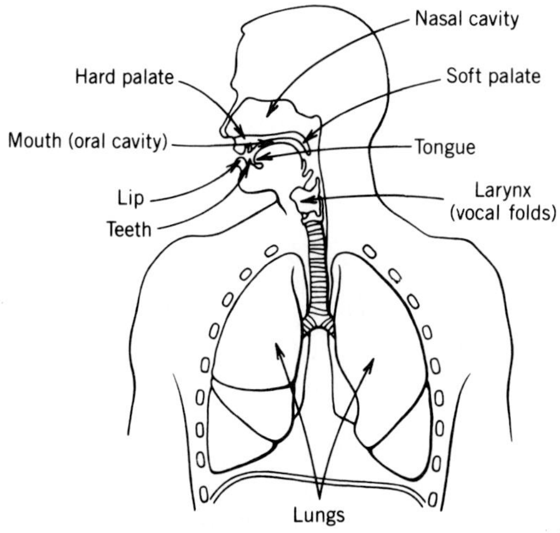

FIGURE 2.2   The Speech Mechanism. (Adapted from *Basic Anatomy and Physiology of Speech and Hearing: A Learning Guide,* 2nd ed. [p. 2], by Vicki Reed, 1982, Austin, TX: PRO-ED. Copyright 1982 by PRO-ED. Used with permission.)

ward the mouth. If a hand is placed lightly against the front of the neck as consonants such as /p/, /t/, and /s/ are said, no vibration is felt. However, during production of all vowels and the remaining consonants, the vocal folds vibrate, causing air passing through the larynx toward the mouth to vibrate. Phonemes that require vocal-fold vibration are termed *voiced sounds.* These vocal-fold vibrations can be felt when a hand is held lightly on the front of the neck as sounds such as /z/, /b/, /d/, and /e/ are said. The size of the vocal folds and the rate at which they vibrate are primary factors in determining the pitch of a person's voice. *Pitch* is the psychological correlate of the physical phenomenon of **frequency** of vibration. Generally, the faster something vibrates, the higher the pitch.

After the exhaled air passes through the larynx, whether or not the phoneme to be produced is voiced, it reaches the mouth area. For production of consonants, the major *articulators* (the lips, tongue, teeth, and palate) impede the flow of outgoing air and create noises. As we recall from chapter 1, the characteristics of the individual consonants depend, in part, on the positions of the articulators and the degrees to which they obstruct the flow of exhaled air. Some obstructions are complete and are then released (e.g., /p/, /t/, /k/), while other obstructions allow for an obstructed but continuous flow of air (e.g., /s/, "sh"). The type of obstruction is called *manner of formation*. The place in the mouth where obstruction occurs (e.g., lips-teeth for /f/ or back of the tongue for /k/) is termed the *place of articulation*. The different positions of the articulators cause sound energy to be concentrated in different frequencies. For example, /s/ has sound energy concentrated in the higher frequencies, whereas /f/ has sound energy concentrated in the lower frequencies. Because voiceless consonants have no vocal-fold vibrations, the sounds are only the result of mouth noise created by the articulators. If a consonant is voiced, such as /z/, the mouth noises created by the articulators are superimposed on the vibrations of the vocal folds. Therefore, voiced sounds have a fundamental frequency from the vocal-fold vibrations, which is comparatively low, and concentrations of sound energy in certain higher frequencies (mouth noises) because of the obstructions of the articulators.

For most English vowels and consonants the exhaled air is directed into the mouth. To accomplish this, the soft palate, which is the mobile end of the palate, is able to move up and back to close the opening into the nasal cavity. However, production of three English phonemes ("m," "n," and "ng") requires that the air be directed into the nasal cavity to create a nasal resonance (**nasalization**). For these phonemes, the soft palate lowers and allows the air to pass into the nasal cavity. The effect of the air in the nasal cavity can be felt if an index finger is placed lightly along the bony side of the nose while saying a prolonged /n/. As all three nasal sounds are voiced, the nasal resonance is superimposed on the vocal-fold vibrations.

All vowels are voiced, and in contrast to consonants, the articulators place few obstructions in the way of the exhaled air. Instead, movement of the articulators, primarily the tongue, changes the internal shape of the mouth cavity in order to give each vowel its unique sound. These changes in the internal shape of the mouth also concentrate sound energy in different fre-

quencies. For each vowel, energy concentration occurs in identifiable bands at different frequencies, including the low-frequency one associated with the vocal-fold vibrations. The frequency location of the higher-frequency bands of energy gives each vowel its unique acoustic features. The bands of energy are called *formants*; these will be discussed further in chapter 9 in relation to their importance in hearing impairment.

The Nervous System

Two major divisions of the nervous system are integrally involved in speech and language: the central nervous system (brain and spinal cord) and the peripheral nervous system (cranial and spinal nerves). A third division, the autonomic nervous system, regulates the presumably involuntary bodily functions, such as stomach and bowel contractions and heart-beat. Since this last system affects speech and language only indirectly, it will not be discussed here.

The Central Nervous System (CNS)   At its superior end, the spinal cord forms a structure known as the *brain stem,* composed of the medulla, the pons, and the midbrain (Figure 2.3). The cerebrum (often

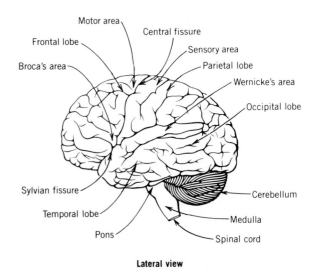

Lateral view

FIGURE 2.3   The Brain.

referred to as the *brain*) sits on top of the brain stem and surrounds it, much as a mushroom top surrounds the upper stem of a mushroom. The wrinkled outer surface of the cerebrum is the *cortex*. The cerebellum is located below the cerebrum and behind the brain stem. Like the cerebrum, the cerebellum also has a wrinkled outer surface called the cortex. The wrinkles of both structures are the result of folds in the surfaces. Each ridge created by these folds is known as a *gyrus,* or *convolution,* and each indentation caused by the folds is called a *sulcus,* or *fissure.* These convolutions and fissures provide us with landmarks in order to describe the brain.

Both the cerebellum and the cerebrum are divided into right and left hemispheres. Each cerebral hemisphere is further divided into four lobes. The most anterior lobe is known as the *frontal lobe.* The *parietal lobe* lies behind the frontal lobe and is separated from it by the *central fissure.* Behind the parietal lobe is the *occipital lobe.* The *temporal lobe* is on the side and separated from the frontal lobe by the *Sylvian fissure.*

As the result of studies investigating the effects of damage to parts of the brain on neurological functions and, more recently, studies using newer neuroimaging techniques (blood flow rates, positron emission tomography, magnetic resonance imaging, event-related electrophysiological procedures), we know that certain functions in adults are generally related to different parts of the cerebral cortex. The *motor area* is located in the frontal lobe in front of the central fissure. Neural impulses are sent from the motor area to various muscles of the body, including those involved in speech production, in order to produce movement. Two motor pathways or *tracts* (the pyramidal and extrapyramidal motor tracts) provide routes for the impulses running from the cortex to nerves of the peripheral nervous system and then to muscles. The *pyramidal tract* provides the most direct route between the motor cortex and the peripheral nervous system, while the *extrapyramidal tract* contains many junctions in its route to the peripheral nervous system. Most neural impulses coursing through these pathways travel to the nerves of the peripheral nervous system on the side of the body opposite the cerebral hemisphere in which the impulses originated. That is,

a neural impulse to the muscles capable of moving the right arm is sent from the motor area of the left hemisphere.

For most adults, despite which hand is dominant, the left cerebral hemisphere is the primary controller of speech and language. In the left frontal lobe in front of the motor area and above the Sylvian fissure is a region known as *Broca's area,* which programs speech production. It coordinates neural signals that then travel to the motor area and subsequently to the articulators. Congruent with the left hemisphere's dominance for speech and language, Broca's area in the left frontal lobe is typically described as more convoluted than the corresponding area in the right hemisphere. Furthermore, for adults, damage to Broca's area in the left hemisphere impairs speech production, whereas damage to the same area in the opposite hemisphere results in no discernible disturbance of speech production.

The sensory area of the cerebrum is located in the parietal lobe just behind the central fissure. This area receives neural impulses from various parts of the body and uses this information to help control functions in those parts of the body.

Many of the functions of the temporal lobe are involved in receiving and processing auditory stimuli. For example, the auditory (vestibulocochlear) nerve, which transmits neural impulses from the ear to the brain, courses toward a cerebral gyrus located on the superior border of the temporal lobe. An area in an adult's left hemisphere especially important for the comprehension of oral language—Wernicke's area— is located partially in the temporal lobe and partially in the parietal lobe. As with Broca's area, the left Wernicke's area is dominant for understanding spoken words. In contrast, processing of other types of sounds, including music, takes place in the right hemisphere. However, there is some evidence that in adults, both the right and left temporal-parietal areas are active when humans listen to speech (Lassen, Ingvar, & Skinhøj, 1978). It may be that although Wernicke's area in the left hemisphere is primarily responsible for processing the phonetic elements of a spoken message, the right hemisphere processes the prosodic (melodic) portions of speech, such as intonation.

Although certain functions can be attributed to specific parts of the cerebral cortex, "there is far greater appreciation today of the interplay among all parts of the brain as a requisite for normal function" (Boone, 1985, p. 374). One way in which the structure of the cerebrum provides for functional interrelationships among cortical areas is via its association fibers (Lieberman, 1990). These fibers, located in the interior of the cerebrum, interconnect various cortical areas. The recognition of this interplay among various parts of the cerebrum is applicable to interhemispheric as well as interlobe interactions (Lieberman, 1990). Wolff (1977) suggests that "the developmental analysis of interhemispheric cooperation and competition may be as critical to an understanding of brain behavior relationships as the study of lateralized function *per se*" (p. 12).

Much of our discussion thus far has centered on the adult nervous system. Care must be taken when attempting to draw parallels between adult and child neurological functioning. The nervous systems of children are immature. It takes many years for a child's nervous system to develop physically and functionally to parallel that of an adult. Children's brains a described as having much more **plasticity** and much less cerebral **localization** and specialization than those of adults. Conseque the effects on language seen

from focal CNS damage in adults may not be seen in children. Damage limited to left hemispheric areas in children appears not to account fully for the presence of developmental, specific language disorders, as opposed to language disorders in children who have acquired language problems as a result of childhood trauma or disease. Instead, bihemispheric involvement seems implicated in developmental, specific language disorders of children who have underlying CNS damage. In summarizing the research, Bashir, Kuban, Kleinman, and Scavuzzo (1983) state:

> It appears that bihemispheric dysfunction underlies central nervous system based developmental language disorders. This may occur as a consequence of direct damage to both hemispheres or damage to one hemisphere when associated with physiologic dysfunction of the contralateral side. We suggest that bihemispheric dysfunction restricts the brain's plasticity and interferes with the mediation of language functions, otherwise potentially available with strictly unilateral damage. (p. 96)

The cerebellum is the last structure of the CNS to be discussed. This structure is integrally involved in coordination of motor activity, although it does not initiate any of the activity. In describing the function of the cerebellum, Zemlin (1981) writes, "In recent years the cerebellum has been likened to a computer, ca-

TABLE 2.2 Seven Cranial Nerves Involved in Language and Speech

Number	Name	Functions
∨	Trigeminal	*Sensory*—face; jaw; mouth *Motor*—jaw; soft palate
VII	Facial	*Sensory*—taste; mucous membrane of soft palate and pharynx *Motor*—face; lips
VIII	Vestibulocochlear (auditory)	*Sensory*—hearing; balance
IX	Glossopharyngeal	*Sensory*—taste; mucous membrane of pharynx, middle ear, and mouth *Motor*—pharynx
X	Vagus	*Sensory*—mucous membrane of pharynx, larynx, soft palate, tongue, and lungs *Motor*—larynx; pharynx
XI	Accessory	*Motor*—soft palate; larynx; pharynx; neck
XII	Hypoglossal	*Sensory*—tongue *Motor*—tongue

pable of rapid analysis of a variety of input information and whose output coordinates the timing and extent of muscle contraction, limb movement, and so forth" (p. 465). These analytic and coordinating functions result in the ability to produce well-timed, smooth movements.

The Peripheral Nervous System (PNS)   The PNS is made up of 12 pairs of cranial nerves and 31 pairs of spinal nerves. The cranial nerves extend from the brain stem primarily to the neck and head areas, and the spinal nerves extend from the spinal cord to the remaining lower parts of the body. Many of the nerves contain both sensory fibers, which travel to the CNS and provide it with information, and motor fibers, which transmit commands from the CNS to various parts of the body. Cranial nerves are identified by both Roman numerals and names. Seven of these 12 pairs of cranial nerves are especially important for speech and language functions (see Table 2.2). These nerves carry the command signals originating in the CNS to the specific muscles of speech production that they innervate. Their sensory fibers then feed back to the CNS information about the performances of muscles. This allows the CNS to monitor the activities and send corrective signals if necessary. Furthermore, information about the acoustic characteristics of a speech signal, sent to the CNS via the auditory nerve, augments other sensory data about an organism's speech and language performance.

THE LANGUAGE LEARNING ENVIRONMENT

We are well aware that different societies speak different languages. However, different sociological groups speaking the same language may well have different styles of language use. The sociological influences in children's language-learning environments play a major role in their acquisition of their respective linguistic codes and the rules that govern how the code is used in context. In chapter 10 these sociological aspects of language are discussed in more detail. Here our discussion focuses on the roles the children and their caregivers play in language learning and briefly examines imitation and reinforcement as they relate to language acquisition.

Because children's caretakers constitute the majority of the children's early environmental interactions, the caretakers have primary roles in influencing language learning (Seitz & Marcus, 1976). However, the influences are not unidirectional. Although caretakers' behaviors can create environments conducive to language acquisition, children's behaviors can affect the caretakers' behaviors. The effects are, therefore, reciprocal.

Children

Certain infant behaviors appear to stimulate adults to respond in specific ways. Among these behaviors is the helplessness of infants, which seems to motivate adults to attend to them and respond to their needs (Carrow-Woolfolk & Lynch, 1982). During these attending patterns, adults tend to talk to infants in special ways (which we discuss later) and to provide a variety of sensory stimulation. Infants' responses to these adult inputs can, in turn, either motivate the adults to continue their language-facilitating behaviors, discontinue them, or modify the behaviors to some less beneficial for language learning (Lasky & Klopp, 1982; Moerk, 1977; Snow, 1977; Wulbert, Inglis, Kriegsmann, & Mills, 1975). It appears that disabled children may not respond to parents' attention in ways that positively reinforce the parents to provide appropriate language stimulation (Emde, Katz, & Thorpe, 1978).

In infancy, children's behaviors that seem to act as **positive reinforcers** of adults' language stimulation include gaze, smiling, and reciprocal touch and vocalization (Lewis & Lee-Painter, 1974; Ramey, Farran, Campbell, & Finkelstein, 1978; Snow, 1977). As children become capable of producing some speech, they provide verbal feedback to adults in terms of what has and has not been comprehended, as well as signal understanding by increasing their attention to the adults' speech (Bohannon & Marquis, 1977; Carrow-Woolfolk & Lynch, 1982; Mahoney, 1975). As Hubbell (1981) states, "In this way children regulate the input they receive and hence the language models that they learn from" (p. 276).

Parents of language-disordered children have sometimes been criticized for not providing adequate and

Mothers' speech to young children is modified in ways that help the children learn language. This unique speech pattern is known as "motherese."

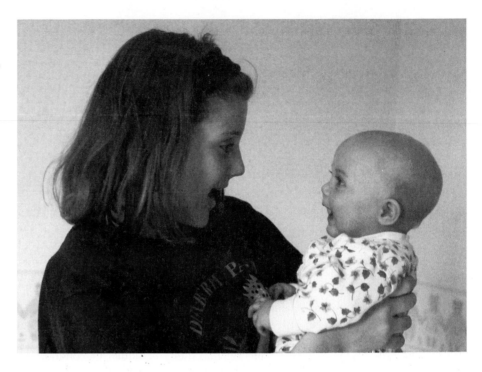

appropriate language stimulation for their children. This may not be a totally fair judgment. For the most part, parents of language-disordered children have been found to provide language stimulation similar to the stimulation that parents of younger, normal language-learning children provide. However, in other instances, parents of language-disordered children may engage in some types of child–adult interactions that are less conducive to language learning. We must be careful, however, not to overgeneralize. In light of our previous discussion, it may be that the children, because of their disorders, do not provide the reinforcement for the parents to engage in appropriate language stimulation activities.

Adults

Most investigations of adults' language to children have focused on mothers' speech rather than fathers' speech. Consequently, our discussion here will be limited to *motherese,* a term sometimes used to describe the unique characteristics of maternal language

patterns to children (Berko Gleason & Weintraub, 1978).

The length and complexity of mothers' utterances addressed to children have consistently been found to vary as a function of the children's ages and language skills (Broen, 1972; Mahoney & Seely, 1977; Moerk, 1976; Phillips, 1973; Snow, 1977). That is, in talking to younger children, mothers use shorter and less complex utterances than in talking to older children or adults. Furthermore, as the children grow older, the speech addressed to them becomes more complex and the utterances longer.

Beyond the effects of children's ages and linguistic competencies on the speech used with them, there appear to be specific characteristics of motherese. Overall, utterances are short (Brown, 1973; Snow, 1972), and although they are syntactically simple, they are grammatically well formed (Berko Gleason & Weintraub, 1978; Broen, 1972). The content of the utterances generally includes more concrete nouns and verbs and fewer modifiers, function words, and pronouns (Brown, 1973; Phillips, 1973). Proper names tend to replace pronouns. Prosodic features of mothers' speech are also modified. Berko Gleason and Weintraub (1978) describe maternal utterances to children as higher-pitched than speech addressed to adults, with a tendency to have rising intonation patterns, rather than falling patterns, at the ends of the utterances. The duration with which words are spoken is longer, and the overall rate of speech is slowed. Broen (1972) has also indicated that obvious pauses occur between individual utterances in mothers' speech. Berko Gleason and Weintraub suggest that utterances often contain more than one stressed word, and according to Brown (1973) these stressed words are typically the substantive words, rather than functional words, in the utterances.

Not only do adults appear to modify their verbal input to children, they also appear to alter the ways they respond to children's utterances. Corrections of young children's inaccurate utterances tend to be corrections of content (semantics) rather than morphosyntactic or phonological corrections. As children grow older, however, mothers begin to correct these latter aspects of their children's utterances. During parent–child communicative interactions, adults have been found to respond to what the children say by using **expansions** and **recasts** of the children's utterances (Conti-Ramsden, 1990; Moerk, 1977), with semantically contingent responses that may be paraphrases of the children's comments. Furthermore, adult responses tend to consist of frequent repetitions of messages (Brown, 1973; Phillips, 1973; Snow, 1972). Snow (1972) concludes that these almost unconscious modifications in adults' speech are "admirably designed to aid children in learning language. This makes it somewhat easier to understand how a child can accomplish the formidable task of learning his native language with such relative ease" (p. 564).

Imitation and Reinforcement

The roles of imitation and reinforcement in language acquisition have been debated. Much of this debate has probably resulted from differing definitions of the terms (Moerk, 1977). Imitation, if viewed as children's exact reproductions of adults' utterances, cannot account fully for the language-learning process. If it

were the entire basis of language and speech acquisition, children would not produce novel utterances. Rather, they would only say things that had been heard previously, and we know that children produce utterances for which no exact models have been provided. On the other hand, if we view imitation in light of Bandura's (1971) concept of social, observational learning, in which adults provide numerous models from which children abstract the key elements to form rules for behavior, then imitation that encompasses the rules, not exact duplications of the models, may well be involved in language learning (Moerk, 1977).

This discussion does not imply that imitation in the form of exact duplications has no role in language learning, although its role may change as a function of age and/or language skill. Young children approaching the end of the sensorimotor stage of cognitive development have been found to produce a high percentage of imitative utterances (Slobin, 1968). However, as productive language skills develop, the number of imitative responses decreases (Bowerman, 1973; Slobin, 1968). That is, children begin to use a higher proportion of unique, spontaneously generated utterances and a lower proportion of imitated responses.

The role of reinforcement in language acquisition is also unclear. Reinforcement, as it is used in conditioning or stimulus-response theories of learning (Skinner, 1957), is not totally sufficient for language learning. Not all children's early utterances are reinforced, and those that are may not be reinforced in a manner conducive to learning to talk. Yet, children do learn to talk. Humans are social beings, and for them "the need to relate is more basic than the need to know. Speech is acquired in a social context, and interpersonal relationships precede verbal speech" (Carrow-Woolfolk & Lynch, 1982, pp. 85–86). If infants find that their early vocalizations and toddlers discover that their early words establish and maintain adults' interactions with them, then we may consider that reinforcement is operating. Furthermore, adults' expansions and paraphrases of children's utterances, in addition to providing language models, probably serve to reinforce verbal behavior since they also maintain the adults' interactions with the children and support language production (Carrow-Woolfolk & Lynch, 1982).

SUMMARY

In this chapter we have seen that:

► Some view language as dependent on cognition, others view cognition and language as separate but sometimes related entities, and still others view language as a mediating factor in cognition; it is possible that relationships between cognition and language change, depending on the types of activities involved and the child's age.

► Metacognition involves conscious analysis, control, planning, and organization of our thinking.

► Information processing focuses on the components involved in dealing with stimuli.

► Auditory processing and the components of auditory processing are seen as factors in language learning, but their relationships to language learning and language disorders in children are not clear or agreed upon.

► The physiological mechanisms that underlie speech and language consist of the ear, parts of the respiratory and digestive systems that form the speech mechanism, and the CNS and PNS.

► Young children engage in certain behaviors that make them active partners in their own language learning.

► Characteristics of caregivers' speech and language to children, known as motherese, facilitate children's language learning.

We began this chapter by indicating that language acquisition comes about as a result of complex interactions among cognitive, physiological, psychological, and sociological factors. Numerous approaches have been taken in attempting to explain these interactions. None alone is sufficient to describe how children learn language. Language is a complicated human behavior that has yet to be explained by any single theory or approach.

REFERENCES

Anderson, B. (1975). *Cognitive psychology.* New York: Academic Press.

Aram, D., & Nation, J. (1982). *Child language disorders.* St. Louis, MO: Mosby.

Atchison, M., & Canter, G. (1979). Variables influencing phonemic discrimination performance in normal and learning-disabled children. *Journal of Speech and Hearing Disorders, 44,* 543–556.

Aten, J., & Davis, J. (1968). Disturbances in the perception of auditory sequence in children with minimal cerebral dysfunction. *Journal of Speech and Hearing Research, 11,* 236–245.

Bandura, A. (1971). *Psychological modeling.* Chicago: Aldine-Atherton.

Bashir, A., Kuban, K., Kleinman, S., & Scavuzzo, A. (1983). Issues in language disorders: Considerations of cause, maintenance, and change. In J. Miller, D. Yoder, & R. Schiefelbusch (Eds.), *Contemporary issues in language intervention.* Rockville, MD: American Speech-Language-Hearing Association.

Bates, E., Benigni, L., Bretherton, I., Camaioni, L., & Volterra, V. (1977). From gesture to the first word: On cognitive and social prerequisites. In M. Lewis & L. Rosenblum (Eds.), *Interaction, conversation, and the development of language.* New York: Wiley.

Bates, E., Benigni, L., Bretherton, I., Camaioni, L., & Volterra, V. (1979). *The emergence of symbols: Cognition and communication in infancy.* New York: Academic Press.

Bates, E., Bretherton, I., Snyder, L., Shore, L., & Volterra, V. (1980). Gestural and vocal symbols at 13 months. *Merrill-Palmer Quarterly, 26,* 407–423.

Beasley, D., Maki, J., & Orchik, D. (1976). Children's perception of time compressed speech on two measures of speech discrimination. *Journal of Speech and Hearing Disorders, 41,* 216–225.

Berko Gleason, J., & Weintraub, S. (1978). Input language and the acquisition of communicative competence. In K. Nelson (Ed.), *Children's language* (Vol. 1). New York: Gardner Press.

Berry, M. (1980). *Teaching linguistically handicapped children.* Englewood Cliffs, NJ: Prentice-Hall.

Bohannon, J., & Marquis, A. (1977). Children's control of adult speech. *Child Development, 48,* 1002–1008.

Boone, D. (1985). Disorders of language in adults. In P. Skinner & R. Shelton (Eds.), *Speech, language, and hearing: Normal processes and disorders* (2nd ed.). New York: Wiley.

Bowerman, M. (1973). *Early syntactic development: A cross-linguistic study with special reference to Finnish.* London: Cambridge University Press.

Brandes, P., & Ehinger, D. (1981). The effects of early middle ear pathology on auditory perception and academic achievement. *Journal of Speech and Hearing Disorders, 46,* 301–307.

Broen, P. (1972). The verbal environment of the language learning child. *Monographs of the American Speech and Hearing Association, 17.*

Brown, A. (1975). The development of memory: Knowing, knowing about knowing, and knowing how to know. In H. Reese (Ed.), *Advances in child development and behavior* (Vol. 10). New York: Academic Press.

Brown, R. (1973). *A first language: The early stages.* Cambridge, MA: Harvard University Press.

Bruner, J. (1964). The course of cognitive growth. *American Psychologist, 19,* 1–15.

Carrow-Woolfolk, E., & Lynch, J. (1982). *An integrative approach to language disorders in children.* New York: Grune & Stratton.

Chalfant, J., & Scheffelin, M. (1969). *Cerebral processing dysfunctions in children.* Washington, DC: U.S. Department of Health, Education and Welfare, National Institute of Neurological Diseases and Stroke.

Chermak, G., & Musiek, F. (1992). Managing central auditory processing disorders in children and youth. *American Journal of Audiology, 1,* 61–65.

Clark, H. (1973). Space, time, semantics, and the child. In T. Moore (Ed.), *Cognitive development and the acquisition of language.* New York: Academic Press.

Conti-Ramsden, G. (1990). Maternal recasts and other contingent replies to language-impaired children. *Journal of Speech and Hearing Disorders, 55,* 262–274.

Costello, M. (1977). Evaluation of auditory behavior using the Flowers-Costello test for central auditory abilities. In R. Keith (Ed.), *Central auditory dysfunction.* New York: Grune & Stratton.

Eimas, P. (1974). Auditory and linguistic processing of cues for place of articulation by infants. *Perception and Psychophysics, 16,* 513–521.

Eisenson, J. (1968). Developmental aphasia: A speculative view with therapeutic implications. *Journal of Speech and Hearing Disorders, 33,* 3–13.

Elliott, L. (1986). Discrimination and response bias for CV syllables differing in voice onset time among children and adults. *Journal of the Acoustical Society of America, 80,* 1250–1255.

Elliott, L., & Busse, L. (1987). Auditory processing by learning disabled young adults. In D. Johnson & J. Blalock (Eds.), *Adults with learning disabilities: Clinical studies* (pp. 107–129). New York: Grune & Stratton.

Elliott, L., Busse, L., Partridge, R., Rupert, J., & DeGraaf, R. (1986). Adult and child discrimination of CV syllables differing in voicing onset time. *Child Development, 57,* 628–635.

Elliott, L., Hammer, M., & Scholl, M. (1989). Fine-grained auditory discrimination in normal children and children with language-learning problems. *Journal of Speech and Hearing Research, 32,* 112–119.

Emde, R., Katz, E., & Thorpe, J. (1978). Emotional expression in infancy II. Early deviations in Down's syndrome. In M. Lewis & L. Rosenblum (Eds.), *The development of affect:* Vol. I. *Genesis of behavior.* New York: Plenum Press.

Flavell, J. (1976). Metacognitive aspects of problem solving. In L. Resnick (Ed.), *The nature of intelligence.* Hillsdale, NJ: Erlbaum.

Flavell, J. (1977). *Cognitive development.* Englewood Cliffs, NJ: Prentice-Hall.

Flowers, A., & Costello, M. (1963). The responses to distorted speech of children with severe articulation disorders. *Journal of Auditory Research, 3,* 133–140.

Grieser, D., & Kuhl, P. (1989). The categorization of speech by infants: Support for speech-sound prototypes. *Developmental Psychology, 25,* 577–588.

Haggerty, R., & Stamm, J. (1978). Dichotic auditory fusion levels in children with learning disabilities. *Neuropsychologia, 16,* 349–360.

Hedrick, D. (1967). *A developmental investigation of children's abilities to respond to competing messages varied in intensity and content.* Unpublished doctoral dissertation, University of Washington, Seattle.

Hirsh-Pasek, K., Nelson, D., Jusczyk, P., Cassidy, K., Druss, B., & Kennedy, L. (1987). Clauses are perceptual units for young infants. *Cognition, 26,* 269–286.

Hubbell, R. (1981). *Children's language disorders: An integrated approach.* Englewood Cliffs, NJ: Prentice-Hall.

Kamhi, A. (1987). Metalinguistic abilities in language-impaired children. *Topics in Language Disorders, 7,* 1–12.

Kamhi, A., Gentry, B., Mouer, D., & Gholson, B. (1990). Analogical learning and transfer in language-impaired children. *Journal of Speech and Hearing Disorders, 55,* 140–148.

Katz, J. (1978). The effect of conductive hearing loss on auditory function. *Asha, 20,* 879–886.

Keith, R. (1984). Central auditory dysfunction: A language disorder? *Topics in Language Disorders, 4,* 48–56.

Kelly, C., & Dale P. (1989). Cognitive skills associated with the onset of multiword utterances. *Journal of Speech and Hearing Research, 32,* 645–656.

Kuhl, P. (1990). Auditory perception and the ontogeny and phylogeny of human speech. *Seminars in Speech and Language, 11,* 77–91.

Kuhl, P., & Meltzoff, A. (1988). Speech as an intermodal object of perception. In A. Yonas (Ed.), *Minnesota symposia in child psychology: The development of perception* (pp. 235–266). Hillsdale, NJ: Erlbaum.

Lahey, M. (1988). *Language disorders and language development.* New York: Merrill/Macmillan.

Langacker, R. (1968). *Language and its structure: Some fundamental linguistic concepts.* New York: Harcourt, Brace & World.

Lasky, E., & Klopp, K. (1982). Parent–child interactions in normal and language-disordered children. *Journal of Speech and Hearing Disorders, 47,* 7–18.

Lassen, N., Ingvar, D., & Skinhøj, E. (1978). Brain function and blood flow. *Scientific American, 239,* 62–71.

Leonard, L. (1982). Phonological deficits in children with developmental language impairment. *Brain and Language, 16,* 73–86.

Leonard, L., McGregor, K., & Allen, G. (1992). Grammatical morphology and speech perception in children with specific language impairment. *Journal of Speech and Hearing Research, 35,* 1076–1085.

Lewis, M., & Lee-Painter, S. (1974). An interactional approach to the mother–infant dyad. In M. Lewis & L. Rosenblum (Eds.), *The effect of the infant on its caregiver.* New York: Wiley.

Lieberman, P. (1990). The evolution of human language. *Seminars in Speech and Language, 11,* 63–76.

Locke, J. (1980a). The inference of speech perception in the phonologically disordered child. Part I: A rationale, some criteria, the conventional tests. *Journal of Speech and Hearing Disorders, 45,* 431–444.

Locke, J. (1980b). The inference of speech perception in the phonologically disordered child. Part II: Some clinically novel procedures, their use, some findings. *Journal of Speech and Hearing Disorders, 45,* 445–468.

Lubert, N. (1981). Auditory perceptual impairments in children with specific language disorders: A review of the literature. *Journal of Speech and Hearing Disorders, 46,* 3–9.

Luria, A. (1961). *The role of speech in the regulation of normal and abnormal processes in the child.* Baltimore: Penguin.

Luria, A., & Yudovich, F. (1971). *Speech and the development of mental processes in the child.* Baltimore: Penguin.

Maccoby, E. (1967). Selective auditory attention in children. In L. Lippsitt & C. Spiker (Eds.), *Advances in child development and behavior* (Vol. 3). New York: Academic Press.

Maccoby, E., & Konrad, K. (1966). Age trends in selective listening. *Journal of Experimental Child Psychology, 3,* 113–122.

Maccoby, E., & Konrad, K. (1967). The effect of preparatory set on selective listening: Developmental trends. *Monographs of the Society for Research in Child Development, 32* (Serial No. 112).

Mahoney, G. (1975). Ethnological approach to delayed language acquisition. *American Journal of Mental Deficiency, 80,* 139–148.

Mahoney, G., & Seely, P. (1977). The role of the social agent in language acquisition. In H. Ellis (Ed.), *International review of research in mental retardation* (Vol. 8). New York: Academic Press.

McCroskey, R., & Thompson, N. (1973). Comprehension of rate-controlled speech by children with learning disabilities. *Journal of Learning Disabilities, 6,* 621–627.

McReynolds, L. (1966). Operant conditioning for investigating speech sound discrimination in aphasic children. *Journal of Speech and Hearing Research, 9,* 519–528.

Mehler, J., Jusczyk, P., Lambertz, G., Halsted, N., Bertoncini, J., & Amiel-Tison, C. (1988). A precursor of language acquisition in young infants. *Cognition, 29,* 143–178.

Menyuk, P., & Looney, P. (1972a). A problem of language disorder: Length versus structure. *Journal of Speech and Hearing Research, 15,* 264–279.

Menyuk, P., & Looney, P. (1972b). Relationships among components of the grammar in language disorder. *Journal of Speech and Hearing Research, 15,* 395–406.

Moerk, E. (1976). Processes of language teaching and training in the interactions of mother–child dyads. *Child Development, 47,* 1064–1078.

Moerk, E. (1977). *Pragmatic and semantic aspects of early language development.* Baltimore: University Park Press.

Moffitt, A. (1971). Consonant cue perception by twenty- to twenty-four-week-old infants. *Child Development, 42,* 717–731.

Morse, P. (1972). The discrimination of speech and nonspeech stimuli in early infancy. *Journal of Experimental Child Psychology, 14,* 477–492.

Muma, J. (1978). *Language handbook: Concepts, assessment, intervention.* Englewood Cliffs, NJ: Prentice-Hall.

Noffsinger, D. (1992). Standardization of test materials for

CHAPTER 2   Bases of Language Functioning: An Overview **59**

central auditory assessment. *American Journal of Audiology, 1,* 10–11.

Northern, J., & Downs, M. (1984). *Hearing in children* (3rd ed.). Baltimore: Williams & Wilkins.

Peck, D. (1977, November). *The effects of presentation rates on the auditory comprehension of learning-disabled children.* Paper presented at the Annual Convention of the American Speech and Hearing Association, Chicago.

Phillips, J. (1973). Syntax and vocabulary of mothers' speech to young children: Age and sex comparisons. *Child Development, 44,* 182–185.

Piaget, J. (1957). *Logic and psychology.* New York: Basic Books.

Pierce, J. (1969). Wither speech recognition. *Journal of the Acoustical Society of America, 49,* 1049–1051.

Ramey, C., Farran, D., Campbell, F., & Finkelstein, N. (1978). Observations of mother–infant interactions: Implications for development. In F. Minifie & L. Lloyd (Eds.), *Communicative and cognitive abilities—Early behavioral assessment.* Baltimore: University Park Press.

Reed, V. A. (1982). *Basic anatomy and physiology of speech and hearing: A learning guide* (2nd ed.). Austin, TX: PRO-ED.

Rees, N. (1973). Auditory processing factors in language disorders: The view from Procrustes' bed. *Journal of Speech and Hearing Disorders, 38,* 304–315.

Rice, M. (1983). Comtemporary accounts of the cognition/language relationship: Implications for speech-language clinicians. *Journal of Speech and Hearing Disorders, 48,* 347–359.

Rosenthal, W. (1970). *Perception of temporal order in aphasic and normal children as a function of certain stimulus parameters.* Unpublished doctoral dissertation, Stanford University, Stanford, CA.

Sanders, D. (1977). *Auditory perception of speech: An introduction to principles and problems.* Englewood Cliffs, NJ: Prentice-Hall.

Seitz, S., & Marcus, S. (1976). Mother–child interactions: A foundation for language development. *Exceptional Children, 42,* 445–449.

Simon, H. (1974). How big is a chunk? *Science, 183,* 482–488.

Sinclair-deZwart, H. (1973). Language acquisition and cognitive development. In T. Moore (Ed.), *Cognitive development and the acquistion of language.* New York: Academic Press.

Skinner, B. (1957). *Verbal behavior.* Englewood Cliffs, NJ: Prentice-Hall.

Slobin, D. (1968). Imitation and grammatical development in children. In N. Endler, L. Boulter, & H. Osser (Eds.), *Contemporary issues in developmental psychology.* New York: Holt, Rinehart and Winston.

Snow, C. (1972). Mothers' speech to children learning language. *Child Development, 43,* 549–565.

Snow, C. (1977). The development of conversation between mothers and babies. *Journal of Child Language, 4,* 1–22.

Stark, J., Poppen, R., & May, M. (1967). Effects of alternations of prosodic features on the sequencing performance of aphasic children. *Journal of Speech and Hearing Research, 10,* 849–855.

Tallal, P. (1976). Rapid auditory processing in normal and disordered language development. *Journal of Speech and Hearing Research, 19,* 561–571.

Tallal, P., & Piercy, M. (1973a). Defects of non-verbal auditory perception in children with developmental aphasia. *Nature, 241,* 468–469.

Tallal, P., & Piercy, M. (1973b). Impaired rate of non-verbal auditory processing as a function of sensory modality. *Neuropsychologia, 11,* 389–398.

Tallal, P., & Piercy, M. (1974). Developmental aphasia: Rate of auditory processing and selective impairment of consonant perception. *Neuropsychologia, 12,* 83–93.

Tallal, P., & Piercy, M. (1975). Developmental aphasia: The perception of brief vowels and extended consonants. *Neuropsychologia, 13,* 69–74.

Tallal, P., & Piercy, M. (1978). Defects of auditory perception in children with developmental dysphasia. In M. Wyke (Ed.), *Developmental dysphasia.* New York: Academic Press.

Tallal, P., Stark, R., Kallman, C., & Mellits, D. (1981). A reexamination of some nonverbal perceptual abilities of language-impaired and normal children as a function of age and sensory modality. *Journal of Speech and Hearing Research, 24,* 351–357.

Thal, D. (1991). Language and cognition in normal and late-talking toddlers. *Topics in Language Disorders, 11,* 33–42.

Thal, D., & Barone, P. (1983). Auditory processing and language impairment in children: Stimulus considerations for intervention. *Journal of Speech and Hearing Disorders, 48,* 18–24.

Tomblin, J. B., & Quinn, M. (1983). The contribution of perceptual learning to performance on the repetition task. *Journal of Speech and Hearing Research, 26,* 369–372.

Trehub, S. (1973). Infant's sensitivity to vowel and tonal contrasts. *Developmental Psychology, 9,* 91–96.

van Kleeck, A. (1984). Metalinguistic skills: Cutting across spoken and written language and problem solving abilities. In G. Wallach & K. Butler (Eds.), *Language learning* disabilities in school-age childen (pp. 128–153). Baltimore: Williams & Wilkins.

Van Tasell, D. (1981). Auditory perception of speech. In J. Davis & E. Hardick, Rehabilitative audiology for children and adults. New York: Wiley.

Vygotsky, L. (1962). Thought and language. Cambridge, MA: MIT Press.

Weener, P. (1974). Toward a developmental model of auditory processes. Acta Symbolica, 5, 85–104.

Weiner, P. (1967). Auditory discrimination and articulation. Journal of Speech and Hearing Disorders, 32, 19–28.

Weiner, P. (1969a). The cognitive functioning of language deficient children. Journal of Speech and Hearing Research, 12, 53–61.

Weiner, P. (1969b). The perceptual level of functioning of aphasic children. Cortex, 5, 440–457.

Wellman, H. (1985). The origins of metacognition. In D. Forrest-Pressley, G. MacKinnon, & T. Waller (Eds.), Metacognition, cognition, and human performance. New York: Academic Press.

Wepman, J. (1960). Auditory discrimination, speech, and reading. Elementary School Journal, 9, 325–333.

Werker, J. (1989). Becoming a native listener. American Scientist, 77, 54–59.

Wiig, E. (1989). Steps to language competence: Developing metalinguistic strategies. San Antonio, TX: Psychological Corporation.

Wiig, E., & Semel, E. (1976). Language disabilities in children and adolescents. New York: Merrill/Macmillan

Witkin, B. (1971). Auditory perception—Implications for language development. Language, Speech, and Hearing Services in Schools, 2, 31–52.

Wolff, P. (1977). Maturational factors in behavioral development. In M. McMillan & S. Henao (Eds.), Child psychiatry: Treatment and research. New York: Brunner/Mazel.

Wulbert, M., Inglis, S., Kriegsmann, E., & Mills, B. (1975). Language delay and associated mother–child interactions. Developmental Psychology, 11, 61–70.

Zemlin, W. (1981). Speech and hearing science: Anatomy and physiology (2nd ed.). Englewood Cliffs, NJ: Prentice-Hall.

· Chapter 3 ·

A Review of Normal
Language Development

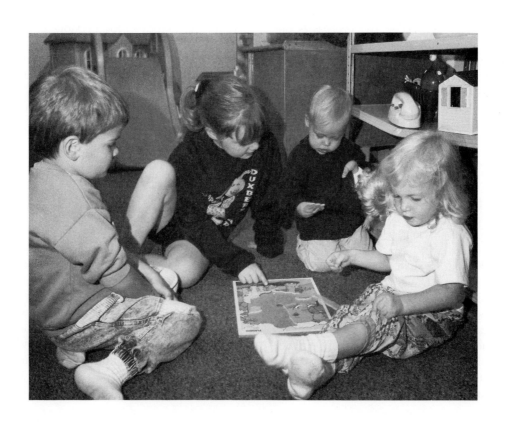

OBJECTIVES

Upon completion of this chapter, the reader should be able to:

▶ Describe the types of words that comprise children's lexicons during the one- and two-word utterance stages, trace the growth in lexicon size during the preschool years, and understand some of the general patterns that influence acquisition of lexical items.

▶ Understand sequences of children's language development from the one-word stage to the basic kernel sentence, as well as negative, question, and compound and complex sentences.

▶ Trace the developmental sequence of specific morphological forms.

▶ Understand developmental patterns related to the functions and intentions of language use, presuppositions and adaptation of messages, turn taking, and topic maintenance.

▶ Identify the developmental sequence for characteristics of narratives.

▶ Understand metalinguistic skills as advanced developmental abilities.

▶ Discuss children's acquisition of speech sounds and use of phonological processes.

Learning to talk is a relatively orderly process. Newly acquired skills are used to modify and augment existing language abilities, and these new abilities are based on earlier learned skills. The process is one of refinement, expansion, and extension. Language learning is synergistic in nature. All components of language—syntax, morphology, semantics, phonology, and pragmatics—interact to evolve gradually into adultlike competence with oral language. Although there is variability in individual children's language acquisition, there is also a great deal of consistency. What may be the most amazing aspect of this process is that by about 7 to 8 years of age, most children have learned to use oral language to communicate in basically adultlike fashion. This does not mean, however, that language development stops at these ages, and we need to be careful not to fall into the trap of thinking that only uninteresting and minor language development occurs beyond 8 years of age. As we see later, especially in chapter 11, some important language skills are not fully acquired until the adolescent years and possibly beyond. Nevertheless, 7- and 8-year-old children typically produce a wide variety of well-formed sentences containing large numbers of different words, with only rare sound production errors. Further, they use these sentence types and words effectively for many different purposes.

In this chapter we will review some of the language developmental achievements of younger children. The discussion is by no means complete. As with the topics introduced in the previous chapters, volumes have been written on children's language development. An extensive discussion is well beyond the scope of this chapter. Language development in adolescence will be discussed in chapter 11, which addresses language disorders, as well as language development, of adolescents.

THE EVOLUTION OF SENTENCES

The First Sentences

The sounds children make during early infancy change in the first year of life from reflexive **vocalizations** to babbling to the emergence of the first word at approximately 12 months of age. In the second year of life, children gradually expand their single-word vocabularies until they have learned to combine two words in one utterance. This first two-word utterance usually occurs at around 18 to 26 months of age. A child's expressive vocabulary at 18 months is about 50 words. Between 18 and 24 months, children experience a lexical growth spurt, and at 24 months of age they typically have a single-word lexicon of 200 to 300

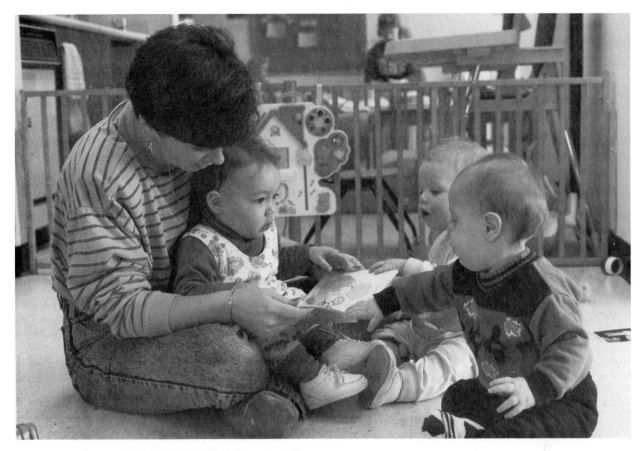

By the time these children are 12 months old they will likely have said their first word.

words (Dale & Thal, 1989; Reich, 1986). However, the vocabulary expansion that occurs from the single-word to the two-word stage is not haphazard. These vocabularies form the foundations that, in part, allow children eventually to use two-word combinations that, in turn, evolve into sentences.

As we recall from chapter 2, children from birth to about 2 years of age are in Piaget's sensorimotor stage of cognitive development. During this period, children learn about the world by acting on it and observing changes and consistencies. One of the resulting cognitive achievements is the concept of **object permanence**, or object constancy, that is, that objects exist in the environment even though they may not be im-

mediately visible. Object permanence is a basis for internal representations of the environment, or mental images or symbols of those objects and events that exist around the children. Many suggest that these internal representations are related to children's ability to use verbal symbols—words.

Lahey (1988) identifies three broad categories of single words that children use to represent what they learn about the environment: substantive, relational, and social. Children use **substantive words** to name objects. Many of the words are used to refer to classes or categories of objects. Some objects look like or act like other objects, and objects that have these similar characteristics are grouped together to form a **class**, or category. As children learn about the perceptual or behavioral consistency of objects, they learn that objects with similarly identified characteristics have the same names. Different balls have similar features and behave in similar ways. Therefore, children learn to use the label "ball" to refer to members of this class of objects. Many of these early words are names for objects on which children can act and produce changes, such as cookie, ball, and shoe, or objects that themselves move (Dale, 1976; Lahey, 1988). Children's information about the substantive words they use includes knowledge of "the ways that objects move and are affected by movement" and "the perceptual attributes of objects that distinguish among different object concepts" (Bloom & Lahey, 1978, p. 108). However, even though knowledge of objects' perceptual features is necessary in order to acquire object permanence and recognize objects as members of a class, children at this stage use fewer **attributives**, words such as color and size words, than names for objects (Goldin-Meadow, Seligman, & Gelman, 1976). Other types of substantive words refer to objects that children believe exist only as one of a kind. There is only one "Mommy"

and one favorite blanket and, to the child, one bottle. In a child's mind, these are unique instances of objects that do not belong to a class of objects.

The second broad category of single-word utterances identified by Lahey (1988) consists of relational words. **Relational words** describe the relationships or characteristics among objects, including movements of objects, or relationships of an object to itself, such as an object that has suddenly disappeared. Some children may use more relational than substantive words (Bloom, 1973; Gopnik, 1981). The types of relational words include existence, nonexistence/disappearance, recurrence, rejection, denial, attribution, possession, action, and locative action (Lahey, 1988). Table 3.1 lists and explains the types of relational words that children use in the single-word stage. It is important to realize that the same word may actually be used to express several different relations. For example, "no" can be used to indicate rejection, denial, or nonexistence/disappearance. "No" is a very functional, versatile, and important word for children. A noun, such as "ball," can be used to mean existence or recurrence or to label the object.

TABLE 3.1   Relations Expressed in Single-Word Utterances

Relation	Explanation
Existence	An object is present in a child's immediate environment, and the child is attending to it. Examples: "this," "that," "there"
Nonexistence/ disappearance	An object is expected to be present but is not. An action is expected to occur but does not. An object has been present but disappears. Examples: "all gone," "no," "bye-bye"
Recurrence	An object reappears. Another object like the one the child is attending to is placed with the first one. An event happens again. Examples: "more," "another"
Rejection	The child does not want an object or an event to occur. Example: "no"
Denial	The child rejects the truthfulness of a previous utterance. Example: "no"
Attribution	The child mentions a characteristic of an object or event, usually not shape or color in this stage. Example: "big," "little"
Possession	The child identifies ownership of an object. Examples: "mine," "my"
Action	The child identifies or requests an action. Examples: "go," "open"
Locative action	The child refers to a change in an object's location. Examples: "here," "there," "in," "up"

Source: Adapted from Lahey (1988).

The last broad category of single-word utterances consists of **social words**, such as "hi" and "bye." These are important words in a child's early repertoire, as they provide a foundation for establishing and maintaining human relationships according to a culture's social code. Although important, these words, unlike substantive and relational words, do not lead to later grammatical complexity.

As children approach their second birthday, several characteristics of their language indicate that two-word utterances may soon emerge. First, rarely does a child begin to use 2-word combinations until a vocabulary of at least about 50 words has been acquired. However, most 2-year-old children have expressive single-word vocabularies four to six times greater than 50 words (Dale & Thal, 1989; Reich, 1986). Children also demonstrate an increase in the number of verbs, a reduction in other types of relational words, and an increase in the number of object-class words used in their language as they approach the two-word stage (Bloom, 1973; Bloom & Lahey, 1978). Some have also suggested that children begin to produce chained single-word productions shortly before they use two-word combinations (Bloom & Lahey, 1978), although not all agree with this suggestion (Branigan, 1979; Owens, 1992). *Chained single-word utterances* are two single words that children use in close succession to each other but, based on stress and intonation patterns, they are used as individual words. These utterances appear to demonstrate that children are beginning to see more than one aspect of an event. That is, the children seem to identify and talk about relations within one event, such as "ball/roll" or "cookie/gone." These successive single-word utterances may form a base for the two-word utterances about to occur, such as "ball roll," "no cookie," and "more juice."

The two-word utterances children typically begin to use at about their second birthday are often described as reflections of *semantic relations* (Bloom, 1970; Brown, 1973). That is, these productions reflect meaning based on different relationships among the words in the utterances. Children can use the utterance "baby ball" to signify possession ("baby's ball") or to signify the actor and the object of an action ("baby [rolls] ball"). An utterance can indicate two different meanings or two separate relations between the words. Table 3.2 lists a number of the more common semantic relations Brown (1973) identified in children's two-word productions. As we can see, different semantic relations can be expressed in the same grammatical form, such as noun + noun (N + N) to signify possession, agent-object, and entity-locative. Another sig-

TABLE 3.2 Common Semantic Relations

Relation	Example	Structure
Nomination	That ball	Demonstrative + N
Nonexistence	No ball	No(allgone) + N
Action-object	Roll ball	V + N
Agent-action	Baby cry	N + V
Recurrence	More cookie	More(another) + N
Action + locative	Jump [on] chair	V + N
	Roll here	V + Loc.
Entity + locative	Ball [in] chair	N + N
	Mommy here	N + Loc.
Possessor-possession	Baby ball	N + N
Agent-object	Baby [roll] ball	N + N
Entity-attributive	Pretty ball	Att. + N
	Ball pretty	N + Att.
Notice	Hi ball	Hi + N
Instrumental	Cut [with] knife	V + N
Action-indirect object	Give [to] doggie	V + N
Conjunction	Coat hat	N + N

Source: Adapted from Brown (1973).

nificant characteristic of this stage of language use is the total absence of morphological endings on the words used. Children do not use the possessive word endings even though their intent is to indicate possession, nor do they use any endings on verbs. Instead, only lexical, or root, forms of words are used.

Brown (1973) has termed this semantic relations period of language development *Stage I*. During this period, children use about an equal number of one- and two-word utterances. If we average the number of words in many of their utterances, we obtain a mean length of about 1.5. The average lengths of young children's utterances are frequently used as measures of their language growth. Although we can average the number of words children use in their responses, such an approach does not tell us whether or not the children are using more complex word endings, such as plural markers. A more common method of arriving at average length is to count the number of morphemes, both free and bound, that occur in the utterances. When children are in Stage I, this averaging procedure also results in a **mean length of utterance** (**MLU**) of about 1.5 because children are not yet using grammatical inflections, or bound morphemes. In the early periods of language learning, as MLU increases, the complexity of children's utterances generally increases. However, when children begin using complex sentence forms, this relationship between length and linguistic maturity does not remain as closely correlated as in the earlier stages of language acquisition (Klee & Fitzgerald, 1985; Scarborough, Wyckoff, & Davidson, 1986; Wells, 1985).

An increase in length comes about through two events. First, children learn to expand their utterances by combining previously separate semantic relations, such as "baby ball" (possessive) and "ball roll" (agent-action) to form "baby ball roll" (Brown, 1973; Lahey, 1988; Wood, 1981). Children do not, however, use any new relations in forming these longer utterances. Only previously expressed two-word semantic relations are combined and expanded. The production of the first true sentences is also derived from this combining process. Agent-action ("baby roll") and action-object ("roll ball") combine to form agent-action-object ("baby roll ball"), the subject + verb + object basic English syntactic rule discussed in chapter 1. Utterance

length also increases because children begin to use grammatical morphemes in their utterances. At this point the child's MLU is about 2.0. (Appendix E gives Brown's [1973] rules for calculating MLU.) Children then progress to Brown's *Stage II,* acquiring the present progressive "-ing" ending for verbs ("ball rolling") and the prepositions "in" and "on" ("kitty in chair" and "cup on table"). It is important to note, however, that acquisition of a grammatical morpheme, as used in relation to Brown's stages, means that a child uses it correctly in at least 90% of the situations in which it is required by adult standards, that is, in 90% of the obligatory contexts. Children may use morphemes such as "in" and "on" before this stage but not at the criterion level set by Brown. Table 3.3 summarizes Brown's (1973) findings about the sequence in which children acquire 14 selected grammatical morphemes and indicates the corresponding stages determined by MLU at which the morphemes are acquired. The process of learning these morphemes occurs over several years, and children are developing other language skills during that time. By the time children are 3 years old, they typically demonstrate the use of negative and interrogative sentences, as well as basic declarative sentences. This does not mean that these sentences are error free. However, it does mean that children have acquired the basic subject-predicate relationship and have learned several early-developing transformations of the kernel sentence.

Negatives

We have just seen how the use of simple declarative sentences evolves from earlier two-word semantic relations. Negative sentences develop in a similar way. In our discussion of the types of single words that children use, we saw that negative words occur very early in the developmental process. Few adults who have been around young children would be surprised to hear that the negative word most commonly used by toddlers is "no." When children begin to combine words, negative utterances are produced by placing the negative marker "no" in front of an element that occurs in the predicate of a sentence, such as a verb or direct object (Bloom, 1970). Utterances like "no milk" and "no go" are typical. Even though children at

TABLE 3.3 Sequence of Acquisition for 14 Grammatical Morphemes

	Morpheme	MLU	Maximum Length in Morphemes	Stage
1.	Present progressive verb ending ("ing")			
2., 3.	"In" and "on"	2.25	7	II
4.	Noun plurals			
5.	Past tense irregular verbs			
6.	Possessive nouns	2.75	9	III
7.	Uncontractible copula ("Here I *am*")			
8.	Articles			
9.	Past tense regular verbs	3.50	11	IV
10.	Regular third-person singular present tense verbs			
11.	Irregular third-person singular present tense verbs			
12.	Uncontractible auxiliary ("He *was* running")			
13.	Contractible copula ("She's big")	4.00	13	V
14.	Contractible auxiliary ("The boy's eating")			

Source: Adapted from Brown (1973).

this stage may produce affirmative sentences with a subject and predicate ("boy roll ball"), the subject is deleted when a negative marker is added (Bloom, Miller, & Hood, 1975). It appears that the use of negation increases the length and complexity of an utterance, which, as a result, can exceed children's linguistic capacities. Perhaps to accommodate these limited capacities, the overall length and complexity of an utterance are reduced to a manageable unit by omitting the subject when a negative is added ("no roll ball"). Furthermore, the subject of a sentence is usually the information shared most between speaker and listener, so its omission tends not to affect communication. Meaning can still be conveyed despite the omission.

Children gradually learn to re-add the subject to produce negative sentences such as "boy no roll ball." However, before these negative sentences can evolve into more complex forms, children need to learn that "no" is the negative word used with nouns and "not" is the negative for verbs. The occurrence of later neg-

ative sentences also depends on the use of a **copula** or **auxiliary verb** ("the ball is not big" and "the boy is not running"). A review of Table 3.3 indicates that the copula and auxiliary verbs are acquired during *Stages III* and *V* (Brown, 1973). For sentences in which an auxiliary verb does not occur ("the boy eats"), an auxiliary in the form of "do" must be added ("the boy does not eat" or "the boy doesn't eat"). Although the use of "do" plus a negative is generally considered to be a reasonably complex language skill, the negative words "don't" and "can't" do appear in children's early language productions. These early occurrences of "can't" and "don't," however, are typically viewed as vocabulary words indicating negation rather than as evidence that children have acquired the operation of adding "do" when an auxiliary is absent. The negatives "won't" and "isn't" also occur in children's early productions, although less frequently than "don't" and "can't" (Klima & Bellugi, 1966; Lee, 1974).

Negatives can be used to express a number of different concepts. For example, with negative utterances, we can reject ("I don't want any"), deny ("That's not a red car"), or signify nonexistence ("It's not here"). A number of investigators have examined the developmental sequence of the purposes for which negatives are used (Belkin, 1975; Bloom, 1970; Bloom, Lightbown, & Hood, 1975). Table 3.4 presents six functions of negatives in a suggested developmental sequence and provides examples of each (Bloom & Lahey, 1978). Denial may be the last to develop because children must deal with two things—knowledge of a correct option and the speaker's utterance that is to be denied (Bloom & Lahey, 1978). The syntactic representation of these negative functions appears to follow this same sequence. That is, children at a specific developmental level will express nonexistence in a fairly complex way ("It isn't here"), while at the same time signifying denial in a less sophisticated manner ("That not a ball") (Bloom & Lahey, 1978).

A listener's comprehension of negative sentences depends, in part, on the word or words that a speaker stresses. The sentence "The ball is not red" could be interpreted in a number of ways if different words are emphasized ("The *ball* is not red" leads us to wonder what object is red; "The ball is not *red*" indicates that the ball is some color other than red). The context in which a negative sentence is uttered also affects comprehension. We could anticipate that the fewer the external cues, the more difficult comprehension would be. Wiig and Semel (1984) list four important factors

that influence the ease or difficulty of comprehending negative sentences:

1. The proximity of and the relationship between the negation *not* and the negated word or phrase.
2. The immediate relevance of the negated feature or features to the child.
3. The prominence of the stress placed on the negated word or phrase.
4. The complexity of the logical operation of subtraction required. (p. 322)

In addition, the grammatical function of the word or phrase being negated and the length of the sentence have been found to affect children's understanding (Wiig, Florence, Kutner, Sherman, & Semel, 1977). As a result of their study, Wiig et al. suggested a hierarchy in understanding negative sentences. Table 3.5 shows this hierarchy, with items ordered from easiest to hardest in terms of the part of speech being negated. All of the factors mentioned here most likely influence the order in which children learn to interpret negative sentences.

Questions

Children's acquisition of **interrogative**, or question, forms tends to lag somewhat behind their negative utterances. However, before discussing the development of questions, we need to review several types of question forms that can occur in English. *Tag ques-*

TABLE 3.4 Suggested Developmental Sequence for Negative Functions	**Negative Function**	**Example**
	Nonexistence/disappearance	No ball (The ball is not in the toy box where it belongs.) No milk (The milk is all gone.)
	Nonoccurrence	No pull (The toy is stuck and cannot be pulled.)
	Cessation	No turn (The top has stopped spinning and has fallen over.)
	Rejection	No juice (The child does not want any juice.)
	Prohibition	No go (The child is telling Mommy not to leave.)
	Denial	No doggie (Having been told the Great Dane is a dog, the child does not believe it belongs to the same class as the toy poodle at home.)

Source: Adapted from Bloom and Lahey (1978).

TABLE 3.5 Hierarchy of Difficulty in Understanding Negative Sentences According to the Part of Speech Being Negated

Part of Speech	Example
Predicate adjective (Easiest)	The ball is not *red*.
Object of the preposition with a copula verb	The ball is not under the *table*.
Predicate	The boy is not *riding* a horse.
Preposition	The ball is not *under* the table.
Indirect object	The girl is not throwing the ball to the *boy*.
Subject	The *boy* is not riding a horse.
Object of the preposition with a noncopula verb	The girl is not sitting on the *table*.
Direct object (Hardest)	The girl is not throwing the *ball* to the boy.

Source: Adapted from Wiig, Florence, Kutner, Sherman, and Semel (1977).

tions use a form in which a subject-verb-object sequence is followed by a query, such as "You can do that, can't you?" or "You can't do that, can you?" When the verb in the first part of the question is affirmative, the verb in the tag is negative, and vice versa. A second type of question is the *yes/no interrogative,* referred to as such because the answer to such a query is "yes" or "no." This interrogative transformation involves moving, or *transposing,* a copula or auxiliary verb to the beginning of the sentence, as in changing the kernel sentence "The boy is running" to "Is the boy running?" If the kernel sentence does not have an auxiliary or copula verb to transpose, as in the sentence "The girl rides the bike," one must be added in the form of "do"; it is then transposed to form the question "Does the girl ride the bike?" Because this transposing operation reverses the usual sequence of subject and verb, the term *interrogative reversal* is also used to refer to this process. Another type of question asks for information other than a yes/no answer and requires that a wh- word, such as "what" or "who," be added to the beginning of an utterance. The process of using a wh- word to start a question form is called *preposing.* However, most wh- question forms involve both a transposing operation and a preposing process, as in transforming the declarative "The boy is riding" into "What is the boy riding?" In using these sentence types, we must not only change the word order of a kernel sentence and add an initial wh- word, but also select a wh- word that reflects the correct meaning of our utterance:

What is the boy riding?

Where is the boy riding?

When is the boy riding?

How is the boy riding?

Therefore, as we look at children's acquisition of questions, we need to consider both the syntactic structures and the specific wh- words that may be used.

In the early stages of learning to ask questions, children mark their yes/no queries only by using rising inflections, such as "mommy go ⤴" (Bellugi, 1965). These children may also use a limited set of wh- questions, although the utterances are not yet in adult form ("What that?" and "Where Mommy going?"). Children learn to prepose with wh- words before they learn to transpose verbs (Brown, 1968). This is a particularly logical pattern because children are not yet using copula and auxiliary verbs in these early stages; therefore, they have nothing in their utterances to transpose.

Although children learn to add copula and auxiliary verbs to their basic kernel sentences, their yes/no questions may continue to be marked by rising intonations ("Mommy is gone ⤴"), although some children may begin with correct transposing (Klee, 1985). The children do prepose for their wh- questions, but they still do not transpose, so their queries sound something like "What Daddy is doing?" or "Where Mommy is going?" If we examine these forms, we see that the children are using a basic kernel sentence that includes the auxiliary "is" and are simply adding the preposed wh- word to the beginning. Gradually, the children begin to transpose for their yes/no questions ("Is the girl eating?") At this stage, however, they may still fail to transpose copula or auxiliary verbs in their wh- questions ("What the girl is eating?"). Children's attempts at negative questions demonstrate the same patterns (Erreich, 1984). Transposing occurs in yes/no questions ("Can't we go?") but not in wh- questions ("Why Daddy can't go?"). Finally, children learn to transpose in their wh- questions ("What is the girl eating?" and "Why can't Daddy go?").

Tag question forms are learned after children acquire declarative and negative sentences and other question forms, and there appear to be several developmental stages (Bloom & Lahey, 1978; Brown & Hanlon, 1970; Reich, 1986). According to Brown and Hanlon (1970), children, in learning to produce tag questions, begin by giving truncated or **elliptical responses** such as "He is" or "He isn't" to questions like "Who is running?" The children then start to use truncated questions such as "Is he?" Finally, the tag forms appear for such utterances as "He isn't running, is he?" or "He is running, isn't he?", although initially the question part of the tag may not be negated appropriately, such as "You want milk, do you?" Although we are discussing normal language acquisition here, it is interesting to note that Wiig and Semel (1984) suggest that "language and learning disabled children tend to find tag questions the easiest question form to interpret and use" (p. 327). This contrasts with what might be expected based on the normal developmental sequence.

The choice of which wh- word to use in wh- question forms requires children to apply semantic concepts. "What" and "who" reflect concepts that differentiate between people and things; "where" involves the concept of location. These semantic concepts develop fairly early in children and, not surprisingly, the wh- words reflecting them are among the first to be used in wh- questions (Brown, 1968; Brown, Cazden, & Bellugi, 1969; Lahey, 1988; Lee, 1974). Children use "when" and "how" in their questions somewhat later, since time and manner concepts are acquired after the three early-developing concepts. Causal relations develop even later. As a result, wh- questions with "why" are among the last to be used meaningfully. The word "meaningfully" is used here because children may ask "Why?" as an attention-getting device before they truly understand the concept of causality and use it accurately in wh- questions.

Wootten, Merkin, Hood, and Bloom (1979) have provided additional evidence that meaning influences the sequence in which wh- words appear. Wh- words that request information about the sentence element they replace occur earlier in children's language than wh- words that ask "for information pertaining to semantic relations among all the constituents of a sentence" (Leonard, 1984, p. 22). As such, questions with "what" or "where" in queries like "What is that?" and "Where is it?" occur before questions with "how" and "why." The semantics of the verbs and the verb types also seem to influence the developmental order of wh- words. Wh- questions with "what," "where," and "who" typically occur with the copula verb or "do" and "go." In contrast, "why" queries tend to occur with verbs indicating states and specific actions. We saw that the former wh- question words are among the earlier-appearing forms, whereas "why" is the last to appear. "How," which is acquired somewhere between these early wh- words and "why," occurs with copula verbs, "go" and "do," and verbs indicating states and specific actions. It is likely, therefore, that the information being sought by specific wh- questions and the semantics of the verbs usually associated with specific wh- words affect the order of occurrence in young children's language.

Pragmatic influences may also affect what we observe about children's uses of wh- questions (Wooten et al., 1979). Wh- questions that are ungrammatical because they lack verbs ("What Mommy doing?") gradually disappear from children's language as the children grow older. In contrast, the occurrences of elliptical, pragmatically appropriate responses to others' comments ("Where?," "How?") increase with age, even though these latter forms also lack verbs.

In chapter 1 we suggested that children sometimes acquire a linguistic form receptively before using it in their utterances. It appears that this pattern is true for at least "what" and "why" questions. Children have been found to ask "what" and "why" questions only after they can answer these question forms appropriately (Hood, 1977; Soderbergh, cited in Bloom & Lahey, 1978). It also appears that the order in which children learn to comprehend wh- questions corresponds closely to the sequence in which they learn to ask them. Children respond adequately to "where," "what," and "who" questions before "when," "how," and "why" queries (Ervin-Tripp, 1970). The earlier forms, "who," "what," and "where," appear to be comprehended at about 3 years of age (Brown, 1968; Brown et al., 1969).

Compound and Complex Sentences

The use of a **compound sentence** (a sentence containing more than one independent clause) or a **complex sentence** (a sentence that contains at least one independent clause and at least one dependent or subordinate clause) involves the expression of two or more ideas or propositions in the one sentence. (A **clause**, in contrast to a phrase, contains a subject and a verb.) These more advanced sentence forms are created by joining two or more clauses together, often with a linguistic form such as a conjunction or a relative pronoun. This clausal joining process usually begins sometime between 2 and 3 years of age when a child's MLU reaches about 3.0 morphemes (Bloom & Lahey, 1978; Miller, 1981). This approximates Brown's Stage IV (Brown, 1973). The first conjunction children learn to use is "and." Bloom, Lahey, Hood, Lifter, and Fiess (1980) indicated that the first appropriate use of "and" appears when a child is about 25 to 27 months old, but it may initially be used for serial naming ("baby and kitty"). For clausal joining, some data suggest that this conjunction is initially employed to conjoin two independent clauses in utterances such as "You do this and I do that" and "The boy runs and the boy jumps" (Lust, 1977; Lust & Mervis, 1980). These types of sentences simply require the children to add on to existing utterances in their language. This addition operation is among the earlier transformations children acquire (Menyuk, 1969). However, because a number of coordinated sentences with "and" contain redundant information, as in "The boy runs and the

boy jumps," the redundant elements can be deleted to form sentences like "The boy runs and jumps." There is other evidence to suggest that children use "and" in sentences where redundant elements have been deleted before using the conjunction in sentences coordinating two independent clauses with all the redundancies (de Villiers, Tager-Flushberg, & Hakuta, 1977). Two terms—*forward deletion* and *backward deletion*—have been used to describe where in these sentences with "and" the deletions of redundant elements occur. *Forward deletions* occur in sentences in which the entire first clause is stated, then the conjunction, and finally, the sentence elements that remain after deletion, as in "The boy runs and [deletion of 'the boy'] jumps." In contrast, *backward deletions* occur in sentences in which the entire clause is stated after the portion of the sentence containing the deletion, as in "The boy [deletion of 'jumps'] and girl jump." Children appear to use "and" sentences with forward deletions before using those with backward deletions (de Villiers et al., 1977; Lust, 1977; Lust & Mervis, 1980). It may be that attaching elements to or modifying the ends of utterances is an easier operation for children than changing or altering elements of internal sentence components. As a result, we may see children use compound objects or verbs in sentences, as in the first example, before we observe them compounding elements such as subjects, as in "The boy and girl jump."

Utterances that contain object complements appear to be the first types of complex sentences children use (Limber, 1973). In sentences with **object complements**, a second basic sentence or clause is used as the object of the verb in the first sentence or clause. For example, in the sentence "I think I have it," the clause "I have it" operates as the object of the verb "think" in the clause "I think." Often included in discussions of object complements are sentences that contain certain types of infinitives. (An *infinitive* is a form of a verb that typically appears with "to," e.g., "to run," "to go.") In these sentences an infinitive and its associated words are used as an object of a verb, as in "I want to run fast." The infinitive "to run" with the word "fast" is used as the object of the verb "want." Both object complement forms—those with a second basic sentence and those with an infinitive—appear in children's utterances at about the same time. Complex sentences in which a second clause is introduced with a wh- adverbial word are acquired shortly after object complement sentences (Limber, 1973). Examples of these sentence types are "I remember *where Mommy is*" and "Daddy knows *when Mommy comes home.*" According to Dale (1976), "clauses referring to location and to time seem to emerge somewhat before other wh- clauses" (p. 113).

Relative clauses, which are clauses serving as modifiers for nouns (and are, therefore, a type of adjectival clause), develop somewhat later (Limber, 1973; Paul, 1981). A relative clause is often introduced by a relative pronoun, such as "what," "who," "which," "whose," or "that" ("I see the boys *who are running*" or "The dog *that has the bone* is growling"). However, in some instances the relative pronoun may be omitted ("That's the bed [that] *we sleep in*"). Children initially use relative clauses to modify predicate nouns ("That is the balloon *that I like*") and objects ("I see the boy *who wears glasses*"). They later begin to modify subjects with relative clauses ("The girl *who wears glasses* sees better"). Again, we see a pattern in which children add to the ends of their sentences before rearranging or adding elements within the sentences. The latter process, termed **embedding,** is one of the later-developing transformational operations (Menyuk, 1969), possibly because it disrupts the usual sequence in which a verb immediately follows a sentence's subject. However, another possible explanation for the delayed appearance of relative clauses modifying subjects in comparison to object relatives is that subjects may frequently be pronouns or proper names, to which relative clauses cannot be attached. In contrast, objects are often inanimate nouns that can be modified by relative clauses (Limber, 1973).

Although Limber (1973) indicates that 3-year-old children demonstrate the use of clauses with object complements, wh- adverbials, and object relatives, Paul (1981) suggests that the use of all of these clause types may not be demonstrated until children are closer to 4 years of age. Embedded relative clauses (subject relatives), having already been identified as later developing, are not used by children at these ages. In one study (Hass & Wepman, 1974), the embedding operation was shown to be a continuing

developmental process in children 5 to 13 years old. Embedding appears to emerge somewhat later than other types of clausal operations, and it continues to develop into adolescence. Furthermore, the use of various types of dependent clauses, as found in complex sentences, continues to increase through 12th grade (Loban, 1976), with a major shift to the use of clausal constructions occurring at about 10 years of age (Naremore & Dever, 1975).

The construction of many compound and complex sentences requires the use of **connective** devices such as conjunctions. The accurate use of these sentences involves both the syntactic operations to combine clauses and the selection of appropriate conjunctions to express the correct meanings. In some instances, the semantic task may be more difficult than the syntactic task. Lee (1974) explained this by comparing different conjunctions in sentence forms with the basic subject-verb-object clause plus a conjunction followed by another subject-verb-object clause. Two of her examples are "Billy found cookies *and* Billy likes cookies" and "Billy looked for cookies *although* Billy was not hungry" (p. 40). Although both sentences contain the same basic syntactic constructions, the second example expresses a much more subtle and complex relation than the first because of the differences in the meanings of the conjunctions. We indicated earlier that the conjunction "and" is the first to be acquired by children. Beyond "and," the exact sequence in which children learn other conjunctions and the ages at which they acquire them are difficult to report. Authors have investigated the use of different conjunctions by children at varying ages and have reported their data in different ways. In one study of children 2 and 3 years old, the sequence in which certain conjunctions appeared in their language was "because," "what," "when," "but," "that," "if," and "so," all, of course, after the emergence of "and" (Hood, Lahey, Lifter, & Bloom, 1978). Clark (1970) looked at the frequency with which 3½-year-old children used various conjunctions. She indicated that the more frequently used conjunctions were "and," "and so," and "then," followed by "when" and "because." "If" occurred less frequently. Although the frequency with which conjunctions occur in children's language may be influenced by context, the types of things children talk about, the opportunity, and the frequency of use may also be related to children's knowledge of and facility with the different conjunctions. As such, the frequency with which conjunctions occur in children's language may provide a clue to their developmental sequence.

In addition to the studies focusing on preschoolers' acquisition of conjunctions, the use of conjunctions by first graders was examined (Menyuk, 1969). As might be expected, 95% of these children produced well-formed sentences with the conjunction "and." In contrast, 35% of them used adequate sentences with "because." The conjunctions "if" and "so" were more difficult. Only 20% and 19% of the first graders produced well-formed sentences with "if" and "so," respectively. These results certainly suggest that children continue their acquisition of conjunctions past the first grade and into middle and late childhood.

Studies investigating school children's comprehension of conjunctions support the suggestion of continuing development into the later grades. Although children use the conjunction "because" prior to second grade, and possibly even before age 4 (Clark, 1970; Hood et al., 1978; Menyuk, 1969), they apparently do not fully comprehend its meaning. Use of the conjunction at these early ages seems to be related to familiar cause–effect situations, and comprehension tends to depend on contextual clues and semantic probability (Emerson, 1979). (*Semantic probability* refers to the aspect of language that makes some utterances logical, based on the interrelationships among the meanings of words, and others illogical because of semantic constraints.) However, when "because" was examined with tasks in which contextual information was removed and the amount of information from semantic probability clues was systematically varied, children's comprehension of the conjunction was not complete until sometime between the ages of 10 and 11 (Emerson, 1979). Children's comprehension of the conjunctions "if," "if/not," "either," "although," "neither/nor," "unless," "either/or," and "but/not" also shows a continuing developmental trend from first through sixth grades (Granowsky, 1976). In support of this developmental trend, Rystrom (1972) suggests that primary school children often misunderstand sentences with the conjunctions "unless," "although," "since," "while," "whether," "after," and "before."

MORE WORDS

After using the first word at about 12 months of age, children acquire an expressive vocabulary of about 10 words at 15 months (Reich, 1986), 50 words at 18 months, 150 words at 20 months (Dale, Bates, Reznick, & Morisset, 1989), 200–300 words at 24 months (Dale & Thal, 1989; Reich, 1986), 1,000 words at 3 years (Owens, 1992; Wehrebian, 1970), 1,500–1,600 words at 4 years (Owens, 1992), 2,100–2,200 words at 5 years, and 2,600–7,000 words at 6 years (Owens, 1992; Zintz, 1970). In light of our previous discussions, it is not surprising that development for lexical comprehension precedes and exceeds development for lexical use. Children comprehend their first words at about 8 to 9 months of age (Benedict, 1979). At about 13 months of age, children comprehend about 50 words (Benedict, 1979). By 6 years of age their comprehension vocabulary is between 20,000 and 24,000 words, and by 12 years of age it is 50,000 or more words (Owens, 1992). The size of a child's vocabulary depends, in part, on the experiences and words to which the child is exposed, which after the early years leads to variability in vocabulary size. Vocabulary size is also difficult to measure.

There seem to be some patterns to the sequence in which children acquire words:

1. How often particular terms are used in children's environments.
2. Overextension and underextension of the meanings of words. As an example of **overextension**, all four-legged animals may be "dogs" for a while. In **underextension**, children associate the meanings of words with specific objects or events and do not realize the broader applications of the words. For instance, "bottle" may only apply to the baby's bottle. Children gradually narrow and broaden word meanings with additional exposure to their environments.
3. A general tendency to label first objects and actions; then words that attach attributes to objects or events ("big"); and finally, words that express temporal, spatial, conditional, and causal relationships.
4. A shift from classifying words on the basis of perceptual or functional characteristics (concrete

classifications) to classifying words according to abstract properties such as temporal-spatial features or animate-inanimate characteristics. This change evolves gradually over the Piagetian cognitive stages from preoperational thinking through formal operations and possibly beyond.

During the single-word utterance stage, there also seems to be a relationship between a child's phonological and semantic development. Children appear to learn more easily and quickly new words that begin with consonants they have used previously in other words than words that begin with consonants they have not yet used (Leonard, Schwartz, Morris, & Chapman, 1981; Schwartz & Leonard, 1982). For children in the single-word utterance stage of development, word type, that is, object or action words, has also been found to affect the phonetic accuracy with which children produce words. Camarata and Schwartz (1985) reported that object words tend to be said more correctly than action words. These findings additionally support the notion of synergism among the various components of language in children's development (Reed, 1992).

Fast Mapping

One way that children appear to learn the meaning of words is with a process known as **fast mapping**, also referred to as *quick incidental learning* (Carey & Bartlett, 1978; Crais, 1992; Dickinson, 1984; Dockrell & Campbell, 1986; Dollaghan, 1985; Heibeck & Markman, 1987). Dollaghan (1987) describes fast mapping as a lexical acquisition strategy "in which a listener rapidly constructs a representation for an unfamiliar word on the basis of a single exposure to it. This initial representation might contain information on the semantic, phonological, or syntactic characteristics of the new lexical item, as well as nonlinguistic information related to the situation in which it was encountered" (p. 218). This first meaning may or may not be complete and/or accurate. It does, however, create a basis for further refinement as additional experiences with the word in context occur. Fast mapping has been documented as a lexical learning strategy that children use (Dickinson, 1984; Dockrell & Campbell, 1986; Dollaghan, 1985; Heibeck & Markman, 1987; Rice,

Huston, Truglio, & Wright, 1990; Rice & Woodsmall, 1988).

Semantic Feature Hypothesis

Another approach to explaining how children learn the meanings of words has been proposed by Clark (1973b). According to this approach, the *semantic feature hypothesis,* meanings of words are composed of sets of individual features or characteristics that are either present (+) or absent (−). Clark provides an example with the word "before." The features that together comprise the meaning are as follows:

+ time (The word has some type of temporal orientation.)
− simultaneous (The word refers to sequence rather than simultaneity.)
+ prior (The word indicates a specific order in which the sequence occurs.)

Clark suggests that children learn the meanings of words by gradually acquiring the features that make up the meanings. The following list (Clark, 1973b) shows that when "before" is contrasted with "after," the last feature (" + " or " − " prior) is the only one that distinguishes meaning. If a child has not yet acquired this last feature, "before" may be used synonymously with "after."

Before	*After*
+ time	+ time
− simultaneous	− simultaneous
+ prior	− prior

Words may be related to each other in meaning. That is, they may share some of the same semantic features. However, one or more of the words will have additional features not included in the meanings of the other words. For example, both "big" and "tall" have elements of largeness in their meanings, although "big" is a more general term and "tall" refers to largeness in a vertical direction. As another example, the word "give" has the features that involve transferring possession of something and specifying the direction of the transfer. The verb "sell" also has these two features of "give," but it adds the three components of obligation, money, and mutual agreement between the parties involved in the transfer (Dale, 1976; Gentner, 1975). "Sell" is, therefore, considered to be more semantically complex than "give" because "sell" has more features. The semantic feature hypothesis predicts that children often learn the meanings for less semantically complex words before more semantically complex ones.

The last aspect of Clark's approach relates to unmarked and marked words in *antonym pairs*. When most of us consider a pair of opposite words ("big"-"little"), we intuitively prefer or gravitate toward one of the words in the pair, and many of us would agree on which is the preferred word. The preferred word is typically considered the more positive, greater, or more expected term and is called the *unmarked word* in an antonym pair. The less positive word in the pair is called the *marked word*. Generally, the unmarked word is learned first, although there may be exceptions to this situation. Because children focus on change, it may be that the word of an antonym pair that represents the most change from the status quo will be the one they acquire first (Greenfield & Smith, 1976).

In many instances of children's semantic development, the semantic feature hypothesis does seem to apply. However, there are data that conflict with the predictions of word acquisition order proposed by this hypothesis (e.g., Barrie-Blackley, 1973; Coker, 1978). Several factors may account for these conflicting reports. As previously mentioned, the frequency with which specific words are used in children's environments and the words that signify the greatest changes from normal conditions affect the order of word acquisition. Differences in research design may account for the conflicting results. In addition, some word meanings may evolve from the specific to the general (Anglin, 1970), in contrast to Clark's (1973b) approach. Other words may simply represent idiosyncratic learning on a child's part.

Spatial, Temporal, and Familial Terms

Children's comprehension of **spatial** (location in space) and **temporal** (location in time) words develops gradually, from about 2 years for "in" as a preposition (Bangs, 1975) to about 11 years for terms such as "before" and "after" (Wiig & Semel, 1974). In Wiig and Semel's study (1974) examining school-age children's understanding of selected spatial and temporal relationships, comprehension of these relationships continued to develop throughout Piaget's concrete operational period (while the children were in Grades 1 through 5 and approximately 7 to 11 years old). Comprehension then seemed to stabilize as the children moved cognitively into the formal operations stage at about 11 years of age. When the children were in Grade 1, their ability to interpret temporal terms was greater than their comprehension of spatial relationships. However, in Grade 2, they were able to understand the spatial terms better than the temporal ones. This difference in skills in favor of spatial relationships continued to Grade 5.

Many conjunctions involve temporal concepts (e.g., "She will leave *when* it is convenient" and "We ate breakfast *before* we went to school"), as does the wh-question word "when." We will not repeat our previous discussions of the development of these forms here. However, a number of these same terms occur as prepositions (e.g., "We ate breakfast *before* school"). Children generally use these temporal terms as prepositions before using them as conjunctions (Coker, 1978). Additionally, terms expressing order of events (e.g., "before" and "after") appear to be learned prior to terms expressing simultaneity (e.g., "while" and "at the same time") (Feagans, 1980).

Spatial relationships are also often expressed by *prepositions*. In attempting to explain the strategies children use in acquiring spatial prepositions, Clark (1973a) and Clark and Clark (1977) suggest that there are three rules children apply:

1. When a container is present, an object belongs in it. ("In")
2. When a supporting surface is present, an object belongs on it. ("On")
3. When two objects are together in space, they should touch each other. ("To")

Clark (1973a) also indicates that the first rule has precedence over the second. These rules imply that "in" will be acquired before "out," that "in" will be acquired before "on," that "on" will be acquired before "off," and that "to" will be acquired before "from." This seems to be true when children's developmental sequences for these terms are examined, although Brown (1973) suggests that "in" and "on" are acquired at the same time. Some of these same words that function as prepositions also occur as part of a *verb particle,* that is, a multiword construction that functions as a verb, as in "She *put up* a good argument." Like prepositions, these words as verb particles emerge early in children's language and by about 4 to 5 years of age are used with reasonable accuracy (Goodluck, 1986; Wegner & Rice, 1988). However, Wegner and Rice (1988) suggest that certain words seem to be used more as prepositions ("in," "on," and "over") and others ("up," "down," and "off") more as verb particles.

Other spatial prepositions (e.g., "in front of" and "next to") are more difficult for children. The referents for these prepositions vary, depending on the children's relationships to objects and the characteristics of the objects. When an object has a front, such as a person, "in front of" relates to the object's front (Owens, 1992). Without a front on an object such as a ball, "in front of" derives its meaning from the relative positions of the speaker and the object—positions that can vary. Furthermore, "next to" can mean "beside," "in back of," or "in front of," all of which can be very confusing for a child. As might be expected, these types of spatial prepositions develop later.

Wiig and Semel's (1974) study also examined children's comprehension of familial terms. In comparison to both spatial and temporal relationships, comprehension and use of familial terms (e.g., "father," "grandmother," and "cousin") were more difficult than both spatial and temporal relationships. When the results of this study are combined with those of Romney and D'Andrade (1964), a sequence of acquisition seems to appear: "mother" and "father," "sister" and "brother," "grandmother" and "grandfather," "aunt" and "uncle," and "cousin."

Deictic Words

Deictic words are terms that have changing referents, depending on who in a communicative dyad is speaking, on the respective locations of objects and people, and on the temporal relationships relative to the speaker and listener. The spatial prepositions dis-

cussed in the preceding section are deictic in nature. As another example, the referents for "I" and "you" shift as the speaker–listener relationship changes. The terms "here" and "there" and "this" and "that" vary, depending on the location of the speaker, listener, and/or objects. Among the deictic verbs are "come," "go," "bring," and "take." Such words must be confusing for young children, although the literature suggests that children demonstrate some use of deictic shifts for first- and second-person pronouns ("I," "you," "me") sometime between approximately 1 and 2 years of age (Bloom, Rocissano, & Hood, 1976; Morehead & Ingram, 1973). Third-person pronouns appear later in children's language, between approximately 2 and 3 years of age, and their development may even continue up to 5 years of age and possibly beyond. Bloom et al. (1976) indicate that, when children's MLUs approach 4.0, they evidence deictic shifts for the terms "here," "there," "this," and "that."

Other deictic words, such as "come," "go," "bring," and "take," tend to be learned later, and complete acquisition may extend into children's school years. According to Bloom and Lahey (1978), the development of these types of words "involves the very complex interplay between children's opportunities for using and hearing others use shifting reference and their linguistic, conceptual, and social development" (p. 225). These authors even describe the learning process as one of "trials and tribulations over a very long period of time" (p. 225).

LEARNING WORD FORMS

Children's acquisition of morphological rules begins in early childhood and continues into the school years. Earlier, we indicated that when children's MLUs reach about 2.0 morphemes, they begin to use grammatical markers on their words (Brown, 1973). Table 3.3 shows that the first of these morphological forms to be acquired is the present progressive "ing" ending on verbs ("rolling"). Other authors have agreed with Brown's finding that "ing" is the earliest-developing and easiest of the grammatical markers (de Villiers & de Villiers, 1973; Newfield & Schlanger, 1968; Wiig, Semel, & Crouse, 1973).

Of the other verb forms Brown (1973) investigated, irregular past tense words such as "ran" and "saw" appeared next in the children's language (see Table 3.3). We must be careful, however, in our interpretation of this sequence. In learning morphological rules, children typically acquire a more general rule first. Gradually, they modify and refine the rule to account for the more specific applications and exceptions (Berko, 1958). Acquiring irregular past tense verb forms before regular ones appears to contradict the usual learning pattern. Rather than interpreting Brown's finding as an indication that children learn the exceptions to the rules for forming past tense verbs before learning the usual rules, it may be that children simply acquire these terms as vocabulary words instead of word form variations derived from lexical verbs. Support for such an interpretation comes from the observation that after children begin to use regular past tense verb forms correctly, they incorrectly apply the rules to irregular verbs previously used accurately. At this stage, utterances such as "He runned" and "I seed a dog" are not uncommon.

Uncontractible forms of the copula "to be" ("Here I am") appear next, followed by regular past tense forms ("She jumped") (Brown, 1973). However, not all variations of regular past tense verbs are acquired at the same time. Verbs to which the past tense allomorph /d/ is added ("played") appear to develop slightly before those to which the allomorph /t/ is attached ("jumped") (Berko, 1958; Moran, 1975; Newfield & Schlanger, 1968; Wiig et al., 1973). Acquisition of the /əd/ allomorph ("painted") occurs somewhat later. As we might expect from our previous discussion of irregular past tense verbs, complete learning of these many variations lags considerably behind that of the regular forms. When the performances of 7- and 8-year-old children were examined, the children gave fewer than 75% correct responses to several types of irregular verbs in which a vowel change was required to arrive at the correct past tense form, such as "ride" to "rode" and "sing" to "sang" (Moran, 1975). These elementary school children provided only about 40% correct responses for irregular verbs formed by changing both a vowel and a final consonant ("catch" to "caught" or "bring" to "brought"). Such data indicate that children continue to refine their morphological usage well past the time they begin school.

According to Brown (1973), the regular forms of third-person singular present tense verbs ("She jumps" and "He swims") emerge after past tense regular forms (see Table 3.3). Shortly thereafter, children begin to use irregular forms of third-person singular present tense verbs ("do" to "does" and "have" to "has"). Of the 14 grammatical morphemes in Brown's investigation, the verb forms involving the contractible copula and auxiliary ("We're big" and "She's running") and the uncontractible auxiliary ("He was running") were the last ones the children acquired.

Bloom, Lifter, and Hafitz (1980) suggest that meanings of verbs affect which verb inflections children are likely to use. For verbs that denote ongoing actions for which there are no obvious results, such as "play," children tend to use the "ing" inflection. In contrast, verbs denoting ongoing actions that leave a more lasting effect, such as "go," are more frequently inflected with a third-person singular present tense verb ("goes"). Verbs whose meanings imply actions that come to an end and leave a relatively obvious effect ("crash" or "bite") are likely to be used in their past tense forms ("crashed" and "bit"). This tendency to use a specific type of inflection with a specific type of action was observed most notably when a verb word was relatively new in the children's vocabularies.

Table 3.3 indicates that children begin to use regular noun plurals after present progressive verb endings and before irregular past tense forms (Brown, 1973). Again, there are various forms of regular noun plurals, and there appears to be a developmental sequence for acquisition of these variations. Children's utterances with the plural allomorph /z/ ("pigs") tend to be more accurate before their utterances containing plural nouns with the /s/ allomorph ("boats") (Berko, 1958; Solomon, 1972; Wiig et al., 1973). Accurate use of the /əz/ plural allomorph is achieved after the /s/ and /z/ plural forms. In fact, 6- and 7-year-old children may still demonstrate problems with plural nouns that require use of the /əz/ ending (Berko, 1958; Solomon, 1972). Although children begin to use some noun plurals early in their language-learning process, the complete acquisition of plural forms takes several years. Koziol (1973) even suggests that an important stage in children's acquisition of plural noun forms occurs at about the kindergarten–first grade period. Furthermore, the learning of irregular noun plurals ("child" to "children") seems to lag behind the acquisition of regular forms by about 2 to 3 years (Koziol, 1973).

Brown (1973) indicates that children begin to use possessive forms of nouns shortly after the appearances of noun plurals and irregular past tense verbs (see Table 3.3). Possessive forms of nouns are derived in basically the same ways as noun plurals, and their sequence of acquisition appears to be essentially similar. Correct use of the /z/ allomorph ("bug's") tends to be achieved somewhat before that of the /s/ allomorph ("bike's"), which, in turn, tends to be acquired before the /əz/ ending ("horse's") (Berko, 1958; Newfield & Schlanger, 1968; Wiig et al., 1973). We note that regular forms of noun plurals, possessives, and third-person singular present tense verbs all use the same word endings—/z/, /s/, and /əz/. Therefore, it is not surprising that Brown (1973) found that once the children in his study correctly added the endings to form any one of the three word types (plurals, possessives, or third-person verbs), they used the other two types within 1 year.

Other morphological forms include comparatives ("bigger") and superlatives ("biggest"), noun and adverb derivations ("painter," "fireman," "violinist," "gently," "quickly"), and prefixes ("preheat," "undone," "miscue"). The results of Berko's (1958) classic study indicated that even by age 7 children had not yet fully acquired the rules for forming comparative and superlative adjectives and for deriving nouns and adverbs. In a similar investigation (Wiig et al., 1973), academic achievers with an average age of 9 years were still giving fewer than 50% correct responses to tasks involving noun and adverb derivations. Prefixing also is a difficult skill to acquire because it requires knowledge of the meanings for both the prefix form and the root word. As we can see, refinement of several morphological rules continues well into the school years.

LANGUAGE USE

Although the realization that language is useful and serves numerous functions for humans is not new, serious study of how children acquire competence in the pragmatic aspects of language is relatively recent. As a result, developmental data in this area are still sketchy and less extensive than for the other aspects of language. There are many factors involved in how people use language and what influences their communicative choices in various speaking situations. In this section, we look at children's developing skills in several of these areas—their changing abilities in the functions for which they use language and what they intend to accomplish by its use, their competencies in maintaining a topic and taking turns during a conversation, their uses of presuppositions, their fluency in delivering their messages, and their evolving narrative skills.

Functions and Intentions

Before children use their first words, they engage in **perlocutionary acts** (Bates, 1976), including such nonverbal behaviors as smiling, crying, laughing, and gazing. Although these behaviors have an effect on the listener, the behaviors themselves lack communicative intent. Children demonstrate **illocutionary acts**, such as showing objects to adults, pointing to items, and giving objects to adults, at approximately 9 or 10 months. In contrast to perlocutionary acts, these illocutionary acts are intentional and seem to indicate the intent to communicate. These behaviors may well be precursors to some of the types of events children first verbalize about when they enter the **locutionary** stage at about 12 months of age and begin to use words.

Halliday (1975) described seven purposes, or functions, of communicative attempts that occur between approximately 9 and 16 or 18 months of age. Table 3.6 lists and explains these seven functions. Because these functions emerge during part of a period in which children have few words, much of the communication may be accomplished in nonverbal ways. For these reasons, Bloom and Lahey (1978) suggest that this stage may be referred to as the *level of primary forms* (p. 202).

Halliday's view of communicative functions considers the listeners' responses. On the other hand, Dore (1975), who concentrated on the period during which children were using single words (approximately 12 to 18–24 months), focuses on children's intention to use these single-word utterances with less emphasis on the listeners' reactions to the intents. As Prutting (1979) explains, Dore provides a way of identifying children's reasons (intentions) for communication, while Halliday furnishes a way of describing how well

TABLE 3.6 Seven Functions of Early Language

Function	Definition
Instrumental	The purpose of this function is to receive material needs, desired objects, or assistance from others.
Regulatory	This function is somewhat related to the previous one, although the emphasis is directed to individuals rather than to desired objects or actions. Here children are attempting to control the behavior of others.
Interactional	In using this function, children are making interpersonal contact with others in their environments to initiate and/or sustain contact with them.
Personal	This is an awareness of self and an expression of one's own feelings and individuality.
Heuristic	Functionally, children attempt to have their environments or events in their environments explained.
Imaginative	This is the pretend or play-acting communicative function.
Informative	Children communicate their experiences or tell someone something.

Source: Adapted from Halliday (1975).

the reasons worked or functioned. Dore's (1975) intentions are as follows:

1. Labeling
2. Answering
3. Requesting action
4. Requesting an answer
5. Calling/addressing
6. Greeting
7. Protesting
8. Repeating/imitating
9. Practicing (language)

Because children at this period are evidencing more consistent uses of words to communicate their intentions, this stage of pragmatic development can be viewed as the *level of conventional forms* (Bloom & Lahey, 1978, p. 203).

During the stage from about 16 or 18 months to 24 months, children use language for different functions. According to Halliday (1974), the earlier instrumental and regulatory functions combine with part of the interactional function to form a new function—the pragmatic function. The *pragmatic* function is basically a controlling one used to satisfy desires and needs while interacting with people at the same time. Some re-

sponse from the listener is expected. The newly acquired mathetic function is derived from the more basic personal and heuristic functions in combination, again, with part of the interactional function. The *mathetic* function focuses on language as a tool for learning more about the environment (e.g., asking the names of objects) and for commenting on the environment. In contrast to the pragmatic function, the mathetic function does not always require a response from the listener. Children use a third function during this period—the informative function. In employing the *informative* function, children actually convey information to the listeners. An important achievement occurs by the end of this stage. Children learn that language can be multifunctional. That is, one utterance can serve more than one function at a time, a characteristic of most adult communications.

By age 3, children's utterances consistently contain more than one function. This is the third, adultlike stage, and the functions that Halliday (1975) has identified in children's communications in this period are the *interpersonal* purpose (used to relate to other people), the *textual* purpose (used to relate to preceding and following utterances in a dialogue), and the *ideational-experiential* purpose (used to express ideas or events to others).

The true intentions and functions of some speech acts do not, however, always match the forms of the utterances or their propositional content. Common uses of these indirectives are hiding the true purposes of utterances in syntactic forms created for the sake of politeness (the interrogative "Can you open the door?" instead of the imperative "Open the door") or hinting at a purpose by employing content different from the true intent (a child's utterance to a babysitter such as "My mommy always lets me stay up late on Fridays" or an adult's remarks, on wishing to have a window closed, "My, it's chilly in here," with no direct reference to the window). In some ways, children's ability to understand and use these indirect speech acts depends partly on their skills in making presuppositions about communicative situations, a topic we discuss in the next section. However, intentions and functions of speech acts are certainly involved.

After about age 3½, children employ these polite devices and hints in their utterances (Ervin-Tripp & Mitchell-Kernan, 1977; Nippold, Leonard, & Anastopoulos, 1982). In the Nippold et al. (1982) study, children steadily improved with age in their ability to regard requests that contained "please" as more polite than those without it. However, their skill at judging interrogative forms as polite (e.g., "Could I have some candy?") developed later than their skill with "please." When the children were asked to determine whether a request in the form of an interrogative with "please" ("Could you give me a nut, please?") was more polite than a request in the form of an imperative with "please" ("Give me a nut, please"), even 7-year-olds had difficulty, although their performances were better than those of the 3- and 5-year-olds in the study. Use of the polite form—interrogative with "please"—increased steadily between 3 and 7 years, the age at which the children's uses of this form approximated the adults'. These findings suggest that although children may begin to use indirectives and polite forms sometime after age 3, it takes at least 4 more years for their use to reach adultlike levels. Furthermore, it appears that any request with "please," despite its syntactic form, may be regarded by children as more polite until sometime after 7 years of age.

Presuppositions

In pragmatics, **presuppositions** refer to the assumptions speakers make about what knowledge is shared between speakers and listeners and about what information listeners need to understand messages. Effective speakers modify the form and content of their utterances based on their presuppositions. Accurate presuppositions about listeners and skill in choosing from among alternative communicative forms result in messages that provide sufficient information for listeners but that do not include excessive redundant knowledge. Wood (1982), in borrowing from Olson and Nickerson (1978), lists five aspects of presupposition:

1. Shared knowledge, inclusive of prior knowledge, world knowledge, and listener-specific knowledge.
2. Shared experiential context of the moment when the utterance is expressed.
3. Preceding utterances in the conversation.
4. Assumed listener biases.
5. Numerous nonverbal clues regarding the speaker's intentions. (p. 34)

Once speakers take these aspects into account, they choose the form and content to encode their messages. When children learn to modify their language by selecting from among alternative ways of achieving the same purposes in order to meet the needs of their listeners, they have achieved the "level of conventional use" (Bloom & Lahey, 1978, p. 203). From this perspective, the use of indirectives, hints, and polite forms could be viewed as part of the presupposition aspect of language use.

It was previously believed that children's egocentricity would prevent them from taking a listener's needs into account as they formulated their messages. Surprisingly, however, there is some evidence that even at the single-word stage, children adapt what limited language they have for their listeners (Greenfield & Smith, 1976). That is, they tend to code "the information that is most needed by the listener to understand the communicative intent" (Prutting, 1979, p. 11). Normal-hearing 2-year-old children of deaf parents have been found to alter the amount of their oral language, the length of their utterances, and the degree to which they use manual communication, depending on whether they are talking with a normal hearing adult or one of their hearing-impaired parents (Schiff, 1976). Furthermore, children between ages 3 and 4 change the amount of information they give to listeners relative to their listeners' prior knowledge of communicative topics and ability to share in immediate communicative contexts (Maratsos, 1973; Menig-Peterson, 1975). The less the listeners know, the more information the children include in their language. The ages of children's communicative partners also influence how 4-year-old children encode their messages. Children at this age use shorter and less complex sentences when talking to younger children than when speaking to their peers or to adults (Shatz & Gelman, 1973). It appears, then, that children even in the sensorimotor stage and the preconceptual period of the preoperational stage of cognitive development are capable of adapting both the form and the content of their language according to their presuppositions about their listeners' needs.

How children differentially encode new and old information in their utterances is another aspect of presupposition. The following example of sequential utterances illustrates what happens as new and old information occurs in the content of a message:

> I got new shoes. They're brown and white. But Billy doesn't like them. He liked the black ones.

In the first sentence, a noun is used to identify the objects. It is new information for the listener. However, in the second sentence, the shoes become old information as the new information regarding color is introduced. As a result, the pronoun "they" is used to refer to the old information. In the third sentence, a new person is introduced and is, therefore, referred to by name, while the old information remains encoded by a pronoun. The last sentence contains old information about the person and shoes, so both are referred to by pronouns. However, because shoes other than the ones initially introduced into the message are being encoded, a different pronoun is used. Basically, new information is emphasized, while old information is deemphasized. As a result of her investigation of the ways in which children refer to old and new information, Greenfield has proposed a *principle of informativeness* (Greenfield, 1978; Greenfield & Smith, 1976; Greenfield & Zukow, 1978). According to this principle, children in the single-word stage will verbalize information that is new or different about an event and ignore redundant information or, at least, not verbalize about it. This principle has been shown to hold true for children in this early period of language development (Greenfield & Zukow, 1978). Children who have advanced to using utterances containing two to four words also tend to verbalize most the words that represent new information in a communicative context (Miller, 1975; Weisenberger, 1976). Developmentally, it appears that children from the single-word to approximately the three- or four-word utterance stages of language learning simply omit old information in their speech and encode information that is new or changing about a situational context. However, as children increase the length of their utterances to approach five words or morphemes, they tend to use pronouns in referring to old information and to name specifically new information (Skarakis & Greenfield, 1982). The children who showed this tendency to pronominalize old information and nominalize new information in the Skarakis and Greenfield investigation ranged from 2 years to 2 years, 10 months of age. These findings appear to correspond to the approximate developmental trends seen for the use of pronouns, discussed in the previous section on deictic words.

Use of the definite ("the") and indefinite ("a" and "an") articles is related to the ways in which new and old information is encoded. Although we see children using articles when their MLUs are about 3.5 and they are approximately 2½ to 3 years old (Brown, 1973), accurate use of articles varies, depending on the context in which they occur, the amount of shared information between listener and speaker, and whether or not the information is new or old. In a sequence of utterances, the indefinite article is used to introduce a new referent and the definite article is employed to encode a previously introduced referent. The following example illustrates this variation:

> I bought *a* new dress. *The* dress is red with ruffles.

Because of the shifting use required for articles, we might anticipate that complete acquisition evolves over a number of years.

Warden (1976) investigated the developmental changes that occur in the use of articles in children 3, 5, 7, and 9 years old and compared their performances to those of adults. All of the children and the adults showed a consistent preference for using the definite article to refer to previously introduced referents. However, the 3-year-old children randomly used either the definite or indefinite article for introducing initial referents. From 3 years on, there was an increase in appropriate use of the indefinite article for initial referents, but it was not until 9 years of age that the children demonstrated a true preference for using the indefinite article for initial referents. In contrast, adults consistently introduced initial referents with the indefinite article.

Turn Taking, Topic Maintenance, and Revisions

Two aspects of engaging in effective dialogues involve taking one's turn appropriately and helping to maintain the topic of conversation. It appears that children even before the age of 9 months demonstrate rudimentary turn-taking skills in the forms of **reciprocal** interactions (Bruner, 1975). By the time children are 18 to 24 months old, they have learned to participate in dialogues and demonstrate ability in applying rules of turn taking in their dialogues (Bloom et al., 1976; Halliday, 1975). However, a number of years are necessary to refine these skills. In contrast to children younger than 4½ years, who have a fair amount of overlap in their conversations with others, 6- to 8-year olds show few overlaps (Leonard, 1984). Being able to time interruptions so that they occur at appropriate places in dialogues is a developmental skill, with younger children having more difficulty than older ones (Leonard, 1984). Ervin-Tripp (1979) also indicates that when three people, as opposed to two, are involved in a conversation, younger children have more difficulty than older ones in timing interruptions.

Beyond turn taking, a person's response must relate in some way to a speaker's previous utterance if a topic of conversation is to be maintained. Somewhat before age 2, approximately 40% of children's responses to adults' utterances were found to maintain a topic of conversation (Bloom et al., 1976). This proportion increased steadily during approximately the next 12 months, and at about 3 years approximately 50% of children's responses in a conversational dyad continued the topic. However, children at these ages tend not to maintain topics with series of several successive related utterances. As a result, topic shifts are frequent during interchanges (Keenan & Schieffelin, 1976). It is not until approximately age 3½ to 4 that children demonstrate skills in maintaining topics through a number of adjacent comments in a dialogue (Bloom et al., 1976). Brinton and Fujiki (1984) reported that the average number of utterances that even 5-year-old children produced on a single topic during a conversational interchange was five. Additionally, these children covered, on the average, 50 topics in 15 minutes of conversation. The type of activity/context may, however, influence children's ability to maintain topics. Schober-Peterson and Johnson (1989) found that 4-year-old children were able to maintain one topic over as many as 13–91 utterances during activities that involved enacting, describing, and problem-solving conversations. Although these children demonstrated considerable topic maintenance skill during activities that promoted these forms of text, 75% of their topic maintenance utterances were still relatively short.

Not only do children show developmental patterns in their turn-taking skill and topic maintenance ability, they also demonstrate changes with age in the devices they use to maintain topics. Two topic maintenance techniques are focus/imitation and substitution/expansion operations (Bloom et al., 1976; van Kleeck & Frankel, 1981). As children grow older, they increasingly add new information to a topic to maintain it. Before age 3, children tend to use *focus/imitation* topic maintenance devices (Bloom et al., 1976; Keenan, 1975). That is, they attend to one or more of the words in a previous utterance and repeat or imitate those portions in their succeeding responses. As children approach age 3, their use of focus/imitation devices decreases and their use of substitution/expansion operations increases (Bloom et al., 1976; Keenan, 1975). In *substitution/expansion*, children add information to the topic of a previous utterance or modify the previous utterance in some way. Van Kleeck and Frankel (1981) suggest that substitution/expansion topic maintenance devices are more complex operations because children must manipulate the semantic-syntactic structures of the previous utterances.

Unfortunately, not all utterances in a conversation are understood by listeners. When confusion occurs, effective speakers revise their messages. Children between the ages of 21 and 29 months have been found consistently to modify their original utterances when their listeners misunderstand (Gallagher, 1977). Initially, children use phonetic modifications (changing word pronunciations) in attempts to clarify their messages. As children mature, they change their revision strategies and use more word substitutions to modify their communicative attempts. However, at 4½ years of age, children tend to increase the length of succeeding utterances when they know their listeners have not adequately received the message (Iwan & Siegel, 1982). Conversely, they decrease the length of succeeding utterances when they are aware that their message has been understood.

Fluency

All speakers revise phrases, repeat words, hesitate, use fillers such as "uh," and make false starts in the delivery of messages. In fact, preschool children typically go through a period of normal disfluency when their language proficiency cannot keep up with their thoughts and their need to communicate. However, most children outgrow this period of normal disfluency, and once they enter school, the degree to which their messages are delivered with a smooth, easily flowing series of words often becomes one of the factors people use, consciously or unconsciously, to evaluate the language proficiency of children (Loban, 1976).

In his longitudinal study of the language development of children in kindergarten through 12th grade, Loban (1976) termed these fluency disrupters **mazes**. Contrary to what we might have expected to see, the overall occurrence of mazes in the children's spoken language did not decrease with age. Twelfth-grade students used virtually the same proportion of mazes as

first-grade children, even though the length and complexity of the students' utterances increased through the grades. That is, as the length and complexity of utterances increased with age, so did the number of maze behaviors. Although the 12th- and 1st-grade children demonstrated the same proportion of fluency disrupters, an interesting phenomenon occurred during the 4th through 9th grades. During this period, the children showed erratic increases and decreases in the number of their maze behaviors. Unfortunately, Loban did not elaborate on the possible reasons for these erratic fluctuations, and we can only speculate that the educational, maturational, linguistic, social, and/or cognitive changes that occur during this period in some way affect the fluency of the students' communications. However, children who were more linguistically competent used fewer and shorter mazes at all ages than did children who demonstrated less language ability.

Narratives

In chapter 1 we indicated that narratives are a common part of language use and are not limited to relating information about movies or storybooks. We use narratives when we describe to officials what happened in an automobile accident or when we recount events that occurred during our summer vacations. Narratives are "decontextualized monologues" (Owens, 1992, p. 302) that place heavy demands on logical structure, temporal and causal sequencing, cohesion, and presuppositional abilities. To relate a narrative, the speaker must pay particular attention to the listener's need for adequate information because rarely is information about the content of a narrative already known to the listener. As such, successful narrative ability is a later-developing language skill in children. Children generally are not successful at producing full narratives until the early school years. However, preschoolers pass through several stages in developing the ability to produce true narratives.

Applebee's (1978) six narrative levels provide a structure with which to discuss children's early development of narratives. Recall from chapter 1 that these levels are heaps, sequences, primitive temporal narratives, unfocused temporal chains, focused temporal or causal chains, and proper narratives. Although children between the ages of 2 and 3 years begin to tell fictional narratives and briefly describe what has happened to them (Sutton-Smith, 1986), these narratives are considered to be protonarratives and are characterized by what Applebee refers to as *heaps*—series of unrelated, unsequential statements. Little, if any, concern for the listener's informational need is present, and beginnings and endings are not obvious. These heaps gradually evolve to sequences. The information in *sequences* is presented in an additive but not a temporal fashion. This means that the utterances can be moved around without affecting the narrative. Only the similarity with regard to events or attributes provides the "theme" (Owens, 1992).

From about 3 to 5 years of age, children begin to relate narratives that show some concern for temporal sequencing of events. Initially, children's narratives represent what Applebee terms *primitive temporal narratives*. Although these narratives still do not contain plots or evidence causality, they do present information in a rudimentary temporal sequence and are focused on a central event. These primitive temporal narratives are gradually replaced with narratives characterized by *unfocused temporal chains*. Narratives of this type contain concrete relationships chained in temporal order. Applebee suggests that the next narrative level is that of *focused temporal or causal chains*. Narratives of this type typically have a main character, and events are presented in a chained manner about the character. Initially, events are chained in a temporal order (Lahey, 1988). Causal chaining generally does not emerge until the early school years, or about 5 to 7 years of age. Focused causal chain narratives are the forerunners of true narratives, which appear at about 7 to 8 years of age (Lahey, 1988). *True narratives* not only have central themes and/or characters but generally include multiple causal chains, as well as temporal organization (Lahey, 1988). When children achieve the true narrative level, the narratives have defined episode structure(s) made up of the multiple focused causal and temporal chains referred to previously (Stein & Glenn, 1979). In chapter 1 we presented the elements of story grammar proposed by Stein and Glenn (1979) (see Table 1.4). All elements except the setting are parts of episode structure. Typically by about 9 years of age, children are producing all elements of story grammar; however, they continue to develop in their ability to include more multiply embedded episode structures. In summary, children's narratives evolve from those presented at about 2 years of age, characterized by heaps of unrelated statements, to those produced in the first 2 or 3 years of school, characterized by several embedded episodes containing causal and temporal patterns.

METALINGUISTICS

We know from chapter 1 that metalinguistic skills refer to the abilities to talk about language, analyze it, see it as an entity separate from its content, and judge it. Young children who are initially learning language do not understand that what they are doing can be something separate from what they are doing. They are simply learning language to communicate. When they begin to ask what an object's name is, comment that they have forgotten the word for something, repair their utterances spontaneously, practice words or sounds, rhyme words spontaneously, or say that somebody did not say something correctly, they are showing the early glimmers of metalinguistic awareness (Kamhi, 1987).

True metalinguistic skills do not, however, appear until the early school years, or about 7 to 8 years of age (Saywitz & Cherry-Wilkinson, 1982). And the degree of metalinguisitic skills depends, in part, on the level of development of the other language components (Owens, 1992). Metalinguistic skills develop well into, if not throughout, the school years (Clark, 1978; Saywitz & Cherry-Wilkinson, 1982). Two aspects of oral language that are related to the development of metalinguistic skills are the ability to detect ambiguities in utterances and the intentional use of figurative language and jokes. Because these are relatively late-developing skills, they are discussed in chapter 11.

SPEECH SOUNDS

Babbling, which is characterized by nonmeaningful sound play that is under some degree of the infant's control, emerges between 4 and 6 months of age. Early babbling often consists of consonant-vowel (CV) and vowel-consonant (VC) combinations, and it may contain sounds that are both representative and not representative of the infant's native language, that is, the language of the infant's environment. At about six months of years, children begin to demonstrate **reduplicated babbling**, which is characterized by repetitions of CV syllables. **Variegated babbling**, in which successive syllables of different CV syllables (e.g., C^1VC^2V) are produced, usually begins at about 8 months of age. Babbled single syllables consist of VCV and CVC forms in which the consonants and vowels are the same in each production (Stark, 1986). Children's early single words typically consist of monosyllabic CV ("my"), VC ("up"), or CVCV ("baby") combinations.

Stoel-Gammon (1987) has found that at approximately 2 years of age, children use a repertoire of 9 to 10 different consonants in the initial position of words. In the final position of words, these children use five to six different consonants. Between 24 and 39 months of age, children use an average of 2.2 consonant **clusters** in the initial position and 1.7 clusters in the final position of words. With advancing age, children's phonological repertoires increase, in terms of both the number of different sounds used and the word positions in which they are used. Most researchers agree that by 7 or 8 years of age, children have fairly well mastered the English phonemes and are producing them correctly in their speech. However, Sax (1972) suggests that some mastery of the more difficult sounds may continue throughout fifth grade, or approximately age 10.

Three classic investigations have contributed significantly to our knowledge of when children learn to produce specific sounds (Poole, 1934; Templin, 1957; Wellman, Case, Mengurt, & Bradbury, 1931). Although differences in research designs and criterion levels prevent exact comparisons among results, several similar trends have emerged from the studies. Generally, children learn to produce nasal sounds, such as /m/,[1] /n/, and /ŋ/; stop consonants, such as /d/, /k/, /g/, /p/, and /b/; and glides, such as /w/, around age 3 or 4.

These phonemes are typically considered early developing and relatively easy sounds. In contrast, fricative sounds, such as /s/, /z/, /ʃ/, and /ʒ/, and affricates, such as /tʃ/ and /dʒ/ are acquired later, often not until age 7 or 8. There was a great deal of variation in the results of these three studies on children's acquisition of the /l/ and /r/ sounds, ranging from acquisition at 4 years of age to past 7. For the most part, the findings of these investigations have been confirmed by other researchers. Stop consonants and nasals are typically learned before fricatives and affricates. Furthermore, children often continue to have difficulties with /r/ and /l/ after they begin school. We must keep in mind, however, that children demonstrate variability in the ages at which they acquire the phonemes (Prather, Hedrick, & Kern, 1975; Sander, 1972).

So far, we have only discussed consonant sound development. Children generally learn to produce the vowels correctly before they acquire the consonant sounds. In fact, vowel production may be mastered by the time children are 3 years old (Metraux, 1950; Templin, 1957). It is unusual to see school-age children making more than occasional errors in their vowel productions.

More recently, attention has been directed to identifying the processes children demonstrate as they attempt to put sequences of sounds together in words. Ingram (1976) has listed several of these processes under the three broad classifications of syllable structure, assimilation, and substitution processes. In *syllable structure* processes, young children tend to omit consonants in the final positions of words or syllables ("ba" for "bat"), delete unstressed syllables in polysyllabic words ("jama" for "pajamas"), and reduce the number of sounds produced in consonant clusters, such as /bl/ ("bu" for "blue"). *Assimilation* processes are those in which one sound in a word affects the production of another sound so that its production is modified. Examples of assimilative processes are "gog" for "dog" or "mam" for "lamb." When children use both a syllable duplication and an assimilative process simultaneously, an utterance such as "gaga" for "doggie" may be produced. Finally, *substitution* processes are employed when children use one group of sounds, such as stops, in place of another group, such as fricatives. It is not uncommon to hear children

---

[1]Because letters of the alphabet can have several pronunciations, symbols of the IPA are used in this discussion to prevent confusion. The IPA is shown in Appendix A.

say "toap" for "soap." Another substitution process involves changing the place in the mouth where a sound is produced. Often children will replace a sound produced in the back of the mouth with one produced in the front of the mouth, such as /t/ for /k/, resulting in "tub" for "cub."

As children grow older, they modify their early phonological processes so that they approximate those used by adults. Because this learning process takes time, however, any one word may go through several stages in pronunciation. Consequently, just because a child is capable of saying a sound correctly in one word, this does not mean that the sound will be said correctly in all words that contain it if different phonological processes are operating in the production of the other words.

SUMMARY

In this chapter we have seen that:

▶ In the one- and two-word stages, children learn the names for objects and relations in their environments.

▶ Vocabulary growth begins slowly, spurts ahead between 18 and 24 months of age, and continues to grow thereafter.

▶ Children's early one- and two-word utterances systematically develop into basic kernel, negative, and question sentences and later into compound and complex sentences.

▶ Semantic as well as syntactic factors are involved in sentence development.

▶ Several patterns influence word learning, and children seem able to form hypotheses about word meaning with only limited exposure to the words.

▶ Children acquire specific grammatical morphemes in a developmental sequence related to increasing MLU.

▶ The functions and intentions of language use change as children grow older; utterances change from those containing one function to those containing more than one function.

▶ Young children adapt the form of their language for their listeners; this ability to adapt grows more refined as children become better able to make accurate presuppositions about their listeners.

▶ Turn taking, topic maintenance, and revision skills improve gradually throughout the preschool years.

▶ Children's narratives develop from those produced at about 2 years of age, characterized by heaps of unrelated statements, to those produced in the first 2 or 3 years of school, characterized by multiply embedded episodes with causal and temporal patterns.

▶ Speech sound acquisition takes a number of years to reach adultlike levels of correctness, and during the developmental period, several phonological processes are evident in the ways children pronounce words.

As this review of normal language and speech development illustrates, there are many skills that children must acquire in the process of learning to talk. We have seen, however, that the process follows developmental patterns. A summary of many of these language and speech developmental milestones can be found in Appendixes B, C, and D. Often these developmental patterns become a basis for planning intervention programs for children who have impaired language skills. These same developmental sequences also provide one way of identifying children who are not progressing appropriately in acquiring their language.

REFERENCES

Anglin, J. (1970). *The growth of word meaning*. Cambridge, MA: MIT Press.

Applebee, A. (1978). *The child's concept of story*. Chicago: University of Chicago Press.

Bangs, T. (1975). *Vocabulary comprehension scale.* Hingham, MA: Teaching Resources.

Barrie-Blackley, S. (1973). Six-year-old children's understanding of sentences adjoined with time adverbs. *Journal of Psycholinguistic Research, 2,* 153–165.

Bates, E. (1976). *The emergence of symbols: Cognition and communication in infancy.* New York: Academic Press.

Belkin, A. (1975). *Investigation of the functions and forms of children's negative utterances.* Unpublished doctoral dissertation, Columbia University, New York.

Bellugi, U. (1965). The development of interrogative structures in children's speech. In K. Riegel (Ed.), *The development of language functions* (Report No. 8). Ann Arbor: University of Michigan Language Development Program.

Benedict, H. (1979). Early lexical development: Comprehension and production. *Journal of Child Language, 6,* 183–200.

Berko, J. (1958). The child's learning of English morphology. *Word, 14,* 150–177.

Bloom, L. (1970). *Language development: Form and function in emerging grammars.* Cambridge, MA: MIT Press.

Bloom, L. (1973). *One word at a time: The use of single-word utterances before syntax.* The Hague: Mouton.

Bloom, L., & Lahey, M. (1978). *Language development and language disorders.* New York: Macmillan.

Bloom, L., Lahey, M., Hood, L., Lifter, K., & Fiess, K. (1980). Complex sentences: Acquisition of syntactic connectives and the semantic relations they encode. *Journal of Child Language, 7,* 235–262.

Bloom, L., Lifter, K., & Hafitz, J. (1980). Semantics of verbs and the development of verb inflection in child language. *Language, 56,* 386–412.

Bloom, L., Lightbown, P., & Hood, L. (1975). Structure and variation in child language. *Monographs of the Society for Research in Child Development, 40* (Serial No. 160).

Bloom, L., Miller, P., & Hood, L. (1975). Variation and reduction as aspects of competence in language development. In A. Pick (Ed.), *Minnesota symposia on child psychology* (Vol. 9). Minneapolis: University of Minnesota Press.

Bloom, L., Rocissano, L., & Hood, L. (1976). Adult–child discourse: Developmental interaction between information processing and linguistic knowledge. *Cognitive Psychology, 8,* 521–552.

Branigan, G. (1979). Some reasons why successive single word utterances are not. *Journal of Child Language, 6,* 411–421.

Brinton, B., & Fujiki, M. (1984). Development of topic manipulation skills in discourse. *Journal of Speech and Hearing Research, 27,* 350–357.

Brown, R. (1968). The development of wh questions in child speech. *Journal of Verbal Learning and Verbal Behavior, 7,* 279–290.

Brown, R. (1973). *A first language: The early stages.* Cambridge, MA: Harvard University Press.

Brown, R., Cazden, C., & Bellugi, U. (1969). The child's grammar from I to III. In J. Hill (Ed.), *Minnesota symposia on child psychology* (Vol. 2). Minneapolis: University of Minnesota Press.

Brown, R., & Hanlon, C. (1970). Derivational complexity and order of acquisition in child speech. In J. Hayes (Ed.), *Cognition and the development of language.* New York: Wiley.

Bruner, J. (1975). The ontogenesis of speech acts. *Journal of Child Language, 2,* 1–19.

Camarata, S., & Schwartz, R. (1985). Production of object words and action words: Evidence for a relationship between phonology and semantics. *Journal of Speech and Hearing Research, 28,* 323–330.

Carey, S., & Bartlett, E. (1978). Acquiring a single new word. In *Papers and reports on child language development* (Vol. 15, pp. 17–29). Stanford, CA: Stanford University.

Clark, E. (1970). How young children describe events in time. In G. Flores d'Arcais & W. Levelt (Eds.), *Advances in psycholinguistics.* New York: American Elsevier.

Clark, E. (1973a). How children describe time and order. In C. Ferguson & D. Slobin (Eds.), *Studies of child language development.* New York: Holt, Rinehart and Winston.

Clark, E. (1973b). Non-linguistic strategies and the acquisition of word meanings. *Cognition, 2,* 161–182.

Clark, E. (1978). Awareness of language: Some evidence from what children say and do. In A. Sinclair, R. Jarvella, & W. Levelt (Eds.), *The child's conception of language.* New York: Springer-Verlag.

Clark, H., & Clark, E. (1977). *Psychology and language: An introduction to psycholinguistics.* New York: Harcourt Brace Jovanovich.

Coker, P. (1978). Syntactic and semantic factors in the acquisition of "before" and "after." *Journal of Child Language, 5,* 261–277.

Crais, E. (1992). Fast mapping: A new look at word learning. In R. Chapman (Ed.), *Processes in language acquisition and disorders.* St. Louis, MO: Mosby Year Book.

Dale, P. (1976). *Language development: Structure and function* (2nd ed.). New York: Holt, Rinehart and Winston.

Dale, P., Bates, E., Reznick, S., & Morisset, C. (1989). The validity of a parent report instrument of child language at twenty months. *Journal of Child Language, 16,* 239–250.

Dale, P., & Thal, D. (1989, November). *Assessment of language in infants and toddlers using parent report.* A short course presented at the Annual Convention of the American Speech-Language-Hearing Association, St. Louis, MO.

de Villiers, J., & de Villiers, P. (1973). A cross-sectional study of the acquisition of grammatical morphemes in child speech. *Journal of Psycholinguistic Research, 2,* 331–341.

de Villiers, J., Tager-Flushberg, H., & Hakuta, K. (1977). Deciding among theories of the development of coordination in child speech. *Papers and Reports on Child Language Development, 13,* 118–125.

Dickinson, D. (1984). First impressions: Children's knowledge of words gained from a single experience. *Applied Psycholinguistics, 5,* 359–374.

Dockrell, J., & Campbell, R. (1986). Lexical acquisition strategies in the preschool child. In S. Kuczaj & M. Barrett (Eds.), *The development of word meaning: Progress in cognitive development research* (pp. 121–154). New York: Springer-Verlag.

Dollaghan, C. (1985). Child meets word: "Fast mapping" in preschool children. *Journal of Speech and Hearing Research, 28,* 449–454.

Dollaghan, C. (1987). Fast mapping in normal and language-impaired children. *Journal of Speech and Hearing Disorders, 52,* 218–222.

Dore, J. (1975). Holophrase, speech acts, and language universals. *Journal of Child Language, 2,* 21–40.

Emerson, H. (1979). Children's comprehension of "because" in reversible and nonreversible sentences. *Journal of Child Language, 6,* 279–300.

Erreich, A. (1984). Learning how to ask: Patterns of inversion in yes/no and wh- questions. *Journal of Child Language, 11,* 579–592.

Ervin-Tripp, S. (1970). Discourse agreement: How children answer questions. In J. Hayes (Ed.), *Cognition and the development of language.* New York: Wiley.

Ervin-Tripp, S. (1979). Children's verbal turn-taking. In E. Ochs & B. Shieffelin (Eds.), *Developmental pragmatics.* New York: Academic Press.

Ervin-Tripp, S., & Mitchell-Kernan, C. (Eds.). (1977). *Child discourse.* New York: Academic Press.

Feagans, L. (1980). Children's understanding of some temporal terms denoting order, duration, and simultaneity. *Journal of Psycholinguistic Research, 9,* 41–57.

Gallagher, T. (1977). Revision behaviors in the speech of normal children developing language. *Journal of Speech and Hearing Research, 20,* 303–318.

Gentner, D. (1975). Evidence for the psychological reality of semantic components: The verbs of possession. In D. Norman, D. Rumelhart, & the LNR Research Group (Eds.), *Explorations in cognition.* San Francisco: Freeman.

Goldin-Meadow, S., Seligman, M., & Gelman, R. (1976). Language in the two-year-old: Receptive and productive stages. *Cognition, 4,* 189–202.

Goodluck, H. (1986). Children's knowledge of prepositional phrase structure: An experimental test. *Journal of Psycholinguistic Research, 15,* 177–188.

Gopnik, A. (1981). The development of non-nominal expressions: Why the first words are not about things. In D. Ingram & P. Dale (Eds.), *Child language: An international perspective.* Baltimore: University Park Press.

Granowsky, S. (1976). *Oral language comprehension of children in grades one through six.* Unpublished doctoral dissertation, Duke University, North Carolina.

Greenfield, P. (1978). Informativeness, presupposition and semantic choice in single-word utterances. In W. Waterson & C. Snow (Eds.), *Development of communication: Social and pragmatic factors in language acquisition.* London: Wiley.

Greenfield, P., & Smith, J. (1976). *The structure of communication in early language development.* New York: Academic Press.

Greenfield, P., & Zukow, P. (1978). Why do children say what they say when they say it? An experimental approach to the psychogenesis of presupposition. In K. Nelson (Ed.), *Children's language* (Vol. 1). New York: Gardner Press.

Halliday, M. (1974). A sociosemiotic perspective on language development. *Bulletin of the School of Oriental and African Studies, 37,* Part 1.

Halliday, M. (1975). *Learning how to mean: Explorations in the development of language.* London: Edward Arnold.

Hass, W., & Wepman, J. (1974). Dimensions of individual difference in the spoken syntax of school children. *Journal of Speech and Hearing Research, 17,* 455–469.

Heibeck, T., & Markman, E. (1987). Word learning in children: An examination of fast mapping. *Child Development, 58,* 1021–1034.

Hood, L. (1977). *A longitudinal study of the development of the expression of causal relations in complex sentences.* Unpublished doctoral dissertation, Columbia University, New York.

Hood, L., Lahey, M., Lifter, K., & Bloom, L. (1978). Observational descriptive methodology in studying child language: Preliminary results on the development of complex sentences. In G. Sackett (Ed.), *Observing behavior: Vol. I. Theory and applications in mental retardation.* Baltimore: University Park Press.

Ingram, D. (1976). *Phonological disability in children.* London: Edward Arnold.

Iwan, S., & Siegel, G. (1982). The effects of feedback on referential communication of preschool children. *Journal of Speech and Hearing Research, 25,* 224–229.

Kamhi, A. (1987). Metalinguistic abilities in language-impaired children. *Topics in Language Disorders, 7,* 1–12.

Keenan, E. (1975). Evolving discourse—The next step. *Papers and Reports on Child Language Development, 10,* 80–87.

Keenan, E., & Schieffelin, B. (1976). Topic as a discourse notion: A study of topic in the conversations of children and adults. In C. Li (Ed.), *Subject and topic.* New York: Academic Press.

Klee, T. (1985). Role of inversion in children's question development. *Journal of Speech and Hearing Research, 28,* 225–232.

Klee, T., & Fitzgerald, M. (1985). The relation between grammatical development and mean length of utterance in morphemes. *Journal of Child Language, 12,* 251–269.

Klima, E., & Bellugi, U. (1966). Syntactic regularities in the speech of children. In J. Lyons & R. Wales (Eds.), *Psycholinguistic papers. Proceedings of the Edinburgh conference.* Edinburgh: Edinburgh University Press.

Koziol, S. (1973). The development of noun plural rules during the primary grades. *Research in the Teaching of English, 7,* 30–50.

Lahey, M. (1988). *Language disorders and language development.* New York: Merrill/Macmillan.

Lee, L. (1974). *Developmental sentence analysis.* Evanston, IL: Northwestern University Press.

Leonard, L. (1984). Normal language acquisition: Some recent findings and clinical implications. In A. Holland (Ed.), *Language disorders in children.* San Diego, CA: College-Hill Press.

Leonard, L., Schwartz, R., Morris, B., & Chapman, K. (1981). Factors influencing early lexical acquisition: Lexical orientation and phonological composition. *Child Development, 52,* 882–887.

Limber, J. (1973). The genesis of complex sentences. In T. Moore (Ed.), *Cognitive development and the acquisition of language.* New York: Academic Press.

Loban, W. (1976). *Language development: Kindergarten through grade twelve.* Urbana, IL: National Council of Teachers of English.

Lust, B. (1977). Conjunction reduction in child language. *Journal of Child Language, 4,* 257–288.

Lust, B., & Mervis, C. (1980). Development of coordination in the natural speech of young children. *Journal of Child Language, 7,* 279–304.

Maratsos, M. (1973). Nonegocentric communication abilities in preschool children. *Child Development, 44,* 697–700.

Menig-Peterson, C. (1975). The modification of communicative behavior in preschool-aged children as a function of the listener's perspective. *Child Development, 46,* 1015–1018.

Menyuk, P. (1969). *Sentences children use.* Cambridge, MA: MIT Press.

Metraux, R. (1950). Speech profiles of the pre-school child 18 to 54 months. *Journal of Speech and Hearing Disorders, 15,* 37–53.

Miller, J. (1981). *Assessing language production in children.* Baltimore: University Park Press.

Miller, M. (1975). *Pragmatic constraints on the linguistic realization of "semantic intentions" in early child language ("telegraphic speech").* Paper presented at the Third International Child Language Symposium, London.

Moran, M. (1975). *Verb inflections of normal and learning disabled children.* Unpublished doctoral dissertation, University of Kansas, Lawrence.

Morehead, D., & Ingram, D. (1973). The development of base syntax in normal and linguistically deviant children. *Journal of Speech and Hearing Research, 16,* 330–352.

Naremore, R., & Dever, R. (1975). Language performance of educable mentally retarded and normal children at five age levels. *Journal of Speech and Hearing Research, 18,* 82–95.

Newfield, M., & Schlanger, B. (1968). The acquisition of English morphology by normal and educable mentally retarded children. *Journal of Speech and Hearing Research, 11,* 693–706.

Nippold, M., Leonard, L., & Anastopoulos, A. (1982). Development in the use and understanding of polite forms in children. *Journal of Speech and Hearing Research, 25,* 193–202.

Olson, D., & Nickerson, N. (1978). Language development. In K. Nelson (Ed.), *Children's language* (Vol. 1). New York: Gardner Press.

Owens, R. (1992). *Language development: An introduction* (3rd ed.). New York: Merrill/Macmillan.

Paul, R. (1981). Analyzing complex sentence development. In J. Miller, *Assessing language production in children.* Baltimore: University Park Press.

Poole, E. (1934). Genetic development of articulation of consonant sounds in speech. *Elementary English Review, 11,* 159–161.

Prather, E., Hedrick, D., & Kern, C. (1975). Articulation development in children aged two to four years. *Journal of Speech and Hearing Disorders, 40,* 179–191.

Prutting, C. (1979). Process: The action of moving forward progressively from one point to another on the way to completion. *Journal of Speech and Hearing Disorders, 44,* 3–30.

Reed, V. A. (1992). Associations between phonology and other language components in children's communicative performance: Clinical implications. *Australian Journal of Human Communication Disorders, 20,* 75–87.

Reich, P. (1986). *Language development.* Englewood Cliffs, NJ: Prentice-Hall.

Rice, M., Huston, A., Truglio, R., & Wright, J. (1990). Words from "Sesame Street": Learning vocabulary while viewing. *Developmental Psychology, 26,* 421–428.

Rice, M., & Woodsmall, L. (1988). Lessons from television: Children's word learning when viewing. *Child Development, 59,* 420–429.

Romney, A., & D'Andrade, R. (1964). Cognitive aspects of English kin terms. In A. Romney & R. D'Andrade (Eds.), *American Anthropologist: Transcultural Studies in Cognition, 66,* 146–170.

Rystrom, R. (1972). Language patterns and the primary child. *The Reading Teacher, 26,* 149–152.

Sander, E. (1972). When are speech sounds learned? *Journal of Speech and Hearing Disorders, 37,* 55–63.

Sax, M. (1972). A longitudinal study of articulation change. *Language, Speech, and Hearing Services in Schools, 3,* 41–48.

Saywitz, K., & Cherry-Wilkinson, L. (1982). Age-related differences in metalinguistic awareness. In S. Kuczaj (Ed.), *Language development: Vol 2. Language, thought and culture.* Hillsdale, NJ: Erlbaum.

Scarborough, H., Wyckoff, J., & Davidson, R. (1986). A reconsideration of the relationship between age and mean utterance length. *Journal of Speech and Hearing Research, 29,* 394–399.

Schiff, N. (1976). *The development of form and meaning in the language of hearing children of deaf parents.* Unpublished doctoral dissertation, Columbia University, New York.

Schober-Peterson, D., & Johnson, C. (1989). Conversational topics of 4-year-olds. *Journal of Speech and Hearing Research, 32,* 857–870

Schwartz, R., & Leonard, L. (1982). Do children pick and choose? An examination of phonological selection and avoidance in early lexical acquisition. *Journal of Child Language, 9,* 319–336.

Shatz, M., & Gelman, R. (1973). The development of communication skills: Modifications in the speech of young children as a function of listener. *Monographs of the Society for Research in Child Development, 38* (Serial No. 152).

Skarakis, E., & Greenfield, P. (1982). The role of new and old information in the verbal expression of language-disordered children. *Journal of Speech and Hearing Research, 25,* 462–467.

Solomon, M. (1972). Stem endings and the acquisition of inflections. *Language Learning, 22,* 43–50.

Stark, R. (1986). Prespeech segmental feature development. In P. Fletcher & M. Garman (Eds.), *Language acquisition* (2nd ed.). New York: Cambridge University Press.

Stein, N., & Glenn, C. (1979). An analysis of story comprehension in elementary school children. In R. Freedle (Ed.), *New directions in discourse processing* (Vol. 2). Norwood, NJ: Ablex.

Stoel-Gammon, C. (1987). The phonological skills of two-year-olds. *Language, Speech, and Hearing Services in Schools, 18,* 323–329.

Sutton-Smith, B. (1986). The development of fictional narrative performances. *Topics in Language Disorders, 7,* 1–10.

Templin, M. (1957). *Certain language skills in children: Their development and interrelationships.* Minneapolis: University of Minnesota Press.

van Kleeck, A., & Frankel, T. (1981). Discourse devices used by language disordered children: A preliminary investigation. *Journal of Speech and Hearing Disorders, 46,* 250–257.

Warden, D. (1976). The influence of context on children's use of identifying expressions and references. *British Journal of Psychology, 67,* 101–112.

Wegner, J., & Rice, M. (1988, November). *The acquisition of verb–particle constructions: How do children figure them out?* Paper presented at the Annual Convention of the American Speech-Language-Hearing Association, Boston.

Wehrebian, A. (1970). Measures of vocabulary and grammatical skills for children up to age six. *Developmental Psychology, 2,* 439–446.

Weisenberger, J. (1976). A choice of words: Two-year-old speech from a situational point of view. *Journal of Child Language, 3,* 272–281.

Wellman, B., Case, I., Mengurt, I., & Bradbury, D. (1931). Speech sounds of young children. *University of Iowa Studies in Child Welfare, 5.*

Wells, G. (1985). *Language development in the preschool years.* New York: Cambridge University Press.

Wiig, E., Florence, D., Kutner, S., Sherman, B., & Semel, E. (1977). Perception and interpretation of explicit negatives by learning-disabled children and adolescents. *Perceptual and Motor Skills, 44,* 1251–1257.

Wiig, E., & Semel, E. (1974). Logio-grammatical sentence comprehension by learning disabled adolescents. *Perceptual and Motor Skills, 38,* 1331–1334.

Wiig, E., & Semel, E. (1984). *Language assessment and intervention for the learning disabled* (2nd ed.). New York: Merrill/Macmillan.

Wiig, E., Semel, E., & Crouse, M. (1973). The use of morphology by high-risk and learning disabled children. *Journal of Learning Disabilities, 6,* 457–465.

Wood, B. (1981). *Children and communication: Verbal and nonverbal language development* (2nd ed.). Englewood Cliffs, NJ: Prentice-Hall.

Wood, M. (1982). *Language disorders in school-age children.* Englewood Cliffs, NJ: Prentice-Hall.

Wootten, J., Merkin, S., Hood, L., & Bloom, L. (1979). *Wh-questions: Linguistic evidence to explain the sequence of acquisition.* Paper presented to the Society for Research in Child Development, San Francisco.

Zintz, M. (1970). *The reading process.* Dubuque, IA: William C. Brown.

Part Two

Language Disorders of Children

· Chapter 4 ·

An Overview of Children's Language Disorders

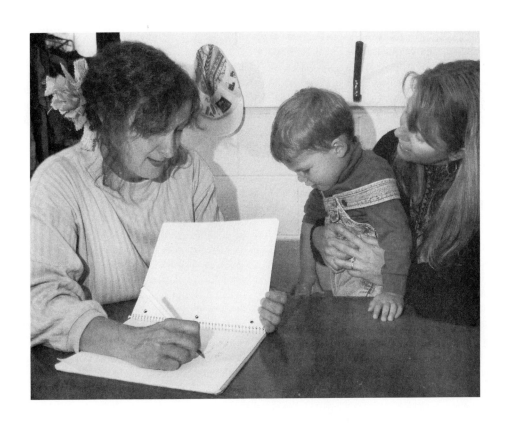

Upon completion of this chapter, the reader should be able to:

▶ Describe historical developments in the study of children's language and their impact on approaches to language-disordered children.

▶ Discuss issues involved in and approaches to identifying children with language problems.

▶ Describe federal laws that have influenced services for language-disordered children.

▶ Discuss the issues surrounding different approaches to classifying and categorizing children with language disorders.

▶ Describe three of the more commonly used approaches to children's language disorders.

Compared to many other areas of study, systematic study of children's language disorders is relatively new. In this chapter, we review historical developments related to children's language disorders and the contributions made to the present state of knowledge. We also discuss one of the unresolved issues in the study of children's language disorders—the identification of children with language problems. Because federal laws related to the education of children with disabilities have influenced the nature of services for language-disordered children, we review several of these laws. The classification and categorization of children with language disorders is another unresolved and somewhat controversial issue. In this chapter, we present some of the varying perspectives surrounding this issue. Models can help simplify complex phenomena, make them more understandable, and provide ways of dealing with them. Language is most certainly a complex phenomenon. For this reason, three of the more popular approaches to children's language disorders are presented.

AN HISTORICAL PERSPECTIVE

The current approaches to assessment of and intervention for children's language disorders are rooted in developments that have taken place primarily in the last 30 to 40 years. Prior to the late 1950s, little information was available regarding children's language development and their language disorders. Although some professionals working with children's communication skills (mostly in the areas of articulation, voice, and stuttering) recognized that many children's problems involved more than speech difficulties, the label applied to these problems was often something like *delayed speech.* This label reflected the orientation to speech and the lack of organized knowledge about language.

The 1950s

In the late 1950s, several theories that were to have tremendous impacts on the area of child language were published. One of these was Chomsky's (1957) theory of *generative transformational grammar.* As we recall from chapter 1, his was a linguistic theory that differentiated between a deep structure of language and the mapping of deep structures by surface structures, or observable linguistic forms. He proposed that use of these structures could be explained by implicit knowledge of a set of rules that govern how sentences or phrases can be put together and how they can be transformed systematically by additional sets of rules. To account for the way children acquire this implicit knowledge of linguistic rules, Chomsky suggested that children are born with an innate *language acquisition device* (LAD) that provides the basis for mapping the syntactic surface structures onto deep structures. His approach became known, therefore, as a *nativist theory.*

In contrast to Chomsky's approach was Skinner's (1957) theory of **behaviorism,** in which language learning was viewed as a process whereby children's verbal behaviors were systematically shaped by selective reinforcement. This approach focused attention on antecedent events (stimuli)-responses-reinforcements, and it proposed that verbal behaviors could be modified by changing and controlling the stimuli and reinforcements. This approach also provided the background for the delineation of sequenced behavioral objectives and the documentation of progress through charting, seen today in many intervention plans.

Osgood's (1957) behavioral approach expanded on Skinnerian behaviorism by adding to the stimulus–response model an emphasis on the *internal mediations* that take place in an organism between the presentation of a stimulus and the overt response. That is, responses to stimuli are mediated mentally, and the mediation affects what the responses will be and what stimuli will elicit responses in the future.

The 1960s

The 1960s extended these three theories into the research, assessment, and intervention arenas. The *Illinois Test of Psycholinguistic Abilities* (ITPA), first published in 1961 by Kirk and McCarthy, was based heavily on Osgood's model. The ITPA focused attention on the presumed specific deficits children might exhibit in processing and encoding language, and it implied that remediation of these deficits would result in improved language performance. With this emphasis came intervention approaches such as improving auditory sequential memory in order to assist children in decoding auditory-linguistic stimuli.

Chomsky's linguistic theory provided analytic techniques for studying children's syntactic development and describing deviant syntactic performance. In addition to the intervention approaches influenced by the ITPA, intervention began to emphasize teaching language-disordered children the syntactic rules that they apparently had not learned. Strategies for language teaching generally involved using behavioral techniques that stemmed from Skinner's work. Stimuli and reinforcements were systematically controlled and varied, and stimulus and response generalization were promoted.

The 1970s

The approaches used in the 1960s were not sufficient to explain the complex phenomenon of language acquisition, and voids in assessment and intervention remained. Three developments that occurred primarily in the 1970s came to influence further professionals'

ideas about and practices in children's language development and language disorders.

In the late 1960s and during the 1970s, Bandura's (1971, 1977) *social learning theory* began to influence approaches to children with language disorders. Bandura's theory introduced the notion that children can learn by observing the behaviors of others and the effects (reinforcements) of those behaviors and by abstracting from those observations commonalities that lead to either desirable or undesirable results. The behaviors of others that the children observe were seen as providing *models*. Although the concepts of stimuli and reinforcements from Skinner's behavioral approach remained in Bandura's social learning theory, they were modified to include aspects such as motivation and vicarious reinforcement. These concepts placed the children in more active roles as learners than did the strict behavioral approach.

In the early 1970s, emphasis also shifted to semantics. The shift was sparked by the work of such people as Bloom (1970) and Brown (1973). The basic tenets of the *semantic theories* were that children learn first about meaning and that it is meaning they first attempt to convey. Syntactic development was viewed as an outgrowth of attempts to express meaning. Researchers proposed sets of *semantic intentions, semantic relations,* and *semantic functions* that were integrated into assessment and intervention procedures. With the shift to semantics came the question of how children learn the concepts behind the words. Linguistic answers focused on children's learning of semantic features (e.g., Clark, 1973). Other researchers turned to the work of Piaget in looking for the answers, and a cognitive emphasis emerged with the semantic focus.

With the work of the early and mid-1970s came the realization that not all identical utterances meant the same thing all the time. The same sequences of words or the same syntactic structures were used to convey one meaning at one time and another meaning at another time. Meaning and grammatical structure were, therefore, influenced by the speaker's intentions in communicating. This realization was one of the factors behind yet another paradigm shift—the shift to the functions that language serves and an emphasis on communicative pragmatics. The context in which communication occurred was recognized as influencing the ways in which messages were delivered. The move to pragmatics began primarily in the mid- and late 1970s through the writings of people such as Bates (1976), Halliday (1975), Dore (1975), and Rees (1978).

The 1980s

In the 1980s the emphasis on communicative pragmatics continued. A broadening notion of pragmatics extended attention to the interactions among participants in communicative situations, the rules that guided the interactions, and the ways in which the contexts of communication affected what was said and how it was said. Some have labeled this an interactional approach to language. Writings of people such as Fey (1986) and Duchan (1986) reflect this emphasis on context and interaction in approaches to language learning and disorders, an emphasis that has continued into the 1990s.

Prompted in part by the need to respond to the implications of federal mandates regarding provision of special services to disabled children in the schools, including children with language disorders, researchers and professionals began to focus more attention on language development into and throughout the school years and the relationships among language proficiency or disability, educational performance, and literacy. With this focus, the "metas" began to emerge in the literature—*metalinguistics, metapragmatics, metacognition,* and *metaphonology.* Concern grew about children's ability to use language in nonliteral ways and to infer meaning from cohesive series of utterances in which information was not explicitly stated. These emphases were reflected in the works of people such as Wiig and her colleagues (Wiig, 1989; Wiig & Secord, 1989; Wiig & Semel, 1984), Nippold (1988), and Simon (1985).

Although the 1970s saw a shift away from syntax and grammar, a resurgence of interest in these topics occurred in the early 1980s when Chomsky (1981) published a description of government-binding theory. As we saw in chapter 1, in *government-binding theory* "knowledge of language can be characterized by a formal system of rules and principles of well-formedness" (Leonard & Loeb, 1988, p. 515). Government-

binding theory is currently being used to guide some of the research in language development and disorders (e.g., Leonard, Sabbadini, Leonard, & Volterra, 1987; Leonard, Sabbadini, Volterra, & Leonard, 1988; Loeb & Leonard, 1991). As such, the validity of the theory is being tested.

> The long-term value of such research will be defined in part by the ultimate success or failure of the theory itself. Should the theory prove inadequate, much of the data resulting from this research might have only descriptive value, contributing relatively little to an explanation of the processes of language learning and disruption. Should the theory be on the right track, applied research within the GB [government-binding] framework will be highly revealing. (Leonard & Loeb, 1988, p. 523)

The 1990s

When we look at our current practices in assessment and intervention, it is common to see elements of several of these theories, approaches, and emphases. Table 4.1 summarizes these developments of the past four decades. No one approach, however, yet accounts for all the variations encountered by professionals working with language-disordered children or provides the answers to all the questions that arise (Kamhi, 1993). There is no doubt that in the 1990s as well as in the next decade, we will see further refinements of previous approaches, attempts to blend the various theories, research into the adequacy or inadequacy of the newer theories, and ongoing work and debate in trying to understand an extremely complex ability. Two directions some of this work is taking have resulted in a resurgence of interest in causal factors. One has come about because of new medical technologies (e.g., neuroimaging) that are improving our ability to understand human functioning. The other has come about as we continue to challenge our conceptions and, as a result, rethink our notions of causality as a combination and interaction of factors. A third direction involves improving our predictive abilities with regard to children who demonstrate language problems, and a fourth direction focuses on improving and documenting the effectiveness and efficiency of intervention. As professionals working with language-disordered children, we must keep abreast

TABLE 4.1 Summary of Historical Developments in Children's Language in the Past Four Decades

Decade	Historical Developments
1950s	Generative transformational grammar Behaviorism Mediated behaviorism
1960s	Psycholinguistic testing (ITPA) Syntactic analyses of and intervention for language disorders Behavioral intervention objectives and procedures
1970s	Social learning theory Semantic approach Cognitive approach Pragmatic approach
1980s	Interactional/conversational approach The "metas" Figurative/inferential language Literacy/"educational" language Government-binding theory

of the knowledge, changes, and paradigm shifts, as these potentially add to our information about children's language development and disorders and assist us in helping language-disordered children.

IDENTIFICATION OF LANGUAGE-DISORDERED CHILDREN

It may seem strange to think of identifying children with language problems as a major issue. One might think that identifying children with language problems would be straightforward. Certainly, a child whose language performance does not correspond to that of children of the same age might be considered to have language problems. However, several questions arise. We know that children who are acquiring language normally can show marked variability in language development. If a child's performance does not correspond to that of other children of the same age, does the difference reflect normal variation or a problem? How do we determine if the difference is normal variation or problematic? If the difference is considered not to be a reflection of normal variability, how much of a difference from expectations constitutes a real problem versus a slowed pattern within normal limits? If a child demonstrates above-average development in

areas other than language, such as cognition/intelligence or motor skills, but only average development in language, should we consider the child to have a language impairment? A related issue is how we think about infants who are **preverbal**, so that oral language performance cannot be observed, or about children who at a particular point in time demonstrate adequate language skills but who have background factors, such as intermittent hearing losses, birth difficulties, or environmental deprivations, that may place them at risk for later language problems? Should these children be considered to have language impairments? These are only a few of the questions. The answers to these questions influence which children "shall be called language disordered" (Lahey, 1990, p. 619), who may and may not receive intervention, and what the forms of intervention may be.

We will not embark on a full discussion of the issues surrounding identification here. These issues are not yet resolved, although they are currently receiving a great deal of attention and debate in the literature. We will, however, discuss a few of the issues. The discussion will first address those children who demonstrate language performance differing from that expected of same-age children. We will then turn our attention to the at-risk children.

Given normal variability in children's language development and in their language performances from one communicative context to another, the standard to which we compare an individual child's performance and the conditions under which we observe that performance are important factors in identification. The latter factor requires that a child's language performance be observed in a variety of contexts, a topic that will be discussed later in this book. Although language developmental milestones provide relevant information about whether a child's performance is similar to or different from these milestones, they provide very little information about the significance of any variations that might be observed. It is the significance attached to the variations that leads to identification of a child as having a language problem. However, deciding on the significance of the variations depends, in part, on the standard to which we compare the performance.

The two standards of comparison that have commonly been used are mental age (MA) and chronological age (CA). **Mental age** refers to the age level at which a child is functioning on cognitive/intellectual tasks. In using MA as the standard, children's language performances are compared to those of children with similar MAs. The assumption is that normal children's language performance does not generally differ markedly from their nonverbal cognitive ability. When language performance is lower than MA, a language impairment is presumed to be present. That is, there is a gap between MA and LA (language age). There are, however, several problems with this approach:

1. Some children may have language skills that are higher than their cognitive skills (Leonard, 1983).
2. The exact relationship between cognition and language has not been established (see chapter 2). Therefore, it cannot be assumed that cognitive abilities will set the limits for or determine language performance (Lahey, 1990).
3. There may be different "types of intelligence," and a theoretical relationship between these and language has not been demonstrated (Lahey, 1990).

4. It is possible that many mentally retarded children would not be identified as language disordered because there may be no gap between MA and LA. As a result, these children may not receive language intervention services even though intervention might benefit them (Fey, 1986).

One advantage of this approach is that children who have above-average cognitive skills but language skills below their cognitive levels could be identified as language impaired.

The second approach uses CA as the standard to which language performance is compared. "With CA referencing, language impairment is defined as a clinically significant departure from what is expected for children of the child's own CA" (Fey, 1986, p. 36). That is, there is a gap between CA and LA. Although this approach resolves the concern about the still unestablished relationship between cognition/MA and language performance, it has certain problems:

1. Children whose cognitive level exceeds their CA but whose language performance corresponds to their CA may not be identified as having language problems. These might be very bright or gifted children whose language abilities may prevent achievement at the level that might be expected from their cognitive level. This topic is discussed in chapter 13.
2. The number of children identified as having language problems may be so large that it strains the professional resources available to serve them.
3. This approach implies that the ultimate goal of intervention for any child identified as language disordered "would be to bring the child's communicative abilities to an age-equivalent level. . . . Unfortunately, this is frequently an unrealistic expectation for many of the children" (Fey, 1986, p. 36).

Despite the problems associated with the CA–LA gap approach to identifying the children, Lahey (1990) suggests that these are less serious than the problems related to the MA–LA comparison. She advocates the use of the CA as the standard for comparison.

We now return to the issue of what constitutes an important variation from the standard we use. Even though Lahey (1990) suggests that CA is a more relevant standard for comparison, she, as well as others (e.g., Carrow-Woolfolk, 1985; Lawrence, 1992; McCauley & Demetras, 1990; McCauley & Swisher, 1984; Salvia & Ysseldyke, 1988), caution against using age-equivalency measures, that is, relating a child's performance to a language age, such as LA referred to in the preceding discussion. One reason for this caution is that the same delay in terms of age-equivalent performance may not have the same importance for children of different ages. For example, a 1-year delay in language performance for a 10-year-old child does not likely carry the same significance as a 1-year delay for a 3-year-old child. Lahey (1990) argues that a more appropriate approach describes a child's "relative standing with peers" (p. 615), so that normal variability from an average is considered. Such descriptions include standard scores, standard deviations from the mean, and percentile ranks.

However, even these types of scores do not tell us when a child might have language problems that seriously affect academic and/or social achievements, and there is some arbitrariness in deciding what the cutoff point will be. That is, a child whose language performance is at the 10th percentile might be considered language disordered, whereas one whose performance is at the 15th percentile might not. It may be that the child at the 15th percentile will experience just as many or more difficulties because of language problems than the one at the 10th percentile. Such circumstances do occur. This approach also has the danger of leading professionals to depend too heavily on norm-referenced, standardized tests of language for identifying language-disordered children, a topic discussed in chapter 14.

There may be a third standard of comparison to consider, that is, a social standard. In using this standard, societal values placed on the degree of language facility and on the degree of success for life functions that are dependent on language facility (e.g., educational success, social success) become important in identifying children. Children whose language performances are evaluated as being sufficiently poor to cause potential problems in succeeding within the conditions of societal values could then be seen to have language impairments. Tomblin's (1991) model, illustrated in Figure 4.1, attempts to bring together the notions of factors causing language impairments and social evaluation of language performance. Although this standard is harder to measure in numerical terms, it may overcome some of the difficulties inherent in the CA and MA standards for identification discussed earlier. This may be particularly true if a societal standard is used in combination with one of these more

FIGURE 4.1   A Schematic Model of the Primary Causal Factors in Developmental Language Disorder. (From "Examining the Cause of Specific Language Impairment" by J. B. Tomblin, 1991, *Language, Speech and Hearing Services in Schools, 22*, p. 70. Copyright © 1991 by the American Speech-Language-Hearing Association. Reprinted by permission.)

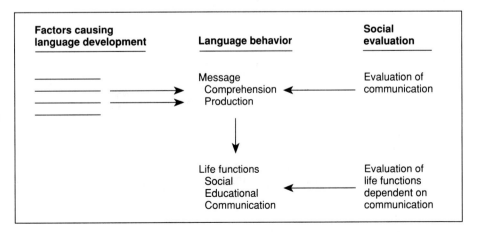

traditional standards. It also has the potential to provide a framework for approaching language and language impairments in multilingual/multicultural children.

None of the preceding discussions addresses the identification of children who appear to be able to communicate adequately but who have subtle language problems that potentially interfere with academic performance or social interactions. These children may obtain scores on standardized language tests that place them within normal limits, and they may be able to converse adequately in casual interchanges (Lahey, 1990). Yet, they may experience difficulty with academic skills closely related to oral language abilities, such as reading, spelling, and writing. These factors have implications for the procedures we use in identifying these children. For this reason, Lahey (1990) suggests that identification should be made under conditions that stress the child's language performance, "so that difficulties with performance would most likely be evident" (p. 618).

Identification also involves predicting which children will ultimately experience problems related to language. There are very young and, therefore, primarily nonverbal children (e.g., below 1 or 1½ years of age) who may be at risk for language development problems, and there are preschool and school-age children who may not have observable language problems at a specific time but who have a history or other problems that place them at risk for the emergence of later language difficulties. Tomblin and his colleagues (Tomblin, Hardy, & Hein, 1991) suggest that it might be possible to assign neonates to an at risk for language problems category based on criteria related to prenatal and perinatal events. The children's development could then be monitored and intervention begun as soon as any problems with language emerged. It might also be possible to institute "preventive intervention" for these children, even before actual language problems are identified, through parent/caregiver training programs. For older children who have histories or other problems that place them at risk for the emergence of language difficulties, preventive intervention through parental and/or teacher training programs might also be effective.

These approaches depend, of course, on determining what factors place children at risk for language disorders. Some birth factors (e.g., **anoxia**, hyperbilirubinemia, **kernicterus**), chromosomal syndromes (e.g., Down syndrome), and known neurological or physical conditions (e.g., cerebral palsy, hearing loss, cleft palate) have been linked to potential language problems. Additionally, risk for language problems has been associated with socioeconomic factors and environmental deprivation. Although some have suggested that prematurity may place an infant at risk for later language problems (e.g., Hubatch, Johnson, Kistler, Burns, & Moneka, 1985), Menyuk and her colleagues found that for certain early lexical and cognitive developmental skills, only infants with very low birth weights, as opposed to premature infants generally, differed from their full-term peers (Menyuk, Liebergott, Schultz, Chesnick, & Ferrier, 1991). In contrast, Aram and her colleagues concluded that children with very low birth weights were at no greater risk for later language problems unassociated with other developmental problems, such as lowered cognitive level, neurological abnormalities, and hearing impairments (Aram, Hack, Hawkins, Weissman, & Borawski-Clark, 1991). When language problems occurred in association with other developmental problems, however, the very-low-birth-weight children had significantly lower language performances than normal-birthweight children (Aram et al., 1991).

When these more obvious factors are absent, there may be other factors that can place children at risk for later language problems. Certain variables have been discussed in the literature that seem to be more predictive of future language disorder than others. Among these may be (1) a family history of communication problems, particularly among members of the immediate family; (2) birth order, with later birth indicating a greater risk; (3) parents' levels of education; and (4) gender of the child, with males appearing to be more at risk than females (e.g., Lewis & Thompson, 1992; Neils & Aram, 1986; Paul, 1991; Tallal, Ross, & Curtiss, 1989; Tomblin, 1989; Tomblin et al., 1991). In interpreting these factors for placing children at risk, some caution is needed. It is likely that not all factors have been fully determined, that the factors just listed are not invariably associated with later language difficulties (e.g., Whitehurst, Arnold, Smith, Fischel, Lonigan, & Valdez-Menchaca, 1991), and that their interrelationships with other factors have yet to be explained.

Despite the limits on the current information, Tomblin et al. (1991) suggest that using an at-risk procedure that places children in a developmental monitoring program in combination with a language screening procedure may aid the identification process. However, if we apply Lahey's (1990) idea, the screening procedure should include tasks that stress the child's language performance. The notion of using high-risk factors with monitoring combined with

screening programs is consistent with Lahey's (1990) suggestion that perhaps two identification categories should be devised. One is for those children who show problems with language, and the other is for children at risk for language problems.

Table 4.2 summarizes some of the issues we have raised with regard to identifying children with language problems. Although the issues remain, Fey (1986) offers a practical definition of "who shall be called language disordered" (Lahey, 1990, p. 619) that is based on one presented in 1983 by Tomblin:

A child may be viewed as language impaired when the pattern of communicative performance exhibited en-

TABLE 4.2 Issues in Identification of Children with Language Problems

Issues	Examples	Problems
Standards of Comparison	Mental age (MA): language performance compared to expectations for child's mental (cognitive) age	▷Children with language performance higher than MAs ▷Relationship between cognition and language not fully established ▷Different forms of intelligence and relationship with language not established ▷Mentally retarded children excluded from being considered language impaired
	Chronological age (CA): language performance compared to expectations for child's chronological age	▷Excludes children with above-normal cognitive abilities but average or below-average language performance ▷Too many children identified as having language problems for resources available ▷Implication that goal of intervention is always to achieve age-equivalent language performance
Measures of Performance	Age equivalency (language age = LA)	▷Same amount of delay in terms of age equivalence not equally important at different CAs ▷Normal variation in language performance not considered
	Variance measures (e.g., standard scores, percentile ranks, standard deviations)	▷Cutoff point not descriptive of actual problems in real-life language functioning ▷Danger of excessive dependence on norm-referenced, standardized language tests
Identifying Subtle Language Problems	Stress on language performance	▷Casual language performance and/or standardized language performance may appear normal unless performance stressed to reveal subtle problems ▷Subtle problems can affect language-related academic skills (e.g., reading, spelling)
Predicting Future Language Problems	Identifying children at risk for language difficulties; supplement screening programs	▷At-risk factors not completely identified ▷Relationships between factors not understood

ables a clinician to predict continued deficits in language development *and* in the social, cognitive, educational or emotional developments which rely heavily on language skills. Furthermore, infants who have biological or behavioral conditions that are commonly associated with future impairments in communicative functioning (e.g., Down's syndrome, profound hearing impairment, autistic symptoms) may be viewed as language impaired even before the age at which language forms typically begin to appear. The degree of confidence that a clinician can place in this prediction will determine the severity rating for the child's impairment. (p. 42)

We would add that children with other factors that may place them at risk for language impairment would be identified as "at-risk for language-related problems" (Lahey, 1990, p. 618) and placed in language developmental monitoring programs.

PUBLIC LAWS AND CHILDREN'S LANGUAGE DISORDERS

Over approximately the last 20 years, several federal laws have been passed that have had important implications for the services offered to children with disabilities, including those with language disorders. Here we will review three of these.

The Education for All Handicapped Children Act, Public Law (PL) 94-142, was passed in 1975 by the U.S. Congress. This law had far-reaching impacts on the services to be made available for all school-age children up to 21 years of age. In essence, the law mandated that all children had the right to free and appropriate education provided by the educational system, regardless of their disabling conditions and special needs. Additionally, the services provided for the children were to be tailored to their individual needs, planned as a result of multidisciplinary input, and delivered in the least restrictive educational environment appropriate for each child. This latter aspect of the law placed the emphasis on **mainstreaming**, or placing children with special needs in the regular educational environment, and provided part of the impetus for specialists to begin to work more closely with regular educators and each other in collaborative and team approaches to service delivery. The law mandated not only that services were to be made available

for the children but also that the educational system was responsible for identifying children in need. That is, the educational system was required to engage actively in finding the children to receive the services. Under the law, parents were seen as active participants in giving permission for assessment and evaluation, planning educational strategies for their children, reviewing their children's progress, and revising educational plans to meet their needs. These mandates applied to children with speech and/or language problems occurring in isolation of other problems and to children with speech and/or language problems associated with other disabling conditions. The law also intended to extend special services that had traditionally been available only in elementary school to secondary school and even into early adulthood, that is, up to 21 years of age.

In the 1980s, a series of directives known as the *Regular Education Initiative* (REI) was issued by the U.S. Department of Education. The REI grew out of PL 94-142 and reinforced the ideas of least restrictive environment and mainstreaming for special children. Concepts of collaboration and consultation among professionals, and of collaborative models and consultative models of service, were also reinforced. However, professionals' interpretations of the REI and, more specifically, how the intent of the REI should be put into practice in service delivery strategies and models are currently not clear (Lieberman, 1990). One extreme position is that all children with special needs, regardless of their individual differences, should be served in the regular classroom through a *collaborative* or *consultative model* in which the specialist assists the regular educator, who is the primary agent in the intervention for the handicapped children. This position seems to have forgotten the words "appropriate" and "individual," which are key elements of PL 94-142. That is, what is appropriate for one child may not be for another, and what is appropriate for a child at one time may not be at another time. Fortunately, most professionals have not adopted this extreme position and have instead tried to expand the variety of approaches for different children at different times, including the variety of service delivery models and strategies employed to serve children with language disorders.

Federal laws have significantly impacted on services for language-disordered children.

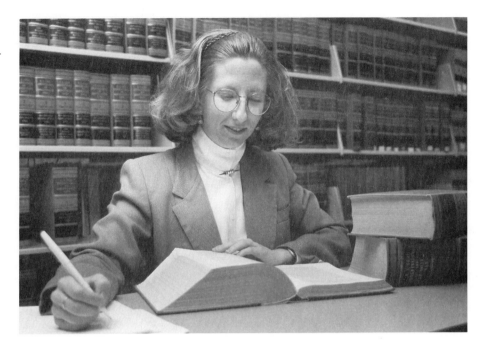

Another federal law influencing the services for language-disordered children was the Education of the Handicapped Act Amendments of 1986, or PL 99-457. Like PL 94-142, these amendments included children with speech and/or language disorders. Early intervention, as well as early identification, was a significant emphasis of this law, and it extended the public educational system's responsibilities to infants and toddlers. As a result, the implementation of infant and toddler screening programs was an outgrowth of PL 99-457. This is one of the reasons for the recent interest in establishing at-risk registers and developmental monitoring programs referred to in the previous section on identification. The early intervention mandate of the law also resulted in increased awareness of the need for professionals to become involved in parent/caregiver training programs to enhance young disabled children's development. PL 99-457 had particular relevance for language-disordered children. Apart from the presence of obvious physical abnormalities or syndromes at birth, delay in acquiring language is often the first indication that children may have problems.

With the 1990 passage of the Education of the Handicapped Act Amendments, the name became *Individuals with Disabilities Education Act* (IDEA), or PL 101-476. An obvious change involved a semantic shift that replaced the descriptor *handicapped* with *disabled.* The law also extended the definition of children with disabilities to include children with autism and traumatic brain injury, but it did not include attention deficit disorder (ADD) as a separate category in the definition of disability. It also placed greater emphasis on *transition services,* which promote disabled students' smooth progress from school to postschool activities such as vocational training, employment, and postsecondary education. This aspect of the law has important implications for services for language-disordered adolescents that aim to help them develop the necessary communication skills to move from high school into postsecondary pursuits. The law also placed greater emphasis on meeting the needs of ethnically and culturally diverse children with disabilities and promoted the development of early intervention programs for children exposed prenatally to maternal substance abuse.

TABLE 4.3   Three Federal Laws and Some Aspects of the Laws Having Implications for Services for Language-Disordered Children

Law	Year	Some Aspects of the Laws
PL 94–142	1975	▷Free, appropriate education for all handicapped children, including those with language disorders. ▷Individualized educational and intervention plans to address children's special needs. ▷Services for children in the regular educational setting (least restrictive environment) as much as possible. ▷Emphasis on interdisciplinary strategies and collaboration for assessment and service delivery. ▷Parental involvement. ▷Active programs to identify children needing special services. ▷Services to be provided for secondary students up to 21 years of age, as well as elementary students.
PL 99–457	1986	▷Extension of services to include infants and toddlers. ▷Early identification and early intervention. ▷Parent training programs.
PL 101–476	1990	▷Change of name to replace *handicap* with *disability*. ▷Included autism and traumatic brain injury but continued to exclude attention deficit disorder. ▷Increased emphasis on transition services from school to postschool activities. ▷Increased emphasis on services for disabled children from ethnically/culturally diverse backgrounds.

Table 4.3 summarizes a number of the implications these federal laws have had for services for disabled children. Several of the current trends in serving language-disordered children have arisen from the impetus provided by these laws. Among these trends are the involvement of parents/caregivers in facilitating the children's language abilities and the emphasis on parent/caregiver education; interdisciplinary collaboration in implementing intervention programs for language-disordered children in a variety of settings, including the regular classroom; integration of oral language into educational curricula; and early identification and intervention.

CLASSIFICATION AND CATEGORIZATION

One approach to classifying language disorders of children has focused on the causes of the disorders. This approach has been referred to as the *causative* or *etiological* orientation, with some of the traditional etiological categories being mental retardation, hearing loss, emotional disturbance, and developmental (childhood) aphasia. In this orientation, knowing the etiology of a language disorder is an important factor in planning intervention. In fact, in its purest form, this approach presumes that specific causative factors result in specific types of language disorders with unique characteristics, and that the unique characteristics of each type require different intervention techniques. It also presumes that specific causes of language disorders can be identified.

In reality, neither of these last two statements is always correct. A specific causative factor does not fully account for the range, individual variation, and unique characteristics seen in the language patterns of children whose language disorders are described as stemming from that etiology. Many professionals who have subscribed unyieldingly to this approach have unfortunately failed to provide intervention that considers the individual variation of children within each etiological category. Instead, broadly developed intervention plans have been used indiscriminately, without attention to children's individual differences. Additionally, some of the language characteristics observed in children in one etiological category are often seen in children in other etiological categories (Lahey, 1988; Leonard, 1982). That is, there is not necessarily a one-to-one relationship between etiology and language patterns. In other instances, specific causes of some children's language deficits cannot always be identified; nevertheless, the intervention for language problems of these children must be provided.

Another problem with the causative approach has been the inaccurate interpretation of these categories as the actual etiologies of the language disorders (Hubbell, 1981; Lahey, 1988). As Hubbell (1981) points out, terms such as *mental retardation, hearing loss,* or *emotional disturbance* "are second-level causal factors. That is, they are conditions that are associated with language disorders in children, but strictly speaking, they are not causal factors. Rather, they themselves result from other factors, sometimes with a heavy genetic or disease influence, sometimes from more amorphous origins" (p. 121).

Because of these difficulties, some professionals have argued that the etiologies, or causes, of children's language disorders are irrelevant. These opponents of the causative approach propose that it is the language behavior of an individual child, not the etiological category, that is relevant in planning intervention. This approach emphasizes description of each child's language strengths and weaknesses and, in its purest form, discounts attempts to search for causative factors. Working with a child's presenting language skills and deficits is the critical element of intervention. Unfortunately, this orientation obscures two facts: (1) there are certain shared language characteristics of children whose communication problems stem from a specific causative factor and (2) there are different language characteristics among the various etiological groups of children. This problem parallels the problems with the causative approach, which clouds the facts there are similarities in the language of children

in different groups, as well as individual variations in the language of children in the same group. In explaining the noncausative approach, Hubbell (1981) writes:

> No matter what conclusions are made about etiology, we will concentrate on communicative functioning of the child. In this sense, the etiology becomes irrelevant; we simply "stick to the behaviors." At the same time, such reasoning has led to disastrous blunders in which, for example, hearing-impaired children are misclassified as retarded, disturbed, or aphasic. (p. 127)

We see, then, that there are real dangers in totally avoiding references to the causes. Such opposition to the causative approach may result in "throwing the baby out with the bathwater." Avoiding references to causes also ignores the fact that many educational systems require a disability/causative label to place children in special services programs and that funding for these services is tied to such labeling (Bernstein & Tiegerman, 1993; Lahey, 1988).

Terms such as *language disordered* or *language impaired* have been proposed to classify children whose linguistic performances are inadequate. These are umbrella terms, however. To explain the range of deviant language behaviors seen in children, additional subclassification systems have been suggested (e.g., Bashir, Kuban, Kleinman, & Scavuzzo, 1983; Bloom & Lahey, 1978; Carrow-Woolfolk & Lynch, 1982; Fey, 1986). Although these systems focus on the communication patterns of children rather than on the causes of the problems, they can still mask the need to specify the precise language skills and deficits of any individual child. For example, to say that a child has primary problems with the "form" of language, drawing from Bloom's (1988) model, describes nothing about the specific aspects of form, such as plural nouns, the auxiliary "is," or conjoining sentences, that may be present or absent in the child's repertoire. Additionally, these subclasses are not mutually exclusive. We do not see the absence of overlap in the language patterns of children in the various classifications and the lack of variability in the language behaviors of children with the same classification that would be expected of ideal classification systems.

What we observe is the replacement of one classification system with another, with neither fully sufficing. As Bashir and his colleagues (1983) clearly point out: "Language disorders is a general term that designates a heterogeneous group of problems characterized by varying degrees and types of deficits in the comprehension, production, and use of language. The disorders are associated with a diverse group of developmental problems and medical conditions" (p. 92). Any one classification system is, therefore, likely to be too simplistic when working with individual children. The specific language behaviors of each child need to be identified if intervention for any one child is to be effective. However, this specification needs to be done while also recognizing that certain behaviors can be characteristic of certain groups of children, that some characteristics can overlap, and that any child can demonstrate **idiosyncratic** language behaviors. At the same time, attempting to identify a cause, even a second-level cause, can prevent serious errors in providing appropriate, coordinated, interdisciplinary services for a child.

Some of the titles of subsequent chapters in this book may appear to be closely aligned with an etiological classification system. This is not the intent, however. We believe that there are special groups of children who can have language problems or whose language behaviors can present unique considerations. Sometimes we see language problems in association with or as part of the child's special status. In other instances, what may make the child special is the age group. We would hardly refer to "adolescents" as an etiological classification. It is the children's language we will be considering, and to lump them and their language behaviors together would cloud the discussions.

APPROACHES TO CHILDREN'S LANGUAGE DISORDERS

In light of our previous discussions, the statement that children with language disorders are not members of a **homogeneous** group likely comes as no surprise. In the same way that language is a behavior or skill that results from a complex interplay of physiological, cognitive, psychological, linguistic, environmental, and social factors, children's language disorders present a complex array of problems. Children with language disorders are indeed a **heterogeneous** group!

Several approaches have been developed in attempts to explain the complexities and variations of children's language disorders. One approach, proposed by Carrow-Woolfolk and Lynch (1982), presents a theoretical, four-dimensional description of language disorders that emphasizes the interrelationships among the dimensions. It is, therefore, referred to as an *integrative* approach that considers the cognitive, linguistic, environmental, and performance factors involved in disordered language. Another approach is that of Bloom and Lahey (1978), an approach reiterated later by Lahey (1988). These authors take the perspective that the intersection of three major components of language—content, form, and use—comprises language knowledge and that language knowledge is *language competence*. Children's language disorders are described in terms of the three components that are deficit or disrupted. A third approach is described by Fey (1986), who views language from an *interactionist* perspective, which appears to have its roots in Bloom and Lahey's perspective. Fey classifies language-disordered children into four subgroups based on their social-conversational patterns.

Although these approaches represent differing views of how to address children's language disorders, they are among the ones more widely adopted by professionals working with language-disordered children. For this reason, we will present these approaches here. We must remember, however, that none has yet been fully validated in the literature. Furthermore, the state of the art is such that any one approach is likely too limited to explain the range, the variation, and all of the factors involved in children's language disorders.

Carrow-Woolfolk and Lynch's Integrative Approach

Carrow-Woolfolk and Lynch's (1982) *integrative approach* focuses on the complex interplay of factors that can be involved in children's language disorders

Children who have language disorders represent a very heterogeneous group.

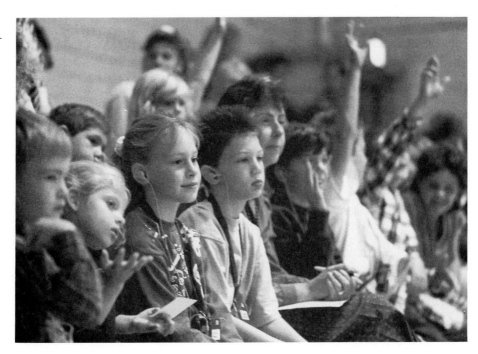

(Figure 4.2). According to these authors, language is composed of four interrelated dimensions:

1. The *cognitive* dimension, which involves the sensory, perceptual, mnemonic, conceptual, representational, and symbolistic skills that provide the ability to learn the linguistic rules and meaning of language.
2. The dimension of *linguistic knowledge,* which involves the acquisition of the semantic, syntactic, morphological, phonological, and pragmatic rules that comprise the language.
3. The dimension of *language performance,* which involves what a child does behaviorally with a knowledge of the language in terms of speech perception, comprehension, language formulation, and speaking.
4. The dimension of *communicative environment,* which involves the external or environmental stimulation and reinforcement that encourage and maintain interpersonal relationships via language and a child's internal needs, desires, and

motivations that lead to communicative attempts and language learning.

As indicated by the arrows in Figure 4.2, Carrow-Woolfolk and Lynch stress the interaction of these dimensions in language functioning. When one or more dimensions, or units within any of the dimensions, are deficient, other aspects of language functioning are affected. This perspective is consistent with our earlier statements regarding the interrelationships of the various components of language.

In using this approach to explain children's language disorders and the effects a deficit in one area may have on other aspects of language, Carrow-Woolfolk and Lynch suggest that deficits in units that comprise the cognitive dimension can have significant impacts on all of the other dimensions. For example, disorders of perception can affect the ways in which concepts are acquired and can result in the learning of faulty semantic rules. Subsequently, the language performance dimension is affected. The meanings of words are not accurately comprehended, nor are the

FIGURE 4.2 The Integrative Model of Language. (From E. Carrow-Woolfolk and J. Lynch, *An Integrative Approach to Language Disorders in Children* [p. 102]. Copyright © 1981. Reprinted by permission of Allyn and Bacon.)

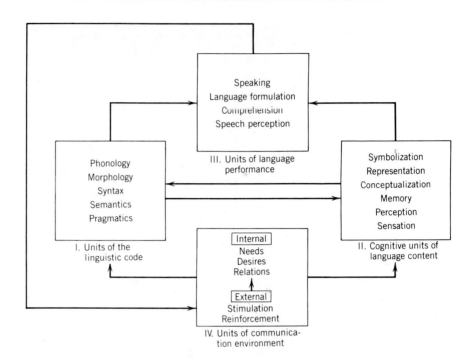

words used appropriately when a child is speaking. Deficits in memory impose limits on the amount of information a child can retain for processing, which leads to inaccurate concept acquisition, faulty learning of the linguistic code, and disorders in the performance dimension. Because concepts are at the heart of meaning, conceptual problems can significantly affect all aspects of the linguistic knowledge dimension, not only semantics, because each of these aspects is used to express underlying concepts. Deficits in comprehension and production are additional consequences of conceptual problems. Carrow-Woolfolk and Lynch point out that because adults modify their language input to a child with a conceptual problem, the dimension of communicative environment is also affected. Deficit representations and symbolization have a severe impact on the semantic aspect of language because a child cannot extend the meanings of words from the concrete to the abstract. Furthermore, because representations and symbolizations are needed to acquire the pragmatic rules governing language, this aspect of the code is impaired, as is language performance.

Within the dimension of linguistic knowledge, language-disordered children may demonstrate problems with one or more aspects of pragmatics, phonology, semantics, and syntax and morphology because the rules that govern the linguistic code have not been learned properly. When deficits occur in the dimension of linguistic knowledge, the dimension of language performance is always affected. Children who have not acquired appropriate syntactic and morphological rules may demonstrate their lack of grammatical knowledge in many ways. Among these are faulty word order in multiword utterances, incorrect use of grammatical inflections, such as plurals or verb-tense markers, and omission of certain grammatical elements, such as the copula verb. A semantic disorder may sometimes appear as a concept disorder. However, children with semantic disorders may acquire appropriate concepts and their meanings, but "the wrong words or the wrong grammatic forms may be associated with specific meanings" (Carrow-Woolfolk & Lynch, 1982, p. 217). In some instances, the words for acquired concepts may not have been learned at all. Pragmatic disorders are reflected in children who have not learned the rules governing what can be said to whom under what circumstances. Like the other linguistic rules, these pragmatic skills must be learned by abstracting from communicative models the similarities and differences in the circumstances and developing the general rules that govern the behaviors. We see, then, an excellent example of how failure to acquire the rules for one aspect of linguistic knowledge can affect language performance. A child with an inadequate set of pragmatic rules is likely to say the wrong thing to the wrong person in the wrong situation. When a child has failed to learn the rules that govern what speech sounds make up the language and/or how these sounds can be combined sequentially, the child demonstrates a phonological disorder. Such a disorder can reduce the intelligibility with which the cognitive underpinnings of language and the other linguistic rules are expressed.

Carrow-Woolfolk and Lynch indicate that even though a child may acquire accurate concepts and an adequate system of linguistic rules, the child may still experience problems with language performance. Among these problems are difficulties in understanding input, resulting in impaired ability to decipher stimuli and difficulty in formulating and executing the linguistic symbols to impart the code. We have also seen that deficits in the cognitive and/or linguistic dimensions can affect language performance.

The fourth dimension that may be involved in children's language disorders is the communication environment. Carrow-Woolfolk and Lynch divide this dimension into two aspects: factors that relate to the internal motivations and needs of the child in communicating and factors in the communication environment that are external to the child. These authors explain that a child who has little or no desire to communicate, or who has his or her needs met in an environment that does not expect communicative attempts, has no reason to talk. Conversely, if a child who is motivated to communicate and who makes attempts at communication does not have those attempts appropriately reinforced, further attempts at communication can diminish. Here we see how an environmental factor external to the child affects language. Other external factors can include inadequate or inappropriate stimulation for language learning and/or poor language models on the part of the child's primary caregivers.

We have previously described the reciprocal influence of a child's language skills and an adult's language stimulation. In viewing the communicative environment, it is important to remember that besides the environment affecting the child, a language disorder stemming from problems in one or more of the other dimensions will affect the external aspects of the child's language environment. An additional factor that must be considered is the dialect or language spoken by a child's caregivers and in the child's linguistic community. In chapter 10 we discuss the topic of discriminating between aspects of a child's language that reflect disorders of the communicative environment and aspects of a child's language that reflect differences resulting from the communicative environment.

Bloom and Lahey's Language Competence Approach

In Bloom and Lahey's (1978) approach, language competence results from the intersection of three aspects of language knowledge: knowledge of the form of the language, knowledge of the content, and knowledge of language use. Bloom's (1988) illustration of the intersection of these three aspects of language knowledge is shown in Figure 4.3. *Form,* as used by Bloom and Lahey, refers to the syntactic, phonological, and morphological components of language described in chapter 1. *Content* is the meaning of messages, or the semantic aspect of language, and *use* refers to the pragmatic component. According to these authors, "language consists of some aspect of content or meaning that is coded or represented by linguistic form for some purpose or use in a particular context" (Bloom & Lahey, 1978, p. 11). In Figure 4.3 the intersection of these three components shows language competence indicated by the shaded area D in the center.

Basing her discussion on her earlier writing with Bloom (Bloom & Lahey, 1978), Lahey (1988) suggests that this approach can be used to describe the ways in which individual components or the interaction among components can be disrupted in children's language. Accordingly, six types of disruption are identified. Although one component or its interaction with

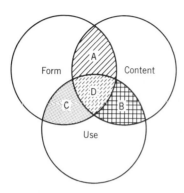

FIGURE 4.3   The Interaction of Content, Form, and Use in Language. (Reprinted with the permission of Macmillan Publishing Company from *Language Disorders and Language Development* [p. 18] by Margaret Lahey. Copyright © 1988 by Macmillan Publishing Company.)

the others may be the most deviant, it is possible that the other components or interactions are also impaired, but to a lesser extent. Lahey (1988) writes that the six subgroups represent "broad characterizations that are helpful in emphasizing the way language functions as a system and the ways in which that system can be disrupted" (p. 23).

The first of these subgroups includes children who are acquiring the aspects of form, content, and use in the normal sequence, and who are developing adequate interactions among the components, but are doing so at rates slower than those of other children. These are the children who might be described as *language delayed.*

Other children can demonstrate *disorders of form.* The concepts, representations, and pragmatic skills of these children are superior to their ability to use linguistic forms to communicate their ideas in appropriate contexts. Children with disorders of form may communicate with gestures and tantrums. Their attempts at oral communication may be unintelligible; may contain frequent sound errors because of aberrant phonological rules; may consist of only a few words because of reduced MLU; may demonstrate confused word order or omission of words because of limited or inaccurate knowledge of syntactic rules; and/or may show morphological errors, again because of the use of inadequately learned rule systems to en-

code ideas. Included in the subgroup of children with form disorders are those who have word-finding or word retrieval problems. For these children, the concepts and even the words to convey the concepts are known, but the ability to access the words quickly on demand is impaired.

The third subgroup consists of children with *disorders of content.* Their weakest area of language appears to be in the acquisition of concepts that form the meanings behind utterances. These children may use relatively well-formed utterances to communicate in social interactions, but the content of their communications evidences distorted, inaccurate, or delayed notions about objects, events, or relations. Although this pattern of language disorder may be less common than other patterns, there are some children whose primary language problems appear to be content disorders. Among these are visually impaired children who may have faulty spatial concepts (Warren, 1981) and hydrocephalic children who may demonstrate a verbal phenomenon labeled *cocktail party speech* after the hyperverbal, social behavior of adults talking in well-formed sentences without saying anything (Schwartz, 1974; Swisher & Pinsker, 1971).

Disorders of use refer to problems in the ways language is employed for human interactions. Examples of these problems include abrupt topic shifts, a limited repertoire of language functions, absence of appropriate presuppositions about a conversational partner, and deficits in reciprocal behaviors that underlie conversational turn taking. Young children may not even attempt to communicate with oral language but, instead, may use gestures. When these children are prodded to talk, the form and content of their productions are often far superior to their skills in using language. For some children, disorders of use are reflected in language that is employed primarily for intrapersonal rather than interpersonal purposes.

The children in the fifth subgroup have *distorted interactions of form, content, and use.* With weakened interactions among the three components, relatively advanced forms and complex concepts may be used with the intent to communicate. However, there may be a mismatch between the content of the message and the form used to express it. Or there may be a contradiction between the way a message is used and its content. In other instances, the form may not correspond adequately to either the meaning or the communicative context.

Just as there are children with weakened or distorted interactions among form, content, and use, as just described, there are other children for whom no interactions among the components appear to be present. Children with *separations of form, content, and use* comprise the sixth subgroup of language-disordered children. For these children, the linguistic structure of utterances, the meaning of the utterances, and the communicative intents of the messages are disjointed. Stereotypic utterances may be produced in inappropriate contexts, without regard for the content of utterances. Some emotionally disturbed children may demonstrate these fragmentations of form, content, and use.

Fey's Language Interactionist Approach

Fey's *interactionist approach,* that is, his emphasis on the importance of the interaction of content, form, and use in approaching children's language disorders, is similar to that of Bloom and Lahey. However, Fey expands on the idea that language-disordered children may differ among themselves, as well as from children with normal language, primarily in how they use or do not use language. That is, Bloom and Lahey's (1978) aspect of use predominates in Fey's approach. Accordingly, Fey proposes four subgroups of language-disordered children based on their social-conversational interaction patterns. These groups arise from considering two continua related to conversational variables. One continuum deals with children's *assertiveness* in conversation, that is, the degree to which they initiate conversational acts or turns. The second continuum refers to the degree of children's *responsiveness* to their conversational partners' needs. For both of these continua, children can be high or low in the variable, depending on the frequency with which their conversational acts display assertive or responsive behaviors.

Figure 4.4 illustrates the four groups/patterns that emerge. One consists of children who are both conversationally assertive and responsive (+assertive, +responsive). Fey refers to these children as *active conversationalists.* Children who may be assertive

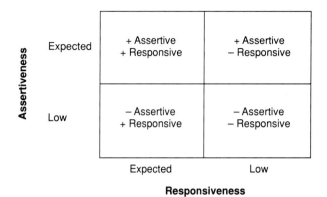

FIGURE 4.4   A Scheme for Profiling Children According to Their Levels of Social-Conversational Participation. (From Marc E. Fey, *Language Intervention with Young Children* [p. 70]. Copyright © 1986 by Allyn and Bacon. Reprinted by permission.)

in conversation but unresponsive to their partners' conversational needs (+assertive, −responsive) comprise the second group, that is, *verbal noncommunicators.* In the third group, the previous pattern is reversed. These children, referred to as *passive conversationalists,* are nonassertive in conversation but responsive to their partners' needs (−assertive, +responsive). The fourth group, *inactive communicators,* consists of children who are neither conversationally assertive nor responsive (−assertive, −responsive).

Fey suggests that this classification system is a "clinically useful scheme" (1986, p. 69) because it leads to a determination of *basic intervention goals* for language-disordered children who differ in their conversational interactions, that is, in how they use language. Within each of the groups, children may differ in linguistic abilities, or children in different groups may exhibit similar linguistic abilities. Children's specific linguistic abilities, therefore, need to be taken into account in planning intervention. Because the language available to the children for use in social-conversational activities may differ, *specific intervention goals* also need to be determined. What the four patterns may provide is information on the emphases that need to be placed on the situations in which specific goals may be targeted.

SUMMARY

In this chapter, we have seen that:

▶ Current approaches to assessment of and intervention for children's language disorders have their roots in the study of children's language and language disorders that has occurred primarily in the last 30 to 40 years, with several paradigm shifts occurring during this period.

▶ Despite the large amount of knowledge that has been gained, no one historical perspective fully accounts for the range and variation seen in language-disordered children.

▶ Identification of children with language problems is currently an issue under debate and depends, in part, on the standards to which children's language performances are compared and the ways in which variations from the standards are measured.

▶ Identification involves not only targeting children who evidence language problems but also predicting which young children are at risk for future language problems; variables that place children at risk for later language problems are being suggested but are still unconfirmed.

▶ Several federal laws have significantly influenced the services provided for language-disordered children, including the increased involvement of parents/caregivers, the settings in which services are delivered, collaboration and cooperation among various disciplines, and emphasis on early identification and intervention.

▶ Classification and categorization of children with language problems have generally centered on two approaches—etiological and nonetiological/descriptive—and remain controversial issues.

▶ Carrow-Woolfolk and Lynch's, Bloom and Lahey's, and Fey's views of language-disordered children are among those commonly adopted by professionals working with language-disordered children, with each view suggesting a somewhat different approach to these children.

This chapter has highlighted some of the unknown factors and unresolved issues in the study of children's language disorders, as well as some of those that are known and agreed upon. Children with language disorders must be viewed as a heterogeneous group, and any satisfactory explanation of their language difficulties will likely reflect the complexity associated with language itself.

REFERENCES

Aram, D., Hack, M., Hawkins, S., Weissman, B., & Borawski-Clark, E. (1991). Very-low-birthweight children and speech and language development. *Journal of Speech and Hearing Research, 34,* 1169–1179.

Bandura, A. (1971). *Psychological modeling.* Chicago: Aldine-Atherton.

Bandura. A. (1977). *Social learning theory.* Englewood Cliffs, NJ: Prentice-Hall.

Bashir, A., Kuban, K., Kleinman, S., & Scavuzzo, A. (1983). Issues in language disorders: Considerations of cause, maintenance, and change. In J. Miller, D. Yoder, & R. Schiefelbusch (Eds.), *Contemporary issues in language intervention.* Rockville, MD: American Speech-Language-Hearing Association.

Bates, E. (1976). Pragmatics and sociolinguistics in child language. In D. Morehead & A. Morehead (Eds.), *Normal and deficient child language.* Baltimore: University Park Press.

Bernstein, D., & Tiegerman, D. (1993). *Language and communication disorders.* (3rd ed.). New York: Merrill/Macmillan.

Bloom, L. (1970). *Language development: Form and function in emerging grammars.* Cambridge, MA: MIT Press.

Bloom, L. (1988). What is language? In M. Lahey, *Language disorders and language development.* New York: Merrill/Macmillan.

Bloom, L., & Lahey, M. (1978). *Language development and language disorders.* New York: Macmillan.

Brown, R. (1973). *A first language: The early stages.* Cambridge, MA: Harvard University Press.

Carrow-Woolfolk, E. (1985). *Test for auditory comprehen-*

sion of language—revised. Allen, TX: DLM Teaching Resources.

Carrow-Woolfolk, E., & Lynch, J. (1982). *An integrative approach to language disorders in children.* New York: Grune & Stratton.

Chomsky, N. (1957). *Syntactic structures.* The Hague: Mouton.

Chomsky, N. (1981). *Lectures on government and binding.* Dordrecht, Holland: Foris.

Clark, E. (1973). Non-linguistic strategies and the acquisition of word meanings. *Cognition, 2,* 161–182.

Dore, J. (1975). Holophrase, speech acts, and language universals. *Journal of Child Language, 2,* 21–40.

Duchan, J. (1986). Language intervention through sense-making and fine tuning. In R. Schiefelbusch (Ed.), *Language competence: Assessment and intervention.* San Diego, CA: College-Hill Press.

Fey, M. (1986). *Language intervention with young children.* Boston: Little, Brown.

Halliday, M. (1975). *Learning how to mean: Explorations in the development of language.* London: Edward Arnold.

Hubatch, L., Johnson, C., Kistler, D., Burns, W., & Moneka, W. (1985). Early language abilities of high-risk infants. *Journal of Speech and Hearing Disorders, 50,* 195–207.

Hubbell, R. (1981). *Children's language disorders: An integrated approach.* Englewood Cliffs, NJ: Prentice-Hall.

Kamhi, A. (1993). Research into practice: Some problems with the marriage between theory and clinical practice. *Language, Speech, and Hearing Services in Schools, 24,* 57–60.

Kirk, S., & McCarthy, J. (1961). *Illinois test of psycholinguistic abilities.* Urbana: University of Illinois Press.

Lahey, M. (1988). *Language disorders and language development.* New York: Merrill/Macmillan.

Lahey, M. (1990). Who shall be called language disordered? Some reflections and one perspective. *Journal of Speech and Hearing Disorders, 55,* 612–620.

Lawrence, C. (1992). Assessing the use of age-equivalent scores in clinical management. *Language, Speech, and Hearing Services in Schools, 23,* 6–8.

Leonard, L. (1982). Early language development and language disorders. In G. Shames & E. Wiig (Eds.), *Human communication disorders: An introduction.* Columbus, OH: Merrill.

Leonard, L. (1983). Defining the boundaries of language disorders in children. In J. Miller, D. Yoder, & R. Schiefelbusch (Eds.), *Contemporary issues in language intervention.* Rockville, MD: American Speech-Language-Hearing Association.

Leonard, L., & Loeb, D. (1988). Government-binding theory and some of its applications: A tutorial. *Journal of Speech and Hearing Research, 31,* 515–524.

Leonard, L., Sabbadini, L., Leonard, J., & Volterra, V. (1987). Specific language impairment in children: A cross-linguistic study. *Brain and Language, 32,* 233–252.

Leonard, L., Sabbadini, L., Volterra, V., & Leonard, J. (1988). Some influences on the grammar of English- and Italian-speaking children with specific language impairment. *Applied Psycholinguistics, 9,* 39–57.

Lewis, B., & Thompson, L. (1992). A study of developmental speech and language disorders in twins. *Journal of Speech and Hearing Research, 35,* 1086–1094.

Lieberman, L. (1990). REI: Revisited . . . again. *Exceptional Children, 56,* 561–562.

Loeb, D., & Leonard, L. (1991). Subject case marking and verb morphology in normally developing and specifically language-impaired children. *Journal of Speech and Hearing Research, 34,* 340–346.

McCauley, R., & Demetras, M. (1990). Identification of language impairment in the selection of specifically language-impaired subjects. *Journal of Speech and Hearing Disorders, 55,* 468–475.

McCauley, R., & Swisher, L. (1984). Use and misuse of norm-referenced tests in clinical assessment: A hypothetical case. *Journal of Speech and Hearing Disorders, 49,* 338–348.

Menyuk, P., Liebergott, J., Schultz, M., Chesnick, M., & Ferrier, L. (1991). Patterns of early lexical and cognitive development in premature and full-term infants. *Journal of Speech and Hearing Research, 34,* 88–94.

Neils, J., & Aram, D. (1986). Family history of children with developmental language disorders. *Perceptual and Motor Skills, 63,* 655–658.

Nippold, M. (1988). *Later language development: Ages nine through nineteen.* Boston: Little, Brown.

Osgood, C. (1957). A behavioristic analysis of perception and language as cognitive phenomena. *Contemporary approaches to cognition.* Cambridge, MA: Harvard University Press.

Paul, R. (1991). Profiles of toddlers with slow expressive language development. *Topics in Language Disorders, 11,* 1–13.

Rees, N. (1978). Pragmatics of language: Application to normal and disordered language development. In R. Schiefelbusch (Ed.), *Bases of language intervention.* Baltimore: University Park Press.

Salvia, J., & Ysseldyke, J. E. (1988). *Assessment in special and remedial education* (4th ed.). Boston: Houghton Mifflin.

Schwartz, E. (1974). Characteristics of speech and language development in the child with myelomeningocele and hydrocephalus. *Journal of Speech and Hearing Disorders, 39,* 465–468.

Simon, C. (1985). *Communication skills and classroom success: Therapy methodologies for language-learning disabled students.* San Diego, CA: College-Hill Press.

Skinner, B. (1957). *Verbal behavior.* Englewood Cliffs, NJ: Prentice-Hall.

Swisher, L., & Pinsker, E. (1971). The language characteristics of hyperverbal hydrocephalic children. *Developmental Medicine and Child Neurology, 13,* 746–755.

Tallal, P., Ross, R., & Curtiss, S. (1989). Familial aggregation in specific language impairment. *Journal of Speech and Hearing Disorders, 54,* 167–173.

Tomblin, J. B. (1983). An examination of the concept of disorder in the study of language variation. *Proceedings from the Fourth Wisconsin Symposium on Research in Child Language Disorders.* Madison: University of Wisconsin Press.

Tomblin, J. B. (1989). Familial concentration of developmental language impairment. *Journal of Speech and Hearing Disorders, 54,* 287–295.

Tomblin, J. B. (1991). Examining the cause of specific language impairment. *Language, Speech, and Hearing Services in Schools, 22,* 69–74.

Tomblin, J. B., Hardy, J., & Hein, H. (1991). Predicting poor-communication status in preschool children using risk factors present at birth. *Journal of Speech and Hearing Research, 34,* 1096–1105.

Warren, D. (1981). Visual impairments. In J. Kauffman & D. Hallahan (Eds.), *Handbook of special education.* Englewood Cliffs, NJ: Prentice-Hall.

Whitehurst, G., Arnold, D., Smith, M., Fischel, J., Lonigan, C., & Valdez-Menchaca, M. (1991). Family history in developmental language delay. *Journal of Speech and Hearing Research, 34,* 1150–1157.

Wiig, E. (1989). *Steps to language competence: Developing metalinguistic strategies.* San Antonio, TX: The Psychological Corporation.

Wiig, E., & Secord, W. (1989). *Test of language competence—expanded edition.* San Antonio, TX: The Psychological Corporation.

Wiig, E., & Semel, E. (1984). *Language assessment and intervention for the learning disabled* (2nd ed.). New York: Merrill/Macmillan.

· Chapter 5 ·

Toddlers and Preschoolers with Specific Language Impairments

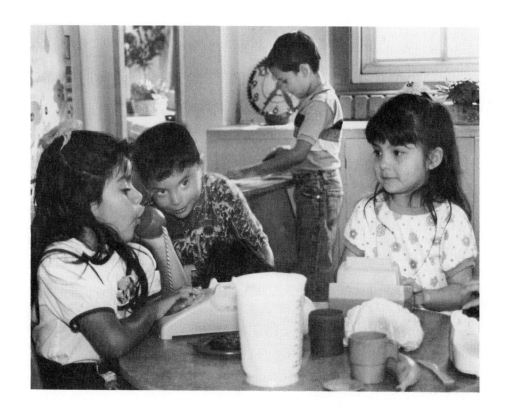

Upon completion of this chapter, the reader should be able to:

▶ Discuss issues related to whether the language problems of children with specific language impairments represent language delays or language disorders.

▶ Recognize the heterogeneous nature of children with specific language impairments and discuss whether or not subgroups of these children exist.

▶ List the various labels that have been used to describe this population of children, identify the issues related to causation, and discuss the relationship between these issues and the various labels.

▶ Discuss the prevalence figures that have been presented for youngsters with specific language impairments and the implications of the figures.

▶ Identify factors that may indicate which youngsters may outgrow early language problems and which may not.

▶ Recognize the relationship between language problems in the preschool years and later academic difficulties.

▶ Describe the various possible language and related characteristics of toddlers and preschoolers with specific language impairments.

▶ Discuss assessment and intervention considerations for toddlers and preschoolers with specific language impairments.

Although intense study of the language disorders of children is relatively new, copious information about language acquisition and children's language disorders has been amassed in the last 30 to 40 years. Despite the knowledge explosion, however, we still do not have a fully integrated and agreed-upon framework within which to discuss children and their language disorders. This is particularly true for toddlers and preschool children who show language problems in the apparent absence of other clearly identifiable problems. This chapter is about these young children who have language problems but who appear to be essentially normal in all other respects. We have chosen to use the phrase "specific language impairments" in the chapter title. This was done after much pondering. The decision was ultimately guided by a desire to distinguish as much as possible the topic of this chapter from the topics of subsequent chapters in this text. Using the phrase "specific language impairments" was not an easy choice because of several unanswered questions, one of which is whether these young children with language problems demonstrate language disorders or language delays. Another is the possibility that there may be subgroups of these children. How

we answer these questions can affect what labels we use when children demonstrate language problems not readily associated with other problems. Two other issues concern the prevalence data for preschool children with language impairments without obvious concomitant problems and our ability to predict who will outgrow early language problems. The intervention implications of these issues must also be considered. These are topics we address in this chapter. We also discuss language characteristics seen in some of these young children, and we introduce assessment and intervention considerations. It is becoming increasingly clear that language problems in the preschool years signal the real possibility of later academic, vocational, and social failures, topics taken up further in chapters 7 and 11.

AN OVERVIEW OF SPECIFIC LANGUAGE IMPAIRMENT

Delay versus Disorder

To say that a child demonstrates a *language delay* implies that specific language skills are slow to emerge or develop but that the child acquires the skills in the same sequence seen in normal children (Leonard, 1972, 1979). It further implies that the degree of delay is basically the same for all features or aspects of language (Kemp, 1983; Leonard, 1979). In contrast, the term *language disorder* implies a deviation from the usual rate and sequence with which specific language skills emerge. This deviation can include differences in the rate of acquisition of skills within one aspect of language (e.g., semantics or syntax), inordinate difficulties with certain features within one aspect of language, differences in the rate of acquisition among various aspects of language (e.g., pragmatic development related to syntactic development), and/or age-appropriate skills in one or more aspects, but with lags in acquisition of other aspects of language. Because of **asynchrony** in the rate of acquisition within and across various language parameters, the normal developmental sequence is disrupted. Despite the differences in these definitions, some children with language-learning problems have been referred to as *language delayed,* while others with similar language characteristics have been termed *language disordered.*

The issue of disorder versus delay has not been resolved by the research in this area. In the area of pragmatics, many authorities suggest that language-impaired youngsters are more similar to than different from normal language-learning children. For example, children with language impairments have been described as using the same range and variety of functions and intentions seen in normally developing children (e.g., Leonard, Camarata, Rowan, & Chapman, 1982; Rowan, Leonard, Chapman, & Weiss, 1983; Skarakis & Greenfield, 1982), but the language-impaired children may begin to use them more slowly. That is, compared to children of the same CA, children with language impairments are behind, but compared to normal language-learning children at the same language level, children with language impairments appear similar in their use of functions and intentions. Such findings are consistent with notions of delay in language development. However, others have suggested that there are differences in the frequency with which young language-impaired children use certain functions and intentions (Paul, 1991; Rom & Bliss, 1981; Snyder, 1975,

1978). This asynchrony suggests a deviance or disorder in these children's pragmatic development.

How we interpret these apparently conflicting results affects what we might conclude about delay versus disorder. If we interpret the findings as representing asynchrony in development, either within or across aspects of language, then we might conclude that this signals a disorder in pragmatic development. In contrast, others might conclude that pragmatic development was delayed if these findings are seen as reflecting constraints in other aspects of language (i.e., the children do not use a specific function frequently because their language abilities hinder them from encoding the function semantically or syntactically). However, if there is a delay because of other linguistic constraints, the question can be asked about the nature (delayed or disordered) of these constraints. This brings us to consider the areas of semantics and linguistic form (syntax, morphology, and phonology).

In the area of semantic development, or content of the language, children with specific language difficulties are frequently late in using their first words and slow in acquiring additional words (Leonard, 1988; Leonard, Bolders, & Miller, 1976; Morehead & Ingram, 1973; Paul, 1991; Rice, Buhr, & Nemeth, 1990). These findings are consistent with the characteristics we would expect to see in language delay, a position supported by others who have examined lexical acquisition of children with language-learning problems (Chapman, Leonard, Rowan, & Weiss, 1983). However, language-impaired children have sometimes been noted to code certain types of semantic relations more frequently than others typically coded by normal language-learning children (Bloom, 1980). Children with language impairments may also have special difficulties in learning quickly the meanings of particular classes of words that normal children generally acquire with ease (Rice et al., 1990). Furthermore, children with specific language impairments can have inordinate and persisting difficulties with certain types of words and expressions and their meanings, such as temporal and spatial terms, deictic words, figurative expressions, propositional meanings, and other words with abstract meanings (Johnston & Kamhi, 1984; Wiig, 1982; Wiig & Semel, 1976, 1984; Wood, 1982). Wiig

(1982) writes that children with language problems can "present striking and specific lags in vocabulary knowledge and use. Analysis of their patterns of errors on vocabulary comprehension tasks frequently indicates islands of specific difficulties in acquiring adequate meanings for selected word categories" (p. 266). These types of difficulties suggest a language disorder rather than a language delay. As we can see, the area of semantics does not help us resolve the issue, although Lahey (1988, p. 56) suggests that there are "more similarities than differences" in the semantic patterns of children with specific language impairments and those learning language normally.

Difficulties with aspects of language form may represent a particular problematic area for children with specific language impairments and in the later preschool years may differentiate them most noticeably from normally developing children (Leonard, 1989; Loeb & Leonard, 1991; van der Lely & Harris, 1990; Watkins & Rice, 1991). Lahey (1988) writes, "By far the most outstanding characteristic of this group of children [children with specific language impairments], and one that they all share, is late and slow development of form with better development of content and use interactions" (pp. 59–60). However, as with pragmatics and semantics, studies regarding the form of language (morphology, syntax, and phonology) have resulted in conflicting interpretations about whether the children demonstrate language delays or disorders.

In an early study, Menyuk (1969) observed that children with language difficulties produced syntactic sequences unlike those observed in children who were acquiring language normally. Examples of these utterances were "No ride feet" for an early-developing but more normal sequence "Ride no feet," "Big the dog" for "Dog big," and "Any more not pictures?" for "No more pictures?" Menyuk concluded:

> In some of the sentences that the children in the deviant speaking population produce there is also some evidence that they may be using rules or forming hypotheses about the structure of the language which are different from those of the normal-speaking population. Nevertheless, these utterances also seem to reflect the fact that certain types of generalizations are being made about their language by these children, although, in some instances, they are different from those made by normal-speaking children. (p. 134)

Such a conclusion about syntactic development supports the language disorder position. Others have found differences in the syntactic skills of children with specific language impairments that suggest disorder, not just delay (e.g., Grimm & Weinert, 1990; van der Lely & Harris, 1990). There is also a suggestion in the literature that children with specific language impairments may differ from normally developing children in the types of learning situations they need to acquire morphological or syntactic forms (Connell, 1987; Connell & Stone, 1992; Weismer & Murray-Branch, 1989). This, too, tends to support the notion of disorder. Young children who are slow in beginning to talk and preschoolers who have been identified as language impaired have also been shown to differ qualitatively in their phonological development (e.g., Paul & Jennings, 1992; Wetherby, Yonclas, & Bryan, 1989), a factor lending further support to the disorder perspective.

In contrast, others suggest that the syntactic development of language-impaired children represents a delay, not a disorder (e.g., Curtiss, Katz, & Tallal, 1992; Eisenson & Ingram, 1972; Leonard, 1979; Morehead & Ingram, 1973). With regard to grammatical morphemes, Johnston and Schery (1976) reported that children with language difficulties learned these linguistic features in the same sequence as normal children but at a much slower rate. These findings support the language delay position. Other positions regarding phonological skills are also conflicting and do not help reconcile the disorder–delay issue (e.g., Grunwell, 1980; Ingram, 1976; Leonard, 1982b; Schwartz, Leonard, Folger, & Wilcox, 1980).

One reason for these conflicting interpretations is that a problem with any one aspect or component of language will affect other aspects, so that the entire language performance appears disturbed. Carrow-Woolfolk and Lynch (1982) explain that "a simplification of the language code is the expected result of a problem in any specific language area" (p. 297). *Although we may talk about the components of language separately, in actuality all components interact at one time, with one component, therefore, affecting others* (e.g., Campbell & Shriberg, 1982; Lahey, 1988;

Leonard et al., 1982; Masterson & Kamhi, 1992; Nelson & Bauer, 1991; Paul, 1992; Paul & Shriberg, 1982; Reed, 1992; Schwartz et al., 1980). Generally, all we see is the total performance. Unless research designs of investigations of children's language address the possible synergistic effects among language components, results regarding delay versus disorder can be very difficult to interpret. Research design issues may, therefore, confound our ability to resolve this ongoing debate.

In light of the unresolved issue of delay versus disorder, the usefulness of *specific language impairment* as a construct has recently been questioned. Leonard (1987, 1991) suggests that the language abilities seen in children with specific language impairment may simply be those observed at the lower end of a continuum of normal variation. Rather than having a language disorder, the children simply are not as good at learning and using language as other children, in the same way that other children may not be as good at learning and using musical skills, for example. In following through with this analogy, the children on the low end of musical skill performance would likely not be seen to have a disorder, but rather would reflect the normal variation in performance within and across individuals. Similarly, the children on the low end of language skill performance would not be seen to have a disorder, but rather would reflect the normal variation within and across individuals. Some children are just better at some things than others, and children differ in what they are strong or weak at learning and doing. From this perspective, it is only because language abilities are so highly regarded in Western societies, and because language abilities are so intimately tied to the Western process of formal education and academic success, which are also highly regarded in these societies, that weaker skills in language may be considered a disorder.

Others reject this view or at least are not ready to accept it and/or its implications (e.g., Aram, 1991; Johnston, 1991; Lahey, 1988; Tomblin, 1991). Lahey (1988) writes that "some children who fit this syndrome [specific language impairment] have such severe difficulties with language learning that if this same degree of difficulty were apparent in motor impairment, for example, they might well be classified as having a disorder or disability" (p. 54). This counter-perspective suggests that the inordinate problems some of these children have in learning and generalizing certain language skills, and their continuing difficulties with language, cannot be viewed as anything but a disability. It is possible that we have erred in our research by grouping all children with "specific language impairment" together. That is, there may be subgroups within this population (Aram, 1991), and children in different subgroups may reflect different language patterns, have different reasons for their language problems, progress differently in language acquisition, and have different outcomes of their language difficulties.

Subgroups of Young Children with Specific Language Impairments?

In the previous chapter, three approaches to children's language disorders were presented. Two of them (Bloom & Lahey, 1978; Fey, 1986) included subgroups of children, and the third included subcategories of language dimensions (Carrow-Woolfolk & Lynch, 1982). Although these approaches addressed language performance and language disorders of children generally, rather than focusing particularly on toddlers and preschoolers with specific language impairments, each approach divided children's language disorders into parts or placed children into different categories. To understand young children with specific language impairments more fully, we may need to consider the possibility that subgroups of these children exist. If this is the case, we need to ask what the relevant subgroups may be.

Some children described as specifically language impaired have difficulties with both language comprehension and expression. Other children have problems with language expression but normal or near-normal comprehension. Still others have comprehension problems alone. Three likely subgroups are, therefore, implicated (Lahey, 1988):

1. Both comprehension and expression difficulties.
2. Expression difficulties only.
3. Comprehension difficulties only (although this pattern appears to occur less frequently than the first two).

This model for subgroups may, however, be too simplistic. Phonological problems have been found to co-occur frequently with syntax problems (e.g., Ekelman & Aram, 1983; Paul, 1991; Paul & Shriberg, 1982). Additionally, differences in gestures representing **symbolic play** have been associated with early language difficulties (Thal & Bates, 1988; Thal, Tobias, & Morrison, 1991). Paul, Looney, and Dahm (1991) also found a relationship between early language deficits and certain socialization characteristics. On the basis of their findings, they proposed four subgroups:

1. Deficits in expression only.
2. Deficits in expression and socialization, with normal comprehension.
3. Deficits in expression, comprehension, and socialization.
4. Deficits in expression and comprehension, with normal socialization.

Of the subjects in this study, one third fell into the first category (expressive deficits only) and about 38% fell into the second (deficits in both expression and socialization, with normal comprehension). Together these two categories accounted for approximately 70% of the children in their study.

If we consider only the five potential deficit areas mentioned thus far (comprehension, expression, pho-

nology, socialization, symbolic play gestures), we can see in Table 5.1 some, but not all, of the combinations that might lead to possible subgroups of children. If we break down expression into the possible specific aspects of language (e.g., semantics, pragmatics, syntax, morphology) that may be problematic, we see even greater complexity in the possible combinations. Furthermore, it may not be valid to separate some of these factors because of the overlaps, interrelationships, and associations that are known to operate across linguistic components and among and across other behaviors (e.g., relationships between measures of socialization and use of communicative intentions/ functions). Our factors or areas of deficit might not be correct and/or discrete. Other factors and associations have also been implicated in specific language disorders (e.g., behavioral difficulties). Additionally, we would likely need to consider possible causal factors, as well as the relative degree of skill (or deficit) in each possible area. It is possible that the combinations could change with CA in an individual child. The syndrome we refer to as *specific language impairment* may be too large and inclusive to account for the heterogeneity seen in these children. It may be that "children with specific language impairment do not represent a single clinical entity, but rather are a cluster of subgroups whose overlapping and defining fea-

TABLE 5.1   Examples of Areas of Deficit Leading to Some Possible Subgroups of Children with Specific Language Impairments

Subgroups	Expression	Comprehension	Phonology	Socialization	Symbolic Play via Gesture
1	X	X	X	X	X
2	X	X		X	X
3	X	X	X		X
4	X		X	X	
5	X		X		
6	X	X			X
7	X			X	
8	X				
9		X			X
10		X	X	X	X
11		X		X	X

ture is that of a language impairment" (Aram, 1991, p. 84). However, our present knowledge does not allow us to identify valid subgroups, even though this task is currently receiving a great deal of research interest.

A Label for It and Its Causes

In the introduction to this chapter, the dilemma regarding its title was raised. Many terms have been used in the literature to label the condition in which language difficulties appear to be the sole problem of these children. Among these terms are *specific language impairment* (SLI), *specific language disability, specific language disorder, developmental aphasia, developmental dysphasia, language delay, developmental language disorder, expressive* and/or *receptive language delay, clinical language disorder, language disorder,* and *slow expressive language development* (SELD), although this last term tends to be used with toddlers more frequently than with older preschool children. When these children go to school and their language problems begin to cause academic difficulties, a situation that is likely to occur, the children may be referred to as *learning disabled* or *language-learning disabled.*

Part of the terminology problem relates to our discussion in the preceding chapter on classification and categorization and to our previous discussion in this chapter on disorder versus delay. Use of the term *delay* or *disorder* in the label depends largely on one's orientation, and as we have seen, this issue has not been resolved. We also indicated in the previous chapter that the cause(s) of a language problem cannot always be identified, a situation that has added to the terminology confusion when children's problems seem confined to language. These children typically have adequate hearing sensitivity at the time of testing, normal nonverbal intelligence test scores, apparently no severe emotional problems, no gross neurological deviations, and apparently adequate environmental opportunities to learn language.

Without obvious hearing, intellectual, cognitive, emotional, neurological, or environmental deficits, the search for explanations has sometimes turned to other, more subtle reasons for the language difficulties. Some authors and researchers have proposed that, in the absence of gross neurological problems,

the children's language difficulties must stem from mild central nervous system dysfunction; thus the terms *minimal brain dysfunction* and *minimal brain injury* have been suggested. In the past, however, no conclusive link was identified between abnormal brain function measurements and the language problems of children. The general superiority of the left cerebral hemisphere over the right in adults' language functioning has been well established. However, in chapter 2 we pointed out that early damage to the left hemisphere in children has not been shown to account for the severity or persistence of their language impairments. Damage to or dysfunction of both the left and right hemispheres has been implicated in the language difficulties of these children (Bashir, Kuban, Kleinman, & Scavuzzo, 1983; Johnston, Stark, Mellits, & Tallal, 1981), although definitive data are still lacking. More recently, advances in technology leading to neuroimaging (e.g., positron emission tomography, magnetic resonance imaging) and event-related electrophysiological procedures have begun to be used with children with language impairments (Cohen, Campbell, & Yaghmai, 1989; Stefanatos, Green, & Ratcliff, 1989). These applications are still in their infancy but, based on early findings regarding anatomical and/or brain functioning, they may hold promise in investigations of causal factors. However, because the terms *developmental aphasia* and *developmental dysphasia* tend to suggest neurological involvement and because the existence of central nervous system dysfunction still has not been unequivocally substantiated, these terms are not used as frequently as several of the other labels.

Another area of investigation in the search for a causal factor involves how children process information in their external environments (Grimm & Weinert, 1990; Leonard, 1989; Tallal, Stark, Kallman, & Mellits, 1981). Much of this attention has been directed to processing of auditory information and auditory perceptual functioning. A basis for this focus is the idea that these children do not handle information in their environments in the same way as normal language-learning children. In chapter 2 we discussed the complexities of the interactions between auditory perception, auditory processing, and language. The question of possible deficits in these areas as causal factors in children's language problems remains unresolved.

Issues regarding information processing deficits generally remain unresolved. Additionally, the question of the underlying reasons for perceptual or processing problems (if they exist when a child has a language problem) suggests the possibility of neurological dysfunction, and as we have just discussed, that question, too, is unanswered. Recurring ear infections that interfere directly with children's language learning or indirectly with language performances by affecting auditory perceptual/processing development have been offered as still other possible explanations for children's language difficulties. Although some children with language problems do have a history of ear infections, as discussed in chapters 2 and 9, this does not explain the presence of impaired language abilities in children with no histories of ear infections or of adequate language skills in other children with frequent ear infections.

Still another suggestion is that children with language problems have difficulty accessing language information that they already know (e.g., Connell & Stone, 1992; German, 1979, 1982; Leonard, Nippold, Kail, & Hale, 1983). That is, the children can take information in but have trouble tapping it for use. This suggestion raises the question of what causes the access problem in the first place. Another question is, how can an access problem account for those children who demonstrate comprehension problems?

Although language-impaired children may demonstrate normal nonverbal intelligence skills, specific deficits in cognitive functioning, such as symbolic play, hypothesis formation and testing, and representational thought, have been suggested as causing language problems or, at least, correlating with them. If this is the case, the terms *specific language impairment, specific language disability,* and *specific language disorder* may be inappropriate (Leonard, 1982a). However, deficit cognitive functioning has not always been found in language-impaired children. Even if it were, this raises the question of the underlying reasons for the cognitive deficits. Studies of the language-learning environments and the emotional development of language-impaired children have yielded equally equivocal results. Given the lack of substantive data and the conflicting evidence about the causes of language impairments in children whose problems *appear* to be

confined to language functioning, it is no wonder that some professionals have opted for a noncausative approach and that disagreement on what to call the problem continues. As Lahey (1988) has stated:

> The question about the cause (or causes) of a language-learning problem in a particular child remains an intriguing and usually an unanswerable question. If we understood how the non-language-disordered child learns language and the relative role of, for example, cognitive, social, and environmental factors, we would have clearer hypotheses about why some children do not learn language easily. Clearly, the lack of an agreed-upon theory of language development hinders our search for an understanding of developmental language disorders. (p. 45)

The question about causation may not have to remain unanswered forever. We are beginning to rethink our approaches. For example, studying children with specific language impairments may help us understand more about normal language learning. In using some of the findings regarding weaknesses of children with specific language impairments, Johnston (1991) suggests that these results may show us what abilities are required to learn language normally:

▷ perception of short duration, sequenced acoustic events, AND
▷ a responsive, anticipatory attentional mechanism, AND
▷ the ability, maybe even vision, to use symbols, AND
▷ the ability to invent syntax, AND
▷ enough mental energy to do this all at once. (p. 77)

Furthermore, if there are subgroups of children with specific language impairment, as discussed earlier, there may be different causal factors for each subgroup. Aram (1991) suggests that to progress in our search for causal factors, "we need to recognize the heterogeneity of observable language behavior and the heterogeneity of potential causal factors. We will not progress if our aim is to identify *the* cause for *the* category of specific language disorder" (p. 86).

Tomblin (1991) presents two possible models of the relationship between causal factors and language performance. In Figure 5.1, deficits in language performance result from "missing, different, or maybe additional variables" (p. 71) or causal factors. This is the

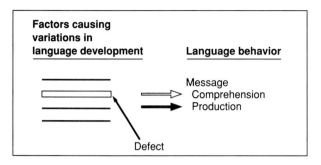

FIGURE 5.1 A Schematic Model of Language Disorder in Which Variation in Language Development Is Produced by Unique Causal Factors or Defects. (From "Examining the Cause of Specific Language Impairment" by J. B. Tomblin, 1991, *Language, Speech, and Hearing Services in Schools, 22*, p. 72. Copyright © 1991 by the American Speech-Language-Hearing Association. Reprinted by permission.)

model that has generally been used in the search for cause(s) and may be the reason for the conflicting or equivocal results. The alternative model, seen in Figure 5.2, approaches possible causal factors in terms of the degree to which each factor may be present in a child. This model views causal factors in relation to each other. Each factor likely operates on a continuum and in relation to each of the other factors. This model has not been used widely to guide research into causes. In using it in combination with the suggestion

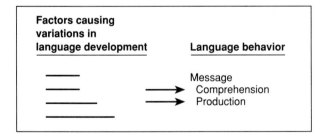

FIGURE 5.2 A Schematic Model of Language Disorder in Which the Causes of Variations in Language Development Differ by Amount, as Represented by the Lengths of the Lines. (From "Examining the Cause of Specific Language Impairment" by J. B. Tomblin, 1991, *Language, Speech, and Hearing Services in Schools, 22*, p. 71. Copyright © 1991 by the American Speech-Language-Hearing Association. Reprinted by permission.)

that subgroups might exist, we could hypothesize that differing combinations of different causal factors in varying amounts could lead to different profiles of language performance. These ideas represent some of the ways in which rethinking the issue of causation in specific language impairment may provide useful avenues for future research that will help in unraveling the puzzle.

Prevalence

If a child has a language delay, we might think that the child will probably catch up with little or no help and, once caught up, would continue to develop much like the peer group. Alternatively, if a child has a language disorder, we might think that the child will not catch up without more than a little help and, even if caught up, may continue to need help to progress at the same rate as the peer group. In reality, some children do catch up and continue to develop, some who appear to catch up fall behind again at older ages, and some have little chance of catching up unless help is provided. Therefore, we may see different **prevalence** figures at different ages.

Vocabulary development is one of the first obvious signs of language growth in very young children. One of the earliest signs that a child may have problems with language is using the first word late or not acquiring many additional words after the first word. Between 18 and 24 months of age, signs that a child may have language problems may include absence of a vocabulary growth spurt, failing to combine words into two-word utterances, and generally talking very little. About 10–15% of 2-year-old children fit this picture (Rescorla, 1989). Yet, some of these toddlers catch up later. These children are often referred to as *late bloomers*.

As we have indicated, however, some of the toddlers who demonstrate *slow expressive language development (SELD)*[1] in their first 2 years continue to lag

---

[1]The current literature on toddlers has so far refrained from using the term *specific language impairment* to refer to these young children. Rather, *slow expressive language development* (SELD) has been the preferred descriptor. In keeping with this trend, SELD will be used in this section of the chapter.

behind in their language development as they grow older. In reviewing the work of several researchers, Paul (1991) suggests that 40–50% of children who are slow in language development at 2 years continue to have expressive language deficits at 3 years, the age at which language skill begins to be measured more by syntactic and morphological abilities than by vocabulary. If we calculate 40–50% of the 10–15% figure given earlier, we arrive at a 4–7.5% prevalence figure for expressive language problems in the 3-year age group. In a study tracking 28 toddlers with SELD, Paul and Smith (1991) found that 57% of these children had persisting expressive language deficits related to narrative skills at 4 years of age. As Paul (1991) points out, this "finding is particularly significant because narrative skills in preschoolers have been shown to be one of the best predictors of school success" (p. 8).

How many of these SELD children will continue to show language problems at 5 years of age? From the results of one study, 5-year-olds who had been slow in their early expressive, but not receptive, language development had expressive vocabulary performances and general verbal fluency skills that were not obviously different from those of their normally developing peers (Whitehurst, Fischel, et al., 1991). Although this study did not include measures of syntactic or pragmatic abilities, the authors reported that if any problems in these areas at 5 years of age did exist, they were "subtle and not apparent" (p. 67). These findings may suggest that the children had caught up to their normally developing peers. Bishop and Edmundson (1987) also found that many SELD children appeared to catch up by school age.

There may be danger in accepting these findings without some evaluation. First, findings such as those of Whitehurst, Fischel, and their colleagues (1991) could be interpreted as suggesting an extremely low prevalence rate by 5 years of age for children who begin with SELD, but the experience of professionals who have worked with young children tells us that this may not be true. Accepting these findings could also cause us to take a "wait and see" approach to providing intervention for SELD toddlers and preschoolers in the belief that they will outgrow the problem. This approach could seriously hinder children who need

early intervention if this finding is wrong. A further concern relates to the measures of language performance employed in the research. It may be that, in contrast to the skills examined in these studies, more in-depth, complex language skills may remain deficit (Paul, 1991). Recall from the previous chapter Lahey's (1990) suggestion that our identification procedures need to examine children's language abilities under conditions that stress the language system. Recall, also, that language form (e.g., syntax, morphology) is often especially problematic for children with specific language impairment and that narrative skills may be predictive of school success. Language deficits may also become more selective or narrow as children grow older (Scarborough & Dobrich, 1990; Whitehurst, Fischel et al., 1991), affecting language performance less globally and more specifically for certain aspects of language. These factors suggest that tasks such as complex sentence usage and narrative skill, in situations that challenge children's language performance, need to be utilized with older preschool children to tap their levels of language competence (Lahey, 1990; Paul, 1991). It is also possible that 2-year-old children who have both expressive and receptive language deficits, rather than expressive vocabulary delays only, will develop differently as they get older.

Another concern relates to a pattern of normal language development in which 5-year-old children seem to plateau but show a language growth spurt again between ages 6 and 7 (Scarborough & Dobrich, 1990). Because normally developing children may plateau at about 5 years of age, 5-year-old children with a history of SELD may appear to catch up (Scarborough & Dobrich, 1990). However, when their peers' language skills move ahead again a year or two later, the children with SELD may be left behind at a time when acquisition of literacy skills, which are heavily dependent on oral language abilities, becomes critical for future academic success. Certain aspects of language behavior may also plateau at different ages (Scarborough & Dobrich, 1990), producing the illusion of recovery for different language skills at different times. This could create an impression of differing profiles of language adequacy in different children at different ages. A final concern relates to what other skills children with SELD may *not* be learning while catching up that their normal language-learning peers can learn because they do not have to use their learning resources to develop more basic language skills.

It is possible that (1) children with a history of SELD give the illusion of recovery and then relapse; (2) if subgroups of young children with language difficulties exist, they may show different patterns of language growth, recovery, and relapse; (3) some language skills may catch up but others do not, and findings may depend on which skills have been measured; and (4) SELD children spend learning resources and learning time catching up and, therefore, miss out on other learning, which may eventually affect their school performances. Paul (1991) writes that the interpretation of findings suggesting that these children catch up by 5 years of age needs to consider the following:

▷ whether the full range of language skills that are important at this age—and not detectable in measures of expressive vocabulary size, general verbal fluency, or unstructured conversation (such as complex sentence use and narrative skill)—is evaluated,

▷ whether any recovery that does appear to be completed by age 5 is stable, or will again be outpaced by development in normal children over the course of the next year or two, when their rate of language growth accelerates, in conjunction with the acquisition of literacy skills, and

▷ even if oral language skills do appear to eventually remain within the normal range by the end of the preschool period, whether the underlying processes that slowed them down at first continue to operate, now influencing primarily the learning of reading, writing, and spelling, as seems to be the case for so many youngsters with a history of language delay. (pp. 9–10)

Until more studies have followed toddlers with SELD into the school years, perhaps we should not wait and see in deciding whether intervention is warranted. The alternative of not intervening when necessary or not monitoring language growth closely may place these children at further risk for failure. The problem with this approach is, of course, that professional resources may be redirected from children who

are most in need to those who might outgrow their slow starts with language development.

As we have indicated, there is no question that preschoolers with continuing language problems in the apparent absence of other problems run the risk of academic failure when they enter school (e.g., Aram & Nation, 1980; Garvey & Gordon, 1973; Tallal, 1988; Vogel, 1977; Weiner, 1985). In fact, in chapter 11 we see that the difficulties created by language problems first evident in the preschool years can continue into and through adolescence and even into adulthood (Aram, Ekelman, & Nation, 1984; Hall & Tomblin, 1978; Tomblin, Freese, & Records, 1992; Weiner, 1974; Wiig & Fleischmann, 1980). Prevalence data on the occurrence of language problems in school-age children are, however, conflicting. Several authors suggest a 3–5% figure (e.g., Silva, 1980; Stevenson & Richman, 1976). In contrast, Leske (1981) gives a prevalence figure of 1%, which represents a considerable drop from the preliminary prevalence data for toddlers and preschoolers. It is this figure that concerned Snyder (1984). Previously, we suggested that the academic difficulties stemming from language deficits may lead to referring to school-age children as *language-learning disabled* or *learning disabled,* a topic taken up in more detail in chapter 7. In combination with a possible false recovery period for oral language skills in the early school years, this relabeling may account for a "great disappearing act" (Snyder, 1984, p. 129). That is, once in school, children with specific language impairments may no longer be seen as language impaired in tallies of children with disabilities. Rather, they are counted in a different category. To support her position, Snyder notes that the prevalence figures for learning disabilities are higher in states where language problems and learning disabilities are combined under one label, *learning disability,* and lower in states where the term *learning disability* is used separately from *language disorder.*

The implications of these prevalence figures raise several questions about intervention for school-age, language-disordered children. One question concerns the legalities and ethics of providing appropriate intervention for these children. If a child demonstrates language deficits with resulting academic difficulties, intervention for both problematic areas would likely be more effective than intervention for either problem alone. Unfortunately, funding issues and the definitional criteria for categorizing disabled children that some educational systems use mean that such a combined approach is not always the situation for these children. A second question concerns professional territorialism. We will not enter the debate of which professional group should serve these children. Instead, we believe that when the children receive intervention for both their learning problems and their underlying language deficits, professional territorialism becomes a nonissue. An issue exists only when intervention for one problem is provided. This may, however, be as much of an ethical and a legal issue as a territorial one. Children whose language problems underlie learning problems need to have their language impairments accurately identified, and they deserve intervention for both the language deficits and resulting academic difficulties.

Prediction

In the previous chapter we presented some of the factors that may place children at risk for language problems. Here we will focus on young children with specific language impairment and on some of their language and behavioral characteristics that may help us predict which ones will catch up permanently and which will not.

PL 99–457, with its emphasis on toddlers and preschoolers, has stimulated considerable research designed to help predict which children with early language delays need early intervention and which "can confidently be left alone to outgrow the problem" (Paul, 1991, p. 1). Although much of this research is still in its infancy, a number of predictive factors may be emerging. For the most part, this research is designed to track children who fail to achieve very early language developmental milestones on a variety of language and nonlanguage factors from 18 to 24 months of age through the preschool years.

Table 5.2 lists several of the factors that may help predict which toddlers and preschoolers are at risk for continuing language problems. These are socialization skills, use of communicative intentions, characteristics

of babble, skill in using symbolic gestures and frequency of gesture use generally, phonological patterns, and behavioral characteristics. Comprehension skills are conspicuously absent from the table. One might think that youngsters who have both expressive and receptive deficits would be more likely to have continuing language problems as they mature than those with only expressive deficits. However, comprehension skills are missing from the table because the current research findings are in conflict. For example, Thal et al. (1991) found that poor vocabulary comprehension in toddlers with expressive language problems was a predictive factor for expressive language problems 1 year later. In contrast, Paul et al. (1991) reported that comprehension delays did not appear to be predictive, although they acknowledged that their data base may have been too small to draw a definitive conclusion. Also absent from the list is MLU, which Thal et al. (1991) found was not a reliable indicator of the future language abilities of toddlers who had had SELD. After initial delays, expressive vocabulary growth in the preschool years also does not appear to predict later expressive language abilities (Paul, 1991; Thal et al., 1991). In fact, there is some evidence that lexical ability is one area where toddlers with early limited expressive vocabularies may eventually catch up (Paul, 1991; Scarborough & Dobrich, 1990; Whitehurst, Fischel, et al., 1991). One difficulty with this suggestion, however, is the way in which lexical skills are measured. Earlier we indicated that children with specific language impairments may have persisting problems with words with abstract or multiple/figurative meanings. If expressive vocabulary is examined primarily for words with concrete meanings, children with early expressive language problems might appear to catch up. Additionally, the ability to retrieve words rapidly is a language skill that needs to be assessed, as there is evidence that this skill may be problematic for specifically language-impaired children. Word retrieval abilities of young children may even predict later reading difficulties in school (Menyuk et al., 1991). Perhaps judgment about the predictive value of expressive vocabulary skills, as well as that of other expressive semantic abilities, should be reserved pending further research.

TABLE 5.2 Factors Potentially Predicting Continuing Language Problems

Factor	Explanation
Socialization (Paul, 1991; Paul et al., 1991)	Possible deficits in social skills (e.g., smiling appropriately, playing social games)
Communicative intentions (Paul, 1991)	Range of communicative intentions appropriate, but frequency of use reduced; particular reduction in frequency of comment/joint attention
Babbling (Whitehurst, Smith, et al., 1991)	Less language growth in children with more vowel babble and greater language growth for children with more consonantal babble; greater language growth also related to greater babble complexity; may be related to phonology (see below)
Gestures (Thal & Tobias, 1992; Thal et al., 1991)	Production of symbolic gestures in familiar script routines (e.g., bathing a teddy bear) reduced; ability to produce symbolic gestures positively related to comprehension vocabulary level; less frequent use of gestures generally (may be related to reduced frequency of communicative intentions produced gesturally)
Phonology (Paul, 1991; Paul & Jennings, 1992; Whitehurst, Fischel, et al., 1991)	Less complex syllable structure (e.g., CV versus CVC versus C_1VC_2V); fewer consonants in phonetic repertoire; continuing phonological difficulties throughout preschool years; may be related to babbling (see above)
Behavior (Paul, 1991; Whitehurst, Smith et al., 1991)	Children described as overly active and difficult to manage; less language growth in children with behavior problems

LANGUAGE CHARACTERISTICS OF CHILDREN WITH SPECIFIC LANGUAGE IMPAIRMENT

In this section, we review a number of the language characteristics observed in toddlers and preschool children with specific language impairment. In approaching this topic, we need to be aware that not all children demonstrate all of these problems and that a problem with one aspect of language can result in problems with other aspects. These potentially diverse patterns reemphasize the fact that specifically language-impaired children represent a heterogeneous group. Additionally, we need to be aware that some of the same problems can be observed in school-age children and adolescents with language disorders, albeit at more advanced language levels.

Some Language Precursors

Recognition of and attention to environmental change are important in language acquisition. Some toddlers and preschoolers seem not to realize when their environments change. Or, if these children recognize such changes, they do not attend to them for a sustained period. In chapter 3, we saw that children often first learn words that represent a change in the environment or that refer to objects they can manipulate and change. Without recognizing change and/or without attending to novel stimuli, a child will not develop the underlying concepts of language. Furthermore, children need to learn that they themselves can be the agents of change, something that certain infants fail to understand. Unless children realize that what they do modifies objects' or people's behaviors, they will be unlikely to learn that language is one of the most effective ways of producing change.

The abilities to participate in reciprocal interactions and to establish joint reference with an adult also appear to be precursors to language. Early child–adult behaviors of give-and-take play routines and repetitive games like pattycake may be prerequisites of conversational turn-taking skills. These activities also teach attention to gestures and speech, anticipation of events, and adaptation of behaviors to contexts. Some preschoolers with specific language impairments fail to learn these reciprocal routines. These children may also not engage frequently in joint attention or learn to utilize cues provided by joint reference with an adult. *Joint reference* refers to an adult's and child's mutual attention either to each other or to some object or event. It can function as a form of social interaction or as an activity used to learn about the environment. One of a child's earliest evidences of the ability to establish joint reference is making eye contact with an adult (**mutual gaze**). Eye contact serves not only as a base for interpersonal interactions but also as a way of indicating attention. Following an adult's visual gaze toward an object or event is another way of indicating joint reference, as is following an adult's pointing gesture. It is from joint reference that a child is able to abstract the salient features of the object or event as the adult provides the linguistic form for the referent. We can see how failure to make joint reference can potentially hinder language development. Table 5.2 indicates that young children with early delayed expressive language who may be at risk for continuing language impairment engage in fewer joint attentional intentions than children without early language delays (Paul, 1991).

Some have suggested that communicative intents in general may be encoded by specifically language-impaired children more by gestures and vocalizations than by verbal means (Caulfield, 1989; Coggins, 1991; Wetherby et al., 1989). The reasons for this pattern are unclear. One possibility is that the nonverbal means of communicating intentions are working for the children, so there is little need to learn verbal means. Another is that they find alternative ways of communicating their intentions because of their reduced verbal skills. In contrast, Table 5.2 suggests that

reduced ability to produce *symbolic* gestures reflecting script routines may presage ongoing problems (Thal et al., 1991). Additionally, Thal and Tobias (1992) found that toddlers about 2 years old with SELD who continued to have language problems 1 year later used fewer gestures generally than either their normal language-learning peers or other toddlers with SELD who appeared to have caught up in language development 1 year later.

In chapter 2, we saw that certain language skills and cognitive abilities emerge in children at about the same time. Two of the co-occurring events often noted are the use of illocutionary acts (intentional preverbal communicative acts) and acquisition of cognitive behaviors seen in the late sensorimotor stage. Data do not presently allow us to state that the relationship between these late sensorimotor stage achievements and the emergence of illocutionary, or performative, acts is causal. Instead, it may be that the relationship is correlative (Bates, Benigni, Bretherton, Camaioni, & Volterra, 1977; Steckol & Leonard, 1981; Thal, 1991), the position proposed by the homologue model of language and cognition. That is, the abilities in both areas appear at approximately the same time, instead of the appearance of one resulting in the emergence of the other. However, unless a child has attained skills corresponding to sensorimotor stage V or possibly late stage IV, the child may not use gestures, vocalizations, and other nonverbal signals for intentional communication. The reverse may also be true. Unless a child uses illocutionary acts, the child may not attain sensorimotor stage V skills. In this sense, we can see how preschoolers who are delayed in achieving either of these developmental milestones may be delayed in achieving the other.

The relationship between babbling and the production of first words is not well understood. However, there is a preliminary suggestion that the phonetic content of babbled vocalizations affects early lexicons and may even be a distinguishing feature of some children with language problems (Stoel-Gammon, 1991; Whitehurst, Smith, Fischel, Arnold, & Lonigan, 1991). In order to produce a variety of single words, one might anticipate that children may need to have several different consonants in their repertoires and use these consonants in different distributions and in combinations with different vowels. In this way, the syllable structure of babble might be a precursor to the use of first words. Several authors have suggested that the consonantal composition and syllabic complexity of babble in children with early expressive language delays are reduced (Paul & Jennings, 1992; Stoel-Gammon, 1991; Whitehurst, Smith, et al., 1991). As we recall from Table 5.2, these characteristics of babbling may also be predictive of later language problems in toddlers and preschoolers.

Phonology

Toddlers and preschoolers with specific language impairments frequently have concomitant phonological problems. By about 2 years of age, normally developing children are moderately intelligible. In contrast, it is not unusual to find 3- and 4-year-old children with specific language impairments who are difficult to understand. However, there is some suggestion in the literature that many of the phonological problems preschoolers with specific language impairments experience may appear to resolve by school age (e.g., Whitehurst, Fischel, et al., 1991).

The relationship between phonological difficulties and specific language impairments has not yet been explained, although we have suggested that early phonological problems may predict later poor language performance. Some have proposed that problems with phonological acquisition simply reflect more general language-learning problems. Others suggest that phonological problems may be characteristics of subgroups within the larger, heterogeneous group of specifically language-impaired children. There may even be subgroups within the group of children with phonological disorders in the apparent absence of concomitant language impairments. Whatever the relationship between specific language impairment and phonological problems, we know that young children with specific language impairments acquire more quickly single words that begin with consonants they use correctly in other words than words that begin with consonants not yet produced correctly (Leonard, Schwartz, et al., 1982). This relationship between phonology and lexical acquisition is consistent with a developmental pattern seen in normally developing

toddlers (Schwartz & Leonard, 1982). Also, one study shows that about 20–30% of the preschool children who experienced phonological difficulties not related to apparently concomitant problems in other areas received special education services when they entered school, even though many of them showed no obvious evidence of phonological difficulties at that time (Shriberg & Kwiatkowski, 1988). This may imply that phonological problems in the preschool years influence children's ability to achieve academically in areas related to linguistic skills, possibly because of phonological processing difficulties (Catts, 1989).

Semantics

Of all the language skill areas in children with specific language impairments, we know the least about their semantic skills (Crystal, 1987; Leonard, 1988; Rice et al., 1990). This is true even though we know that a delay in using the first word (usually at about 12 months of age) and failure to show a spurt in single-word learning between 18 and 24 months of age are frequently the first signs of possible language problems. We have also indicated that children with early delays in vocabulary growth may catch up in terms of vocabulary size, but that this growth must be interpreted carefully because it does not necessarily mean that specifically language-impaired children do not have semantic difficulties. For some children, semantic deficits lie in the classes of words they acquire. The children may learn words for certain classes of concepts but may have trouble learning words for other concept classes, which are often abstract or figurative in nature.

As we recall from chapter 3, normal language-learning children overgeneralize the meanings of words and then gradually learn to narrow the meanings as they acquire new words to represent the more defined concepts. Preschoolers with specific language impairment may continue to use overgeneralizations instead of learning new, more restricted meanings and their corresponding words. In contrast, other words may represent context-specific or item-specific learning (Chapman et al., 1983). This means that specifically language-impaired preschoolers may continue to use words for which the meanings are underextended.

When words and their meanings join with other words and their meanings in multiword utterances, *composite meanings* evolve. For example, children learn that the separate possessor–possession semantic relation ("baby ball") and the agent–action semantic relation ("ball roll") can combine to one utterance ("baby ball roll") that expresses a composite meaning of the two relations. The range of two-word semantic relations described by Brown (1973) provides for a variety of propositional meanings that can be combined into more advanced forms. Although preschoolers with specific language impairments generally appear to acquire the range of semantic relations expressed by normal language-learning children, these children may do so more slowly than their language-normal peers (Freedman & Carpenter, 1976; Leonard et al., 1976). Additionally, specifically language-impaired children may experience difficulties in learning to combine semantic relations into utterances with more advanced composite meanings. It is not completely clear whether this latter difficulty relates primarily to problems with the semantic aspects of language or to problems in acquiring syntactic and/or morphological patterns.

In chapter 3 we discussed normal children's ability to learn a lot about a word's meaning from very few and fleeting exposures to the word in context. We referred to this ability as *fast mapping* or *quick incidental learning*. Young children with specific language impairments have been found to demonstrate at least some fast mapping abilities (e.g., Dollaghan, 1987; Rice, Buhr, & Oetting, 1992; Rice et al., 1990). In one study utilizing a highly structured situation, young children with specifically impaired language learned the name of a novel object as readily as normal children (Dollaghan, 1987). However, in a study that involved the more challenging task of learning the meanings of words embedded in an ongoing narrative situation, the children with specific language impairments comprehended the meanings of fewer target words than the normal children. These two findings together suggest that specifically language-impaired children may be able to fast-map the meanings of words but may have difficulty in doing so when novel words occur in connected discourse, as is typical of the stream of language that occurs in everyday situations. Although specifically language-impaired children may be able to fast-map the meanings of words in highly structured situations, such as those similar to the task used in Dollaghan's study, inserting a pause before occurrences of novel words when they are embedded in a narrative may not be helpful (Rice et al., 1992).

When these children are successful in gleaning word meanings from limited exposures, this does not necessarily result in their using the words. The children may learn to comprehend the meanings of words, but they may still have problems using the words appropriately (Dollaghan, 1987). Dollaghan has proposed that these children's problems in using words for which meanings had been learned result from difficulty in accessing or retrieving the words for production rather than from a failure in storing the words in memory. The specifically language-impaired children in her study recognized a newly fast-mapped word when another person used it, even though they could not produce it when asked.

The suggestion that children with language problems have difficulties in retrieving known words or have word-finding problems is not new (e.g., German, 1979, 1982, 1987; German & Simon, 1991; Kail, Hale, Leonard, & Nippold, 1984; Leonard et al., 1983; MacLachlan & Chapman, 1988). In fact, many specifically language-impaired children are described as having word-finding problems. These difficulties can show up when children are asked to name pictures, particularly in rapid naming tasks, or in their connected speech. The connected speech of children with language problems is often characterized by hesitations, dysfluencies, reformulations, word substitutions, and fillers that may be related to word retrieval difficulties. Additionally, the children may use a substantially higher number of words without clear referents, such as "thing," "this," "that," "here," and "there." Some have proposed that these difficulties in accessing known words may be related to a less elaborate and extensive knowledge of the word meaning (Kail & Leonard, 1986; McGregor & Leonard, 1989) rather than to the use of "less efficient algorithms for retrieving word names" (McGregor & Leonard, 1989, p. 141). If this is the case, it would be somewhat similar to the notion of underextension and context-specific/item-specific word learning discussed in previous chapters.

It is not known whether some specifically language-impaired youngsters have semantic difficulties in the absence of problems with other aspects of language. Scarborough and Dobrich's (1990) results suggest not. In describing the children they had followed from 2½ to 5 years of age, these authors stated that when the children reached age 5, "no child ever showed a purely lexical deficit. Instead, residual phonological and syntactic problems, in combination and in isolation, were seen in most cases" (p. 80). If these findings prove to be correct, we suspect that most, if not all, children with semantic difficulties will be found to have other language problems as well. Additionally, as we will see in the next section, these other problems are likely to include deficits in syntax and morphology.

Syntax and Morphology

Even though semantic difficulties may be the first evidence of language problems for toddlers, deficient syntactic and morphological skills are almost classic characteristics of preschoolers with language impairments. At about 3 years of age, evidence of syntactic and/or morphological problems may emerge as children's MLUs, sentence complexity, and use of morpho-logical markers are expected to increase. As examples of the difficulties that are observed in these young-sters, we tend to see (1) shorter utterances (MLU) than those of same-age peers; (2) limited types of transfor-mations used, including limited use of subordination; (3) omissions and/or confusions of grammatically obligatory elements, such as the copula verbs "is" and "are," articles, and plural morphemes; and (4) subject case marking problems, as in "him" for "he" and "her" for "she" when the pronouns serve as the subjects of sentences. In fact, several authors suggest that the morphological aspect of language is especially problematic for children with specific language im-pairments. Table 5.3 lists some of the common problematic morphemes for specifically language-impaired children (Leonard, McGregor, & Allen, 1992).

One possible reason these children demonstrate in-ordinate difficulties with certain morphemes is that the morphemes have "low phonetic substance" (Leonard et al., 1992, p. 1077). This is similar to the view that these children have difficulties processing rapidly changing auditory stimuli, that is, they have an audi-tory processing deficit. As Leonard et al. (1992) ex-plain, these problematic morphemes are unstressed, which means that they have shorter durations in con-nected speech than adjacent morphemes. They are also nonsyllabic segments, and they often have lower fundamental frequencies and amplitude, which means

	Morpheme	Examples
TABLE 5.3 Some Trouble-some Grammatical Morphemes for Specifically Language-Impaired Children	Plural -s	boys; coats
	Possessive 's	baby's; cat's
	Past -ed	played; liked
	Third person singular -s	plays; likes
	Articles a and the	a boy; the cat
	Copula	The baby is big
	On	on the floor; put on the coat
	Auxiliary be	The baby is crying; The girls are playing
	Irregular past tense	ate; went; drank
	Complementizer to	I'm going to (go); gonna (go)

Source: Adapted from Leonard et al. (1991).

that they may seem to be lower-pitched and less loud. In essence, these morphemes may be auditorily less salient than the surrounding morphemes in the connected speech that specifically language-impaired children hear in everyday situations.

Others have proposed that perceptual difficulties alone cannot explain the problems and that some degree of semantic, grammatical rule learning, and/or accessing process is involved. For example, Watkins and Rice (1991) examined specifically language-impaired preschoolers' acquisition of certain prepositions (e.g., "in," "up") and these same words when they occurred as part of a verb particle (e.g., a multiword construction that functions as a verb, such as "climb up"). Given that the same word in these different grammatical functions has the same meaning and carries a similar level of auditory salience, any differences in acquisition should be primarily grammatically or morphosyntactically based. The children had more difficulty with verb particles than with prepositions, suggesting that "semantic and syntactic factors have greater influence than is acknowledged by processing accounts" (Watkins & Rice, 1991, p. 1139). Similarly, Loeb and Leonard (1991) found a developmental link between specifically language-impaired youngsters' acquisition of two morphological features—correct use of the proper pronoun case for pronouns functioning as subjects of sentences (e.g., "She is eating" versus "Her is eating") and correct use of verbs (e.g., copula "is," auxiliary "is," third person singular -s inflection). Correct use of subject case marking correlated with correct verb formation. Perceptual salience alone could not account for this apparent grammatical learning link. These results are similar to Connell's (1986) suggestion of an acquisition link between subject case pronouns and verb morphology, further implicating an influence of morphosyntactic rule induction.

Connell and Stone's (1992) later work, however, suggests that specifically language-impaired children may be able to induce morphological rules as well as normal children, but that the language-impaired children cannot use the morphemes in their own speech unless they have been asked to produce them during a teaching task. These authors concluded that specifically language-impaired children's difficulties with

morphology relate to accessing rules that have been induced rather than to their learning of the rules in the first place. This conclusion counters the notions of problems in inducing grammatical rules or in perceiving the grammatical morphemes in the speech of others.

A semantic factor may also be involved. The grammatical elements that children omit tend to be ones that are often not critical to the meanings of utterances. That is, children seem to preserve the meanings of utterances even though morphosyntactic problems are present (Cole, 1976; Menyuk, 1969; Wood, 1976). Many grammatical elements are redundant in meaning. In the utterance "Three girls are fishing" there are three markers to indicate plurality: the word "three," the plural morpheme "girls," and the use of "are." Omission of the plural inflection and the auxiliary "are" would still preserve the meaning of the utterance ("Three girl fishing"). Therefore, grammatical morphemes may sometimes be less semantically salient than high-content words.

One suspects that "multiple sources of vulnerability for mastery of grammatical form classes are implicated" (Watkins & Rice, 1991, p. 1139), including the possibility of limited resource capabilities (Leonard et al., 1992). If one or more areas of functioning are fragile for whatever reason, increased demands, complexity, or operations may overload the system in such a way as to cause loss or breakdown, with fewer resources to direct to the other operations. This perspective is consistent with a synergistic view of language functioning and research findings that document trade-offs between linguistic components, especially when one or more components are stressed.

Pragmatics

Although "not all language-disordered children have pragmatic deficits that go beyond their problems with language structure and content" (Rowan, Leonard, Chapman, & Weiss, 1983, p. 103), some toddlers and preschoolers with specific language impairments do show difficulty with the pragmatic aspect of language. For example, Snyder (1975, 1978) has reported that young language-impaired children use fewer declarative and imperative functions than normal children.

Similarly, Rom and Bliss (1981) found fewer uses of the acknowledging function and more uses of the answering function by language-impaired children. Rom and Bliss' finding that language-impaired children make increased use of the answering function is consistent with that reported by Leonard, Camarata, Rowan, and Chapman (1982). When these researchers analyzed the language of children at the one-word stage of production, the language-impaired children were found to use more answering functions than their normal counterparts. More recently, Paul (1991) reported on the work she and Shiffer had completed on toddlers with SELD. These toddlers used fewer comment or joint attentional intentions and generally engaged in fewer communicative initiations, including those communicated with gesture or vocalizations, than their normal peers. It would seem, then, that language-impaired youngsters may demonstrate differences in their use of functions when compared to normal language-learning children. Wilcox (1984) suggests that the differences may lie in functions that are child initiated rather than in functions initiated by conversational partners. Language-impaired youngsters may use fewer functions that initiate and more that involve responding. Paul (1991) commented that the toddlers with language problems she examined simply appeared to be "less interested in interacting with others, even nonverbally" (p. 6). This impression is similar to Fey's (1986) description of children who are low on the conversational assertiveness continuum (chapter 4). Passivity in communicative interactions is not uncommon among specifically language-impaired youngsters.

Differences in frequency of use of other functions and intentions have also been identified. The language-impaired children in the Leonard, Camarata, et al. (1982) study used fewer statement functions involving naming than did the normal children, a finding somewhat similar to Snyder's. Rom and Bliss (1981) also reported a reduction in the number of descriptive functions used by language-disordered children.

Rowan et al. (1983) indicate that the size of the expressive lexicon may affect the children's uses of functions and intentions. As the lexicon increases, the child may develop more flexibility in using certain types of communicative functions that are more difficult to express nonverbally, such as descriptive functions. In the Rowan et al. study, language-impaired preschoolers demonstrated skills similar to those of normal preschoolers in the use of imperative and declarative performative intents. When these authors attempted to explain the disparity between their results and Snyder's, one of the factors cited was that the children in the Rowan et al. study had larger vocabularies than the children in Snyder's (1975) investigation.

Conversational pragmatics that involve, in part, the ability to initiate and sustain a verbal interaction and to adapt messages to the needs of a conversational partner have also been investigated in language-impaired children. Although much of the research has been conducted with school-age children and older preschoolers, younger preschoolers may exhibit similar problems. These children may have difficulty in using appropriate methods to gain a listener's attention and may attempt to initiate conversations at the wrong times (Dukes, 1981; Lucas, 1980). Once conversations are initiated, the children may not be able to sustain the topic over several conversational turns due, in part, to their problems with turn taking; inserting noncontingent, irrelevant comments; switching topics abruptly; and failing to ask for clarifications (e.g., Brinton & Fujiki, 1982; Donahue, Pearl, & Bryan, 1980; Dukes, 1981; Lucas, 1980). For example, normal language-learning youngsters are less likely to respond to their specifically language-impaired peers' attempts to initiate communicative interactions (Hadley & Rice, 1991). In turn, specifically language-impaired children are less likely to respond to their normal language-learning peers' initiations (Hadley & Rice, 1991). Using Fey's (1986) definitions, this latter behavior places the children low on the conversational responsiveness continuum. The two factors together result in breakdowns in the conversational interactions of specifically language-impaired children.

Rice, Sell, and Hadley (1991) also found that preschoolers with specific language impairments tended to address their communicative attempts to adults more than to their peers, possibly because of a history of unsuccessful communicative interactions with their peers and/or because of a history of having had their communicative initiations ignored by their peers. Rice et al. (1991) suggest that "children are sensitive to their relative communicative competence, or incompetence, at an early age" and that "as young as 3 years of age, children adjust their social interactions to take into account their communication abilities relative to those of others" (p. 1304). These early breakdowns in communicative interactions may be the beginning "of a negative interactive spiral generated by a child's history of communicative failure wherein a child becomes less likely to respond as he or she experiences failure in peer interactions and peers become less likely to attend to the child's initiations" (Hadley & Rice, 1991, p. 1315). The long-standing failures in and problems with peer interactions that have been well documented for language-impaired children and adolescents seem to have their roots in early childhood.

One rule of conversation obligates listeners to signal a lack of understanding to their conversation partners. Yet, specifically language-impaired children may fail to do so. Until recently, it was not known whether this occurred because the children did not recognize that they did not understand; did not know that they should send a signal; were too passive and/or unresponsive to give an indication; and/or did not know how to signal. The findings of Rice and her colleagues, however, seem to indicate that young language-impaired children are aware not only of their communication weaknesses but also that they do not understand the messages of others. This conclusion is confirmed by the research findings of Skarakis-Doyle, MacLellan, and Mullin (1990). Not only did the language-impaired children in this study recognize their lack of comprehension, they indicated it through subtle nonverbal behaviors, although, as the authors suggested, this occurred at a preintentional, nonverbal level. Compared to the language-normal children in the study, the language-impaired children had a limited repertoire of nonverbal behaviors that they used to indicate their comprehension failures, most often using changes in eye contact following noncomprehension of utterances. When a message was not understood, the children tended to look at the examiner's face rather than at the stimulus item. Even though the children had rudimentary awareness of their comprehension failure, they rarely produced a **clarification**

request or indicated verbally their lack of comprehension.

Conflicting results have been found regarding specifically language-impaired children's ability to adapt their messages to the communication context and to their listeners. Snyder's (1975, 1978) results suggest that young language-impaired preschoolers do not verbally encode the most informative elements of messages as frequently as language-normal preschoolers do. Language-impaired children are just as apt to convey uninformative elements as informative ones, whereas normal children more consistently encode the informative elements of messages. These findings were partially confirmed by Skarakis and Greenfield's (1982) study of older preschool and young school-age children with language problems. With older preschoolers, Shatz, Bernstein, and Shulman (1980) found that language-impaired children did not use prior linguistic information and context to determine whether to interpret question forms with "Can you . . ." as indirect requests or as true questions. In a study of both preschoolers and elementary school-age children, Prinz and Ferrier (1983) similarly noted that language-impaired children have difficulty varying their use of polite devices, as well as problems interpreting direct and indirect requests as more or less polite.

In contrast, the language-impaired children in the Fey, Leonard, and Wilcox (1981) study were able to adapt their messages to their listeners and to the communicative context. A later investigation by Fey and Leonard (1984) supported the findings of the earlier study. The language-impaired preschoolers and elementary school-age children in this study were able to modify their language based on their conversational partner's age. Similarly, Gallagher and Darnton (1978) found that the language-impaired children in their study revised previous utterances when it was apparent that they had not been understood. The children's repertoires of revision strategies were, however, more limited than those of the normal children, and the language-impaired children rarely used revisions involving substitutions of one syntactic or semantic element for an equivalent. Although there is conflicting information about this aspect of communication, it may be a problematic area for some language-impaired pre-schoolers and serves to remind us of the heterogeneity of children with specific language impairments.

Socialization and Psychosocial Factors

Although specific language impairments generally occur in the absence of *severe* emotional disturbances, there has recently been increased recognition of a possible relationship between some degree of behavioral/emotional involvement and language impairment (Baltaxe & Simmons, 1988; Mack & Warr-Leeper, 1992; Prizant et al., 1990). It is difficult, however, to separate information about behavioral/emotional factors from some pragmatic characteristics seen in children with specific language impairments and from the recent information on the social and adaptive behaviors of these toddlers and preschoolers. In some respects we may have a "chicken and egg" dilemma. Communicative failures may result in psychosocial difficulties, or psychosocial difficulties may be a part of the syndrome of specific language impairment, or early psychosocial difficulties may be manifested in terms of language problems. We at least suspect a reciprocal, if not a cyclical, relationship. As Rice et al. (1991) write:

> To the extent that experiencing success in social interactions is central to a child's sense of self-esteem and social role, children with communication limitations are at risk for the development of social competencies. Limited social interactions would in turn limit their opportunities to learn communication skills from their peers, especially in the development of discourse skills. (p. 1305)

The degree to which repeated failures in social interactions because of impaired language skills and decreased opportunities to learn communicative interactional skills lead to long-term psychosocial difficulties is unknown. However, we suspect that these problems have negative effects on the children. For example, Gualtieri and colleagues found that of 40 consecutive patients admitted to a child psychiatric unit, 20 had language problems (Gualtieri, Koriath, Van Bourgondien, & Saleeby, 1983). In another study of approximately 300 successive intakes of children to

a community-based speech and language clinic, 95% of the children with expressive language problems had some form of psychosocial difficulty, according to 1980 criteria used by the American Psychiatric Association (Baker & Cantwell, 1982). Finally, Prizant et al. (1990) reported that 67% of the children consecutively admitted to an inpatient facility with behavioral/emotional problems failed a speech and language screening. In chapter 11, we will see further references to psychosocial difficulties in adolescents with language disorders.

In Table 5.2 we saw that the occurrence of behavior problems in toddlers with SELD may be a predictive factor for whether or not their language delays will resolve with increasing age (Paul, 1991; Whitehurst, Smith, et al., 1991). Additionally, in Paul's (1991) study, 62% of the toddlers with expressive language problems received adaptive behavior scores at least 6 months below their age level. She suggested that "slowness in language growth and poor socialization are both related to an underlying decrement in motivation to interact. These children may experience somewhat less drive for interaction than other toddlers, which could result in less need to acquire language, even when the potential to do so exists" (p. 5). Although Paul indicates that this suggestion is preliminary and speculative, a follow-up study of the children at 3 years of age showed that about half of them continued to have socialization problems (Paul et al., 1991). These problems continued even though some of the expressive language difficulties had apparently resolved. Recall also that the toddlers in Paul's (1991) work generally attempted fewer communicative interactions than normal children.

It is possible that as early as 2 years of age, children with language problems show problems in the psychosocial arena. These problems may continue, and in fact become exacerbated, as the children continue to have communicative interaction failures as they grow older. Baker and Cantwell (1983) would likely support this suspicion. They state that "since language is a uniquely human quality, it is therefore not unexpected that a disorder in language development might have far reaching consequences for other areas of early childhood development" (p. 51).

Narratives

Skill in relating understandable, complete narratives is important in school achievement, and school-age children with language problems frequently have difficulty in telling cohesive narratives. Because narratives are generally discussed in terms of school-age children's language skills, chapter 7 reviews some of the characteristics of narratives seen in children with learning disabilities associated with language disorders. Although narratives are typically thought of as later-developing language skills, preschoolers do use early forms of narration. They relate rudimentary accounts of things that have happened to them, and they retell favorite stories from children's books that they have been read.

There is evidence that preschoolers with specific language impairments demonstrate difficulties with narrative skills. We have previously indicated that the quality of language-impaired preschoolers' narrative skills is a strong predicting factor for their later school success (Bishop & Edmundson, 1987). The narratives of children with specific language impairments tend to contain less information generally and less information per utterance than preschoolers with normal language skills (Paul, 1992). Paul reports that these language-impaired youngsters may, in fact, repeat information already encoded in their own utterances. As such, the story lines of their narratives may unfold slowly. It may take the language-impaired children several utterances to impart the same amount of information that normal language-learning children convey in one utterance (Paul, 1992). One explanation for the limitations on the information these youngsters encode may relate to the linguistic features they bring to the task. An efficient method used to encode more than one proposition per utterance is complex sentence usage. Children whose language is limited to simple sentences or even to compound sentences are not efficient in conveying multiple pieces of information. Contrast "When he hit the water he started to sink, so he closed his mouth" with "He hit the water. He started to go down in the water. He closed his mouth." Good, tightly composed narratives also depend on the use of high-content words with appropriate semantic choices to signal old and new information. Children who have difficulties with certain abstract words, such as temporal and deictic words, and children who have difficulty retrieving words quickly and who instead use low-content words (e.g., "thing"), will encounter problems in producing narratives. Production of narratives generally challenges most aspects of a language-impaired child's language system. Thus, difficulties with one aspect of language may overload the child in such a way that either other aspects of language are affected or the whole system breaks down (Paul, 1992). For this reason, even preschoolers who may appear to have adequate conversational language skills or who score within normal limits on standardized language tests may evidence language problems when they are asked to relate narratives.

IMPLICATIONS FOR INTERVENTION

Assessment

Specific language impairment in toddlers and preschoolers appears to be manifested in different ways at different times. It follows, therefore, that assessment considerations may need to differ at different times.

Toddlers

Predictive Factors in Assessment.   In chapter 4 we discussed factors that might place infants and young children at risk for language impairments. The presence of any of these factors in a child's background needs to be considered part of an assessment process. In this chapter, we also identified some of the factors that may place a toddler with SELD at risk for continuing language problems (see Table 5.2). Beyond assessing expressive language, the following possible predictive factors suggest aspects of toddlers' performances that professionals would want to assess: (1) socialization; (2) phonological composition of vocalizations and babbling, as well as **verbalizations**; (3) use of gestures, particularly symbolic play gestures expressing script routines; and (4) behavior. Assessment of toddlers needs to be multifaceted. Although language comprehension skills were not included in Table 5.2 because they have not yet been unequivocally established as

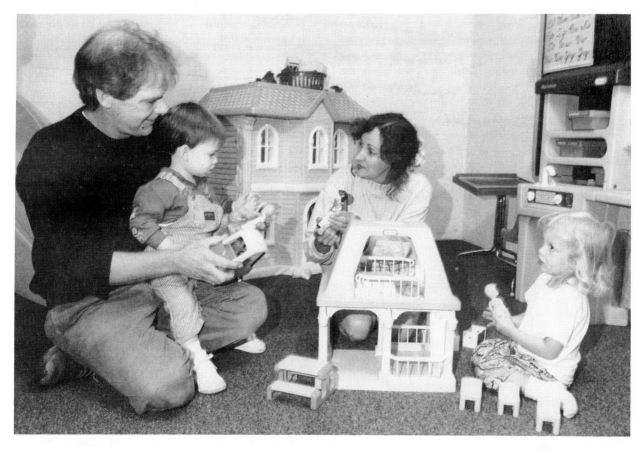

Accurate and early identification of toddlers with slow expressive language development is essential in providing early intervention for those who will not outgrow their early language delays.

predictors of continuing language problems, these skills should be included in an assessment process. There is evidence that many toddlers with expressive language problems have comprehension problems even though, on superficial observation, they may appear to understand quite well (e.g., Paul et al., 1991; Thal et al., 1991). Information about a toddler's comprehension skills is important in planning intervention, as well as in providing additional assessment documentation of language problems.

Another predictive factor in Table 5.2 was communicative intentions. Young children's uses of such intentions, produced through gestures and vocal-

izations, can be assessed even before they use their first words. Coggins (1991) discusses how to manipulate the assessment environment to identify children's uses of communicative intentions. He suggests that the children should be assessed under conditions of both minimal and maximal support for producing intentions. Table 5.4 gives examples of the ways in which contextual variables might be manipulated to influence children's performances in producing intentions. Any differences in performance under these conditions can be identified and may indicate the children's potential for change (Coggins, 1991; Platt & Coggins, 1990). The ability to modify behavior quickly

TABLE 5.4 Manipulating Contextual Variables That Influence Performance

Variable	Minimal Contextual Support	Maximal Contextual Support
Nonlinguistic		
Interaction	Naturalistic	Contrived tasks
Materials	No toys or props	Familiar and thematic
Interactor	Clinician	Mother/caregiver
Activities	Novel	Event routines
Linguistic		
Cuing	Indirect model	Elicited imitation

Source: Reprinted from T. Coggins, Bringing Context Back Into Assessment, in *Topics in Language Disorders*, Vol. 11:4, pp. 43–54, with permission of Aspen Publishers, Inc., © 1991.

under various conditions of support often has prognostic value and can provide valuable information about strategies that might be included in intervention plans.

Early Language Milestones.   Early language developmental milestones provide additional guidelines for assessment. A quick review of some of these milestones is in order. Recall from chapter 3 that children produce their first word at about 12 months of age. At about 15 months, expressive vocabulary approximates 10 words (Reich, 1986) and at about 18 months, 50 words. Between 18 and 24 months, children demonstrate an expressive vocabulary spurt, so that at about 20 months of age they are using over 150 words and at 24 months of age over 200 words (Dale, Bates, Reznick, & Morisset, 1989; Reich, 1986). Also, between 18 and 24 months of age, children begin to combine single words into two-word combinations. At 24 months MLU generally falls between 1.5 and 2.4 (Miller, 1981). Phonological development is such that by about 24 months of age, children are fairly intelligible to those who know them. Comprehension vocabulary typically exceeds production, so that children often comprehend their first word at about 8 to 9 months of age and comprehend about 50 words slightly beyond 12 months of age. Using these milestones as guidelines, several authors suggest that SELD can be identified at least at 24 months of age. These children are not yet using lexicons of 50 single words

and/or are not yet combining words into two-word combinations (e.g., Coplan, Gleason, Ryan, Burke, & Williams, 1982; Rescorla, 1989). Children who are not yet reasonably intelligible would also be suspect.

Assessment Instruments and Parental Report.   A number of developmental instruments are available to assess infants and toddlers. Among these are the *Bayley Scales of Infant Development* (Bayley, 1969), the *Denver Developmental Screening Test* (Frankenburg, Dodds, Fandal, & Kazuk, 1975), the *Minnesota Child Development Inventory* (Ireton & Thwing, 1974), and the *Vineland Adaptive Behavior Scales* (Sparrow, Balla, & Cicchetti, 1984). These instruments examine a range of developmental areas (e.g., gross motor, fine motor, personal-social), including communication skills. In addition to these more general assessment tools, several others focus specifically on early communication skills. Among these are the *Early Language Milestone Scale* (Coplan, 1987) and the *Clinical Linguistic and Auditory Milestone Scale* (Capute et al., 1986). These are screening tools that are used most often in identifying severe developmental delays in children (Rescorla, 1991).

The use of parental reports of young children's communicative behaviors for assessing their language abilities has recently increased in popularity. Although their accuracy has been questioned, parental reports have the following features that make them an attractive method of assessment: (1) parents have many opportunities to observe their children's language, so they may know more about what the children do with their communication than a professional can learn in an assessment session; (2) parental reports can be obtained before professionals see the children and can, therefore, be used to help plan assessment sessions; and (3) parental reports are cost-effective (Dale, 1991; Rescorla, 1991).

Several authors have suggested that the concerns about accuracy of parental report can be overcome by structuring the form of parents' reports (Dale et al., 1989; Rescorla, 1989, 1991). Specifically, a recognition format, in which the tool presents parents with communicative behaviors and asks them to identify those that apply to their children, is a valid and reliable technique for soliciting information from parents (Dale, 1991; Rescorla, 1989). Two parental report instruments that use this technique and are designed to tap toddlers' communication skills are the *MacArthur Communicative Development Inventory: Toddlers*[2] (CDI) (Dale, 1991) and the *Language Development Survey* (LDS) (Rescorla, 1989). Both instruments focus on expressive vocabulary and the emergence of syntactic skills. Of the two, the CDI is more extensive, requiring about 30 minutes for parents to complete. In contrast, the LDS is designed "as a quick and efficient ... screening tool for the identification of language delay in 2-year-old children" (Rescorla, 1991, p. 17). The LDS takes about 10 minutes for parents to complete. Both instruments provide a list of vocabulary words and ask parents to indicate which ones their children use. In the section that addresses syntactic development, the CDI uses a forced-choice method. For each item, parents are given two multi-word utterances that contrast a specific morphosyntactic feature and asked to indicate which one better describes the child. The LDS asks parents whether or not the child combines words and requests them to list three of the child's longest and best multiword utterances. Rescorla (1991) suggests that the LDS can be used for initial identification of the child, followed by the CDI if the child's language appears delayed.

Several other instruments are available for professionals to use in assessing toddlers. Space limitations preclude a comprehensive list. Additionally, any such list would be immediately outdated, as new instruments are continuously being developed. However, some of the more commonly used instruments are the *Sequenced Inventory of Communication Development* (SICD) (Hedrick, Prather, & Tobin, 1975), the *Preschool Language Scale-3* (PLS-3) (Zimmerman, Steiner, & Pond, 1992), the *Receptive-Expressive Emergent Language Test–Second Edition* (REEL-2) (Bzoch & League, 1991), and the *Bracken Basic Concept Scale* (BBCS) (Bracken, 1984). A number of these instruments include a parental report, as well as direct professional–child interaction. General aspects of assessing children's language and factors involved in selecting and using standardized instruments are discussed in chapter 14.

Parent/Caregiver–Child Interactions. An important part of assessment involves the interactions between primary caregivers and their children (MacDonald & Carroll, 1992; Sparks, 1989). As we know from chapter 2, parents'/caregivers' interactions with their language-impaired children are, for the most part, not greatly different from the interactions of other parents/caregivers with their younger normal language-learning children. That is, the parents/caregivers seem to respond more to the child's language level than to the child's CA. The few problematic areas that have sometimes been noted generally relate to (1) the degree of directiveness, with parents/caregivers of language-impaired children tending to use more directive language, such as commands, rather than responses to their children's initiations, and (2) a reduction in the frequency of semantically contingent responses when parents/caregivers reply to their children's utterances. Somewhat related to the latter factor is how quickly parents/caregivers respond. Roth (1987) has suggested that a 1-second interval between a child's production and a parent's/caregiver's response is the time frame in which a 1-year-old child can pick up on the contingency of the response. However, care must be taken in interpreting these findings. Although some research has suggested that there may be a few differences, these findings have not been substantiated by other

---

[2]Earlier versions were known as the *Early Language Inventory.*

studies (e.g., Lahey, 1988; Paul & Elwood, 1991). Recall also the statement in chapter 2 that a child's language behavior itself may modify an adult's mode of interaction, so that interactions may be less appropriate and stimulating. The communicative interactions likely have reciprocal effects. However, some of these adult behaviors, once established possibly because of previous adult–child interactions, may maintain slowed language development in a child. The purpose of assessing parent/caregiver–child interactions is not to judge the adult. Rather, it is to identify possible factors that can be modified or included in interactive routines to enhance and facilitate a child's language learning.

One tool that has been developed to examine parent–child interactions is the assessment component of the *Ecological Communication Model* (ECO) (Mac-Donald & Gillette, 1989). Four basic premises undergird the ECO assessment approach:

1. Children learn to interact, play, communicate, talk, and have conversations from their natural interactions with primary social partners.
2. Adults can alter the structural, cognitive, and social aspects of their natural interactions to help the child actively learn to communicate; when using certain strategies, they can influence the child's communicative development.
3. Children have sharply differential needs in their communication learning before and beyond language itself; one or more of at least five areas may be the source of the problem; action knowledge, interactions, communication, language, and conversation. An adequate program needs to identify the critical problem areas for the child, rather than merely target the most apparent delay.
4. A child learns how to communicate with others; the adult's strategies in interacting with the child are the primary tools we have to make the child more communicative and less isolated. (MacDonald & Carroll, 1992, p. 114)

This assessment **protocol** evaluates child–caregiver interactions in three different interactive contexts (play with objects, play with people alone, and spontaneous interactions during caretaking) for five aspects of communication development: social play partnerships, turn-taking partnerships, nonverbal communication

partnerships, language partnerships, and conversation partnerships. From six to nine behavior items are used to assess more specifically the interactions for each of the five communication areas. The entire protocol, consisting of 40 items divided across the five areas, is used. After observing interactions, each item is rated on a 1 (low/poor) to 9 (high/outstanding) scale. The completed protocol provides a profile of strengths and weaknesses in child–caregiver interactions. MacDonald and Carroll (1992) suggest that the profile allows identification of possible areas for parent/caregiver training.

Preschoolers

General Guidelines. For preschoolers, many more standardized language instruments are available, and it is easier to obtain reliable test results from preschoolers than from toddlers. However, professionals still need to be alert to the fact that considerable variability in preschoolers' communicative performance can occur. As with toddlers, in assessing preschoolers it is important to assess caregiver–child interactions and a variety of behaviors. Language developmental milestones continue to be important guidelines, although MLU may no longer be a consistently reliable indicator of language growth (e.g., Klee & Fitzgerald, 1985; Klee, Schaffer, May, Membrino, & Mougey, 1989; Scarborough, Wyckoff, & Davidson, 1986; Wells, 1985). Additionally, gross measures of expressive vocabulary size may also be less reliable indicators of language skill with preschoolers than with toddlers. Previously, we suggested that delays in expressive vocabulary acquisition may appear to resolve during the later preschool years (Paul, 1991; Whitehurst, Fischel, et al., 1991). This is not to say that expressive vocabulary should be omitted from the assessment process. Rather, the assessment needs to include the child's use of words with more abstract meanings. Comprehension vocabulary is also part of the assessment process. Again, however, abstract vocabulary words need to be included.

Because syntax and morphology are especially troublesome areas for preschoolers with specific language impairments, children's performances in these areas should be thoroughly assessed. Of particular importance is the use of complex sentences. As we have seen, this affects children's skills with narratives, and narrative skills, in turn, may predict later school success. In assessing complex sentence usage, the range of subordinate conjunctions in these sentences also needs to be examined. The use of grammatical morphemes, per Table 5.3, should also be included in the assessment. Measures need to be fine-grained rather than global and general (Paul, 1991).

Illusionary Recovery.   If preschoolers appear to recover from deficits in certain aspects of language behavior at different times, this has implications for assessment. Language performance needs to be assessed in a way that reduces the possibility of obtaining *false negative* results—that is, results indicating that no problem exists when, in fact, it does.

One way to address the problem of illusionary recovery is to ensure that assessment is comprehensive, that is, that many aspects of communication are assessed, as well as behavioral aspects known to be associated with specific language impairments, such as those listed in Table 5.2. It may be appropriate to assess over several sessions and in a variety of settings, including the child's home and in situations where the child interacts with other children.

Another way to address the problem is to stress or challenge the child's language performance (Lahey, 1990). It is not enough to know what a child *does* with language; we also need to know what a child *can do*. Earlier we indicated that narrative production, in particular, challenges a child's language performance. Asking a child to relate a narrative should probably be a standard part of a preschooler's language assessment, not only to stress the system but for its predictive value as well. However, professionals should avoid basing decisions about a child's language abilities only on the production of stereotyped narratives such as fairy tales. These may be "rehearsed" narratives because they have occurred frequently in the child's environment. Rather, novel narratives should be elicited, either by asking the child to repeat a story after hearing it from the examiner or by requesting a spontaneous narrative. The former method is more frequently used, as it allows the examiner to compare the child's production against the known standard.

However, an important factor to consider in the retelling is the amount of prior knowledge the listener/examiner has. Children are apt to reduce the complexity of their narratives if they are aware that the listener/examiner already knows the content or if pictures about the narrative are in front of the listener/examiner during the retelling. A method to counter this problem is to ask the child to retell the story to another person, such as the child's primary caregiver, who was not present when the child heard the story and who cannot see any pictures related to it.

Social Communicative Interaction.   Assessing language performance includes an assessment of the child's communication in social interactive situations. For preschoolers, this goes beyond assessment with the primary caregiver alone. Ideally, children should be assessed as they interact in a group with other children, some of whom have normal language. As Rice and her colleagues (Rice, Sell, & Hadley, 1990) point out, however, most systems designed to measure children's social communicative interactions are so complex and cumbersome that they are impractical for routine assessment.

To provide "a quick way of obtaining clinically relevant information about the use of language in natural settings along the social dimension" (p. 7), Rice et al. (1990) developed the *Social Interactive Coding System* (SICS). This instrument focuses on Fey's (1986) assertion/passivity conversational dimension and examines a child's interactions with peers during a variety of typical preschool activities, such as art, dramatic/symbolic play, and free play with toys. Each turn a child takes in an interaction, the nature of each turn (e.g., initiation, response–verbal, response–nonverbal, ignore), and the number of turns in the interaction are recorded on a standardized protocol, which also allows the addressee of the child's interactions to be recorded. The tool incorporates an on-line observational technique in which the professional records all of the child's interactions in a 5-minute period and then takes a 5-minute break to update notations on the protocol. The "5 minutes on/5 minutes off" procedure is repeated three times, for a total of four observational segments. The advantages of the SICS are as follows: (1) it can be completed in the classroom; (2) it is easy to learn; (3) minimal equipment is necessary; and (4) results are immediately available for interpretation. The authors caution, however, that the SICS should not be used as the sole assessment procedure, but rather as a supplement to other forms of assessment.

Chapter 14 provides additional information about assessment of children's language in general. It is relevant to language assessment of toddlers and preschoolers and should be used in conjunction with the information presented here.

Intervention

Decisions About Intervention   The issue of predicting which toddlers and preschoolers will outgrow their early delays in acquiring language without assistance and which will not leads to a main consideration for intervention: That is, under what conditions is intervention recommended, when is it recommended, and what is the nature of the intervention—monitoring, indirect intervention, or direct intervention by a professional? There are no hard and fast answers to these questions (Olswang & Bain, 1991b). The philosophical and theoretical positions of the professional, the philosophical and procedural positions of the organization in which the professional works, and the attitudes and wishes of the caregivers affect the decision. Professionals' decisions are influenced by information about identification of language impairment and standards to which a child's language performance is being compared, predictive and risk factors relevant to a specific child, and the long-term implications of unresolved language impairments. To this, information about a child's potential for language change and the factors important in facilitating the change are added (Coggins, 1991; Olswang & Bain, 1991b; Platt & Coggins, 1990).

An important principle is that whatever initial decision is made, it is reassessed regularly as a child's behavior does or does not change (Bain & Dollaghan, 1991; Campbell & Bain, 1991; Olswang & Bain, 1991a, 1991b). If direct intervention by a professional is not recommended initially, it is possible to use indirect methods, such as parent training and/or preschool enrollment, and monitor the child's progress. If the anticipated progress is not seen in a specified period of time, direct intervention can be implemented. If direct intervention is the initial decision, the child's progress is also monitored regularly. If progress is rapid, the professional may decide to discontinue direct intervention, implement indirect intervention to maintain the level of progress, and monitor the child's behaviors at regular intervals. If progress is not continued, direct intervention can be reinstated. Ongoing monitoring, regular measurements of a child's language performance across many parameters, consistent follow-up, and flexibility in moving from one form of intervention to another are critical in providing effective intervention.

Indirect Intervention   As indicated previously, one aspect of intervention is deciding how services for a specific toddler or preschooler are to be delivered, that is, direct intervention by a professional working with the child or indirect intervention through consultation and collaboration with others. Both methods may be employed. The decision will differ for each child. *No one service delivery model is suitable for all language-impaired youngsters.* However, parents/caregivers play a large role in the early language learning of toddlers and preschoolers, and their participation in intervention is essential. Furthermore, a common recommendation for youngsters with specific language impairments is placement in a preschool program.

Parents/Caregivers.   Toddlers and preschoolers spend most of their time interacting with parents/caregivers. Therefore, these adults are potentially powerful sources of change in children's communicative behavior. Involving parents/caregivers in intervention is not only mandated by federal education laws but generally makes good sense as well. As Olswang and Bain (1991a) point out, the "question is not should the parent be involved in the intervention process, but how" (p. 77). The "how" usually takes one of two forms. The parents/caregivers can augment, expand, and supplement the intervention provided directly by a professional, who is the primary agent of change. Alternatively, the parents/caregivers can serve as the primary agents of change, with the professional developing the initial directions and methods for change and monitoring both the process and the progress.

Whichever strategy is chosen for an individual child, the parents/caregivers need education and training. This generally focuses on two objectives: (1) creating or enhancing the child's environment to facilitate change in the child's language and (2) responding within that environment in a manner that best facilitates language change.

At least two primary aspects are involved in changing or enhancing the child's language-learning environment. One aspect focuses on helping the parents/caregivers recognize and take advantage of language-learning opportunities that occur in the child's daily activities. This approach stresses seizing opportunities and capitalizing on language-teaching moments. These moments can occur during dressing, interactive play, meal or snack time, story time, or any other time during the day when the child's attention is focused on a specific action, object, or event. The parents/caregivers are shown how to identify these moments and how to structure their language and gestural input accordingly. The second aspect involves creating opportunities for language learning. The parents/caregivers are shown how to set up moments in the environment to facilitate the child's use of specific language behaviors and how to encourage the child to use these behaviors during those periods. These moments may or may not be specified, allocated periods. In some instances, the parents/caregivers may be able to observe a situation and know that if they make an immediate and sometimes small change, they will be able to facilitate a desired language behavior. In other instances, short periods may be set aside to facilitate certain communicative behaviors in the child. As with the "opportunistic" approach, the parents/caregivers are shown how to structure their communicative behavior to enhance the child's learning.

In helping parents/caregivers respond to the children in ways that best promote language learning, it is important to remember that the aim is likely to help them do more of some things and perhaps less of others. In most instances, it may simply be a matter of changing the frequency of certain behaviors. Earlier we indicated that most parents/caregivers of specifically language-impaired children interact verbally in ways that are similar to those of parents of normally developing children, but that there may be two or three adult behaviors that are worthy of particular at-

tention. One may involve helping the parents/caregivers reduce their frequency of directive speech acts, including commands and demands for responses from the children, and increase their use of (1) responsive speech acts, (2) information-seeking questions when the information presumably is not known to the adult, (3) confirmation requests to affirm that the adult understood the child correctly, and (4) simple recasts of the child's utterances to maintain the content of these utterances but in a form that modifies slightly the one used by the child (e.g., Conti-Ramsden, 1990; Fey, 1986; Paul & Elwood, 1991; Yoder, 1989). Another way in which parents/caregivers may be able to facilitate the child's language learning is to respond more frequently to what the child says, using semantically contingent statements. These responses again maintain the content of the child's utterances and may serve as comments on the child's utterances; for example, to the child's utterance "Big doggie" the adult might say "Yes, it is a big doggie." A third possibility for enhancing a child's language learning may be for parents/caregivers to respond more quickly to the child's utterances.

Preschools. Preschool experiences are often recommended for youngsters with specific language impairments to provide a stimulating language-learning environment and opportunities for social communication. Often the preschool will have both specifically language-impaired and normal language-learning children, with the idea that the normal children will provide models and stimulation for the language-impaired youngsters. However, the simple presence of normal language-learning children does not guarantee that they will be effective facilitators. Special attention may have to be given to how this can be achieved.

One problem is that normal and language-impaired youngsters in preschools do not spend much time in communicative interactions with each other (Hadley & Rice, 1991; Rice et al., 1991; Weiss & Nakamura, 1992). As Hadley and Rice (1991) point out in their study on the conversational interactions of normal and language-impaired preschoolers:

The implications for intervention are somewhat sobering. It seems that placement of these children [with specific language impairments] in an integrated setting, even one in which adults are highly responsive to and encourage the children's initiation attempts, does not necessarily ensure peer interactions.... Preschoolers behave as if they know who talks well and who doesn't, and they prefer to interact with those who do. Therefore, placement of communicatively impaired children in an integrated setting, with normal-language peers and facilitative adults, will not in and of itself establish successful peer interactions in spontaneous interactions. (p. 1315)

It would seem, therefore, that the facilitative adults in these settings need to develop specific strategies to encourage successful peer interactions. It cannot be assumed that these interactions will occur without attention and planning.

A second issue relates to the involvement of parents/caregivers in children's preschool experiences. In one study (Roberts et al., 1989), children who attended a preschool that included parent/caregiver education achieved better conversational skills by 5 years of age than either children who did not attend preschool but whose parents/caregivers did receive education or children who neither attended preschool nor whose parents/caregivers received education. This finding suggests that the combination of parent/caregiver education and preschool programs provides more powerful opportunities for enhancing children's language performances than parent/caregiver education alone.

SUMMARY

In this chapter we have seen that:

▶ The issue of whether specific language impairment in young children represents a delay or a disorder is still debatable.

▶ Some authors suggest that youngsters with specific language impairments represent a large, generic grouping and that there may be subgroups of children with specific language impairments. If there are subgroups, they have not yet been fully identified.

▶ Many different labels to describe these children have been used, but no one label is universally agreed upon.

▶ Causal factors remain elusive.

▶ Some children outgrow early delays in acquiring language; others do not. Predicting who will and who will not catch up is currently an important area of research. Issues related to possible illusionary recovery need to be addressed. Issues of illusionary recovery and prediction influence assessment strategies and intervention decisions.

▶ Children with specific language impairments can exhibit different combinations of communication problems involving some or all parameters of language. One common feature is difficulty with syntax and morphology.

▶ Intervention is a process of ongoing monitoring, regular measurements of the children's language performances, consistent follow-up, and flexibility in moving from direct to indirect intervention modes and vice versa.

▶ Parental/caregiver involvement is important in obtaining assessment information, and parental/caregiver education is an important aspect of intervention.

▶ Placing language-impaired and normal language-learning children in preschools together will not necessarily ensure successful social communicative interactions between them unless these interactions are specifically addressed.

Toddlers and preschoolers with specific language impairments are at risk for academic failure when they begin school. They are also at risk for early social communication failure. Proper and early identification and intervention are critical if a potential cycle of social and academic failure is to be prevented.

REFERENCES

Aram, D. (1991). Comments on specific language impairment as a clinical category. *Language, Speech, and Hearing Services in Schools, 22,* 84–87.

Aram, D., Ekelman, B., & Nation, J. (1984). Preschoolers with language disorders: 10 years later. *Journal of Speech and Hearing Research, 27,* 232–244.

Aram, D., & Nation, J. (1980). Preschool language disorders and subsequent language and academic difficulties. *Journal of Communication Disorders, 13,* 159–170.

Bain, B., & Dollaghan, C. (1991). The notion of clinically significant change. *Language, Speech, and Hearing Services in Schools, 22,* 264–270.

Baker, L., & Cantwell, D. (1982). Psychiatric disorder in children with different types of communication disorders. *Journal of Communication Disorders, 15,* 113–126.

Baker, L., & Cantwell, D. (1983). Developmental and behavioral characteristics of speech and language disordered children. In S. Chess & T. Thomas (Eds.), *Annual progress in child development* (pp. 205–216). New York: Brunner-Mazel.

Baltaxe, C., & Simmons, J. (1988). Communication deficits in preschool children with psychiatric disorders. *Seminars in Speech and Language, 8,* 81–90.

Bashir, A., Kuban, K., Kleinman, S., & Scavuzzo, A. (1983). Issues in language disorders: Considerations of cause, maintenance, and change. In J. Miller, D. Yoder, & R. Schiefelbusch (Eds.), *Contemporary issues in language intervention.* Rockville, MD: American Speech-Language-Hearing Association.

Bates, E., Benigni, L., Bretherton, I., Camaioni, L., & Volterra, V. (1977). From gesture to the first word: On cognitive and social prerequisites. In M. Lewis & L. Rosenblum (Eds.), *Interaction, conversation, and the development of language.* New York: Wiley.

Bayley, N. (1969). *Bayley scales of infant development: Birth to two years.* San Antonio, TX: Psychological Corporation.

Bishop, D., & Edmundson, A. (1987). Language-impaired 4-year-olds: Distinguishing transient from persistent impairment. *Journal of Speech and Hearing Disorders, 52,* 156–173.

Bloom, L. (1980). Language development, language disorders, and learning disabilities: LD3. *Bulletin of the Orton Society, 30,* 115–133.

Bloom, L., & Lahey, M. (1978). *Language development and language disorders.* New York: Wiley.

Bracken, B. (1984). *Bracken basic concept scale (BBCS).* San Antonio, TX: Psychological Corp.

Brinton, B., & Fujiki, M. (1982). A comparison of request-response sequences in the discourse of normal and language-disordered children. *Journal of Speech and Hearing Disorders, 47,* 57–62.

Brown, R. (1973). *A first language: The early stages.* Cambridge, MA: Harvard University Press.

Bzoch, K., & League, R. (1991). *Receptive-expressive emergent language test* (2nd ed.). Austin, TX: PRO-ED.

Campbell, T., & Bain, B. (1991). How long to treat: A multiple outcome approach. *Language, Speech, and Hearing Services in Schools, 22,* 271–276.

Campbell, T., & Shriberg, L. (1982). Associations among pragmatic forms, lexical stress, and phonological processes in speech-delayed children. *Journal of Speech and Hearing Research, 25,* 547–553.

Capute, A., Palmer, F., Shapiro, B., Wachtel, R., Schmidt, S., & Ross, A. (1986). Clinical linguistic and auditory milestone scale: Prediction of cognition in infancy. *Developmental Medicine and Child Neurology, 28,* 762–771.

Carrow-Woolfolk, E., & Lynch, J. (1982). *An integrative approach to language disorders in children.* New York: Grune & Stratton.

Catts, H. (1989). Phonological processing deficits and reading disabilities. In A. Kamhi & H. Catts (Eds.), *Reading disabilities: A developmental language perspective.* Boston: College-Hill Press.

Caulfield, M. (1989). Communication difficulty: A model of the relation of language delay and behavior problems. *SRCD Abstracts, 7,* 212.

Chapman, K., Leonard, L., Rowan, L., & Weiss, A. (1983). Inappropriate word extensions in the speech of young language-disordered children. *Journal of Speech and Hearing Disorders, 48,* 55–62.

Coggins, T. (1991). Bringing context back into assessment. *Topics in Language Disorders, 11,* 43–54.

Cohen, M., Campbell, R., & Yaghmai, R. (1989). Neuropathological abnormalities in developmental dysphasia. *Annals of Neurology, 25,* 567–570.

Cole, P. (1976). *The influence of certain semantic factors on syntax of normal and language disordered children.* Unpublished doctoral dissertation, University of Texas, Austin.

Connell, P. (1986). Teaching subjecthood to language-disordered children. *Journal of Speech and Hearing Research, 29,* 481–493.

Connell, P. (1987). An effect of modeling and imitation teaching procedures on children with and without specific language impairment. *Journal of Speech and Hearing Research, 30,* 105–113.

Connell. P., & Stone, C. A. (1992). Morpheme learning of children with specific language impairment under controlled instructional conditions. *Journal of Speech and Hearing Research, 35,* 844–852.

Conti-Ramsden, G. (1990). Maternal recasts and other contingent replies to language-impaired children. *Journal of Speech and Hearing Disorders, 55,* 262–274.

Coplan, J. (1987). *Early language milestone scale.* Austin, TX: PRO-ED.

Coplan, J., Gleason, J., Ryan, R., Burke, M., & Williams, M. (1984). Validation of early language milestone scale in a high-risk population. *Pediatrics, 70,* 677–683.

Crystal, D. (1987). Teaching vocabulary: The case for a semantic curriculum. *Child Language Teaching and Therapy, 3,* 40–56.

Curtiss, S., Katz, W., & Tallal, P. (1992). Delay versus deviance in the language acquisition of language-impaired children. *Journal of Speech and Hearing Research, 35,* 373–383.

Dale, P. (1991). The validity of a parent report measure of vocabulary and syntax at 24 months. *Journal of Speech and Hearing Research, 34,* 565–571.

Dale, P., Bates, E., Reznick, S., & Morisset, C. (1989). The validity of a parent report instrument of child language at twenty months. *Journal of Child Language, 16,* 239–250.

Dollaghan, C. (1987). Fast mapping in normal and language-impaired children. *Journal of Speech and Hearing Disorders, 52,* 218–222.

Donahue, M., Pearl, R., & Bryan, T. (1980). Learning disabled children's conversational competence: Responses to inadequate messages. *Applied Psycholinguistics, 1,* 387–403.

Dukes, P. (1981). Developing social prerequisites to oral communication. *Topics in Learning and Learning Disabilities, 1,* 47–58.

Eisenson, J., & Ingram, D. (1972). Childhood aphasia: An updated concept based on recent research. *Acta Symbolica, 3,* 108–116.

Ekelman, B., & Aram, D. (1983). Syntactic findings in developmental verbal apraxia. *Journal of Communication Disorders, 16,* 237–250.

Fey, M. (1986). *Language intervention with young children.* Boston: Little, Brown.

Fey, M., & Leonard, L. (1984). Partner age as a variable in the conversational performance of specifically language-impaired and normal-language children. *Journal of Speech and Hearing Research, 27,* 413–423.

Fey, M., Leonard, L., & Wilcox, K. (1981). Speech style modifications of language-impaired children. *Journal of Speech and Hearing Disorders, 46,* 91–96.

Frankenburg, W., Dodds, J., Fandal, A., & Kazuk, E. (1975). *Denver developmental screening test* (rev. ed.). Denver: Denver Developmental Materials.

Freedman, P., & Carpenter, R. (1976). Semantic relations used by normal and language-impaired children at stage I. *Journal of Speech and Hearing Research, 19,* 784–795.

Gallagher, T., & Darnton, B. (1978). Conversational aspects of the speech of language-disordered children: Revision behaviors. *Journal of Speech and Hearing Research, 21,* 118–135.

Garvey, M., & Gordon, N. (1973). A follow-up study of children with disorders of speech development. *British Journal of Disorders of Communication, 8,* 17–28.

German, D. (1979). Word-finding skills in children with learning disabilities. *Journal of Learning Disabilities, 12,* 176–181.

German, D. (1982). Word-finding substitutions in children with learning disabilities. *Language, Speech, and Hearing Services in Schools, 13,* 223–230.

German, D. (1987). Spontaneous language profiles of children with word-finding problems. *Language, Speech, and Hearing Services in Schools, 18,* 217–230.

German, D., & Simon, E. (1991). Analysis of children's word-finding skills in discourse. *Journal of Speech and Hearing Research, 34,* 309–316.

Grimm, H., & Weinert, S. (1990). Is the syntax development of dysphasic children deviant and why? New findings to an old question. *Journal of Speech and Hearing Research, 33,* 220–228.

Grunwell, P. (1980). Developmental language disorders at the phonological level. In F. Jones (Ed.), *Language disability in children.* Baltimore: University Park Press.

Gualtieri, L., Koriath, U., Van Bourgondien, M., & Saleeby, N. (1983). Language disorders in children referred for psychiatric services. *Journal of the American Academy of Child Psychiatry, 22,* 165–171.

Hadley, P., & Rice, M. (1991). Conversational responsiveness of speech- and language-impaired preschoolers. *Journal of Speech and Hearing Research, 34,* 1308–1317.

Hall, P., & Tomblin, J. B. (1978). A follow-up study of children with articulation and language disorders. *Journal of Speech and Hearing Disorders, 43,* 227–241.

Hedrick, D., Prather, E., & Tobin, A. (1975). *Sequenced inventory of communication development.* Seattle: University of Washington.

Ingram, D. (1976). *Phonological disability in children.* London: Edward Arnold.

Ireton, H., & Thwing, E. (1974). *Manual for the Minnesota child development inventory.* Minneapolis: Behavior Science Systems.

Johnston, J. (1991). The continuing relevance of cause: A reply to Leonard's "Specific Language Impairment as a Clinical Category." *Language, Speech, and Hearing Services in Schools, 22,* 75–79.

Johnston, J., & Kamhi, A. (1984). The same can be less: Syntactic and semantic aspects of the utterances of language impaired children. *Merrill-Palmer Quarterly, 30,* 65–86.

Johnston, J., & Schery, T. (1976). The use of grammatical morphemes by children with communication disorders. In D. Morehead & A. Morehead (Eds.), *Normal and deficient child language* (pp. 239–258). Baltimore: University Park Press.

Johnston, R., Stark, R., Mellits, E. D., & Tallal, P. (1981). Neurological status of language impaired and normal children. *Annals of Neurology, 10,* 159–163.

Kail, R., Hale, C., Leonard, L., & Nippold, M. (1984). Lexical storage and retrieval in language-impaired children. *Applied Psycholinguistics, 5,* 37–49.

Kail, R., & Leonard, L. (1986). Word-finding abilities in language-impaired children. *ASHA Monographs* (No. 25). Rockville, MD: American Speech-Language-Hearing Association.

Kemp, J. (1983). The timing of language intervention for the pediatric population. In J. Miller, D. Yoder, & R. Schiefelbusch (Eds.), *Contemporary issues in language intervention.* Rockville, MD: American Speech-Language-Hearing Association.

Klee, T., & Fitzgerald, M. (1985). The relation between grammatical development and mean length of utterance in morphemes. *Journal of Child Language, 12,* 251–269.

Klee, T., Schaffer, M., May, S., Membrino, I., & Mougey, K. (1989). A comparison of the age–MLU relation in normal and specifically language-impaired preschool children. *Journal of Speech and Hearing Disorders, 54,* 226–233.

Lahey, M. (1988). *Language disorders and language development.* New York: Merrill/Macmillan.

Lahey, M. (1990). Who shall be called language disordered? Some reflections and one perspective. *Journal of Speech and Hearing Disorders, 55,* 612–620.

Leonard, L. (1972). What is deviant language? *Journal of Speech and Hearing Disorders, 37,* 427–446.

Leonard, L. (1979). Language impairment in children. *Merrill-Palmer Quarterly, 25,* 205–232.

Leonard, L. (1982a). Early language development and language disorders. In G. Shames & E. Wiig (Eds.), *Human communication disorders: An introduction.* Columbus, OH: Merrill.

Leonard, L. (1982b). Phonological deficits in children with developmental language impairment. *Brain and Language, 16,* 73–86.

Leonard, L. (1987). Is specific language impairment a useful construct? In S. Rosenberg (Ed.), *Advances in applied psycholinguistics: Volume 1. Disorders of first-language development* (pp. 1–39). New York: Cambridge University Press.

Leonard, L. (1988). Lexical development and processing in specific language impairment. In R. Schiefelbusch & L. Lloyd (Eds.), *Language perspectives: Acquisition, retardation, and intervention* (2nd ed.) (pp. 69–87). Austin, TX: PRO-ED.

Leonard, L. (1989). Language learnability and specific language impairment in children. *Applied Psycholinguistics, 10,* 179–202.

Leonard, L. (1991). Specific language impairment as a clinical category. *Language, Speech, and Hearing Disorders, 22,* 66–68.

Leonard, L., Bolders, J., & Miller, J. (1976). An examination of the semantic relations reflected in the language usage of normal and language-disordered children. *Journal of Speech and Hearing Research, 19,* 371–392.

Leonard, L., Camarata, S., Rowan, L., & Chapman, K. (1982). The communicative functions of lexical usage by language-impaired children. *Applied Psycholinguistics, 3,* 109–126.

Leonard, L., McGregor, K., & Allen, G. (1992). Grammatical morphology and speech perception in children with specific language impairment. *Journal of Speech and Hearing Research, 35,* 1076–1085.

Leonard, L., Nippold, M., Kail, R., & Hale, C. (1983). Picture naming in language-impaired children. *Journal of Speech and Hearing Research, 26,* 609–615.

Leonard, L., Schwartz, R., Chapman, K., Rowan, L., Prelock, P., Terrell, B., Weiss, A., & Messick, C. (1982). Early lexical acquisition in children with specific language impairment. *Journal of Speech and Hearing Research, 25,* 554–564.

Leske, M. (1981). Speech prevalence estimates of communicative disorders in the U.S. *Asha, 23,* 229–237.

Loeb, D., & Leonard, L. (1991). Subject case marking and verb morphology in normally developing and specifically language-impaired children. *Journal of Speech and Hearing Research, 34,* 340–346.

Lucas, E. (1980). *Semantic and pragmatic language disorders: Assessment and remediation.* Rockville, MD: Aspen.

MacDonald, J., & Carroll, J. (1992). A social partnership model for assessing early communication development: An intervention model for preconversational children. *Language, Speech, and Hearing Services in Schools, 23,* 113–124.

MacDonald, J., & Gillette, Y. (1989). *ECO scales manual.* San Antonio, TX: Special Press.

Mack, A., & Warr-Leeper, G. (1992). Language abilities in boys with chronic behavior disorders. *Language, Speech, and Hearing Services in Schools, 23,* 214–223.

MacLachlan, B., & Chapman, R. (1988). Communication breakdowns in normal and language learning-disabled children's conversation and narration. *Journal of Speech and Hearing Disorders, 53,* 2–9.

Masterson, J., & Kamhi, A. (1992). Linguistic trade-offs in school-age children with and without language disorders. *Journal of Speech and Hearing Research, 35,* 1064–1075.

McGregor, K., & Leonard, L. (1989). Facilitating word-finding skills of language-impaired children. *Journal of Speech and Hearing Disorders, 54,* 141–147.

Menyuk, P. (1969). *Sentences children use.* Cambridge, MA: MIT Press.

Menyuk, P., Chesnick, M., Liebergott, J., Korngold, B., D'Agostino, R., & Belanger, A. (1991). Predicting reading problems in at-risk children. *Journal of Speech and Hearing Research, 34,* 893–903.

Miller, J. (1981). *Assessing language production in children: Experimental procedures.* Baltimore: University Park Press.

Morehead, D., & Ingram, D. (1973). The development of base syntax in normal and linguistically deviant children. *Journal of Speech and Hearing Research, 16,* 330–352.

Nelson, L., & Bauer, H. (1991). Speech and language production at age 2: Evidence for tradeoffs between linguistic and phonetic processing. *Journal of Speech and Hearing Research, 34,* 879–892.

Olswang, L., & Bain, B. (1991a). Intervention issues for toddlers with specific language impairments. *Topics in Language Disorders, 11,* 69–86.

Olswang, L., & Bain, B. (1991b). When to recommend intervention. *Language, Speech, and Hearing Services in Schools, 22,* 255–263.

Paul, R. (1991). Profiles of toddlers with slow expressive language development. *Topics in Language Disorders, 11,* 1–13.

Paul, R. (1992). Speech–language interaction in the talk of young children. In R. Chapman (Ed.), *Processes in language acquisition and disorders.* St. Louis, MO: Mosby Year Book.

Paul, R., & Elwood, T. (1991). Maternal linguistic input to toddlers with slow expressive language development. *Journal of Speech and Hearing Research, 34,* 982–988.

Paul, R., & Jennings, P. (1992). Phonological behavior in toddlers with slow expressive language development. *Journal of Speech and Hearing Research, 35,* 99–107.

Paul, R., Looney, S., & Dahm, P. (1991). Communication and socialization skills at ages 2 and 3 in "late-talking" young children. *Journal of Speech and Hearing Research, 34,* 858–865.

Paul, R., & Shriberg, L. (1982). Associations between phonology and syntax in speech-delayed children. *Journal of Speech and Hearing Research, 25,* 536–547.

Paul, R., & Smith, R. (1991). *Narrative skills in four year olds with normal, impaired, and late-developing language.* Paper presented at the biennial meeting of the Society for Research in Child Development, Seattle.

Platt, J., & Coggins, T. (1990). Comprehension of social-action games in prelinguistic children: Levels of participation and effects of adult structure. *Journal of Speech and Hearing Disorders, 55,* 315–326.

Prinz, P., & Ferrier, L. (1983). "Can you give me that one?": The comprehension, production and judgment of directives in language-impaired children. *Journal of Speech and Hearing Disorders, 48,* 44–54.

Prizant, B., Audet, L., Burke, G., Hummel, L., Maher, S., & Theadore, G. (1990). Communication disorders and emotional/behavioral disorders in children and adolescents. *Journal of Speech and Hearing Disorders, 55,* 179–192.

Reed, V. A. (1992). Associations between phonology and other language components in children's communicative performance: Clinical implications. *Australian Journal of Human Communication Disorders, 20,* 75–87.

Reich, P. (1986). *Language development.* Englewood Cliffs, NJ: Prentice-Hall.

Rescorla, L. (1989). The language development survey: A screening tool for delayed language in toddlers. *Journal of Speech and Hearing Disorders, 54,* 587–599.

Rescorla, L. (1991). Identifying expressive language delay at age two. *Topics in Language Disorders, 11,* 14–20.

Rice, M., Buhr, J., & Nemeth, M. (1990). Fast mapping word-learning abilities of language-delayed preschoolers. *Journal of Speech and Hearing Disorders, 55,* 33–42.

Rice, M., Buhr, J., & Oetting, J. (1992). Specific-language-impaired children's quick incidental learning of words: The effect of a pause. *Journal of Speech and Hearing Research, 35,* 1040–1048.

Rice, M., Sell, M., & Hadley, P. (1990). The social interactive coding system (SICS): An on-line, clinically relevant descriptive tool. *Language, Speech, and Hearing Services in Schools, 21,* 2–14.

Rice, M., Sell, M., & Hadley, P. (1991). Social interactions of speech- and language-impaired children. *Journal of Speech and Hearing Research, 34,* 1299–1307.

Roberts, J., Rabinowitch, S., Bryant, D., Burchinal, M., Koch, M., & Ramey, C. (1989). Language skills of children with different preschool experiences. *Journal of Speech and Hearing Research, 32,* 773–786.

Rom, A., & Bliss, L. (1981). A comparison of verbal communicative skills of language impaired and normal speaking children. *Journal of Communication Disorders, 14,* 133–140.

Roth, F. (1987). Temporal characteristics of maternal verbal styles. In K. Nelson & A. van Kleeck (Eds.), *Children's language* (Vol. 6). Hillsdale, NJ: Erlbaum.

Rowan, L., Leonard, L., Chapman, K., & Weiss, A. (1983). Performative and presuppositional skills in language-disordered and normal children. *Journal of Speech and Hearing Research, 26,* 97–106.

Scarborough, H., & Dobrich, W. (1990). Development of children with early language delay. *Journal of Speech and Hearing Research, 33,* 70–83.

Scarborough, H., Wyckoff, J., & Davidson, R. (1986). A reconsideration of the relation between age and mean utterance length. *Journal of Speech and Hearing Research, 29,* 394–399.

Schwartz, R., & Leonard, L. (1982). Do children pick and choose? An examination of phonological selection and avoidance in early lexical acquisition. *Journal of Child Language, 9,* 319–336.

Schwartz, R., Leonard, L., Folger, M., & Wilcox, M. J. (1980). Evidence for a synergistic view of linguistic disorders: Early phonological behavior in normal and language disordered children. *Journal of Speech and Hearing Disorders, 45,* 357–377.

Shatz, M., Bernstein, D., & Shulman, M. (1980). The responses of language-disordered children to indirect directives in varying contexts. *Applied Psycholinguistics, 1,* 295–306.

Shriberg, L., & Kwiatkowski, J. (1988). A follow-up study of children with phonologic disorders of unknown origin. *Journal of Speech and Hearing Disorders, 53,* 144–155.

Silva, P. (1980). The prevalence, stability, and significance of developmental language delay in preschool. *Developmental Medicine and Child Neurology, 22,* 768–777.

Skarakis-Doyle, E., MacLellan, N., & Mullin, K. (1990). Nonverbal indicants of comprehension monitoring in language-disordered children. *Journal of Speech and Hearing Disorders, 55,* 461–467.

Skarakis, E., & Greenfield, P. (1982). The role of new and old information in the verbal expression of language-disordered children. *Journal of Speech and Hearing Research, 25,* 462–467.

Snyder, L. (1975). *Pragmatics in language-deficient children: Their prelinguistic and early verbal performatives and presuppositions.* Unpublished doctoral dissertation, University of Colorado, Boulder.

Snyder, L. (1978). Communicative and cognitive abilities and disabilities in the sensorimotor period. *Merrill-Palmer Quarterly, 24,* 161–180.

Snyder, L. (1984). Developmental language disorders: Elementary school age. In A. Holland (Ed.), *Language disorders in children.* San Diego, CA: College-Hill Press.

Sparks, S. (1989). Assessment and intervention with at-risk infants and toddlers: Guidelines for the speech-language pathologist. *Topics in Language Disorders, 10,* 43–56.

Sparrow, S., Balla, D., & Cicchetti, D. (1984). *Vineland adaptive behavior scales.* Circle Pines, MN: American Guidance Service.

Steckol, K., & Leonard, L. (1981). Sensorimotor development and use of prelinguistic performatives. *Journal of Speech and Hearing Research, 24,* 262–268.

Stefanatos, G., Green, G., & Ratcliff, G. (1989). Neurophysiological evidence of auditory channel anomalies in developmental dysphasia. *Archives of Neurology, 46,* 871–875.

Stevenson, J., & Richman, N. (1976). The prevalence of language delay in a population of three year old children and its association with general retardation. *Developmental Medicine and Child Neurology, 18,* 431–441.

Stoel-Gammon, C. (1991). Normal and disordered phonology in two-year-olds. *Topics in Language Disorders, 11,* 21–32.

Tallal, P. (1988). Developmental language disorders. In J. Kavanagh & T. Truss (Eds.), *Learning disabilities: Proceedings of the national conference.* Parkton, MD: York Press.

Tallal, P., Stark, R., Kallman, C., & Mellits, D. (1981). A reexamination of some non-verbal perceptual abilities of language-impaired and normal children as a function of age and sensory modality. *Journal of Speech and Hearing Research, 24,* 351–357.

Thal, D. (1991). Language and cognition in normal and late-talking toddlers. *Topics in Language Disorders, 11,* 33–42.

Thal, D., & Bates, E. (1988). Language and gesture in late talkers. *Journal of Speech and Hearing Research, 31,* 115–123.

Thal, D., & Tobias, S. (1992). Communicative gestures in children with delayed onset of oral expressive vocabulary. *Journal of Speech and Hearing Research, 35,* 1281–1289.

Thal, D., Tobias, S., & Morrison, D. (1991). Language and gesture in later talkers: A 1-year follow-up. *Journal of Speech and Hearing Research, 34,* 604–612.

Tomblin, J. B. (1991). Examining the cause of specific language impairment. *Language, Speech, and Hearing Services in Schools, 22,* 69–74.

Tomblin, J. B., Freese, P., & Records, N. (1992). Diagnosing specific language impairment in adults for the purpose of pedigree analysis. *Journal of Speech and Hearing Research, 35,* 832–843.

van der Lely, H., & Harris, M. (1990). Comprehension of reversible sentences in specifically language-impaired children. *Journal of Speech and Hearing Disorders, 55,* 101–117.

Vogel, S. (1977). Morphological ability in normal and dyslexic children. *Journal of Learning Disabilities, 10,* 35–43.

Watkins, R., & Rice, M. (1991). Verb particle and preposition acquisition in language-impaired preschoolers. *Journal of Speech and Hearing Research, 34,* 1130–1141.

Weiner, P. (1974). A language-delayed child at adolescence. *Journal of Speech and Hearing Disorders, 39,* 202–212.

Weiner, P. (1985). The value of follow-up studies. *Topics in Language Disorders, 5,* 78–92.

Weismer, S., & Murray-Branch, J. (1989). Modeling versus modeling plus evoked production training: A comparison of two language intervention methods. *Journal of Speech and Hearing Disorders, 54,* 269–281.

Weiss, A., & Nakamura, M. (1992). Children with normal language skills in preschool classrooms for children with language impairments: Differences in modeling styles. *Language, Speech, and Hearing Services in Schools, 23,* 64–70.

Wells, G. (1985). *Language development in the pre-school years.* New York: Cambridge University Press.

Wetherby, A., Yonclas, D., & Bryan, A. (1989). Communicative profiles of preschool children with handicaps: Implications for early identification. *Journal of Speech and Hearing Disorders, 54,* 148–158.

Whitehurst, G., Fischel, J., Lonigan, C., Valdez-Menchaca, M., Arnold, D., & Smith, M. (1991). Treatment of early expressive language delay: If, when, and how. *Topics in Language Disorders, 11,* 55–68.

Whitehurst, G., Smith, M., Fischel, J., Arnold, D., & Lonigan, C. (1991). The continuity of babble and speech in children with specific expressive language delay. *Journal of Speech and Hearing Research, 34,* 1121–1129.

Wiig, E. (1982). Language disabilities in the school-age child. In G. Shames & E. Wiig (Eds.), *Human communication disorders: An introduction.* Columbus, OH: Merrill.

Wiig, E., & Fleischmann, N. (1980). Knowledge of pronominalization, reflexivization, and relativization by learning disabled college students. *Journal of Learning Disabilities, 13,* 571–576.

Wiig, E., & Semel, E. (1976). *Language disabilities in children and adolescents.* New York: Merrill/Macmillan.

Wiig, E., & Semel, E. (1984). *Language assessment and intervention for the learning disabled* (2nd ed.). New York: Merrill/Macmillan.

Wilcox, M. J. (1984). Developmental language disorders: Preschoolers. In A. Holland (Ed.), *Language disorders in children.* San Diego, CA: College-Hill Press.

Wood, M. (1976). *An analysis of selected morphemes in the spontaneous speech of normal and language-impaired children.* Unpublished doctoral dissertation, University of Texas, Austin.

Wood, M. (1982). *Language disorders in school-age children.* Englewood Cliffs, NJ: Prentice-Hall.

Yoder, P. (1989). Maternal question use predicts later language development in specific-language-disordered children. *Journal of Speech and Hearing Disorders, 54,* 347–355.

Zimmerman, I., Steiner, V., & Pond, R. (1992). *Preschool language scale—3.* San Antonio, TX: Psychological Corporation.

Chapter 6

Language and Children with Mental Retardation

Steven H. Long and Susan T. Long

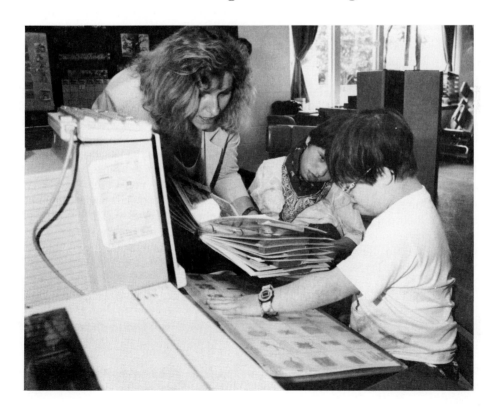

OBJECTIVES

Upon completion of this chapter, the reader should be able to:

▶ Understand the definitions and etiological categories of mental retardation.

▶ Discuss how research on children with mental retardation is conducted.

▶ Understand the distinction between children with Down syndrome and children with mental retardation due to other causes.

▶ Discuss the characteristics of the language of children with mental retardation.

▶ Discuss the principles of language intervention for children with mental retardation.

In the study of language disorders, it is conventional to discuss children with mental retardation as a group. This chapter will not break with that practice but will try to show how diverse these children really are. We find among children with mental retardation a wide range of physical conditions and behaviors. Some children may show mild intellectual deficits but few other problems: They look like their peers, attend school and interact well with typically developing children, do not have seizures or other neurophysiological disorders, and speak intelligibly and effectively. Other children with mental retardation may present a totally different picture: They have physical disabilities and attend a special school with other severely handicapped children. One child may occasionally scream and scratch himself; another may wear a helmet to protect her head when she falls during a **seizure**; and a third may not communicate with speech. When you read about research on children with mental retardation, it is important to ask questions: What kind of children were studied? How old were they? What did they look like? How severe was their intellectual impairment? How severe were their physical, social, and educational problems? By challenging the information in this way, you will not fall into the trap of thinking about children with mental retardation as being all the same.

AN OVERVIEW OF MENTAL RETARDATION

Definition

There is no official definition of mental retardation, and not everyone is careful to say precisely what he or she means by the term. The most influential definition is that of the American Association on Mental Retardation (AAMR)[1]:

> Mental retardation refers to significantly subaverage general intellectual functioning existing concurrently with deficits in adaptive behavior and manifested during the developmental period. (Grossman, 1983, p. 1)

What does this mean? An individual's "general intellectual functioning" is determined from the results of an **intelligence quotient** (**IQ**) test, and "significantly subaverage" functioning is defined as "approximately IQ 70 or below." The AAMR deliberately uses the word *approximately* to allow for differences in the reliability of various IQ tests (Grossman, 1983). The number 70 is the cutoff recommended by the AAMR, but each state is allowed to set its own guidelines for identifying children with mental retardation. As of 1985–86, the majority of states (59%) had established IQ cutoffs of either 70 or 75, consistent with the AAMR definition. Many states (26.8%), however, had not set IQ cutoffs, and the remainder varied from the AAMR recommendation (Frankenberger & Harper, 1988).

A number of tests are used to measure intelligence, depending on the age and verbal ability of the child:

▷ The *Stanford-Binet Intelligence Scale* (Terman & Merrill, 1973) has a long history and is still used with children of all ages.

---

[1]Formerly called the American Association on Mental Deficiency (AAMD).

154

▷ The *Wechsler Intelligence Scale for Children–Revised* (Wechsler, 1974) is another test used commonly with children of school age.

▷ As detection and intervention efforts increasingly focus on infants and preschoolers, the *Bayley Scales of Infant Development* (Bayley, 1969) has come into widespread use.

▷ For nonspeaking individuals, tests that do not require verbal responses are needed, such as the *Leiter International Performance Scale* (Leiter, 1979).

There are still other IQ tests with specific uses and advantages. What all IQ tests have in common, however, is that they yield a mental age (MA), an estimate of the individual's level of cognitive functioning. The MA is expressed as an IQ by dividing it by the individual's chronological age (CA), that is, IQ = MA/CA.

Though the IQ scale is a continuous set of numbers, it is the practice of professionals in the field to describe four levels of impairment. In recent years two sets of labels have been used, one from the AAMR and the other derived from traditional practice in educational placement. Table 6.1 presents these labels, along with their corresponding IQ ranges and prevalence. The preferred practice now is to use the AAMR classification system. If the IQ of a child has not been or cannot be determined, it is common practice for the child to be identified by etiological category (e.g., Fragile X syndrome) or labeled as *developmentally disabled* (Taylor & Kaufmann, 1991).

Another term in the AAMR definition of mental retardation is **adaptive behavior,** the ability to act as independently and responsibly as other people of the same age and cultural background. Adaptive behavior is harder to measure than IQ. Examiners rely on their own clinical judgment, as well as standardized scales such as the AAMR *Adaptive Behavior Scales* (Grossman, 1983) or the *Vineland Social Maturity Scale* (Doll, 1965). It is important to note that the AAMR definition requires evidence of subaverage intelligence *and* adaptive behavior deficits. Also, the term *mental retardation* is used only when these deficits appear during the *developmental period,* that is, up to 18 years of age.

In the literature on exceptional children, several other terms are used whose meaning is similar to that of mental retardation. *Developmental disability* is one such term. This label is used in federal law to describe mental or physical disabilities, or both, that appear before age 22, are likely to continue indefinitely, and result in substantial functional limitations in self-care, language, learning, mobility, self-direction, capacity for independent living, and economic self-sufficiency. There is great, though not total, overlap between the categories of mental retardation and developmental disability. The differences occur at the upper end of the retarded intellectual range (e.g., an IQ of 65), where an individual may receive a diagnosis of mental retardation but *not* developmental disability (Grossman, 1983).

Autism is another term that has substantial overlap with mental retardation. Approximately 70% of children with autism have IQ scores within the retarded range (Grossman, 1983). Both researchers and practitioners, however, have tended to treat children with autism as a distinct group. Therefore a separate chapter in this text (chapter 8) is devoted to them.

Learning disability is a category of impairment that is defined in federal law PL 94–142. Children with mental retardation are specifically excluded from this category. In practice, though, there is a relationship

TABLE 6.1   Levels of Impairment of Individuals with Mental Retardation

AAMR Classification	Traditional Label	IQ Range	Percentage of Persons with Mental Retardation[1]
Mild	Educable	50–55 to 70	89%
Moderate	Trainable	35–40 to 50–55	7%
Severe	Custodial	20–25 to 35–40	3%
Profound	Life support	Below 20–25	1%

[1]President's Committee on Mental Retardation, 1967.

between learning disability and mental retardation. In the 7 years following the enactment of PL 94–142, a 19% decrease was reported in the number of children receiving special education services who were identified as mentally retarded. In actuality, however, this decrease may have reflected a shift in labeling practices, with many of the individuals with mild mental retardation being reclassified as learning disabled (Frankenberger & Harper, 1988).

Causes of Mental Retardation

In the preceding discussion, test performance was used to distinguish different levels of retardation. Differentiation by level of performance is important to educators and administrators because it serves to place children with mental retardation into programs

and allocate funds to those programs (Jones & Payne, 1986). Other differences are frequently more important, however, to researchers who are interested in uncovering the causes of mental retardation.

Research findings from many sources suggest that there are two broad categories of retardation: *organic* retardation, which results from major chromosomal, genetic, or traumatic causes, and *familial* retardation, which has no known cause but tends to run in families. Table 6.2 summarizes the general characteristics of the two etiological categories.

The causes of organic retardation are commonly identified by their period of occurrence: before pregnancy (**genetic**), during pregnancy (**prenatal**), or during delivery (**perinatal**). Several types of chromosomal or other genetic abnormalities produce **congenital** syndromes associated with mental retardation (Sanger,

TABLE 6.2   General Characteristics of Individuals with Organic and Familial Retardation

Organic Retardation	Familial Retardation
IQ most often below 50	IQ rarely below 50
Demonstrable organic etiology	No demonstrable organic etiology; parents may have this same type of retardation
Found at all socioeconomic levels	More prevalent at lower socioeconomic levels
Siblings usually of normal intelligence	Siblings often have subnormal intelligence
Often accompanied by severe health problems	Health within normal range
Appearance often marred by physical stigmata	Normal appearance
Mortality rate higher (more likely to die at a younger age than the general population)	Normal mortality rate
Often dependent on care from others throughout life	With some support, can lead an independent existence as adults
Unlikely to marry and often infertile	Likely to marry and produce children of low intelligence
Unlikely to experience neglect in the home	More likely to experience neglect in the home
High prevalence of associated physical handicaps (e.g., epilepsy, cerebral palsy)	Less likely to have other physical handicaps

Source: Adapted from Zigler and Hodapp (1986), p. 53.

Stick, Sanger, & Dawson, 1984). Down syndrome[2] and Fragile X syndrome are the more common disorders of this type. Prenatal events, such as physical injury or substance abuse, may cause injury to the fetus and lead to retardation. Fetal alcohol syndrome (FAS), caused by excessive drinking during pregnancy, is estimated to occur in 1/750 live births (Sparks, 1984b). During the actual delivery, there is a risk of **hypoxia**—inadequate oxygen going to the brain of the baby—that may result in brain damage and retardation.

While organic retardation is frequently studied and appears to have clear subtypes, it is less evident how familial retardation should be viewed. One proposal (Burack, 1990; Zigler & Hodapp, 1986) is that there are three subtypes:

1. Either or both parents of a child with retardation are themselves retarded, about 35% of all individuals with retardation.
2. The parents are not retarded but the retardation is genetically inherited, another 35% of the total. In contrast to organic retardation, which may also be genetic, inherited familial retardation is not associated with a syndrome and produces less severe developmental disabilities.
3. Retardation is due to extreme environmental deprivation, about 5% of the total.

Types and subtypes of retardation are distinguished on the basis of what is presently known about genetic and environmental phenomena. As more becomes known, it is likely that our classifications will continue to shift. For example, Fragile X syndrome is a chromosomal abnormality with characteristics that place it between the organic and familial categories. Though it is clearly a chromosomal disorder, it also runs in families, produces moderate retardation, and is sometimes inherited from a mother who has the syndrome (Dykens & Leckman, 1990). Future research may decide in which category this syndrome should be placed or it may show that the two-group model is inadequate to describe all causes of retardation.

---

[2]This chapter observes the convention that names of syndromes omit the possessive form (Gerber, 1990). Hence we use *Down syndrome* rather than *Down's syndrome*.

Of all the known or suspected causes of mental retardation, Down syndrome is unique because it can be identified from birth and has a clearly organic etiology. Fragile X syndrome and FAS are two other conditions that are now beginning to be studied as biologically well-defined subgroups. However, these conditions are currently harder to diagnose from observation and laboratory tests. Consequently, children with Down syndrome have been the most intensively studied population of children with mental retardation. This is especially true of early-developing behaviors. Because our information base is so much greater for Down syndrome, a separate section of this chapter will be devoted to a discussion of these children.

Associated Problems

Many children with mental retardation show differences in appearance and have physical handicaps and health problems much more frequently than their non-retarded peers. As noted in Table 6.2, these problems are more frequent in children with organic retardation. Few studies, however, have reported separate findings for the organic and familial populations. Table 6.3 summarizes information on associated problems as they have been reported for children with Down syndrome and for children with other retardation syndromes or retardation of unspecified cause.

The high prevalence of hearing loss is an important factor in understanding the language impairment of children with mental retardation. Hearing impairment serves to multiply rather than just add to the handicaps of individuals with mental retardation: Learning is made more difficult, which delays cognitive development; and the delays in cognitive development diminish the use of auditory information and cause further retardation (Stewart, 1978).

The causes of **sensorineural hearing loss** are often the same as the causes of retardation: genetic factors, pre- and **postnatal** trauma, and diseases such as **rubella** and **meningitis** (Kropka & Williams, 1986; Lloyd & Reid, 1967; Newby, 1972). **Conductive hearing loss**, on the other hand, is attributable to several organic and environmental factors. Congenital malformation of the middle ear is more common among children with retardation. Estimates of abnormal middle ear

TABLE 6.3 Associated Problems of Appearance, Physical Handicaps, and Health Problems in Children with Mental Retardation

Condition	All Children with Mental Retardation	Children with Down Syndrome
Appearance		
Deviations in head size	Microcephaly and hydrocephaly	
Deviations in orofacial structure	Small eyes and poor head and midface growth are characteristic of children with FAS (Sparks, 1984b)	Upward-slanting eyes, prominent epicanthal folds, a small nose and chin, and a flattened bridge of the nose (Sparks, 1984a)
Physical Handicaps		
Epilepsy (seizures)	15–30% (McLaren & Bryson, 1987)	
Cerebral palsy and other motor impairments	20–30% (McLaren & Bryson, 1987)	
Behavioral and/or psychiatric problems	30–40% (McLaren & Bryson, 1987) Frequent aggressive outbursts, hyperactivity, and self-injurious behavior in children with Fragile X syndrome (Dykens & Leckman, 1990; Reiss & Freund, 1990)	Less intense affect compared with typically developing children of similar developmental level, possibly due to difference in neurological arousal systems (Cicchetti & Ganiban, 1990) 13% exhibit short attention span, hyperactivity, low frustration tolerance, periodic emotional distress (Menolascino, 1967, cited in Baroff, 1986)
Sensory impairments (see also discussion in text)	10–20% (McLaren & Bryson, 1987)	Visual: 50% Auditory: findings range from 39% to 85% (Kropka & Williams, 1986)
Low muscle tone (hypotonia)		Causes hyperextension of joints (double jointedness) (Sparks, 1984a)
Health Problems		
Cardiac defects		30–60% (Sparks, 1984a)
Other problems		Increased prevalence of leukemia, endocrine disorders, and diabetes (Sparks, 1984a); thyroid problems affect about 40% of these children and may lead to obesity or decreased intellectual functioning Upper respiratory infections (Lloyd & Fulton, 1972) Abnormally high incidence of Alzheimer's disease in middle age (Thase, 1988)

function range from 30% to 63%, with the greatest problems found in individuals with severe retardation (Givens & Seidemann, 1977; Lloyd & Fulton, 1972; Nolan, McCartney, McArthur, & Rowson, 1980). In addition, poor self-care habits may exacerbate hearing problems (Lloyd, 1970).

Hearing loss appears to be especially prevalent in the Down syndrome population (Dahle & McCollister, 1986). For example, one study found abnormal hearing in 69% of subjects with Down syndrome compared with 47% in a group of adults and children with other types of retardation (Nolan et al., 1980). The risk of hearing impairment is high in infancy and continues into adulthood (Fulton & Lloyd, 1968; Gordon, 1987; Kaga & Marsh, 1986; Keiser, Montague, Wold, Maune, & Pattison, 1981; Northern & Downs, 1984). One reason children with Down syndrome are so prone to hearing loss is that they frequently have abnormally small outer ear canals, muscular hypotonia, and skull defects that inhibit middle ear drainage (Fulton & Lloyd,1968; Lloyd & Fulton, 1972; Schwartz & Schwartz, 1978).

COGNITIVE DEVELOPMENT AND THE COGNITION-LANGUAGE RELATIONSHIP

We cannot understand the language impairment of children with mental retardation without first considering the nature of their intellectual deficits. It is not enough merely to say that children with mental retardation are less intelligent. The questions we must try to answer are these:

▷ How does the intelligence of children with mental retardation vary from that of typically developing children?

▷ What is the impact of a cognitive deficit on the rate, sequence, and extent of language development?

The answers to these questions influence the types of intervention programs we develop for these children. For example, if we believe that a child with mental retardation thinks differently than a typically developing child, we may need to develop a style of teaching that is unlike conventional intervention and is also unlike the way we intervene with other language-impaired children.

Different researchers have studied the structure of cognition, the relationship between cognition and language in typically developing children, and this same relationship in children with mental retardation. Much of this work has framed questions around opposing points of view, which are set out in Table 6.4. You may want to refer to this table during the discussion of what these oppositions mean.

The Piagetian View

The Piagetian view is that cognitive development consists of a series of qualitative changes in the way children perceive and structure information about the world. In chapter 2 we saw that in typically developing children these changes occur in a predictable order that has been described as a series of stages.

We also saw that part of the Piagetian view is the so-called *cognitive hypothesis,* the belief that cognition

TABLE 6.4 Opposing Viewpoints in Research on Mental Retardation	Piaget's Stage Model of Cognitive Development		Vygotsky-Luria's Verbal Mediation Model of Cognitive Development
	Strong form of cognitive hypothesis *or*	Weak form of cognitive hypothesis vs.	Cognition and language are somewhat independent in children with mental retardation
	Cognition and language development reach a plateau vs.		Cognition and language advances can occur independently of one another
	Delay vs.		Difference
	Quantitative vs.		Qualitative

and language are linked developmentally, and that the cognitive hypothesis has been stated in two forms. The "strong" form of the cognitive hypothesis maintains that certain cognitive achievements are prerequisite to the emergence of certain language behaviors. The strong form is commonly endorsed by those who take a "delay" or "quantitative" view of mental retardation (see Table 6.4 and the following discussion). However, it is also possible that the language of children with mental retardation is quantitatively different from that of typical children but is not fully consistent with the cognitive level. This "weak" form of the cognitive hypothesis, also called the *interactionist* hypothesis, maintains that language and cognition influence one another but that other social and linguistic factors also play important roles (Kamhi & Johnston, 1982). Put another way, the weak form of the cognitive hypothesis holds that cognitive changes make certain meanings available for expression but that, to express these meanings in language, there must also be specific linguistic capabilities. Thus, language development depends on cognition but also has linguistic sources (Cromer, 1991).

Several studies of sensorimotor development in children with mental retardation suggest that their cognitive learning follows the same developmental sequence as that of typically developing children but at a delayed rate. The correlations between early cognitive achievements (e.g., object permanence) and linguistic achievements (e.g., first meaningful words) are comparable to those seen in typically developing children (Greenwald & Leonard, 1979; Kahn, 1975, 1978, 1984; Mahoney & Snow, 1983; Martin, McConkey, & Martin, 1984). Other research has cast doubt on this conclusion, especially for individuals with severe and profound retardation (Finch-Williams, 1984). In those cases, the language–cognition relationship appears to be less close. Language may not develop to the level that would be predicted from cognitive achievements.

It is sometimes suggested, as part of the Piagetian view of mental retardation, that cognitive development reaches a plateau and cannot continue further. Naturally, language development is also said to be arrested at this point. Tempering this view, however, are two other claims: (1) it appears possible to accelerate the acquisition of cognitive skills associated with the late sensorimotor period in some children with mental retardation (Kahn, 1978, 1984); and (2) there is evidence that limited cognitive development continues into early adulthood, even for some individuals with profound and severe retardation (Silverstein et al., 1982).

The Vygotsky-Luria View

In contrast to the Piagetian interpretation of the language–cognition relationship is the view that language has a lead role and assists the development of cognition (Vygotsky, 1962). After studying children with and without mental retardation, Luria (1961, 1963) proposed a three-stage theory concerning the development of verbal control of motor behavior. In the first stage (0–3 years) children use language to communicate but not to control their behavior. In the second stage (3–4½ years) speech is used in an **asemantic** way to promote desired actions or prevent undesired ones. For example, a child may say "hit hit" when punching a bag or may say "no no" in order to keep from touching a forbidden object. The role of speech is very primitive at this stage and appears to require little cognitive processing. In fact, the meaning of the words used is not very important: A child could say "hit hit" or "me me" or "dog dog" with equal effect. In the third stage (beyond 4½ years), however, it is the meaning of the language that directs a child's behavior in one direction or another. Thus a child may say aloud "Okay, now you can do it" or "No, wait a minute" to impel or inhibit an action.

From this perspective of cognition and language, children with mental retardation are seen to suffer from a deficit in verbal mediation ability due to the inactivity of the verbal system and its **dissociation** from the motor system (Luria, 1963). In terms of the three-stage model, they are thought to be arrested at the second stage. The implication is that children with mental retardation should be able to use language to control their performance of basic all-or-none actions (standing up, pushing objects, sweeping, etc.) but that they will have difficulty in "talking themselves through" more intricate problem-solving tasks (sorting, calculating, etc.).

There is some limited experimental evidence to support Luria's hypothesis. In an investigation comparing teenagers with organic and familial retardation to typically developing preschoolers, 91% of the teenagers performed at Luria's second stage, while only 63% of the preschoolers did, despite the fact that all subjects were of comparable MA (Rotundo & Johnson, 1981). On the other hand, Milgram and Furth (1968) found that adolescents with moderate mental retardation were better able to find hidden objects when they followed instructions to verbalize aloud as they searched. This suggests that some third-stage development was present but that, without prompting, the children with retardation simply failed to apply their ability.

The Delay–Difference Controversy

A fundamental issue in mental retardation research over the years has been the *delay–difference controversy,* that is, whether the cognitive and linguistic processes of individuals with and without mental retardation are the same. No one disputes that the *achievements* of children with retardation are lower. The debate focuses on the *explanation* for that lower achievement and whether it requires us to invoke the idea of specific qualitative differences in how these children develop. The argument is more intense for children with familial retardation, about 75% of those identified as retarded, who show no evidence of central nervous system dysfunction. In those cases there are no "hard signs" to suggest that a qualitative difference does exist (Zigler & Balla, 1982).

To investigate the delay–difference controversy, researchers have applied the scientific method of making and testing predictions. These predictions have relied on the technique of matching subjects with and without retardation according to their CA, MA, or language age (LA). Examples of this matching are shown in Table 6.5. Only by comparing subjects matched according to one or another of these variables has it been possible to explore the issue of delay versus difference without misinterpretation.

Supporters of the difference position point to three findings, any or all of which may be areas of qualitative difference in individuals with mental retardation:

1. They suffer from a deficit in verbal mediation ability, discussed earlier.

2. They are inherently more rigid in their behavior.
3. They have inadequate short-term memory (also called *working memory*) function (Zigler & Balla, 1982).

The notion of *rigidity* is hard to pin down, but it is most often illustrated by studies that show a deficit in abstract thinking. Children with Down syndrome, for example, have been found to classify objects by their common perceptual attributes (size, shape, color) rather than by abstract categories (fruit, clothing, furniture) (Cornwell, 1974). They seem to have difficulty with hierarchical thinking, that is, recognizing that entities can be thought about at several levels. For example, the family pet has a proper name, "Rudy"; has a basic-level name, "dog"; has a subordinate name, "dachshund"; and has several superordinate names: "mammal," "quadruped," and "animal." It may be hard for these children to accept that all of these names provide accurate descriptions of the same dog but at different levels of thinking.

Deficits in working memory have been offered as an explanation for a range of problems commonly seen in children with mental retardation. It is generally believed that these children rarely employ strategies in situations that require active problem solving but that they can be taught to do so. However, the strategies taught for one task do not usually transfer spontaneously to other tasks. Most studies of problem solving, as well as most clinical descriptions, indicate that the performance of children with mental retardation varies widely from one situation to the next. It has been suggested that this variation is due to limitations in functional working memory, which, in turn, may be the result of slowness in information processing (Ferretti & Cavalier, 1991). The problem should not be thought to extend to all memory functions. Research on long-term memory has been conducted on young children with mild mental retardation. Though the data base is still small, most studies suggest that there is no qualitative difference in the long-term memory functions of this population (Turnure, 1991).

In response to this evidence of differences, the delay position draws attention to the distinction between cognition and achievement (Zigler & Balla, 1982). Some of the performance differences observed in fa-

TABLE 6.5 Examples of Subject Matching by CA, MA, and LA

	Typical Development				Mental Retardation		
Subject	CA	MA	Language Test	Subject	CA	MA	Language Test
CA Matching[1]							
A	36	36	36	A	36	20	20
B	36	36	36	B	36	20	20
C	36	36	36	C	36	20	20
D	36	36	36	D	36	20	20
E	36	36	36	E	36	20	20
MA Matching[2]							
A	36	36	36	A	54	36	30
B	36	36	36	B	54	36	30
C	36	36	36	C	54	36	30
D	36	36	36	D	54	36	30
E	36	36	36	E	54	36	30
LA Matching[3]							
A	36	36	36	A	46	30	36
B	36	36	36	B	46	30	36
C	36	36	36	C	46	30	36
D	36	36	36	D	46	30	36
E	36	36	36	E	46	30	36

[1]Subjects are matched by CA. Used to determine whether children with mental retardation are delayed in specific language behaviors.

[2]Subjects are matched by MA as determined by an IQ test. Used to determine whether the language deficits of children with mental retardation are attributable to their overall cognitive delay.

[3]Subjects are matched by LA as determined by MLU or other language measure. Used to determine whether children with mental retardation are delayed in specific domains of language (e.g., syntax) even though they show generally comparable communication abilities to the matched typically developing subjects.

milial retardation may be simply due to lack of experience that results in deficits of knowledge. Other performance differences may be attributed to motivational differences in individuals with retardation. Research has found persons with retardation to be responsive to social reinforcement but at the same time wary of strange adults. They may be less likely to rely on their own cognitive resources and instead tend to problem-solve imitatively. They may have an expectancy of failure based on experience and therefore may be more motivated to avoid failure than to achieve success. They respond better to tangible reinforcement and often exhibit *learned helplessness,*

that is, not doing things even though they know how. Although mental retardation is viewed primarily as a cognitive disorder, it may have associated with it the noncognitive characteristic of *passivity,* that is, not initiating the use of certain strategies known to be available to them. It is unknown why a cognitive disorder should have a motivational trait associated with it (Rosenberg, 1982).

Even without considering the motivational differences of children with mental retardation, the majority of research evidence on cognitive development seems to favor the delay position. In 1982, Weisz, Yeates, and Zigler reviewed the results of Piagetian experiments conducted with retarded and nonretarded subjects. They found that both longitudinal and cross-sectional studies provided overwhelming evidence that subjects with mental retardation traverse Piagetian stages in the same sequence as normal children. Their review of 104 group comparison studies showed that when organically impaired subjects were not part of the group with retardation, the findings consistently showed similar cognitive structures in the two groups. On the other hand, studies of retarded subjects with organic involvement tended to show differences between these and normal MA-matched individuals.

LANGUAGE CHARACTERISTICS OF CHILDREN WITH MENTAL RETARDATION

It can be regarded as a truism that all children with mental retardation exhibit some form of language impairment. The AAMR specifies that one component of the adaptive behavior deficits seen in all mental retardation is communication disability, and federal government reports indicate that speech or language disability combined with mental retardation is the most common of all dual disabilities (Grossman, 1983). Consequently professionals can expect that children with mental retardation may need some form of language or communication intervention (Miller, 1984). It is important to note, however, that language impairment is caused by mental retardation and not by a developmental syndrome in itself. One should be certain not to assume that developmental syndromes, such as De Lange syndrome, always result in communicative impairment (Cameron & Kelly, 1988).

Research Issues

One of the most consistent findings of research on the language of children with mental retardation is that the findings are inconsistent. This inconsistency can be frustrating to professionals who want clear guidelines, but it is not surprising that research outcomes have differed, nor is it destined to always be the case. Some of the inconsistency may be attributed to the different methods of evaluation used by various investigators. For example, a study of comprehension that uses standardized tests may find that few children with

severe or profound retardation respond appropriately to the structured format of the tests (Gould, 1976). Yet, if comprehension were evaluated in these children using observational methods, there would likely be evidence of comprehension in certain familiar situations (Abbeduto, 1991). It may also be that children with retardation are especially likely to test poorly (Zigler & Balla, 1982). In particular, some researchers have asserted that verbal performance in children with Down syndrome may be suppressed under the stress of testing (McCune, Kearney, & Checkoff, 1989).

An even greater impediment to language studies has been the tendency of researchers to treat all individuals with mental retardation as a homogeneous group (Abbeduto, 1991; Fowler, 1990; Rondal, 1988). In the future, we are likely to see more studies that adhere to the practice of using biologically well-defined subgroups (e.g., those with Down syndrome, Fragile X syndrome, or FAS) as subjects (Fowler, 1990). Research with Down syndrome has already developed into a line of investigation distinct from other studies on children with mental retardation. For this reason, in the following review, we have frequently separated those studies in which the subjects were exclusively children with Down syndrome.

Pragmatics

The study of pragmatics in individuals with mental retardation has examined behaviors in six areas: the development and use of speech acts, the ability to establish referents, the ability to repair conversational breakdowns, conversational turn taking, topic management, and generalization of language use from one setting to another.

Speech Acts   As in other areas, much of the research in pragmatics has not carefully differentiated between types of children with mental retardation. An exception has been the study of early speech act development, where identification of Down syndrome at or shortly after birth has resulted in the use of these children as subjects. Compared to nonretarded children matched for MLU, children with Down syndrome produce the same number and type of various speech acts but do so at a rate that is chronologically delayed

(Coggins, Carpenter, & Owings, 1983; McCune et al., 1989; Owens & MacDonald, 1982; Sinson & Wetherick, 1982). The early stages of speech act development have not been studied in other types of children with retardation, but it appears that by adulthood, nearly all individuals with mild or moderate mental retardation develop a full repertoire of speech acts (Abbeduto & Rosenberg, 1980; Owings & McManus, 1980).

Assertive communicative acts, such as requests for information, directives to perform an action, or unsolicited comments and statements, are the "ice breakers" we use to begin conversations. However, children with retardation, especially those who are severely impaired, rarely use language to initiate social contact and tend to maintain responsive communicative roles (Bedrosian & Prutting, 1978; Beveridge, 1976; Calculator & Dollaghan, 1982; Eheart, 1982). As a result, unless they are in some way prodded, children with mental retardation tend to show less peer interaction when placed in groups (Beveridge, 1976; Sinson & Wetherick, 1982). The distinction between the prompted and spontaneous pragmatic behavior of children with retardation can be clinically important. Unlike other children, they may show a considerable gap between the number of speech act types in their repertoire and the number of speech act tokens actually produced in conversation.

To get along socially and communicate information effectively, all individuals modify their style of speech in different situations. For example, typically developing children may select different vocabulary and may vary the syntactic form to make a request sound polite, or they may speak more simply to children who are younger. Studies of children and adolescents with mild to moderate retardation indicate that they too learn to vary the linguistic forms of their utterances in response to contextual cues but that they are delayed in this ability compared to nonretarded children of the same CA (Abbeduto, 1991). In one investigation, Guralnick and Paul-Brown (1986) compared children with mild retardation to typically developing children roughly matched in MA. They found that both groups made similar adjustments in language content, form, and use when talking to children with moderate and severe retardation. That is, the children with mild retardation were sensitive to the fact that their conversational partners were even more impaired intellectually, and they adjusted their own language accordingly.

Referential Communication Although studies of speech style suggest that children with mental retardation do consider the comprehension abilities of their listeners, other research indicates that they frequently fail to take account of informational needs. This problem has been studied in terms of the children's abilities to establish referents, that is, to make it clear who or what they are talking about. The experimental task most often used to study this ability has been the **barrier task**. For example, two children with mental retardation will sit on opposite sides of a screen that allows them to hear but not see each other. Both children will be given identical sets of pictures of unusual geometric forms. One child will be asked to select a picture and then describe it so that the other child will be able to select the same picture from his or her set. The barrier prevents the child from gesturing or from using deictic language. The child must use specific vocabulary that provides an adequate amount of detail. Investigations using the barrier task to study adolescents with mild and moderate retardation have shown consistently that they fail to provide sufficient information (Longhurst, 1972, 1974; Rueda & Chan, 1980). The difficulties do not appear to be due entirely to cognitive delay, as the subjects with mental retardation performed more poorly than typically developing children matched for MA (Longhurst, 1972). It was also clear from these studies that the problems in communication were the fault of the speaker, not the listener. The subjects with mental retardation were able to select the correct pictures when the speaker was a nondisabled adult.

In another type of study on referential communication, subjects were given commands that were ambiguous unless they made use of background information. For example, the experimenter would announce that he was looking for a gift for a child and then would ask the child to "show me that cup." The correct response was to choose a child's small cup rather than an adult's cup. Children with mild to moderate retardation were found to perform these tasks as well as MA-matched, typically developing children (Abbeduto, Davies, Solesby, & Furman, 1991). Taken together, studies of referential communication ability present a mixed picture. On some tasks, children with mental retardation appear to function at a level consistent with their cognitive status; on others, they have more difficulty than would be predicted from intelligence alone.

Conversational Repair   One of the findings of experiments on referential communication is that children and adolescents with mental retardation do a poor job of repairing breakdowns in communication. They rarely make requests for clarification when presented with an inadequate message. Additionally, when others make requests for clarification to children with mental retardation, the children rarely respond (Abbeduto et al., 1991; Longhurst, 1972; Rueda & Chan, 1980). In natural communication settings as well, children with Down syndrome respond less frequently to requests for clarification than their nonretarded peers (Coggins & Stoel-Gammon, 1982). It is unclear whether the problem of making requests for clarification is due to inability or merely social reluctance, especially when the conversational partner is a nondisabled adult (Abbeduto, 1991). As for responding to such requests, it appears that persons with mild to moderate mental retardation do develop this ability by the time they reach adulthood, though they may still fail to respond to subtle, especially nonverbal, requests for clarification (Abbeduto & Rosenberg, 1980; Longhurst & Berry, 1975; Paul & Cohen, 1984).

Turn Taking   Normal conversations are characterized by finely tuned systems for taking turns and avoiding interruptions. It is thought that these behaviors have their origins in very early parent–child interactions involving feeding and reciprocal vocalization. Because infants with Down syndrome are identified early in life, it has been possible to study their early patterns of interaction. Some of these studies have found higher rates of *vocal clashing*—that is, simultaneous vocalization—than is the case with typically developing infants and their mothers (Berger & Cunningham, 1983; Jones, 1977). However, this difference does not seem to foreshadow later problems with turn taking. Young children with Down syndrome show no difference in the rate of turn-taking errors when they are compared to typically developing children (Tannock, 1988). A low rate of turn-taking errors has also been found in a heterogeneous group of preschoolers with mental retardation (Davis, Stroud, & Green, 1988). Thus, turn-taking difficulties are not considered to be generally characteristic of children with mental retardation, even though certain individuals may exhibit problems with this aspect of conversation.

Topic Management   It is one thing for children not to interrupt and to take their turn in a conversation. It is another for them to take a good turn. Research on what is called *discourse management* suggests that individuals with mental retardation learn how to take a turn without adding significantly to a conversation (Abbeduto, 1991). They are able to maintain topics in conversations—that is, not change the subject—but they do so primarily with acknowledgments (e.g., "yeah," "uh-huh," "okay"). They remain deficient in their ability to extend topics by providing new information or new shading on the current subject of discussion. There are several possible explanations for this deficit. Individuals with retardation may simply lack the requisite knowledge for making topic extensions; they may not understand that topic maintenance is socially valued; or they may lack the cognitive ability to link information available to them to the current topic. Future research may help clarify which of these factors is most potent.

Generalization   The quality of any language learning must be measured by how much the language is really used. An opinion commonly held is that children with mental retardation do not generalize behaviors well outside the teaching environment. Two studies of nonverbal children with severe retardation illustrate the point. Calculator and Dollaghan (1982) observed the behavior of children at school and found that they used their communication boards in one-to-one sessions with a speech-language pathologist but used them much less frequently in classroom interactions. In another study, a child with severe retardation was taught to use Bliss symbols by his classroom teacher and to sign by his speech-language pathologist. He reportedly used both systems effectively but only in the settings in which they were taught (Nietupski, Scheutz, & Ockwood, 1980). These examples indicate that although children with mental retardation can acquire new communication skills, the amount of functional improvement attained may be quite limited due to poor generalization of learning.

Comprehension

The language comprehension of children with mental retardation has been studied from three vantage points: as a measure of information processing ability; as a component of linguistic competence; and as a test of contextual understanding.

Information Processing   Psychologists have long been interested in the efficiency with which individuals can derive knowledge from incoming stimuli. By varying the speed of different messages, they have found that adolescents with mild mental retardation require more time to encode incoming verbal information than nonretarded individuals of equal MA (Bilsky, 1985; Merrill & Mar, 1987). That is, it takes longer after hearing a sentence before it makes sense to children with retardation so that they can answer questions about it or identify pictures that match it. Various experiments suggest that the problem occurs at the semantic-analytic rather than at the phonological level. Words are heard as individual units of sound, but they do not quickly form a meaning in the mind of the listener.

Linguistic Competence   Language comprehension can also be considered in relation to the delay–difference controversy. Do children with retardation understand language at a level that is consistent with their cognitive abilities, or are they selectively impaired in comprehension? In a study involving a broad cross section of children and adolescents with retardation, Miller and Chapman (1984) found that only about one fourth of the subjects had receptive language delays that exceeded their cognitive delays. But another team of investigators studied a similar group of subjects and found that almost half of them showed receptive language levels that were 1 year or more below the level corresponding to their nonverbal MA

(Abbeduto, Furman, & Davies, 1989). From this evidence it appears that many, but not all, children with mental retardation may have language comprehension difficulties that exceed their cognitive delays.

Many different types of comprehension errors occur in children with retardation, but it is not clear whether these errors signal a qualitative difference in language acquisition. In one comparison, 6-year-old children with mild mental retardation and 3-year-old typically developing children performed similarly on tasks requiring comprehension of sentences containing contrasting syntactic forms, such as past versus present tense verbs and affirmative versus negative statements (Lovell & Dixon, 1967). Other studies have found similar patterns, suggesting that children with retardation learn to comprehend syntactic structures in approximately the same sequence as typically developing children (Berry, 1972; Dewart, 1979; Lamberts & Weener, 1976; Wheldall, 1976). Nevertheless, sentence comprehension deficits are found even when subjects with and without retardation are matched for LA (Dewart, 1979; Wheldall, 1976). At this point in our research, it is therefore unwise to draw sweeping conclusions. Studies limited to children with Down syndrome (discussed later) are providing more detail about this population, and future research will probably concentrate on other biological subgroups. There is also some indication that children with retardation show similar patterns of comprehension learning up to, but not beyond, a certain developmental level. In children who have reached MAs of 7 and 9 years, comprehension problems have been found to be concentrated in particular syntactic forms, such as passives and comparatives (Abbeduto et al., 1989).

Contextual Understanding   Formal evaluations of information processing or language comprehension may not accurately predict how well children with mental retardation will comprehend in real situations, which provide redundancy and contextual cues to meaning. Both observational and experimental studies suggest that children with mental retardation comprehend requests—even ones made indirectly—at a level comparable to MA- and LA-matched, typically developing children (Abbeduto et al., 1989; Hanzlik &

Stevenson, 1986; Leifer & Lewis, 1984). What is more important, there is evidence that adolescents and adults with mild to moderate retardation learn to respond appropriately to speech acts produced within routine activities (Abbeduto, 1991). They appear to be aided by the predictability of these settings, which makes it unnecessary for them to analyze fully the content of a speaker's request. Thus, individuals with mental retardation may often function more adequately in everyday activities than formal testing or performance in nonroutine situations would lead us to expect.

Semantics

Children with mental retardation have long been characterized as having **concreteness** in their thinking and, consequently, in their learning and use of vocabulary (Karlin & Strazzula, 1952). One of the clearest expressions of lexical concreteness is in the comprehension of idioms (e.g., "got cold feet," "broke her heart"), which rely on nonliteral interpretation. Idiom understanding is significantly poorer in 9-year-old children with mild mental retardation than in typically developing children of the same age (Ezell & Goldstein, 1991a). Is this concreteness a unique feature of mental retardation or is it merely associated with younger MA? Rosenberg (1982), based on a review of studies conducted up to 1980, concluded that the learning of concrete words and semantic relations follows the same course as in typically developing children but moves at a slower pace in children with mental retardation. When language samples produced by children with retardation were compared with typically developing children matched for MA, no significant differences were found in the number of semantic relations produced (Kamhi & Johnston, 1982). Thus concreteness is probably best attributed to cognitive delay and can be expected to be greater in individuals with more severe retardation.

It should be noted that our picture of semantic development is far from complete. Although we believe that children with retardation are delayed in their learning of concrete semantic categories, there is little evidence to indicate whether the acquisition of abstract semantic knowledge is similarly delayed (Rosenberg, 1982). It is possible, though not yet demonstrated, that there is a level above which semantic development may not continue for these children.

Syntax

Any generalizations about the syntactic deficits of children with mental retardation should be treated cautiously. Much of the recent research on children with Down syndrome has highlighted their syntactic difficulty, but similar conclusions do not yet appear warranted for other subgroups (Fowler, 1990; Stoel-Gammon, 1990). In addition, the majority of studies on syntactic development of non–Down syndrome children have been done with high-functioning individuals. Studies with low-functioning children suggest that patterns of syntactic learning may differ, depending on the severity of retardation (Bliss, Allen, & Walker, 1978).

The general conclusion drawn in the past was that syntactic functioning in children with retardation shows a developmental lag and that MA is therefore a better predictor of syntactic performance than CA (Rosenberg, 1982). For example, language samples gathered from adolescents with mild to severe retardation showed a high correlation between MA and the length and syntactic complexity of their sentences (Graham & Graham, 1971).

The interpretation of delay appears to hold regardless of the level of syntax that is measured. Compared to typically developing children, children with mild mental retardation master bound morphemes in approximately the same order but at a slower rate (Newfield & Schlanger, 1968). The number of inflectional errors occurring in language samples is about the same in children with mild mental retardation and typically developing children (Kamhi & Johnston, 1982). A finding inconsistent with the delay position was reported by Lovell and Bradbury (1967), who studied the inflections produced by 14- and 15-year-old English children with mild retardation. When the results were compared to those from typically developing American first graders, the English children's scores were significantly lower, despite their higher MAs. However, this finding may have been due to cultural differences or to the test that was used, which employs nonsense words and has been found to overestimate morphological errors (Berko, 1958; Dever, 1972).

The acquisition of phrase structures appears to follow a similar developmental pattern in children with and without retardation, even though the rate of learning is significantly different. On a sentence imitation task, children with mental retardation who had an MA of 5 years performed like typically developing children who were 3 years of age (McLeavey, Toomey, & Dempsey, 1982). This suggests that phrasal learning follows the typical developmental sequence but is even more delayed than MA would predict. On the other hand, Kamhi and Johnston (1982) measured spontaneous production of pronouns, noun phrases, verb phrases, and negatives and found differences between children with and without retardation that were consistent with their MA differences. It may be that the discrepancy in results is attributable to differences between imitative and spontaneous language production.

The area of syntactic development that does provide some evidence of a difference rather than a delay is the acquisition of clause structures. The same two studies described in the preceding paragraph (Kamhi & Johnston, 1982; McLeavey et al., 1982) both found significant differences in the production of subordinating conjunctions, for example, "who" introducing a relative clause or "because." In spontaneous speech, children with retardation relied on "and" as the only form of clausal linkage. They also produced significantly fewer question forms (interrogative reversals and wh- questions) and used only developmentally simple question forms, such as copula reversal and "what" questions. As a whole, these findings indicate that a difference in clausal syntax development may exist among children with retardation but that it may emerge only in the later stages of language acquisition.

Speech Production

Among all subgroups of children with mental retardation, there is evidence that speech production problems are more prevalent than among typically developing children. It has been estimated that 70% of all children with mental retardation have some form of speech production problem (Fristoe & Lloyd, 1979). Some of the factors that contribute to speech difficulties are the high prevalence of hearing impairment and the neuromotor deficits and orofacial anomalies that are associated with certain developmental syndromes. These factors do not explain, however, why speech production problems are common among children with nonorganic retardation. In one study on this issue, words produced by 5-year-old children with mild retardation were compared to those of preschool groups of communicatively handicapped and typically developing children (Klink, Gerstman, Raphael, Schlanger, & Newsome, 1986). All subjects were roughly matched for MLU. It was discovered that problems occurring as a result of phonological processes were significantly more frequent in the children with retardation and communicative handicap but that the profile of process usage (types of processes used) was comparable across all three groups. The only characteristic that distinguished the children with retardation was the presence of the final consonant **devoicing** process (e.g., "ca*p*" for "ca*b*"). This evidence, though limited, suggests that at least some children with retardation should be considered to have specific phonological delays that are inconsistent with their general level of language development.

LANGUAGE CHARACTERISTICS OF CHILDREN WITH DOWN SYNDROME

Because Down syndrome is the most common chromosomal cause of retardation and because it can usually be identified from birth, this subgroup is the best-studied of all subgroups of children with mental retardation (Gerber, 1990). Many studies also indicate that children with Down syndrome are especially impaired in their development of language compared with other groups of children with mental retardation (Fowler, 1990). They are consistently below CA expectations and frequently show deficits that are incommensurate with other areas of development. To be sure, a major issue in research on children with Down syndrome has become the extent to which some language domains (e.g., phonology, syntax, and vocabulary) may be specifically impaired, that is, lower than MA would predict.

Children with Down syndrome may have more difficulties with some aspects of language than other children with mental retardation.

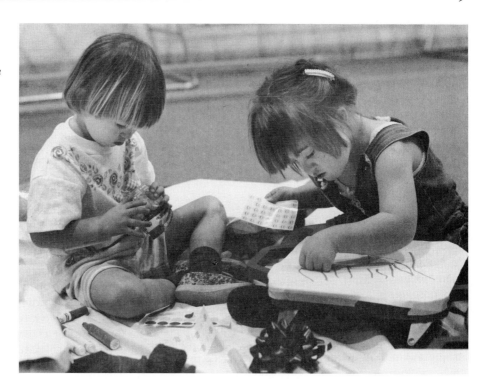

Comprehension

Although the comprehension of children with Down syndrome is clearly delayed, research has not yet indicated conclusively whether it is specifically impaired. Some reviewers have claimed that specific language deficits observed in Down syndrome affect production but not comprehension (Lynch & Eilers, 1991; Stoel-Gammon, 1990). Others see the impairment affecting both aspects of language development (Fowler, 1990). Still others confine themselves to the statement that comprehension abilities often exceed production abilities (Mahoney, Glover, & Finger, 1981; Miller, 1988).

Another question that can be asked about comprehension is whether children with Down syndrome are equally competent at all levels of language. To find an answer, Chapman, Schwartz, and Kay-Raining Bird (1991) compared the lexical and syntactic comprehension test scores of children and adolescents with Down syndrome with those of an MA-matched group of typically developing children. They found that what

distinguished the two groups was the difference between lexical and syntactic test scores. The subjects with Down syndrome achieved age-equivalent scores on the vocabulary test that were nearly a year better than their syntax scores. Moreover, this gap widened steadily with age. During the period from 5 to 8 years the scores were nearly equal, but by 16 to 20 years they were over 2 years apart. Consistent with this finding, children and adolescents with Down syndrome were found to have fast-mapping ability comparable to that of typically developing children matched for MA (Chapman, Kay-Raining Bird, & Schwartz, 1990). Together these studies suggest that comprehension should not be regarded as a singular ability in these children. The evidence indicates that syntactic comprehension is most likely to be specifically impaired compared to vocabulary comprehension.

Semantics

We have just reviewed the relationship between vocabulary and syntax for comprehension. From the perspective of production, a similar pattern can be seen. When children with Down syndrome and typically developing children are matched for MA, speech samples obtained from the children with Down syndrome are found to contain a smaller number of different words. However, when the children are matched for MLU, the result is reversed and the samples from children with Down syndrome show more diverse vocabulary (Miller, 1988; Miller, Budde, Bashir, & LaFollette, 1987). Parent reports reveal that children with Down syndrome show spurts of vocabulary growth but fall steadily behind their typically developing peers (Miller, 1992). These comparisons suggest that vocabulary development lags behind what would be predicted from MA but is superior to syntactic development.

In the area of relational semantics, very limited research suggests that the behavior of children with Down syndrome should be described as delayed but not different. Coggins (1979) studied the spontaneous language production of four children with Down syndrome and mild retardation whose MLUs ranged from 1.22 to 2.06. He found that the frequency and distribution of semantic relations were comparable to those reported for typically developing children at the same level of language development.

Syntax

The notion of a specific language impairment in children with Down syndrome is best supported in the domain of syntax. Researchers have followed the development of cognition, language comprehension, and language production in a group of young (11 to 58 months) children with Down syndrome (Miller, 1988). When measures were first taken, the children fell into three groups: Half of the children were in Group 1, which showed comprehension and production skills that were consistent with MA; the other children were divided between Groups 2 and 3. The children in Group 2 exhibited deficits in production compared to comprehension and MA, while the children in Group 3 showed deficits in both comprehension and production relative to MA. Twenty-four months later, however, the proportions had changed: 75% of the children were in Groups 2 and 3, most of them in Group 2. Therefore, it appears that, over time,

the language production skills of children with Down syndrome fall behind both their cognitive and comprehension abilities.

Speech Production

Research on the phonetic and phonological development of children with Down syndrome has produced a set of inconsistent findings. The early phonetic behaviors of infants with Down syndrome seem to unfold in a pattern similar to that of typically developing children. It is presently unclear, however, whether the rate of learning is the same or slower in infants with Down syndrome. A study of infants enrolled in an early intervention program found that they produced similar vocalizations, had a similar age of onset for reduplicated babbling, and showed similar patterns in place of articulation of consonantlike sounds (Smith & Oller, 1981). But a more recent study of infants with Down syndrome not receiving intervention found that the average age of onset for adultlike syllables was later than that of typically developing children and that mature syllable production was less consistent through the end of the first year (Lynch, Oller, Eilers, & Basinger, 1990, cited in Lynch & Eilers, 1991). Early intervention appears to have played a role in producing these contradictory findings, but further study of the issue is needed.

As meaningful speech begins, the order of phoneme acquisition has been found to be very similar between children with Down syndrome and mild retardation and typically developing children matched for MLU (Stoel-Gammon, 1980). The phonetic inventories of the children with Down syndrome included nearly all of the sounds that were simplified in spontaneous production, showing that their problems are due to phonological delay rather than to phonetic impairment resulting from anatomical or physiological differences. Furthermore, the specific patterns of sound omission and substitution produced by children with Down syndrome are comparable to those found in typically developing children (Bleile & Schwarz, 1984; Smith & Stoel-Gammon, 1983; Stoel-Gammon, 1980).

Not all the research, however, has been consistent with the interpretation of phonological delay. Dodd (1975) compared children with Down syndrome and an average age of 9 years to a CA- and MA-matched group of children with mental retardation but not Down syndrome. She found that while the children with Down syndrome were better at recognizing real and nonsense words, they were poorer at repeating them after delays of 15 and 30 seconds. This finding was interpreted as evidence of a specific motor disability that impeded correct articulation. In another study, Dodd (1976) found a higher frequency of phonological errors in children with Down syndrome than in MA-matched groups of non–Down syndrome children with retardation and typically developing children. This finding is inconsistent with later studies of the same population (Bleile & Schwarz, 1984; Stoel-Gammon, 1980). Dodd's data were taken from older children and were elicited through picture naming rather than spontaneous speech, but a final explanation of the discrepancy awaits further research.

Rate of Language Learning

One of the most interesting findings to emerge from studies of children with Down syndrome is that they do not appear to learn language at a constant rate. Table 6.6 summarizes the general findings from several different types of investigations: longitudinal studies in which the same individuals are followed over a period of months or years; training studies in which children are taught new language forms over a period of months; and cross-sectional studies in which individuals of varying ages are compared to determine their developmental trends. The broad pattern revealed by this research is that children with Down syndrome show strong development during the infant and toddler years, especially when facilitated by early intervention programs. In many cases, these children perform at levels comparable to those of their typically developing peers. Thereafter, language development continues at a slightly slower pace into the early school years. During these years, comparisons with typically developing children begin to reveal more gaps in language ability. From roughly 8 years of age until the middle or end of adolescence, many children with Down syndrome appear to reach a plateau in development. What little language change occurs tends to be growth in vocabulary, so the discrepancy between lexical and syntactic abilities becomes larger

during this time. In early adulthood there appears to be some slight additional growth in language.

Not all scholars agree that individuals with Down syndrome show a developmental ceiling, beyond which it is difficult or impossible for their language to advance. Though some evidence exists in support of this notion, it is unclear whether the ceiling is attributable to physical changes associated with aging or to some type of cognitive limitation. One interpretation of the available information is that individuals with Down syndrome do not progress further than the language level associated with a mental age of 5 years (Fowler, 1988).

Use of Imitation

It sometimes seems that children with Down syndrome use gesture and verbal imitation more often than typically developing children, especially during the early stages of language development. However, a carefully controlled study of 12- to 26-month-old typically developing children and MA-matched children with Down syndrome found the groups to be highly similar, using equal amounts of speech and gesture (McCune et al., 1989).

As for verbal imitation, some studies have found it to be delayed in children with Down syndrome but others have found no difference in its frequency (Coggins & Morrison, 1981; Mahoney et al., 1981; McCune et al., 1989; Owens & MacDonald, 1982). Conclusions are made even more difficult by the fact that subjects in these studies have often been enrolled in language therapy. Thus, the findings may be contaminated by changes in imitative behavior caused by intervention (McCune et al., 1989). When Tager-Flusberg and Calkins (1990) compared the spontaneous and imitative utterances of children with Down syndrome, they found them to be comparable in length and complexity. This suggests that imitation is not a crucial language learning mechanism for these children.

Explanations for Specific Language Deficit in Children with Down Syndrome

It is now well established that children with Down syndrome are delayed in language acquisition. It also appears likely that they are specifically impaired in

TABLE 6.6 Developmental Language Profile of Children with Down Syndrome

CA	MA	Type of Research	Language Profile
0–12 months		Longitudinal	Vocalizations are similar to those of typically developing children. Onset of adultlike syllables may be slightly delayed (Lynch, Oller, Eilers, & Basinger, 1990, cited in Lynch & Eilers, 1991; Smith & Oller, 1981).
20–36 months	13–21 months	Training	Comprehension and production vocabularies are the same as those of typically developing children (Cardoso-Martins, Mervis, & Mervis, 1985).
	24–36 months	Cross-sectional	Productive syntax (as measured by Developmental Sentence Scoring) is consistent with MA (Wiegel-Crump, 1981).
	3:0–6:11 years	Longitudinal	Productive syntax increasingly falls below MA expectations (Fowler, 1988).
3–6 years		Longitudinal	Steady increase in the CA–LA gap in phonological development (Smith & Stoel-Gammon, 1983).
4–8 years		Longitudinal	Rapid constant growth in MLU up to a level of 3.5 morphemes. Syntactic and lexical comprehension are comparable (Chapman et al., 1991; Fowler, 1988).
8–15 years		Longitudinal	Little language change (Fowler, 1988).
13–19 years		Cross-sectional	Steady increase to an MLU of 4.0. Syntactic comprehension is significantly poorer than lexical comprehension (Chapman et al., 1991; Rondal, 1988).
20–26:6 years		Cross-sectional	Slight additional increase in MLU (Rondal, 1988).
	5+ years	Longitudinal	No further language growth. Not all children with Down syndrome reach this level of language development, for reasons that are not well understood (Fowler, 1988).

syntactic development, and perhaps in other language domains, even when compared to MA. How do we account for the special language problems of this subgroup? Table 6.7 provides a short account of some possible explanations and some of the flaws of those explanations. As the table suggests, none of these explanations provides a completely satisfactory answer to the question. Certain accounts are logically flawed, and others must await further research before they can be stated in precise terms.

TABLE 6.7 Explanations for Specific Language Impairment in Children with Down Syndrome

Explanation	Critique
They are less motivated than other children to perform linguistically. In institutions and even at home, their needs are met without requiring them to use language.	This argument ignores the fact that motivation does not explain normal language development, which requires children to learn forms that do not necessarily improve their ability to express needs and wants. We would also expect that there would have been some motivational improvement as institutionalization has decreased. Yet studies have shown no differences in syntactic development between home-reared and institutionalized children with Down syndrome (Fowler, 1990).
Parents of children with Down syndrome do not provide a good language learning environment.	Studies indicate that once children with Down syndrome talk, their mothers interact with them in the same way they interact with non-handicapped children at comparable language levels. It is not clear whether differences in maternal behavior during the prelinguistic period may influence language development (Fowler, 1990).
There are neurological differences in children with Down syndrome that are responsible for the observed language deficits. Dichotic listening tests have found that many children with Down syndrome do not show a right-ear advantage, as typically developing children do (Fowler, 1990). Also, infants and children with Down syndrome may show difficulty in processing some of the acoustic cues that signal the difference between consonants (Lynch & Eilers, 1991).	These studies are methodologically complicated and hard to interpret.
There is a maturational plateau, either an MA or a linguistic stage, beyond which language learning, and syntactic learning in particular, becomes much more difficult (Fowler, 1990).	The neurological mechanisms responsible for such a plateau are not understood.
Hearing loss produces impairment of both language and nonverbal cognition (Lynch & Eilers, 1991; Stoel-Gammon, 1990).	Does not suffice as an explanation. The level of hearing loss observed among individuals with Down syndrome does not produce marked impairment when it occurs in individuals without retardation. Hearing loss is therefore best thought of as a contributory factor.
Structural differences in the speech mechanism, such as a small maxilla, missing teeth, small oral cavity, high palate, or tongue hypertrophy (Stoel-Gammon, 1981, 1990), are responsible for a speech-specific motor difficulty.	Difficult to understand why this would produce a specific syntactic deficit. It is best thought of as a contributory factor.

IMPLICATIONS FOR INTERVENTION

Each child with mental retardation presents a unique pattern of communicative abilities and difficulties, which must be identified as a result of a thorough individual assessment. There is, therefore, no one intervention prescription for children with retardation. There is, however, a set of general principles and considerations that apply to all intervention efforts.

Social and Legislative Influences

Recall from chapter 4 that federal legislation has mandated equal educational opportunity for the disabled. This has led to the end of institutionalization for all but the most severely impaired children with mental retardation and to the mainstreaming of disabled children into regular classrooms. To help these children and their teachers, specialists are increasingly being asked to serve as classroom consultants as part of their role as interventionists. This consultant role involves skills in assessing communicative needs, developing intervention strategies, training personnel who will administer programs, and developing methods of reviewing and improving the treatment programs (Cipani, 1989). The shift to community integration of children with mental retardation also means that an increasing number of intervention strategies are designed to promote interaction with peers (e.g., Goldstein & Ferrell, 1987) and to increase the communicative experiences of the children in public places such as shopping malls, museums, and sports arenas (e.g., Gullo & Gullo, 1984).

Nonspeech Options

Logically, one of the first and most important intervention decisions is whether a child with mental retardation will be taught to communicate by speaking or by manual or electronic means. Most experts in the field recommend that alternative/augmentative communication be initiated only after natural communication systems have been thoroughly tried. With alternative/augmentative communication, the opportunities for incidental learning will be limited because the child will be acquiring a specialized form of communication that not everyone will understand. The child's family will have to learn to sign or understand nonspeech communication, which may increase stress in the home but may also open up avenues of communication (Swift & Rosin, 1990).

Owens and House (1984) reviewed research concerning the cognitive, social, and receptive language prerequisites to alternative/augmentative communication training. If these prerequisites are met and motor speech evaluation does not indicate overwhelming difficulties, they suggest that speech therapy be tried for at least 1 year. If little improvement occurs, then alternative/augmentative approaches should be tried. *Alternative/augmentative communication* consists of naturally occurring behaviors that fall short of speech. Home and school observations of individuals with moderate to severe retardation have identified a number of alternative behaviors, such as vocalization, gesture, and physical manipulation. These behaviors serve a variety of communicative functions: answering, greeting, negating, and so forth. When professionals plan to introduce alternative/augmentative communication systems, they should also consider the role of extant alternative/augmentative communication behaviors (Romski, Sevcik, Reumann, & Pate, 1989). Such behaviors may either complement or interfere with the alternative/augmentative system being considered.

Research on children with mental retardation suggests that speech and sign language are both learned more easily than graphic symbol systems. Children with Down syndrome learn their first signs more easily than their first words, as do typically developing children, but the sign advantage drops out before the onset of syntax (Fowler, 1990). Total communication (simultaneous teaching of speech and sign) and speech training alone have been compared in two groups of preschoolers with Down syndrome. Following a 5-month program, the children in the total communication group successfully acquired signs, but there were no significant differences between the groups in their rate of language and cognitive development (Weller & Mahoney, 1983). In a comparison of alternative/augmentative approaches, Hodges and Schwethelm (1984) found that 52 children with profound retardation learned significantly more ASL signs than graphic symbols when exposed to both communication systems. Studies such as these suggest that sign language can serve an important adjunctive role in intervention, especially with children who lack speech. For children with the motoric ability to produce signs, it is probably more easily learned than other graphic communication systems.

Reduction of Inappropriate Behaviors

Many children with mental retardation produce verbal or nonverbal behaviors that may interfere either with communication itself or with professionals' efforts to teach new communication skills. For example, a child who screams or hits to gain attention will deter many potential communication partners. Aberrant behaviors such as these fall into two categories: escape behaviors maintained by negative reinforcement and attention-seeking behaviors maintained by positive reinforcement (Carr & Durand, 1985). Sometimes the teaching of a new language behavior will empower the children so that they are able to avoid previously aversive conditions (e.g., hunger, a dirty diaper, a need to be held). This, in turn, will reduce the frequency of the undesirable behavior that they formerly used to avoid the aversive conditions. In one study, nondisabled peers were used to enhance the number of communicative interactions entered into by developmentally disabled preschoolers. A side benefit of this program was that it led to a decrease in two undesirable behaviors, nonsocial utterances and interruptions of the teacher (Goldstein & Ferrell, 1987). In sum, it may occasionally be necessary to reduce certain inappropriate behaviors before other language intervention procedures can be implemented. In those instances, professionals should consider teaching alternative behaviors to replace those regarded as undesirable.

Intelligibility

Because a high percentage of children with mental retardation have a speech production problem, it is important to consider whether articulatory and phonological impairments will hinder efforts to change other aspects of language. Fey (1986) argues that improvements in intelligibility will allow children to display linguistic abilities without frustration. This will improve conversational interaction and promote faster language learning. In addition, we should always recall that language production teaching requires us to judge children's attempts at target forms. If those attempts are unintelligible, we cannot reinforce or even respond appropriately; under these circumstances, treatment will languish.

In some instances, attempts have been made to improve intelligibility through surgery rather than therapy. Children with Down syndrome often exhibit tongue hypertrophy, which has been thought to contribute to their articulatory difficulties. However, pre- and postsurgical evaluation of a tongue reduction procedure performed on 18 children with Down syndrome found no significant differences in the number of consonant errors produced on a single-word articulation test (Parsons, Iacono, & Rozner, 1987). This suggests that surgery alone will not produce an improvement in intelligibility. Intervention should instead be based on a child's phonetic repertoire, phonological profile, and cognitive level, as is generally recommended in cases of poor intelligibility (Creaghead, Newman, & Secord, 1989).

Facilitating versus Compensatory Intervention

We noted earlier in this chapter (see Table 6.4) that scholars who view children with retardation as delayed rather than as different also believe that these children reach a developmental plateau beyond which they show relatively few gains. We have also reviewed longitudinal evidence from children with Down syndrome (see Table 6.6) that language learning is most rapid during the early years of life, and that the rate and extent of learning appear to slow dramatically in later childhood and thereafter. Considering these findings, we may need to distinguish between early and late developmental periods and develop different intervention strategies for the two stages. In the early years, the professional role may be to facilitate language by providing and fostering greater cognitive and language stimulation. In the later years, the role may be to teach compensatory strategies that will help both the children and those who interact with them to communicate more functionally (cf. Crystal, 1984). For example, a program for infants and toddlers with mental retardation may provide intensive general stimulation.

As the children grow older, increasingly specific language forms and functions may be targeted so that ultimately, in the adolescent and adult years, communicative intervention is designed to teach abilities that will improve performance in a particular school or job setting.

Developmental versus Remedial Logic

One of the clearest areas of disagreement regarding intervention is found in response to the question "Should children with retardation be taught like typically developing children?" This dispute has been described as a contrast between developmental and remedial logic (Fey, 1986). In simple terms, *developmental logic* argues that language targets should be presented to children with retardation in the same order that they are acquired by typically developing children (Miller & Yoder, 1974). This is consistent with the delay view of mental retardation, which emphasizes that the developmental processes of these children show far more similarities to than differences from those of typically developing children.

On the other hand, *remedial logic* makes the straightforward point that children with retardation are by definition not developing typically (Guess, Sailor, & Baer, 1978); therefore, nondevelopmental approaches are required to assist them. There is, moreover, some research evidence to suggest that children with mental retardation learn language differently. In particular, they do not show the same kinds of interrelationships between language comprehension and production processes as typically developing children (Ezell & Goldstein, 1989; Guess & Baer, 1973). In the case of children with Down syndrome, syntactic skills may be especially problematic compared to other language abilities (Fowler, 1990).

In intervention, it is likely unnecessary to choose one rationale over the other. The heterogeneity of children with mental retardation makes it impossible to generalize, and the critical point is to select approaches that most effectively help the children. It is apparent, however, that most programs that employ remedial logic (e.g., Guess et al., 1978) are intended for use with severely and profoundly impaired individuals. In contrast, developmental logic is more likely to be the basis of treatment regimens for children with mild to moderate retardation. Miller (1984) points out that all instructional approaches—behavior modification, cognitive learning strategies, and naturalistic ecological models—should be used with children who are mentally retarded. Naturalistic methods may be preferred if there is evidence that the child is doing a lot of incidental learning, that is, acquiring language forms that are not specifically trained. On the other hand, if incidental learning stops, new behaviors might be introduced behaviorally and then generalized through more naturalistic strategies.

Language–Cognition Relationships

To those who regard mental retardation from the delay perspective and who accept the cognitive hypothesis, the presence of a gap between a child's MA and LA is regarded as a positive prognostic sign for intervention. The reason is simple. From this perspective, the ceiling for a child's language development is set by the child's cognitive development; if MA exceeds LA, then a child has room to grow. Another similar interpretation would be that when a child's LA approaches or matches the MA, language development can be expected to plateau. At that point, as noted in the preceding section, a change in intervention tactics may be warranted.

These interpretations of the language–cognition relationship are speculative, and not everyone who intervenes with children with retardation will want to accept them. There is little doubt, however, that to teach language to children with retardation, the cognitive requirements for learning must be evaluated. Generally, for example, children with retardation will require more redundancy in instruction. In a study comparing 3-year-old children with Down syndrome to typically developing children matched for MA, the two groups showed different learning patterns when tested on various self-help and preacademic tasks (pouring, hammering, building block towers, etc.). Verbal teaching alone, even when repeated, was far less effective with the children with Down syndrome. Their performance was better when the verbal instructions were accompanied by a model or physical guidance (Rynders, Behlen, & Horrobin, 1979).

The suggestion has been made that if cognitive development is prerequisite to language acquisition, a good intervention strategy would be to train cognition before attempting to introduce language targets. Curricula exist for training sensorimotor skills to children with moderate and severe retardation (Dunst, 1980, 1981; Robinson & Robinson, 1983). At least one researcher has found that training in *object permanence* and *means–end behaviors* enhanced the learning of referential speech by children with profound retardation (Kahn, 1984). With more cognitively mature individuals in whom language is well established, cognitive training is more likely to focus on developing *strategies* for accomplishing particular language tasks. For example, rehearsal strategies have been successfully taught to adolescents with mild retardation. Subjects were instructed to *rehearse* (repeat to themselves) auditory commands silently before they attempted to carry out the requested action. This strategy led to an improvement in their performance (Milgram & Furth, 1968).

It may be, then, that cognition training can facilitate language learning and language performance in children with retardation. As Finch-Williams (1984) has noted, however, there is a sticky issue attached to cognition training, namely, who should do the training—a speech-language pathologist, a school psychologist, a special education teacher, or another professional? At present there are no guidelines to refer to, so each decision is made on an individual basis, hopefully with consultation of the various professionals involved in assisting a child.

Pragmatic Relevance

Practically minded professionals have long recognized that language intervention for children with mental retardation must result in functional gains. There is little point in teaching a child to produce a new set of words, a new bound morpheme, or new grammatical operation if these forms do not help everyday communication in the short or long term. This concern has been stated even more frequently of late, as the pragmatics revolution has emphasized that language intervention should be done in a natural communicative context and should avoid pragmatically isolated drill.

Fey (1986) suggests that the basic goal of language intervention should be to achieve a balance in the child's ability to respond and to produce assertive communicative acts. Yet, children with mental retardation may be passive (Rosenberg, 1982). Thus they may be likely to fall into Fey's categories of passive conversationalists or inactive communicators. For these kinds of children, Fey (1986) recommends intervention procedures that will increase the range and frequency of assertive behavior. Table 6.8 gives examples of specific goals that might be pursued and some procedures that might be used to implement those goals.

Another important consideration in achieving pragmatic success is that we must achieve a reasonable fit between a child's communicative behavior and the typical conditions of everyday life. If the fit is poor, a behavior tends not to be used. Cipani (1989) suggests that in order to be maintained, a communicative behavior must meet three criteria: (1) it must be fluent, that is, occur within an acceptable time after the stimulus; (2) it must be used neither too little nor too much; and (3) it must occur in response to a variety of natural stimuli. In short, the language behaviors we teach must be sufficiently fine-tuned that they do not give the impression of having been learned as a result of intervention.

Goal Attack Strategy

Deciding how many and in what sequence target behaviors will be introduced to a child is an important intervention consideration. As with any children, the number of goals worked on at one time is determined by factors such as attention span, motivation, cooperation, and rate of learning (Fey, 1986). Compared with their typically developing peers, children with mental retardation generally have problems in all of these areas. This suggests that the number of goals should be limited, possibly even to one at a time for some children (Miller & Yoder, 1974).

Caretaker Interaction

The relationship between adult caretakers and children with retardation has important implications for

TABLE 6.8 Goals and Procedures for Children with Mental Retardation Who Are Inactive Communicators or Passive Conversationalists

Basic Goals (After Fey, 1986)	Example of Specific Goal	Example of the Procedure
Increase the child's frequency of social bids (verbal *and* nonverbal) in a variety of social contexts.	Increase the number of spontaneous vocalizations.	Allow periods of silence during interactions with children who are severely retarded so that they have more opportunity to initiate vocalization (Halle, Hunt, & Bjorenson, 1984).
Increase the frequency of use of available assertive conversational acts in a variety of social contexts.	Increase the number of verbal requests.	Wait 5 seconds after approaching a child who is in need of help and is capable of requesting it. If no request is produced, provide an imitative prompt (Halle, Baer, & Spradlin, 1981).
Increase the child's repertoire of requestive conversational acts, using existing forms, when possible.	Increase the number of requests for action.	Use interactive routines to create both the need and the opportunity for adults with severe or profound retardation to communicate. For example, an individual with retardation can be shown how to operate a radio by using a special stick to turn it on. After repeating the demonstration several times, give the radio to the individual with retardation but without the stick needed to operate it (McLean, McLean, Brady, & Etter, 1991).
Train new linguistic forms that are useful in performing available assertive acts.	Increase the number of verbal forms for requesting action.	Use a combination of focused stimulation and incidental teaching to train the forms "Pass me the _____, please" and "Help me, please."

the development of these children and for intervention efforts. Consequently, this relationship has been frequently studied to determine whether and how parents act differently toward children with retardation, to uncover the causes of any differences, and to see if parents' behavior can be changed with positive effects. Table 6.9 summarizes the results from various studies on this topic. Collectively, this research suggests that parents and teachers act and talk somewhat differently to children with mental retardation. Many of the adults' behaviors, however, appear to be in reaction to the conduct of the children. Regardless of how the interaction begins, it appears possible to modify parental behavior toward children with mental retardation and, by so doing, to achieve developmental gains.

Materials Selection

One of the foremost practical considerations in planning an intervention procedure is selecting materials that will engage children's attention and motivate them to participate in the designed activity. In this regard, we should remember that children with mental retardation are often delayed in other areas of development. Delays in sensory and motor development and social skills, combined with cognitive impairment, make it very difficult to predict a child's level of interest with a particular toy or activity. Neither MA nor CA can be expected to provide an unerring guide. A 7-year-old child with an MA of 3 years is likely to reject many of the toys and games that a typically developing 3-year-old would delight in. On the other hand, the child with mental retardation probably lacks the cognitive abilities and knowledge base to play many of the games that a typical second-grade child would play.

A child's level of retardation may provide another guide to materials selection. For example, Spiegel (1983) found that the rate of language learning, the growth of mean sentence length, and the amount of language generalization for adolescents with severe mental retardation were all significantly greater when real objects and behaviors rather than pictures were

TABLE 6.9 Questions Raised and Answers Given by Research on Interaction Between
Adult Caretakers and Children with Mental Retardation

Question	Research indicates that . . .
Do mothers talk differently to children with retardation?	Some say no. Marshall, Hegrenes, and Goldstein (1973) compared the language of mothers of children with retardation to that of mothers of typically developing children. The children were matched for CA. Despite the clear developmental differences between the two groups of children, they found few differences in the language used by the mothers when talking to their children.
	Others say yes. Mothers were found to produce more frequent but shorter utterances in conversation with children with Down syndrome than with their nonretarded siblings (Buium, Rynders, & Turnure, 1974).
	Mothers of children with Down syndrome often use larger numbers of imperatives than mothers of typically developing children (Cardoso-Martins & Mervis, 1985).
Do parents act differently with children with retardation?	There is evidence that the parents of children with mental retardation (Stoneman, Brody, & Abbott, 1983) and the mothers of children with Down syndrome (Cardoso-Martins & Mervis, 1985; Eheart, 1982; Smith, 1989) are more likely than the parents of typically developing children to take a dominant managerial role in interactions with their children.
Why do parents of children with retardation tend to take a dominant role?	One factor contributing to this tendency may be that children with mental retardation have been found to be less responsive to their parents than typically developing children. It may also be that the parents of Down syndrome children, being aware of their handicap, feel the need to provide additional stimulation or draw their children's attention in certain directions (Lynch & Eilers, 1991; Smith, 1989). Parents of children with Down syndrome are especially concerned with the social acceptability of their children's behavior and tend to be more directive when, for example, the children exhibit nonstandard play with toys (Maurer & Sherrod, 1987).
Can parental behavior be changed?	Girolametto (1988) found that an 11-week parent education course was effective in reducing the directiveness and increasing the responsiveness of mothers of children with developmental delays. The children showed significant gains in both assertive and responsive conversational acts, number of verbal turns, and diversity of vocabulary.
Do changes in parental behavior lead to developmental gains in children with retardation?	Some say no. Girolametto (1988) found that parent education produced no language gains, as measured by the Sequenced Inventory of Communication Development.
	Others say yes. A number of studies (Bidder, Bryant, & Gray, 1975; Ludlow & Allen, 1979; MacDonald et al., 1974) have found that early parent training improves the language development of children with Down syndrome.
What methods of parent training work best?	Researchers have not yet undertaken studies comparing different instructional methods, so we must use the suggestions made from studies of language development in children with Down syndrome (Pruess, Vadasy, & Fewell, 1987).
Do teachers talk differently to children with retardation?	Teachers have been found to modify their speech to children with mental retardation in accord with their perceived communicative level (Hodapp, Evans, & Ward, 1989). The changes are largely functional: They request different kinds of responses (attend, identification or yes/no, labeling, topic-comment) based on each child's immediate linguistic performance. Syntax and vocabulary are not altered.

used. Even for more cognitively advanced children, there may be an advantage in using materials that are relatively concrete. Worrall and Singh (1983) reported success in using iconic materials to teach a basic reading vocabulary to children with moderate mental retardation. This method incorporates a realistic drawing of an object into the standard written representation of the word. For example, the letter *S* in the word "snake" would show a real snake twisted into the form of the letter. Gradually, the drawing would be made more abstract until it was entirely replaced by the letter.

Pragmatics

A logical approach to pragmatics intervention is to concentrate in areas where individuals with mental retardation would be expected to show little development on their own (Abbeduto, 1991). Research to date suggests that conversational turn taking is the most easily acquired pragmatic behavior. Therefore, intervention might have more impact if it is targeted to one of the five other areas discussed earlier: speech acts, referential communication, conversational repair, topic management, and generalization of use.

What kinds of techniques can be used to promote pragmatic development? There are no pat methods for stimulating change in this area. However, research on problem solving indicates that children with retardation will improve their performance when they are prompted to apply a particular strategy (Ferretti & Cavalier, 1991). It is easy to see that many of the behaviors we consider pragmatic involve a type of interpersonal problem solving, for example, judging what a listener needs to know. Therefore, prompting to apply pragmatic knowledge in certain situations may improve performance, just as it has been shown to improve performance in cognitive tasks (Abbeduto, 1991). The simple reminder may be one of the most powerful techniques.

The use of a reminder, of course, assumes that a particular behavior is already within a child's repertoire. If this is not the case, then the behavior must be established. For example, to address a problem of conversational repair, Ezell and Goldstein (1991b) trained five children with mild or moderate retardation to request clarification when they were presented with instructions that were obscured by noise, contained an unfamiliar word, or were too lengthy to be comprehended. The experimenters deliberately created the communication breakdowns and then taught the children how to respond to them. In a similar approach, Fey (1986) has discussed the use of the barrier game, modified to suit the cognitive level of the child, to increase awareness of referential difficulties such as deictic language and provide practice in overcoming them.

Another potentially fruitful approach is to use other children to help promote certain pragmatic skills in children with retardation. Goldstein and Ferrell (1987) used a peer-mediated intervention program to try to facilitate communication development in three preschool children with behavior disorders and developmental delays (not all of the children were mentally retarded). They were successful in training six typically developing peers to use four different strategies for enhancing interaction: (1) establishing eye contact by saying the handicapped child's name or touching the child; (2) suggesting joint play; (3) responding to the handicapped child's speech by repeating it, expanding it, or requesting clarification; and (4) self-talk and shadow talk. Although the program did not achieve all the desired effects and showed limited generalization, it did result in an increase in the handicapped children's responsiveness and a decrease in nonsocial utterances and talking to the teacher. Generalization appears to be a consistent problem in nearly all peer-mediated intervention programs (Fey, 1986). Special procedures to enhance carryover are probably necessary if peer-mediation intervention is to be effective.

Comprehension

Promoting comprehension can take many forms, depending on the intellectual level of the child and on whether there is a significant hearing impairment. In cases where there is a known hearing loss, it is appropriate to assess and perhaps provide training to improve prerequisite auditory behaviors such as sound localization, differentiation of speech messages, and auditory attention span (Ross & Ross, 1972). In all cases, it is important to continue to monitor hearing status in order to ensure the success of comprehension training.

It is clear that **operant conditioning** procedures can be effective in training comprehension of specific language forms. For instance, an operant approach has been used successfully to enhance comprehension of object-location stimuli in children with moderate and severe retardation (Ezell & Goldstein, 1989). Training was improved by having the children imitate commands after they heard them and before they attempted to perform the requested action. Here we again see forms of rehearsal strategies being employed.

Operant techniques may be the method of choice for children with severe or profound mental retardation. The use of operant procedures, however, does not mean that language teaching must occur in sterile surroundings or that it cannot take advantage of certain natural tendencies toward learning. In one study, operant methods were used in two forms to enhance comprehension of agent-action-object and action-object-locative sentences by preschool children with moderate mental retardation (Kim & Lombardino, 1991). In one form, the methods were script based, that is, the sentence stimuli were presented in the context of a meaningful story. In the other form, they were not. The researchers found that the script-based technique resulted in more rapid learning and better generalization to nontraining contexts.

A much different set of methods for facilitating comprehension is found in **child-oriented intervention** approaches. Here the clinician follows the child's lead while enriching the verbal environment through self-talk, parallel talk, repetition, or recasting, techniques that are often used with other children with language disorders. Fey (1986) asserts that these techniques "may be especially useful when general gains in language comprehension are the focus of the intervention program" (p. 203). Intervention studies in which parents were trained to stimulate their children in one of these ways report gains not only in comprehension but in production as well, especially if both parents are involved and the targets are modeled in short, nondirective statements (Cheseldine & McConkey, 1979; McConkey, Jeffree, & Hewson, 1979).

Lexicon

Because of the deficits in syntax shown by children with retardation—especially those with Down syndrome—professionals may target vocabulary as a way of teaching to a strength. But lexical teaching should not be carried out without regard to impairments in other areas of language. It should be integrated with syntactic teaching so that children are able to express a variety of ideas, using the syntactic structures available to them (Miller, 1984). Vocabulary teaching is too often limited to **nominals**. A child who already knows a set of nouns ("bike," "ball," "rope," "car") must learn other words that function syntactically with those nouns: verbs ("ride," "throw," "jump," "drive"), modifiers ("big," "little," "thick," "nice," "blue"), adverbs ("fast," "far," "hard," "safely"), and so on.

Attention should also be paid to the semantic field structure of a vocabulary (Crystal, 1982). For example, a child may possess a vocabulary that is full of words and idiomatic phrases to express semantic fields such as man ("daddy," "sister," "team"), clothing ("shoes," "zipper," "take off"), food ("eat," "sandwich," "stir"), and animals ("dog," "meow," "walk the dog"). These are both common to experience and, for the most part, physically tangible. The vocabulary may be weak, however, in semantic fields such as sight ("look," "blind," "invisible"), smell ("nostril," "whiff," "odor"), and flowers ("petal," "thorn," "rose"). These words are either less common or more abstract or both. Professionals should consider whether their aim is to work within existing semantic fields and merely increase the number of functional words that are available to the child, or whether they want to try to stretch the child cognitively and semantically by introducing areas of the lexicon where the child has not ventured previously. The aim is likely to be different for various children with retardation.

Syntax

Two major types of syntax teaching programs have been used with children with mental retardation, which Fey (1986) has described as hybrid and trainer-oriented approaches. The two types are distinguished primarily by the role of the child. In **hybrid intervention**, situations are structured to encourage a child to make a specific communicative attempt, which then serves as the focus for a teaching interaction between the child and an adult. The following are examples of two hybrid procedures, the mand-model and incidental teaching techniques (Warren & Bambara, 1989).

Mand-Model

CONTEXT: Child is scooping beans with a ladle and pouring them into a pot.

TRAINER: "What are you doing?" (target probe question)

CHILD: No response.

TRAINER: "Tell me." (mand)

CHILD: "Beans."

TRAINER: "Say, 'Pour beans'." (model)

CHILD: "Pour beans."

TRAINER: "That's right, you're pouring beans into the pot." (verbal acknowledgment + expansion)

Incidental Teaching

CONTEXT: Making pudding activity. Trainer gives peer a turn at stirring the pudding as the subject looks on.

CHILD: "Me!" (Child initiates and reaches for ladle.)

TRAINER: "Stir pudding." (model)

CHILD: "Stir pudding."

TRAINER: "Alright. You stir the pudding, too." (verbal acknowledgment + expansion + activity participation)

These approaches have been used successfully to train syntax in several experiments with disadvantaged and specifically language-impaired children, but there are few studies of the procedure with children who are mentally retarded (Warren & Kaiser, 1986). Warren and Bambara (1989) reported on one *milieu teaching* program carried out with three children with borderline to moderate retardation. Using a combination of mand-model, incidental teaching, and systematic commenting (similar to focused stimulation, discussed later) techniques, they were able to train action-object forms. Training was conducted three or four times per week for 15 minutes. The authors observed varying amounts of generalization to other communicative acts but very little generalization to other settings or persons.

In **trainer-oriented intervention**, as the name implies, the procedure is more fully under the control of the professional. Operant procedures are one form of trainer-oriented intervention. Although different in their details, all operant procedures are based on a teaching strategy that introduces new language behaviors in a series of small steps. Following is an example of the steps followed in teaching a child to respond to an open-ended question with an action-object sentence (Guess, Sailor, & Baer, 1974).

Goal: Train action-object sentence

(Trainer shows ball to child)

TRAINER: What's that?

CHILD: Ball.

TRAINER: Point to ball.

(Child points to ball)

TRAINER: Is that a ball?

CHILD: Yes.

TRAINER: What do you want?

CHILD: Want ball.

(Trainer shows cup to child)

TRAINER: What's that? Is that a ball?

CHILD: No.

(Trainer shows cup and ball to child)

TRAINER: What's that? (points to ball)

CHILD: Ball.

TRAINER: What's that? (points to cup)

CHILD: Cup

TRAINER: What do you want?

CHILD: Want ball.

The behaviorist principles of prompting, shaping, and reinforcing are used to elicit a high rate of correct responses from the child. These procedures have been successfully used to teach noun and verb inflections (e.g., Baer & Guess, 1973; Schumaker & Sherman, 1970), simple clauses (e.g., Lutzker & Sherman, 1974), and elements of noun phrase structure (e.g., Smeets & Streifel, 1976). There is no doubt that operant procedures can be used successfully to train behaviors that resemble language. Successful outcomes have been achieved with children at all levels of retardation, though the behaviors taught to children with severe and profound retardation are basic communicative functions such as pointing, vocalizing, or crude signing.

The primary criticism of operant procedures to teach language has been that they are not ecologically valid, that is, that the behaviors learned lack the flexibility and context sensitivity of normal communicative functions (Fey, 1986). The result is that language taught by operant techniques tends not to generalize to situations outside those in which it was taught. In response, it may be said that for some children with mental retardation, the ability to use language in a limited number of situations is a satisfactory result. Furthermore, the failure of certain language behaviors to generalize may merely reflect incomplete teaching—inadequate stimulus generalization, to use behaviorist terms—rather than a fundamental flaw in operant procedures.

An alternative trainer-oriented approach is **modeling**. In the techniques known as **focused stimulation** or *systematic commenting,* the professional bombards the child with contextually relevant models of a target form but the child is not asked to respond (Fey, 1986). Modeling is often used in a modified form with children with retardation. The following procedure (Warren & Bambara, 1989) illustrates how a model might be presented with additional repetition, prosodic emphasis, and direct prompts for response.

Trainer makes frequent comments describing the child's and trainer's activity, placing emphasis on the target form:

TRAINER: "I'm *making cookies. See? Make cookies.*"

Also used as an antecedent to a direct prompt for a target response:

(Trainer shakes baby powder on a doll.)
TRAINER: "Let's *shake powder* on the baby."
(Child attempts to grab the powder away from the adult.)
TRAINER: "What do you want to do?"

These modifications are intended to overcome problems of poor attention and verbal passivity, which are often presented by children with mental retardation. In the *Environmental Language Intervention Program* (ELIP) (MacDonald, Blott, Gordon, Spiegel, & Hartmann, 1974; MacDonald & Horstmeier, 1978), a program used successfully with preschool children

with Down syndrome, a model is presented but the children are then also prompted to use certain language targets and reinforced when they do. The program promotes generalization by using the parents as trainers and requiring responses in conversational and play situations (MacDonald et al., 1974).

Another modeling program, *Interactive Language Development Teaching* (ILDT) (Lee, Koenigsknecht, & Mulhern, 1975), which is described more fully in chapter 15, has been similarly modified for use with children with moderate retardation (McGivern, Rieff, & Vender, 1978). In its modified form, children were provided reinforcement for attending behavior and correct grammatical responses. Only one new language story was introduced each week, and additional time was spent on vocabulary instruction. To assess the success of the program, children in an experimental group received instruction for 30 minutes per day, 4 days a week, for 7 months. Children in a control group received an equal amount of "stimulation" but without a consistent focus on syntactic targets. Investigators found significant improvement in the children's ability to repeat modeled structures, as well as in syntax scores obtained from spontaneous language samples. As used with children with mental retardation, the ILDT program requires the following entrance abilities: (1) spontaneous production of phrases with more than two words and subject-verb clauses; (2) ability to repeat at least two words from a modeled sentence; and (3) ability to attend auditorily for at least 10 minutes when reinforcement is provided.

Speech Production

In most respects, intervention for speech production difficulties is the same for children with and without retardation. As noted earlier, accommodation is made in materials and instructions to suit the cognitive level of the child. Also, because of the oral and facial differences they present, oral motor stimulation and exercises are often recommended for children with Down syndrome to improve sucking, oral awareness, and tone of the lips and tongue, as well as to decrease drooling (Swift & Rosin, 1990).

SUMMARY

In this chapter we have seen that:

▶ Mental retardation is a category of disability defined by testing of intelligence and adaptive behavior.

▶ The major etiological categories of mental retardation are organic and familial. Individuals in the two categories show distinct profiles.

▶ Children with mental retardation frequently show differences in appearance and have more physical handicaps and health problems than typically developing children.

▶ Research has yet to resolve the delay–difference controversy over the nature of the cognitive and linguistic systems in children with mental retardation. At least part of the controversy can be attributed to inadequate research methods. Future refinements in research techniques should help to advance our knowledge.

▶ Compared to their CA peers, children with retardation show impairments at all levels of language: pragmatics, comprehension, semantics, syntax, and speech production.

▶ Compared to children equivalent in MA, children with Down syndrome appear to show a specific impairment of syntax. These children also show a decline in rate of language development as they grow older. The causes of these phenomena are presently unknown.

▶ Intervention for children with mental retardation should be planned with consideration of the legal, cognitive, linguistic, logical, environmental, and motivation factors.

▶ Trainer-oriented, child-oriented, and hybrid approaches to language intervention can all be implemented successfully with children who are mentally retarded.

Children with mental retardation, though discussed as a group, must be treated as individuals. The problems of each child are uniquely complex and require us to consider broad issues of personal development and quality of life. The professional challenge is to find resourceful solutions that extend each individual's capacity for communication and social participation.

REFERENCES

Abbeduto, L. (1991). Development of verbal communication in persons with moderate to mild mental retardation. *International Review of Research in Mental Retardation, 17,* 91–115.

Abbeduto, L., Davies, B., Solesby, S., & Furman, L. (1991). Identifying the referents of spoken messages: The use of context and clarification requests by children with mental retardation and by nonretarded children. *American Journal on Mental Retardation, 95,* 551–562.

Abbeduto, L., Furman, L., & Davies, B. (1989). Relation between the receptive language and mental age of persons with mental retardation. *American Journal on Mental Retardation, 93,* 535–543.

Abbeduto, L., & Rosenberg, S. (1980). The communicative competence of mildly retarded adults. *Applied Psycholinguistics, 1,* 405–426.

Baer, D. M., & Guess, D. (1973). Teaching productive noun suffixes to severely retarded children. *American Journal of Mental Deficiency, 77,* 498–505.

Baroff, G. S. (1986). *Mental retardation: Nature, cause, and management* (2nd ed.). Washington, DC: Hemisphere.

Bayley, N. (1969). *Bayley scales of infant development.* New York: Psychological Corp.

Bedrosian, J., & Prutting, C. A. (1978). Communicative performance of mentally retarded adults in four conversational settings. *Journal of Speech and Hearing Research, 21,* 79–95.

Berger, J., & Cunningham, C. C. (1983). Development of early vocal behaviors and interactions in Down's syndrome and nonhandicapped infant–mother pairs. *Developmental Psychology, 19,* 322–331.

Berko, J. (1958). The child's learning of English morphology. *Word, 14,* 150–177.

Berry, P. (1972). Comprehension of possessive and present continuous sentences by non-retarded, mildly retarded, and severely retarded children. *American Journal of Mental Deficiency, 76,* 540–544.

Beveridge, M. (1976). Patterns of interaction in the mentally handicapped. In P. Berry (Ed.), *Language and communication in the mentally handicapped.* Baltimore: University Park Press.

Bidder, R., Bryant, G., & Gray, O. (1975). Benefits to Down's syndrome children through training their mothers. *Archives of Disease in Childhood, 50,* 383–386.

Bilsky, L. H. (1985). Comprehension and mental retardation. *International Review of Research in Mental Retardation, 13,* 215–246.

Bleile, K., & Schwarz, I. (1984). Three perspectives on the speech of children with Down's syndrome. *Journal of Communication Disorders, 17,* 87–94.

Bliss, L., Allen, D., & Walker, G. (1978). Sentence structures of trainable and educable mentally retarded subjects. *Journal of Speech and Hearing Research, 21,* 722–731.

Buium, N., Rynders, J., & Turnure, J. (1974). Early maternal linguistic environment of normal and Down's syndrome language-learning children. *American Journal of Mental Deficiency, 79,* 52–58.

Burack, J. A. (1990). Differentiating mental retardation: The two-group approach and beyond. In R. M. Hodapp, J. A. Burack, & E. Zigler (Eds.), *Issues in the developmental approach to mental retardation* (pp. 27–48). New York: Cambridge University Press.

Calculator, S. N., & Dollaghan, C. (1982). The use of communication boards in a residential setting: An evaluation. *Journal of Speech and Hearing Disorders, 47,* 281–287.

Cameron, T. H., & Kelly, D. P. (1988). Normal language skills and normal intelligence in a child with De Lange syndrome. *Journal of Speech and Hearing Disorders, 53,* 219–222.

Cardoso-Martins, C., & Mervis, C. B. (1985). Maternal speech to prelinguistic children with Down syndrome. *American Journal of Mental Deficiency, 89,* 451–458.

Cardoso-Martins, C., Mervis, C. B., & Mervis, C. A. (1985). Early vocabulary acquisition by children with Down syndrome. *American Journal of Mental Deficiency, 90,* 177–184.

Carr, E. G., & Durand, V. M. (1985). Reducing behavior problems through functional communication training. *Journal of Applied Behavior Analysis, 18,* 111–126.

Chapman, R. S., Kay-Raining Bird, E., & Schwartz, S. E. (1990). Fast mapping of words in event contexts by children with Down syndrome. *Journal of Speech and Hearing Disorders, 55,* 761–770.

Chapman, R. S., Schwartz, S. E., & Kay-Raining Bird, E. (1991). Language skills of children and adolescents with Down syndrome: I. Comprehension. *Journal of Speech and Hearing Research, 34,* 1106–1120.

Cheseldine, S., & McConkey, R. (1979). Parental speech to young Down's syndrome children: An intervention study. *American Journal of Mental Deficiency, 83,* 612–620.

Cicchetti, D., & Ganiban, J. (1990). The organization and coherence of developmental processes in infants and children with Down syndrome. In R. M. Hodapp, J. A. Burack, & E. Zigler (Eds.), *Issues in the developmental approach to mental retardation* (pp. 169–225). New York: Cambridge University Press.

Cipani, E. (1989). Providing language consultation in the natural context: A model for delivery of services. *Mental Retardation, 27,* 317–324.

Coggins, T. E. (1979). Relational meaning encoded in the two-word utterances of Stage I Down's syndrome children. *Journal of Speech and Hearing Research, 22,* 166–178.

Coggins, T. E., Carpenter, R., & Owings, N. O. (1983). Examining early intentional communication in Down's syndrome and nonretarded children. *British Journal of Disorders of Communication, 18,* 98–106.

Coggins, T. E., & Morrison, J. A. (1981). Spontaneous imitations of Down's syndrome children: A lexical analysis. *Journal of Speech and Hearing Research, 24,* 303–308.

Coggins, T. E., & Stoel-Gammon, C. (1982). Clarification strategies used by four Down's syndrome children for maintaining normal conversational interaction. *Education and Training of the Mentally Retarded, 17,* 65–67.

Cornwell, A. (1974). Development of language, abstraction and numerical concept formation in Down's syndrome children. *American Journal of Mental Deficiency, 79,* 179–190.

Creaghead, N. A., Newman, P. W., & Secord, W. A. (1989). *Assessment and remediation of articulatory and phonological disorders* (2nd ed.). New York: Merrill/Macmillan.

Cromer, R. F. (1991). *Language and thought in normal and handicapped children.* Oxford: Basil Blackwell.

Crystal, D. (1982). *Profiling linguistic disability.* London: Edward Arnold.

Crystal, D. (1984). *Linguistic encounters with language handicap.* Oxford: Basil Blackwell.

Dahle, A. J., & McCollister, F. P. (1986). Hearing and otologic disorders in children with Down's syndrome. *American Journal of Mental Deficiency, 90,* 636–642.

Davis, H., Stroud, A., & Green, L. (1988). Maternal language environment of children with mental retardation. *American Journal on Mental Retardation, 93,* 144–153.

Dever, R. (1972). A comparison of the results of a revised version of Berko's test of morphology with the free speech of mentally retarded children. *Journal of Speech and Hearing Research, 15,* 169–178.

Dewart, H. (1979). Language comprehension processes of

mentally retarded children. *American Journal of Mental Deficiency, 84,* 177–183.

Dodd, B. (1975). Recognition and reproduction of words by Down's syndrome and non–Down's syndrome retarded children. *American Journal of Mental Deficiency, 80,* 306–311.

Dodd, B. (1976). A comparison of the phonological systems of mental age matched normal, severely subnormal, and Down's syndrome children. *British Journal of Disorders of Communication, 11,* 27–42.

Doll, E. (1965). *Vineland social maturity scale.* Circle Pines, MN: American Guidance Service.

Dunst, C. J. (1980). *A clinical and educational manual for use with the Uzgiris and Hunt scales of infant psychological development.* Baltimore: University Park Press.

Dunst, C. J. (1981). *Infant-learning: A cognitive–linguistic intervention strategy.* Hingham, MA: Teaching Resources Corp.

Dykens, E., & Leckman, J. (1990). Development issues in Fragile X syndrome. In R. M. Hodapp, J. A. Burack, & E. Zigler (Eds.), *Issues in the developmental approach to mental retardation* (pp. 226–245). New York: Cambridge University Press.

Eheart, B. (1982). Mother–child interactions with non-retarded and mentally retarded preschoolers. *American Journal of Mental Deficiency, 87,* 20–25.

Ezell, H. K., & Goldstein, H. (1989). Effects of imitation on language comprehension and transfer to production in children with mental retardation. *Journal of Speech and Hearing Disorders, 54,* 49–56.

Ezell, H. K., & Goldstein, H. (1991a). Comparison of idiom comprehension of normal children and children with mental retardation. *Journal of Speech and Hearing Research, 34,* 812–819.

Ezell, H. K., & Goldstein, H. (1991b). Observational learning of comprehension monitoring skills in children who exhibit mental retardation. *Journal of Speech and Hearing Research, 34,* 141–154.

Ferretti, R. P., & Cavalier, A. R. (1991). Constraints on the problem solving of persons with mental retardation. *International Review of Research in Mental Retardation, 17,* 153–192.

Fey, M. E. (1986). *Language intervention with young children.* Boston: College-Hill Press.

Finch-Williams, A. (1984). The developmental relationship between cognition and communication: Implications for assessment. *Topics in Language Disorders, 5,* 1–13.

Fowler, A. E. (1988). Determinants of language growth in children with Down syndrome. In L. Nadel (Ed.), *The psychobiology of Down syndrome* (pp. 217–245). Cambridge, MA: MIT Press.

Fowler, A. E. (1990). Language abilities in children with Down syndrome: Evidence for a specific syntactic delay. In D. Cicchetti & M. Beeghly (Eds.), *Children with Down syndrome: A developmental perspective* (pp. 302–328). New York: Cambridge University Press.

Frankenberger, W., & Harper, J. (1988). States' definitions and procedures for identifying children with mental retardation: Comparison of 1981–1982 and 1985–1986 guidelines. *Mental Retardation, 26,* 133–136.

Fristoe, M., & Lloyd, L. (1979). Nonspeech communication. In N. R. Ellis (Ed.), *Handbook of mental deficiency, psychological theory and research* (2nd ed.). Hillsdale, NJ: Erlbaum.

Fulton, R., & Lloyd, L. (1968). Hearing impairment in a population of children with Down's syndrome. *American Journal of Mental Deficiency, 73,* 298–302.

Gerber, S. E. (1990, September). Chromosomes and chromosomal disorders. *Asha, 32,* 39–41, 47.

Girolametto, L. E. (1988). Improving the social-conversational skills of developmentally delayed children: An intervention study. *Journal of Speech and Hearing Disorders, 53,* 156–167.

Givens, G., & Seidemann, M. (1977). Middle ear measurements in a difficult to test mentally retarded population. *Mental Retardation, 15,* 40–42.

Goldstein, H., & Ferrell, D. R. (1987). Augmenting communicative interaction between handicapped and nonhandicapped preschool children. *Journal of Speech and Hearing Disorders, 52,* 200–211.

Gordon, A. G. (1987). Language deficit and hearing loss in Down's syndrome. *Child: Care, Health, and Development, 13,* 137–139.

Gould, J. (1976). Language development and non-verbal skills in severely mentally retarded children: An epidemiological study. *Journal of Mental Deficiency Research, 20,* 129–146.

Graham, J. T., & Graham, L. W. (1971). Language behavior of the mentally retarded: Syntactic characteristics. *American Journal of Mental Deficiency, 75,* 623–629.

Greenwald, C., & Leonard, L. (1979). Communicative and sensorimotor development of Down's syndrome children. *American Journal of Mental Deficiency, 84,* 296–303.

Grossman, H. J. (Ed.). (1983). *Classification in mental retardation.* Washington, DC: American Association on Mental Deficiency.

Guess, D., & Baer, D. M. (1973). An analysis of individual

differences in generalization between receptive and productive language in retarded children. *Journal of Applied Behavior Analysis, 6,* 311–329.

Guess, D., Sailor, W., & Baer, D. (1974). To teach language to retarded children. In R. Schiefelbusch & L. Lloyd (Eds.), *Language perspectives: Acquisition, retardation, and intervention.* Baltimore: University Park Press.

Guess, D., Sailor, W., & Baer, D. (1978). Children with limited languages. In R. Schiefelbusch (Ed.), *Language intervention strategies.* Baltimore: University Park Press.

Gullo, D. F., & Gullo, J. C. (1984). An ecological language intervention approach with mentally retarded adolescents. *Language, Speech, and Hearing Services in Schools, 15,* 182–191.

Guralnick, M. J., & Paul-Brown, D. (1986). Communicative interactions of mildly delayed and normally developing preschool children: Effects of listener's developmental level. *Journal of Speech and Hearing Research, 29,* 2–10.

Halle, J., Baer, D., & Spradlin, J. (1981). Teachers' generalized use of delay as a stimulus control procedure to increase language use in handicapped children. *Journal of Applied Behavior Analysis, 14,* 389–409.

Halle, J., Hunt, F., & Bjorenson, J. (1984). Effects of two antecedent conditions on vocalization frequency of severely retarded children. *Journal of Speech and Hearing Disorders, 49,* 349–359.

Hanzlik, J. R., & Stevenson, M. B. (1986). Interaction of mothers with their infants who are mentally retarded, retarded with cerebral palsy, or nonretarded. *American Journal of Mental Deficiency, 90,* 513–520.

Hodapp, R. M., Evans, D. W., & Ward, B. A. (1989). Communicative interaction between teachers and children with severe handicaps. *Mental Retardation, 27,* 388–395.

Hodges, P., & Schwethelm, B. (1984). A comparison of the effectiveness of graphic symbol and manual sign training with profoundly retarded children. *Applied Psycholinguistics, 5,* 223–253.

Jones, E., & Payne, J. (1986). Definition and prevalence. In J. Patton, J. Payne, & M. Beirne-Smith (Eds.), *Mental retardation* (2nd ed.) (pp. 33–75). New York: Merrill/Macmillan.

Jones, O. H. M. (1977). Mother–child communication with prelinguistic Down's syndrome and normal infants. In H. R. Schaffer (Ed.), *Studies in mother–infant interaction.* London: Academic Press.

Kaga, K., & Marsh, R. R. (1986). Auditory brainstem responses in young children with Down's syndrome. *International Journal of Pediatric Otorhinolaryngology, 11,* 29–38.

Kahn, J. (1975). Relationship of Piaget's sensorimotor period to language acquisition of profoundly retarded children. *American Journal of Mental Deficiency, 79,* 640–643.

Kahn, J. (1978). Acceleration of object permanence with severely and profoundly retarded children. *American Association for the Education of the Severely/Profoundly Handicapped Review, 3,* 15–22.

Kahn, J. (1984). Cognitive training and initial use of referential speech. *Topics in Language Disorders, 5,* 14–23.

Kamhi, A. G., & Johnston, J. R. (1982). Towards an understanding of retarded children's linguistic deficiencies. *Journal of Speech and Hearing Research, 25,* 435–445.

Karlin, I., & Strazzula, M. (1952). Speech and language problems of mentally deficient children. *Journal of Speech and Hearing Disorders, 17,* 286–294.

Keiser, H., Montague, J., Wold, C., Maune, S., & Pattison, D. (1981). Hearing loss of Down syndrome adults. *American Journal of Mental Deficiency, 85,* 467–472.

Kim, Y. T., & Lombardino, L. J. (1991). The efficacy of script contexts in language comprehension intervention with children who have mental retardation. *Journal of Speech and Hearing Research, 34,* 845–857.

Klink, M., Gerstman, L., Raphael, L., Schlanger, B., & Newsome, L. (1986). Phonological process usage by young EMR children and nonretarded preschool children. *American Journal of Mental Deficiency, 91,* 190–195.

Kropka, B. I., & Williams, C. (1986). The epidemiology of hearing impairment in people with a mental handicap. In D. Ellis (Ed.), *Sensory impairments in mentally handicapped people.* San Diego: College-Hill Press.

Lamberts, R., & Weener, P. (1976). T.M.R. children's competence in processing negation. *American Journal of Mental Deficiency, 81,* 181–186.

Lee, L. L., Koenigsknecht, R. A., & Mulhern, S. T. (1975). *Interactive language development teaching.* Evanston, IL: Northwestern University Press.

Leifer, J. S., & Lewis, M. (1984). Acquisition of conversational response skills by young Down syndrome and nonretarded young children. *American Journal of Mental Deficiency, 88,* 610–618.

Leiter, R. (1979). *Leiter international performance scale.* Chicago: Stoelting.

Lloyd, L. (1970). Audiologic aspects of mental retardation. *International Review of Research in Mental Retardation, 4,* 311–374.

Lloyd, L., & Fulton, R. (1972). Audiology's contribution to communications programming with the retarded. In J. McLean, D. Yoder, & R. Schiefelbusch (Eds.), *Language intervention with the retarded.* Baltimore: University Park Press.

Lloyd, L., & Reid, M. (1967). The incidence of hearing impairment in an institutionalized mentally retarded population. *American Journal of Mental Deficiency, 71,* 746–763.

Longhurst, T. M. (1972). Assessing and increasing descriptive communication skills in retarded children. *Mental Retardation, 19,* 42–45.

Longhurst, T. M. (1974). Communication in retarded adolescents: Sex and intelligence level. *American Journal of Mental Deficiency, 78,* 607–618.

Longhurst, T. M., & Berry, G. W. (1975). Communication in retarded adolescents: Response to listener feedback. *American Journal of Mental Deficiency, 80,* 158–164.

Lovell, K., & Bradbury, B. (1967). The learning of English morphology in educationally subnormal special school children. *American Journal of Mental Deficiency, 71,* 609–615.

Lovell, K., & Dixon, E. (1967). The growth of the control of grammar in imitation, comprehension, and production. *Journal of Child Psychology and Psychiatry, 8,* 31–39.

Ludlow, J. R., & Allen, L. M. (1979). The effect of early intervention and pre-school stimulus on the development of the Down's syndrome child. *Journal of Mental Deficiency Research, 23,* 29–44.

Luria, A. R. (1961). *The role of speech in the regulation of normal and abnormal behavior.* New York: Pergamon Press.

Luria, A. R. (1963). *The mentally retarded child.* Oxford: Pergamon Press.

Lutzker, J., & Sherman, J. A. (1974). Producing generative sentence usage by imitation and reinforcement procedures. *Journal of Applied Behavior Analysis, 7,* 447–460.

Lynch, M. P., & Eilers, R. E. (1991). Perspectives on early language from typical development and Down syndrome. *International Review of Research in Mental Retardation, 17,* 55–89.

MacDonald, J., Blott, J., Gordon, K., Spiegel, B., & Hartmann, M. (1974). An experimental parent-assisted program for preschool language-delayed children. *Journal of Speech and Hearing Disorders, 39,* 395–415.

MacDonald, J., & Horstmeier, D. S. (1978). *Environmental language intervention program (ELIP).* San Antonio, TX: Psychological Corp.

Mahoney, G. J., Glover, A., & Finger, I. (1981). Relationship between language and sensorimotor development of Down syndrome and nonretarded children. *American Journal of Mental Deficiency, 86,* 21–27.

Mahoney, G. J., & Snow, K. (1983). The relationship of sensorimotor functioning to children's response to early language training. *Mental Retardation, 21,* 248–254.

Marshall, N., Hegrenes, J., & Goldstein, S. (1973). Verbal interactions: Mothers and their retarded children vs. mothers and their non-retarded children. *American Journal of Mental Deficiency, 77,* 415–419.

Martin, H., McConkey, R., & Martin, S. (1984). From acquisition theories to intervention strategies: An experiment with mentally handicapped children. *British Journal of Disorders of Communication, 19,* 3–14.

Maurer, H., & Sherrod, K. B. (1987). Context of directives given to young children with Down syndrome and nonretarded children: Development over two years. *American Journal of Mental Deficiency, 91,* 579–590.

McConkey, R., Jeffree, D., & Hewson, S. (1979). Involving parents in extending the language development of their young mentally handicapped children. *British Journal of Disorders of Communication, 14,* 203–218.

McCune, L., Kearney, B., & Checkoff, M. (1989). Forms and functions of communication by children with Down syndrome and nonretarded children with their mothers. In S. von Tetzchner, L. S. Siegel, & L. Smith (Eds.), *The social and cognitive aspects of normal and atypical language development* (pp. 113–127). New York: Springer-Verlag.

McGivern, A. B., Rieff, M. L., & Vender, B. F. (1978). *Language stories: Teaching language to developmentally disabled children.* New York: John Day.

McLaren, J., & Bryson, S. E. (1987). Review of recent epidemiological studies of mental retardation: Prevalence, associated disorders, and etiology. *American Journal of Mental Retardation, 92,* 243–254.

McLean, J. E., McLean, L. K. S., Brady, N. C., & Etter, R. (1991). Communication profiles of two types of gesture using nonverbal persons with severe to profound mental retardation. *Journal of Speech and Hearing Research, 34,* 294–308.

McLeavey, B. C., Toomey, J. F., & Dempsey, P. J. R. (1982). Nonretarded and mentally retarded children's control over syntactic structures. *American Journal of Mental Deficiency, 86,* 485–494.

Merrill, E. C., & Mar, H. H. (1987). Differences between mentally retarded and nonretarded persons' efficiency of auditory sentence processing. *American Journal of Mental Deficiency, 91,* 406–414.

Milgram, N., & Furth, H. (1968). The regulatory role of language in systematic search by trainable retardates. *American Journal of Mental Deficiency, 72,* 620–621.

Miller, J. F. (1984). Mental retardation. In W. H. Perkins (Ed.),

Language handicaps in children. New York: Thieme-Stratton.

Miller, J. F. (1988). The developmental asynchrony of language development in children with Down syndrome. In L. Nadel (Ed.), *The psychobiology of Down syndrome* (pp. 168–198). Cambridge, MA: MIT Press.

Miller, J. F. (1992). Lexical development in young children with Down syndrome. In R. S. Chapman (Ed.), *Processes in language acquisition and disorder.* St. Louis, MO: Mosby Year Book.

Miller, J. F., Budde, M., Bashir, A., & LaFollette, L. (1987). *Lexical productivity in children with Down syndrome.* Paper presented at the American Speech-Language-Hearing Association Annual Convention, New Orleans.

Miller, J. F., & Chapman, R. S. (1984). Disorders of communication: Investigating the development of language of mentally retarded children. *American Journal of Mental Deficiency, 88,* 536–545.

Miller, J. F., & Yoder, D. (1974). An ontogenetic language teaching strategy for retarded children. In R. Schiefelbusch & L. Lloyd (Eds.), *Language perspectives—Acquisition, retardation and intervention.* Baltimore: University Park Press.

Newby, H. (1972). *Audiology* (3rd ed.). New York: Appleton-Century-Crofts.

Newfield, M., & Schlanger, B. (1968). The acquisition of English morphology by normal and educable mentally retarded children. *Journal of Speech and Hearing Research, 11,* 82–95.

Nietupski, J., Scheutz, G., & Ockwood, L. (1980). The delivery of communication therapy services to severely handicapped students: A plan for change. *Journal of the Association for the Severely Handicapped, 5,* 13–23.

Nolan, M., McCartney, E., McArthur, K., & Rowson, V. (1980). A study of the hearing and receptive vocabulary of the trainees of an adult training centre. *Journal of Mental Deficiency Research, 24,* 271–286.

Northern, J. L., & Downs, M. P. (1984). *Hearing in children* (3rd ed.). Baltimore: Williams & Wilkins.

Owens, R. E., & House, L. I. (1984). Decision-making processes in augmentative communication. *Journal of Speech and Hearing Disorders, 49,* 18–25.

Owens, R. E., & MacDonald, J. (1982). Communicative uses of the early speech of nondelayed and Down syndrome children. *American Journal of Mental Deficiency, 86,* 503–510.

Owings, N. O., & McManus, M. D. (1980). An analysis of communication functions in the speech of a deinstitutional-ized adult mentally retarded client. *Mental Retardation, 18,* 309–314.

Parsons, C. L., Iacono, T. A., & Rozner, L. (1987). Effect of tongue reduction on articulation in children with Down syndrome. *American Journal of Mental Deficiency, 91,* 328–332.

Paul, R., & Cohen, D. J. (1984). Responses to contingent queries in adults with mental retardation and pervasive developmental disorders. *Applied Psycholinguistics, 5,* 349–357.

Pruess, J. B., Vadasy, P. F., & Fewell, R. R. (1987). Language development in children with Down syndrome: An overview of recent research. *Education and Training of the Mentally Retarded, 22,* 44–55.

Reiss, A. L., & Freund, L. (1990). Fragile X syndrome, DSM-III-R, and autism. *Journal of the American Academy of Child and Adolescent Psychiatry, 29,* 885–891.

Robinson, C., & Robinson, H. (1983). Sensorimotor training for developmentally delayed children. In M. Snell (Ed.), *Systematic instruction of moderately and severely handicapped.* Columbus, OH: Merrill.

Romski, M. A., Sevcik, R. A., Reumann, R., & Pate, J. L. (1989). Youngsters with moderate or severe mental retardation and severe spoken language impairments I: Extant communicative patterns. *Journal of Speech and Hearing Disorders, 54,* 356–366.

Rondal, J. A. (1988). Down's syndrome. In D. Bishop & K. Mogford (Eds.), *Language development in exceptional circumstances.* New York: Churchill Livingstone.

Rosenberg, S. (1982). The language of the mentally retarded: Development, processes, and intervention. In S. Rosenberg (Ed.), *Handbook of applied psycholinguistics: Major thrusts of research and theory* (pp. 329–392). Hillsdale, NJ: Erlbaum.

Ross, D., & Ross, S. (1972). The efficacy of listening training for educable mentally retarded children. *American Journal of Mental Deficiency, 77,* 137–142.

Rotundo, N., & Johnson, E. (1981). Verbal control of motor behaviour in mentally retarded children: A re-examination of Luria's theory. *Journal of Mental Deficiency Research, 25,* 281–290.

Rueda, R., & Chan, K. (1980). Referential communication skill levels of moderately mentally retarded adolescents. *American Journal of Mental Deficiency, 85,* 45–52.

Rynders, J., Behlen, K., & Horrobin, J. (1979). Performance characteristics of preschool Down's syndrome children receiving augmented or repetitive verbal instruction. *American Journal of Mental Deficiency, 84,* 67–73.

Sanger, D., Stick, S., Sanger, W., & Dawson, K. (1984). Specific syndromes and associated communication disorders: A review. *Journal of Communication Disorders, 17,* 385–405.

Schumaker, J., & Sherman, J. A. (1970). Training generative verb usage by imitation and reinforcement procedures. *Journal of Applied Behavior Analysis, 3,* 273–287.

Schwartz, D. M., & Schwartz, R. H. (1978). Acoustic impedance and otoscopic findings in young children with Down's syndrome. *Archives of Otolaryngology, 104,* 652–656.

Silverstein, A., Pearson, L., Colbert, B., Cordeiro, W., Marwin, J., & Nakaji, M. (1982). Cognitive development of severely and profoundly mentally retarded individuals. *American Journal of Mental Deficiency, 87,* 347–349.

Sinson, J., & Wetherick, N. (1982). Mutual gaze in preschool Down's and normal children. *Journal of Mental Deficiency Research, 26,* 123–129.

Smeets, P., & Streifel, S. (1976). Training the generative usage of article-noun responses in severely retarded males. *Journal of Mental Deficiency Research, 20,* 121–127.

Smith, B. L., & Oller, D. K. (1981). A comparative study of premeaningful vocalizations produced by normally developing and Down's syndrome infants. *Journal of Speech and Hearing Disorders, 46,* 46–51.

Smith, B. L., & Stoel-Gammon, C. (1983). A longitudinal study of the development of stop consonant production in normal and Down's syndrome children. *Journal of Speech and Hearing Disorders, 48,* 114–118.

Smith, L. (1989). Case studies of maternal speech to prelinguistic children in the format of object transfer. In S. von Tetzchner, L. S. Siegel, & L. Smith (Eds.), *The social and cognitive aspects of normal and atypical language development* (pp. 69–93). New York: Springer-Verlag.

Sparks, S. N. (1984a). *Birth defects and speech-language disorders.* San Diego: College-Hill Press.

Sparks, S. N. (1984b). Speech and language in fetal alcohol syndrome. *Asha, 26,* 27–31.

Spiegel, B. (1983). The effect of context on language learning by severely retarded young adults. *Language, Speech, and Hearing Services in Schools, 14,* 252–259.

Stewart, L. G. (1978). Hearing impaired/developmentally disabled persons in the United States: Definitions, causes, effects and prevalence estimates. *American Annals of the Deaf, 123,* 488–495.

Stoel-Gammon, C. (1980). Phonological analysis of four Down's syndrome children. *Applied Psycholinguistics, 1,* 31–48.

Stoel-Gammon, C. (1981). Speech development of infants and children with Down syndrome. In J. Darby, Jr. (Ed.),

Speech evaluation in medicine (pp. 341–360). New York: Grune & Stratton.

Stoel-Gammon, C. (1990, September). Down syndrome. *Asha, 32,* 42–44.

Stoneman, Z., Brody, G., & Abbott, D. (1983). In-home observations of young Down syndrome children with their mothers and fathers. *American Journal of Mental Deficiency, 87,* 591–600.

Swift, E., & Rosin, P. (1990). A remediation sequence to improve speech intelligibility for students with Down syndrome. *Language, Speech, and Hearing Services in Schools, 21,* 140–146.

Tager-Flusberg, H., & Calkins, S. (1990). Does imitation facilitate the acquisition of grammar? Evidence from a study of autistic, Down's syndrome and normal children. *Journal of Child Language, 17,* 591–606.

Tannock, R. (1988). Mothers' directiveness in their interactions with their children with and without Down syndrome. *American Journal on Mental Retardation, 93,* 154–165.

Taylor, R. L., & Kaufmann, S. (1991). Trends in classification usage in the mental retardation literature. *Mental Retardation, 29,* 367–371.

Terman, L., & Merrill, M. (1973). *Stanford-Binet intelligence scale.* Boston: Houghton-Mifflin.

Thase, M. (1988). The relationship between Down syndrome and Alzheimer's disease. In L. Nadel (Ed.), *The psychobiology of Down syndrome* (pp. 345–368). Cambridge, MA: MIT Press.

Turnure, J. E. (1991). Long-term memory and mental retardation. *International Review of Research in Mental Retardation, 17,* 193–217.

Vygotsky, L. (1962). *Thought and language.* Cambridge, MA: MIT Press.

Warren, S. F., & Bambara, L. M. (1989). An experimental analysis of milieu language intervention: Teaching the action-object form. *Journal of Speech and Hearing Disorders, 54,* 448–461.

Warren, S. F., & Kaiser, A. P. (1986). Incidental language teaching: A critical review. *Journal of Speech and Hearing Disorders, 51,* 291–299.

Wechsler, D. (1974). *Wechsler intelligence scale for children–Revised.* New York: Psychological Corp.

Weisz, J. R., Yeates, K. O., & Zigler, E. (1982). Piagetian evidence and the developmental-difference controversy. In E. Zigler & D. Balla (Eds.), *Mental retardation: The developmental–difference controversy* (pp. 213–276). Hillsdale, NJ: Erlbaum.

Weller, E., & Mahoney, G. J. (1983). A comparison of oral and total communication modalities on the language training of young mentally handicapped children. *Education and Training of the Mentally Retarded, 18,* 103–110.

Wheldall, K. (1976). Receptive language development in the mentally handicapped. In P. Berry (Ed.), *Language and communication in the mentally handicapped.* Baltimore: University Park Press.

Wiegel-Crump, C. A. (1981). The development of grammar in Down's syndrome children between the mental ages of 2–0 and 6–11 years. *Education and Training of the Mentally Retarded, 16,* 24–30.

Worrall, N., & Singh, Y. (1983). Teaching TMR children to read using integrated picture cueing. *American Journal of Mental Deficiency, 87,* 422–429.

Zigler, E., & Balla, D. (1982). Introduction: The developmental approach to mental retardation. In E. Zigler & D. Balla (Eds.), *Mental retardation: The developmental–difference controversy* (pp. 3–8). Hillsdale, NJ: Erlbaum.

Zigler, E., & Hodapp, R. M. (1986). *Understanding mental retardation.* New York: Cambridge University Press.

· Chapter 7 ·

Language and Children with Learning Disabilities

Steven H. Long and Susan T. Long

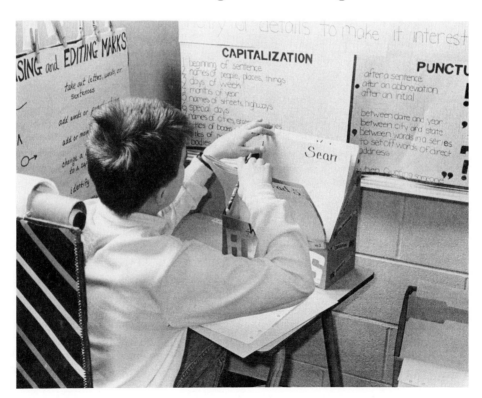

OBJECTIVES

Upon completion of this chapter, the reader should be able to:

▶ Discuss the definitions of learning disabilities and other etiological categories with which learning disabilities overlaps.

▶ Discuss the relationship between language disorders and learning disabilities.

▶ Identify the differences between oral and written language and how these can contribute to learning disabilities.

▶ Understand how research on children with learning disabilities is conducted.

▶ Discuss general characteristics of the language of children with learning disabilities.

▶ Discuss principles of language intervention for children with learning disabilities.

Although it now sounds familiar, the phrase *children with learning disabilities* is of fairly recent origin. The first use of the term by professionals in education was in 1962. It did not appear in federal legislative documents until 1968 (Hammill, 1990). This does not mean, of course, that children with learning problems did not exist until the 1960s. Rather, it reveals a change that has occurred over the last three decades in how we think about and label the problems. It also reflects the influence of the federal government. To a large extent, research on and educational practice with learning disabilities have been guided by actions taken in Washington, D.C. The single most important action was passage of the Education for All Handicapped Children Act (PL 94–142) in 1975. This law provided an official definition of children with learning disabilities. More important, as we recall from chapter 4, it mandated that these children be identified and served by public schools. Another important federal action, beginning in the 1980s, was the Regular Education Initiative (REI), which led the movement in favor of mainstreaming children with learning disabilities, that is, returning them to regular education classrooms for much of their schooling.

To the chagrin of some, legislation alone cannot solve educational problems. Educational service for children with learning disabilities has been required since PL 94-142 was enacted, but the relationship of learning disabilities to other types of behavioral and learning problems is still unclear. Research has not yet determined what is the best model for representing the relationship among various types of speech, read-ing, writing, and learning impairments. Are they the same problem or different problems? If they are different, where is the line drawn between one type of disorder and the next? Because we do not fully understand the nature of the disabilities, it is not surprising that we lack a universally accepted plan for who should educate the children who have them. Consequently, it is a responsibility currently being shared by a number of professionals.

AN OVERVIEW OF CHILDREN WITH LEARNING DISABILITIES

Professionals have struggled for years to develop a definition of learning disabilities that would be satisfactory to everyone. They have not succeeded, though some believe that a consensus view, if not a unanimous one, has evolved (Hammill, 1990). To many practitioners the issue of definition is best left locked up in the ivory towers inhabited by academics. However, definitions are important, inasmuch as they (1) determine how children are placed in our educational systems; (2) influence government decisions about funding (e.g., PL 94-142); (3) influence funding decisions by local school districts; (4) guide professional preparation programs and curriculum design; and (5) assist or hinder discussions among parents, physicians, psychologists, teachers, and other professionals (Murphy & Hicks-Stewart, 1991). If, for example, a specialist attends an educational planning meeting, it must be clear what qualifies a student to receive special assistance for children with learning disabilities. It must also be clear what is meant by terms such as *attention deficit-hyperactivity disorder, specific language impairment,* or *central auditory processing disorder,* all of which are used by certain professionals to describe some children who have learning disabilities.

Labels and Terminology

Various diagnostic labels have been used to refer to children who have trouble learning. Like clothing fashions, labels tend to have a period of general popularity, after which they retain this popularity only with certain professional groups or in certain regions. Some labels are intended to be purely descriptive, whereas others refer to what is presumed to be a cause of a child's learning problems. Following is a list of several terms that are commonly applied by educators and other professionals. We will briefly discuss the meaning of each of these labels.

Descriptive

Learning disabilities

Dyslexia

Slow learner

Attention deficit–hyperactivity disorder

Specific language impairment

Phonological processing disorder

Etiological

Central auditory processing disorder

Minimal brain dysfunction

Developmental apraxia of speech

Learning Disabilities   Since 1962, 11 different definitions of learning disabilities have enjoyed some degree of support by professionals (Hammill, 1990). The two most influential definitions, however, have been those put forward by the National Joint Committee on Learning Disabilities (NJCLD) and the U.S. Office of Education (USOE). These are cited in Table 7.1. It has been noted that the NJCLD definition has "the best chance of becoming the consensus definition" among educational leaders but that, for political reasons, the USOE definition may remain the legal definition (Hammill, 1990, p. 82).

How do the two definitions differ? A careful reading of the two would find that the NJCLD definition is different on three points:

▷ It shifts away from the position that underlying perceptual-motor difficulties ("basic psycholog-

TABLE 7.1   Two Major Definitions of Learning Disabilities

National Joint Committee on Learning Disabilities (1991a, p. 19)	U.S. Office of Education, as Contained in the Education for All Handicapped Children Act of 1975 (PL 94-142)
Learning disabilities is a general term that refers to a heterogeneous group of disorders manifested by significant difficulties in the acquisition and use of listening, speaking, reading, writing, reasoning, or mathematical abilities. These disorders are intrinsic to the individual, presumed to be due to central nervous system dysfunction, and may occur across the life span. Problems in self-regulatory behaviors, social perception, and social interaction may exist with learning disabilities but do not by themselves constitute a learning disability. Although learning disabilities may occur concomitantly with other handicapping conditions (for example, sensory impairment, mental retardation, serious emotional disturbance) or extrinsic influences (such as cultural differences, insufficient or inappropriate instruction), they are not the direct result of those conditions of influence.	[Children with specific learning disabilities are] those children who have a disorder in one or more of the basic psychological processes involved in understanding or in using language, spoken or written, which disorder may manifest itself in imperfect ability to listen, think, speak, read, write, spell, or do mathematical calculations. Such disorders include such conditions as perceptual handicaps, brain injury, minimal brain dysfunction, dyslexia, and developmental aphasia. Such term does not include children who have learning problems which are primarily the result of visual, hearing, or motor handicaps, of mental retardation, of emotional disturbance, or of environmental, cultural, or economic disadvantage.

ical processes") are at the root of all learning disabilities. This change more accurately reflects research findings.

▷ It emphasizes the heterogeneous nature of learning disabilities and the fact that they are not limited to children.

▷ It revises the interpretation of concomitant conditions. The USOE definition is often referred to as *exclusionary* in that it stipulates conditions that *cannot coexist* with learning disabilities, such as mental retardation or economic disadvantage. Under a strict interpretation, this means that children from backgrounds of poverty cannot be diagnosed as having learning disabilities. The wording of the NJCLD definition makes such a diagnosis possible.

Both the NJCLD and USOE definitions make it plain that children with learning disabilities may show problems across a range of skills. What the definitions do not state, but is of intense interest to researchers and practitioners alike, is whether all children with learning disabilities have a single underlying problem or whether they should be regarded as forming subgroups. A number of researchers have attempted to classify learning disabilities into subtypes, using a variety of statistical and analytical methods. Generally, there have been two approaches to classification (Lyon & Risucci, 1988). In a *clinical-inferential approach,* investigators have examined batteries of test scores and identified groups of children with common profiles. Following this method, three subgroups of children with learning disabilities have been distinguished (Mattis, French, & Rapin, 1975):

1. Those with difficulty on language and language-related tasks (40–60% of the population).
2. Those with articulatory and **graphomotor** (handwriting/drawing coordination) deficits (10–40%).
3. Those with **visuospatial perception** deficits (5–15%).

The second approach, used in more recent studies, has been to identify subgroups from *statistical analyses.* For example, researchers have studied children who score poorly on achievement tests despite having average or above-average intelligence (Satz & Morris, 1981). By examining the statistical interrelationships

among scores from a battery of neuropsychological tests, five types of children with learning disabilities were revealed:

1. Those with global language impairment (30% of the population).
2. Those with selective impairment of naming (16%).
3. Those with a mixed deficit of language impairment and difficulty on visual-perceptual-motor tasks (11%).
4. Those with impairment only on nonlanguage visual-perceptual-motor tests (26%).
5. Those with normal performance on all the neuropsychological tests (13%).

Both the clinical-inferential and statistical approaches to classification have used test data to distinguish groups of children. Test data are important, of course, in identifying areas of difficulty. A more important aim of these studies, however, is to identify whether there are specific cognitive, perceptual, or linguistic *processes* that are deficient in children with learning disabilities. If a process or group of processes can be discovered, it might be possible to devise treatment programs tailored to meet the needs of specific students.

Children with learning disabilities can also be differentiated by the age at which their problems are first observed. Three patterns have been identified in these children's language-learning histories (Donahue, 1986):

1. Children diagnosed during the preschool years with obvious language-learning problems.
2. Children who enter school with adequate interpersonal communication skills but soon show poor performance.
3. Children who initially fare well in school but eventually exhibit problems.

All three approaches—clinical-inferential, statistical, and historical—offer insights into the factors that can distinguish one child with learning disabilities from another. None of them, however, represents a canonical view of the disorder that can be used to classify children, place them into different educational settings, or identify particular intervention strategies.

Dyslexia (Reading Disabilities)   Of all the basic skills affected in children with learning disabilities, reading is the most often impaired. Some 60–80% of this population show some impairment in reading decoding or comprehension (Lyon, 1985). The term **dyslexia** (or other terms such as *reading disability* or *specific reading disorder*) is usually used to describe a specific problem—learning to read—of children with learning disabilities. Thus, a child with dyslexia is presumed to be of normal intelligence and without any serious sensory or emotional disorders. One would not refer to a child with mental retardation or autism as also exhibiting dyslexia.

Although problems in reading are found in the majority of children with learning disabilities, the relationship between dyslexia and other kinds of learning deficiency is not clear. Some scholars have argued that children with language impairment and children with reading impairment should be regarded as subgroups of children with learning disabilities. There may be extreme subgroups in both categories, that is, children with marked language impairment but relatively good reading and children with reading impairment but very mild language impairment (Kamhi & Catts, 1986). In support of this claim are findings from longitudinal studies that suggest that dyslexia is a very broad and fluid classification (Shaywitz, Escobar, Shaywitz, Fletcher, & Makuch, 1992). Some children may show reading impairment in first grade but not 2 years later. Other children may seem to be achieving normally in first grade but show problems 2 years later.

Early research into the causes of dyslexia tended to focus on visual perceptual skills. Indeed, as we noted earlier, the USOE definition of learning disabilities refers to problems in "basic psychological processes." That perspective dimmed, however, as researchers failed to find evidence of significant perceptual differences in children with dyslexia. In place of the perceptual deficit model has come what has been called the *developmental language perspective* (Kamhi & Catts, 1991), which emphasizes the connection between reading deficits and problems in other language skill areas: speech production, vocabulary learning, spelling, composition, and so on.

While the majority of recent academic research into dyslexia has concentrated on issues of language competence, considerable public and media attention has focused on reports about a supposedly simple but effective optical remedy for the problem. Beginning in 1983, psychologist Helen Irlen began to treat adults and children with dyslexia by providing them with colored lenses and spectacles (Blakeslee, 1991). These lenses, it was claimed, served to stabilize the visual images on a page, making the perceptual component of reading less taxing. For some individuals, the lenses appeared to have a markedly beneficial effect. Until recently there has been no theory to explain and scant research evidence to support the use of colored lenses. A new study, however, suggests that individuals with dyslexia may have cellular deficits in the portion of the brain that is responsible for low-contrast vision (Livingstone, Rosen, Drislane, & Galaburda, 1991). The use of colored lenses may compensate for this inherent defect and permit the visual system of the impaired reader to function in a more normal manner. Further work is needed to confirm the reported findings, to explore the generality of this visual deficit (do all children with dyslexia have it?), and to study its relationship to other kinds of language impairment that children with dyslexia are known to have.

Slow Learner   It is obvious to any observer that children with learning disabilities do not acquire certain skills easily. However, this cannot be taken to mean that difficulty in learning always signals a learning disability. Learning disability should not be confused with either low achievement or under-achievement (National Joint Committee on Learning Disabilities, 1989). *Low achievement,* the simple failure to learn, may be due to other causes such as mental retardation, sensory impairment, or adverse emotional, social, and environmental conditions. *Underachievement,* the failure of a child to learn up to the level that IQ testing suggests is possible, is a necessary but not sufficient criterion for the diagnosis of learning disabilities. It, too, can result from conditions in a child's environment that reduce the opportunity or motivation to learn.

Behind these definitional distinctions lies a major issue of diagnosis that can determine which children receive special education. In the majority of states today (see the section on "Prevalence"), children are identified as learning disabled by means of an *ability–achievement discrepancy method*. For example, in some states a child's achievement test scores must be two or more standard deviations below the child's IQ score. It has been asserted that the use of a discrepancy definition penalizes children who score poorly on IQ tests because of their cultural background and who are also reading disabled or language impaired. Because these children will *not* show a large discrepancy, they will likely be labeled as slow learners rather than learning disabled (Siegel, 1989). When this assertion was put to the test, it was indeed found that the standard score discrepancy method was more likely to identify children with above-average IQs as learning disabled. An alternative approach, which adjusts statistically for low IQ scores, produced more consistent results across IQ levels (Kamphaus, Frick, & Lahey, 1991). Despite its widespread use, therefore, the discrepancy method of distinguishing between children who are low achieving and learning disabled has been severely criticized. It may not be the most accurate way of differentiating between the two types of problems. For this reason, it is not always applied evenly in states where it is the official criterion for classifying a child as learning disabled (Merrell, 1990).

Attention Deficit-Hyperactivity Disorder Children who have **hyperactivity**, and therefore difficulty in directing and sustaining attention, often are impaired in their ability to learn, especially from formal instruction. They are also likely to interfere with the activities of those around them. For this reason, the American Psychiatric Association considers attention deficit-hyperactivity disorder (ADHD) to be one class of disruptive behavior disorder. The official definition of ADHD is given in Table 7.2.

Professionals who evaluate children for learning disabilities should be well acquainted with ADHD, as it is a common condition. It has been estimated that 10–20% of the school-age population is affected by ADHD (Shaywitz & Shaywitz, 1988). Prevalence figures are even higher for children who present with speech and language disorders, with surveys showing a range

TABLE 7.2 Definition of ADHD	
	The essential features of this disorder are developmentally inappropriate degrees of inattention, impulsiveness, and hyperactivity. People with the disorder generally display some disturbance in each of these areas, but to varying degrees.
	In the classroom . . . inattention and impulsiveness are evidenced by not sticking with tasks sufficiently to finish them and by having difficulty organizing and completing work correctly. The person often gives the impression that he or she is not listening or has not heard what has been said. Work is often messy, and performed carelessly and impulsively.
	Impulsiveness is often demonstrated by blurting out answers to questions before they are completed, making comments out of turn, failing to await one's turn in group tasks, failing to heed directions fully before beginning to respond to assignments, interrupting the teacher during a lesson, and interrupting or talking to other children during quiet work periods.
	Hyperactivity may be evidenced by difficulty remaining seated, excessive jumping about, running in classroom, fidgeting, manipulating objects, and twisting and wiggling in one's seat.

Source: American Psychiatric Association (1987), p. 50.

Note: In the past, other terminology was used to describe children with ADHD. The condition was first described as *brain damage*; the next term in common use was *minimal brain dysfunction* (*MBD*); following this, the label *hyperactivity* was applied. In 1980, the American Psychiatric Association adopted the term *attention deficit disorder* (*ADD*) and described it in two forms: *attention deficit disorder with hyperactivity* (*ADDH*) and *attention deficit disorder without hyperactivity* (*ADD without H*). These terms were revised in 1987, so that what had been termed *ADDH* is now referred to as *attention deficit-hyperactivity disorder* (*ADHD*); what had been labeled *ADD without H* is now referred to as *undifferentiated attention deficit disorder* (Shaywitz & Shaywitz, 1991).

from 22% to 30.4% (Baker & Cantwell, 1982; Beitch-man, Nair, Clegg, & Patel, 1986).

Differentiating ADHD from specific language proc-essing deficits may be difficult. Professionals must ob-serve children at some length to determine whether they are easily distracted in all settings or only in those with verbal stimuli (Prizant et al., 1990). Moreover, the categories of learning disability and ADHD should not be regarded as mutually exclusive. The two conditions are "heterogeneous, overlap frequently, and correlate with a number of other disorders" (Murphy & Hicks-Stewart, 1991, p. 388).

Specific Language Impairment   Both the USOE and NJCLD definitions make it clear that children with learning disabilities commonly exhibit impairments of language. A review of the previous discussion on pos-sible subtypes of learning disabilities illustrates how frequently language problems are seen in children with learning disabilities. In cases where the degree of language impairment is great and seems to be a child's predominant area of difficulty, the label *specific language impairment* (*SLI*) may also be applied. As we saw in chapter 5, there is no universal agreement about this term. *Language-learning disability* is an-other term that may be used. Whether children are described as having learning disabilities, specific lan-guage impairment, or language-learning disabilities often is determined by their age. This point is taken up further later in this chapter.

Phonological Processing Disorder/Develop-mental Apraxia of Speech   The term *phonologi-cal processing disorder* has two senses. In younger language-impaired children it is used as a variant of *phonological disorder* or *phonological disability* to describe a condition in which a child's speech is sys-tematically simplified and, therefore, is less intelligible to listeners. In older language-impaired children the term refers to an individual whose ability to process (i.e., encode and decode) phonological information is impaired, leading to problems in reading, spelling, word retrieval, and other language skills. Although older children with phonological processing disturb-ances may, in fact, have difficulty in saying words and phrases that are phonologically complex (Catts, 1986,

1989), their speech is nearly always intelligible. The problems they exhibit at a phonological level are pri-marily metalinguistic and are seen most clearly on experimental tasks such as phoneme and syllable segmentation (How many sounds are in the word "block"? How many syllables are in the word "cater-pillar"?).

Among children with unintelligible speech, some investigators have identified a subgroup of individuals who present with developmental **apraxia of speech** (*DAS*) (Crary, 1984; Yoss & Darley, 1974). The research evidence for this label has been strongly challenged (Guyette & Diedrich, 1981). However, those who sup-port its use have described the following group of symptoms:

A high incidence of accompanying oral apraxia.

Poor oral imitation ability.

Inconsistent sound substitutions that are often dis-tant from the target, for example, /m/ for /s/.

Exceptional difficulty in producing multisyllabic words.

Poor response to conventional articulation therapy methods.

There appears to be some overlap between the groups of children identified with learning disabilities and with DAS (Yoss & Darley, 1974). It has even been claimed that the children with DAS are identical to those identified in clinical-inferential studies as exhib-iting articulatory and graphomotor coordination defi-cits (Wiig, 1986).

Central Auditory Processing Disorder   The re-lationship between language learning and hearing cannot always be expressed in terms that are satisfy-ingly simple. Many hypotheses have been advanced; some are now well accepted and others are vigorously contested. At one end is a well-studied causal relation-ship between prelingual deafness and impairment in the acquisition of oral language, as we will see in chap-ter 9. At the other end is the incompletely studied and rather controversial set of relationships that have been identified by some professionals as constituting a cen-tral auditory processing disorder (CAPD), a topic in-troduced in chapter 2. The condition of CAPD is not well bounded clinically, and this is one of the reasons it is disputed.

The diagnosis of CAPD requires that the disorder be identified both from performance on a battery of special audiological tests designed to identify central auditory deficits and from a clinical case history (Willeford & Burleigh, 1985). Recall that the audiological tests that are administered to children suspected of having CAPD include auditory figure-ground tasks, dichotic listening, and tests of pitch-pattern sequencing (Keith, 1984). The tests are rarely given to children under age 6 because they are administered through headphones, require sustained attention, measure skills that are not used in everyday communication, and use linguistic stimuli suitable only for school-age children. Given the current means of assessment, the label CAPD can, therefore, only be appropriately assigned only to children who are attending school. The case histories of children identified with CAPD often reveal that they have also been identified as learning disabled or that they display a pattern of school performance very similar to that of children with learning disabilities. A study of 64 children, 7 to 11 years of age, who were referred for CAPD evaluation showed that 55% of them were receiving special services in school (Smoski, Brunt, & Tannahill, 1992). Only half of the children were reading at grade level, but the percentage of those working at grade level in science, spelling, language arts, and math was 69% or higher. Over 92% of the children were rated by their teachers as at least average in general disposition, response to discipline, enjoyment of school, and peer interaction. The only marked behavioral difference was concentration: 56% of the children were rated as below average.

A diagnosis of CAPD is always difficult to make. Even when a child has a case history suggestive of CAPD and shows difficulty on a CAPD test battery, it is hard to untangle cause-and-effect relationships. Many children who exhibit difficulty on figure-ground tasks, for example, may have problems with the attentional rather than the perceptual demands of the task (Keith, 1984). And, as we saw in chapter 2, the relationship between the types of auditory stimuli used as part of central auditory testing and children's language skills complicates interpretation even more.

Minimal Brain Dysfunction In the history of the field of learning disabilities the term *minimal brain dysfunction* (*MBD*) has an important place (Kavale & Forness, 1985). The term *brain-injured* was first used by Strauss and Lehtinen (1947) to describe a child who showed "disturbances in perception, thinking, and emotional behavior" (p. 4). Later it was asserted that brain injury could be diagnosed from behavioral evidence such as perceptual and conceptual difficulties and hyperactivity (Strauss & Kephart, 1955). The notion of "soft signs" as an indication of subtle neurological dysfunction grew out of this contention. Nevertheless, some objected to the use of *brain-injured* to describe a child who had no history of injury and showed no "hard" or "frank" signs of neurological damage. Thus the term slowly changed, first by the addition of the modifier *minimal* and then by the substitution of *dysfunction* for *injury* or *damage*. The resulting label, *minimal brain dysfunction,* was popularized within the medical community in the 1960s. Clements (1966), a physician, wrote an influential report for the Department of Health, Education, and Welfare in which he described children with MBD as "of near average, average, or above average general intelligence with certain learning or behavioral disabilities ranging from mild to severe, which are associated with deviations of functions of the central nervous system" (p. 9). A more specific description of the problem behaviors exhibited by children with MBD is as follows (Wender, 1971):

▷ Motor behavior characterized by high activity level (hyperactivity) and impaired coordination (**dyspraxia**).
▷ Attentional and perceptual-cognitive function characterized by a short attention span and poor concentration (**distractibility**).
▷ Learning difficulties, particularly in learning to read, write, and spell even with normal intelligence.
▷ Impulse control characterized by a decreased ability to inhibit; marked by low frustration tolerance and antisocial behavior.
▷ Interpersonal relations characterized by increased resistance to social demands.
▷ Emotionality characterized by increased lability,

altered reactivity (responses normal in kind but abnormal in degree), increased aggressiveness, increased irritability, depression, and low self-esteem.

As we noted earlier, diagnostic labels tend to change over time as a result of trends in professional opinion. MBD provides a rather straightforward example of this process. The term originated within and was popularized by members of the medical community. However, passage of PL 94-142 had the effect of shifting some of the responsibility for disabled children away from medicine and toward education. It did not take long, therefore, before MBD was criticized within the educational community precisely because it reflected a medical-etiological model rather than an educational model focusing on assessment and remediation (Kavale and Forness, 1985). Most children who display behaviors characteristic of MBD will today be described with other diagnostic labels.

Prevalence

Federal and State Guidelines   The USOE definition of learning disabilities used in PL 94-142 does not state what requirements must be met in order for a child to receive special education. Thus, it is left to the states to set eligibility criteria and establish procedures for diagnosing learning disabilities. The USOE definition of learning disabilities can be considered to have four essential components (Mercer, Hughes, & Mercer, 1985):

1. A process deficit that is manifested in a language disorder.
2. An academic deficit.
3. Exclusion of other primary causes, such as mental retardation, hearing impairment, and emotional disturbance.
4. Neurological deficits.

In recent years, states have moved away from the USOE definition. In particular, as of 1990, almost half of the states had dropped the "neurological" component from their definitions. What is more important, 29% of the states had specified an IQ cutoff that differentiated children with mental retardation and learning

disabilities, and 76% of the states had established specific methods for determining a discrepancy between ability and achievement. The most common method was standard score comparison (e.g., a child's achievement scores must be two or more standard deviations below the IQ score). Statistical analysis has indicated that the effect of these changes in definition by the various states has been to *reduce* the number of students identified as learned disabled (Frankenberger & Fronzaglio, 1991).

General Estimates   Prevalence data gathered by the federal government indicate clearly that PL 94-142 has changed the landscape of publicly funded special education. A major feature of that landscape is now the child with learning disabilities. From 1977 to 1990, the number of children with learning disabilities receiving special education increased from 782,095 to nearly 2 million, a 152% increase over a 13-year period. From 1977 to 1983, the annual rate of increase averaged 14%. Since 1983, the rate has slowed to 2.5% per year, indicating that many states have changed their eligibility criteria to stem the flow of children qualifying for service (U.S. Department of Education, 1990).

Male:Female Ratios   It has long been reported that far more boys than girls are diagnosed with learning disabilities, with reported ratios ranging from 3:1 to 15:1 (Finucci & Childs, 1981). A recent prevalence study conducted in an Alabama school system reported 178 males and 64 females with learning disabilities between the ages of 8 and 12 years (Gibbs & Cooper, 1989). It has been suggested that boys may be identified more often because they tend to exhibit more overt signs of the disorder, such as hyperactivity (Caplan & Kinsbourne, 1974; Gersten & Gersten, 1978). In general, research findings indicate that females with learning disabilities are lower in IQ and have more severe academic deficits in some areas of reading and math but are better in visual-motor abilities, spelling, and handwriting. There is some evidence, however, that past research has been biased in its selection of female subjects (Vogel, 1990). Because girls with learning disabilities are generally less disruptive in school, those with mild deficits may not be selected to receive special education. They would not, therefore, appear as subjects in studies that use school populations.

Risk Factors

The term *risk factor* refers to a condition that increases the likelihood of a particular disease or injury. Thus, high blood pressure is a risk factor for stroke, and playing football is a risk factor for knee injury. In many cases, the causal relationship between a risk factor and a given disease or injury is known. However, even when causes and effects are not clearly understood—as with learning disabilities—it is helpful to be aware of the factors that have been shown to be statistically related to a particular condition. Knowledge of these elements will guide professionals in their decisions about parent counseling, referral for medical or psychological evaluation, and recommendation of speech-language intervention. It must be remembered, however, that if certain conditions such as hearing loss are deemed to be *primarily* responsible for a child's learning difficulties, then by most definitions that child cannot be considered learning disabled. This makes the distinction between risk factor and cause very important to educational placement decisions.

Attention Deficit-Hyperactivity Disorder   We noted earlier that a high percentage of school-age children with speech and language disorders and/or learning disabilities also present with ADHD. It is tempting to infer a causal relationship from this finding, but it is not clear which condition is the cause and which is the effect. Even more to the point, ADHD is not found in all children with learning disabilities, nor does its presence necessarily complicate the problem. Hyperactive and nonhyperactive children with learning disabilities show few differences on tests that measure cognitive maturity and style (Copeland & Weissbrod, 1983).

Hearing Loss   Hearing loss can be regarded as a risk factor for learning disabilities in two ways. First, there appears to be a subpopulation of deaf students (approximately 6–7%) who also have a concomitant learning disability (Bunch & Melnyk, 1989). These stu-dents obviously have special needs that extend well beyond those of hearing students with learning disabilities. The second and more commonly identified risk factor is conductive hearing loss. In surveys of children with learning disabilities, estimates of middle ear pathology range from a low of 15.7% to a high of 49% (Bennett, Ruuska, & Sherman, 1980; Freeman & Parkins, 1979; Gibbs & Cooper, 1989; Masters & March, 1978). Taken as a whole, it is reasonable to expect that one in four elementary school children identified by schools as learning disabled will have experienced recurrent episodes of **otitis media** (ear infections) (Reichman & Healey, 1983). Estimates of the number of children with learning disabilities and measurable conductive hearing loss range from 7.4% to 38% (Bennett et al., 1980; Gibbs & Cooper, 1989). The discrepancy in findings is perhaps due to differences in screening procedures (Gibbs & Cooper, 1989).

Heredity   There has been a long-standing suspicion among professionals that learning disabilities run in families. Previously, there was also limited research to support the suspicion (e.g., Decker & DeFries, 1980). If we take the view that language problems are frequently closely associated with at least some forms of learning disabilities, the risk factors related to a family history of language problems, as discussed in chapter 4, may lend additional support to the suspicion of an hereditary factor in learning disabilities.

The Natural History of Learning Disabilities

The USOE and NJCLD definitions of learning disabilities do not state a minimum age for applying this diagnostic label. Yet, it is rare to hear the term applied to preschool children. A survey of state consultants in special education indicates that programs for preschool children with learning disabilities vary widely. Some states provide no funding for preschoolers with this diagnosis, and there appears to be a great deal of confusion nationwide over appropriate terminology for describing young children with language and learning problems (Esterly & Griffin, 1987).

For many years it has been recognized that the problem in terminology centers on the distinction between what we call *language disorders* and *learning disabilities*. This problem was introduced in chapter 5. In 1984, Wallach and Liebergott offered three possible interpretations of the relationship between these two categories:

1. They are separate problems and a child may have neither, either, or both.
2. A language disorder may be a cause of learning disability in a subset of children.
3. They are a single disorder that manifests itself differently at various points in development.

Most professionals have adopted the last of these interpretations and emphasize that language disorders must be understood in terms of their *natural history* (Bashir, 1989; Bashir & Scavuzzo, 1992). That is, a language disorder is a lasting problem that manifests itself in different ways as a child grows older. The differences in symptoms and levels of severity are the result of changes in communicative contexts and the learning tasks that a child faces. As these children grow older, the language impairment shows up in different ways. As we saw in chapter 5, language impairment among preschool children is typically identified when they have difficulty with the basic communicative functions of talking and understanding speech. Once the children begin school and receive literacy instruction, we begin to identify problems in other aspects of learning that have a language component. These include metalinguistic abilities, narrative and classroom discourse, and figurative language, as well as written language skills.

Although the majority position at this time appears to be that language disorders and learning disabilities represent different points on a developmental continuum, several cautions are warranted. First, the position should not be misinterpreted to mean that all children with learning disabilities are also language impaired. Research on subtypes of learning disabilities, reviewed earlier, suggests that most but not all children with learning disabilities are deficient in some language skill or skills. Second, children with learning disabilities who have no history of spoken language impairment are not immune to language-learning deficits (Lee & Kamhi, 1990). One view of language disorders has it that certain types of problems do not become apparent until the language system is challenged (Lahey, 1990). Thus, children might be able to perform adequately during the preschool years when only oral language is required but find themselves overmatched once they are asked to read and write. Third, it is possible that there are subgroups of children with language-learning disabilities. Children who are identified as language impaired at a young age and later are classified as learning disabled may be the most impaired subgroup of children with learning disabilities (Lee & Kamhi, 1990). The suggestion has also been made that the labels *language disorder* and *learning disability* are applied differentially by professionals, even though they have no formal guidelines for doing so. For example, there is indirect evidence to suggest that children are more likely to be labeled language disordered if they exhibit difficulties with vocabulary (Lapadat, 1991).

As part of their understanding of the natural history of language disorders and learning disabilities, professionals must inevitably address the issue of recovery. Crystal (1984) has framed the question this way:

> Do you believe that, if you had all the time in the world, and all the resources that you needed, the child would be normal one day? (p. 149)

We have already noted that many preschoolers diagnosed with language impairment continue to show that impairment—in different forms—as they grow older. But others do not. However, the issue of *illusionary recovery* (Scarborough & Dobrich, 1990), discussed in chapter 5, may be relevant for these children. Recall that it has been suggested that some preschoolers appear to recover because of the stair-step nature of language development. Typically developing children, it is asserted, show spurts of growth separated by an extended plateau (Scarborough & Dobrich, 1990). The children with language impairment are able to catch up during the normal children's plateau phase, only to fall behind when the normal children spurt again in the early school years.

Another perspective on recovery from language impairment and learning disabilities can be taken at the end of a child's education. To what extent do children—now young adults—show persisting social, educational, and vocational problems as a result of their deficits? Surveys and case records suggest that impairment is persistent. Chapter 11 addresses the problem of continuing language problems in adolescence. With regard to learning disabilities, one sample of college students who had been previously diagnosed with learning disabilities exhibited difficulty in recognizing and producing the proper syntax for complex sentences (Wiig & Fleischmann, 1980). Another sample consisted of 80 adults who referred themselves for evaluation (Blalock, 1982). According to their oral reports, these adults had persistent learning problems, the majority of which were identified before or during elementary school. Learning problems were found in a variety of areas. Reading and writing problems were most frequent, followed by auditory language disturbances and difficulties with math, nonverbal abilities, and attention. Interestingly, the adults were in most cases unaware of the full extent of their problems. The number of problems discovered in every area tested far exceeded the number of complaints. Recently, an extensive follow-up study was reported on students with learning disabilities who had attended vocational-technical programs (Shapiro & Lentz, 1991). The general findings of this survey were that these students

▷ Often did not have future plans when they graduated.
▷ Received most of their help after graduation from friends, family members, and co-workers.
▷ Often (50–60%) worked in areas unrelated to their vocational training.
▷ Remained at low income levels.

These results do little to dispel the notion that learning disabilities, often with concomitant language problems, are likely to remain lifelong disabilities.

The Role of the Professional

The problems experienced by children with learning disabilities are diverse and, therefore, require the expertise of a number of professionals (Table 7.3). Having a number of workers involved in the development and implementation of a child's program can lead to confusion caused by poor understanding and communication of one another's roles. There may even be situations in which professional jealousies develop over the issue of job responsibilities. The boundary lines separating psychology from speech-language pathology from special education are not clearly drawn. Moreover, they are subject to change as ideas evolve within a discipline. For example, speech-language pathologists may be more likely to work with children who are dyslexic as a result of a conceptual shift that views reading impairment as a component of a larger language disorder (Kamhi & Catts, 1991). The National Joint Committee on Learning Disabilities (1985) has recommended that professional educational programs be made interdisciplinary in order to encourage mutual awareness among the different disciplines that treat children with learning disabilities. The ASHA Committee on Language Learning Disorders (American Speech-Language-Hearing Association, 1991) has gone even further, suggesting that speech-language pathologists consider the merits of a *collaborative* service delivery model, in which they would share responsibilities for all aspects of a child's education with a team of educators from different disciplines. This model is discussed further later in this chapter.

LINGUISTIC ISSUES RELEVANT TO LEARNING DISABILITY

As children grow older and advance in school, they are regularly expected to expand and reorganize their language systems. They must come to understand and treat language as a set of tools, as something that can be reflected upon and consciously altered to suit particular educational or social purposes. Children must also deal with a new layer of arbitrary symbolism: the printed word. Not only must they learn to recognize units of written language and their relationship to speech, they must also appreciate the sometimes subtle differences between the written and spoken word and be able to shift smoothly from one language system to another. Upon entering school, children encounter a new world where the rules for communication are designed to promote good conduct and enhance the learning process. And, of course, older children are expected to know more and act more responsibly. Expectations for both the form and content

TABLE 7.3   Professionals Involved in the Assessment and Treatment of Children with Learning Disabilities

Job Title	Job Description
Regular education (classroom) teacher	Organizes and oversees the curriculum in the regular education classroom.
Diagnostic-prescriptive teacher	Following a referral from the classroom teacher, observes and tests students with perceived academic or behavioral problems. Develops recommendations for individual teaching techniques and materials, and then reviews and demonstrates these for the classroom teacher. Carries out periodic follow-up and evaluation.
School psychologist	Conducts psychoeducational evaluations of a child's intelligence, academic achievement, and social interactions and relationships. Consults with parents, classroom teachers, and other personnel regarding issues of cognitive style, cognitive maturity, and group and individual conduct.
Reading specialist	Evaluates problems of reading. Consults with regular education teacher regarding students with relatively mild reading impairments who will benefit from corrective reading instruction delivered in the classroom. Provides intensive remedial instruction to students with more severe reading difficulties.
Resource teacher	Organizes and oversees instruction in a resource room, a common alternative to placement in self-contained special education classrooms. Usually instructs students with mild to moderate educational handicaps for up to half of their school day, spending the other portion of the time in a regular classroom. Some resource teachers are itinerant and provide services in the regular classroom.
Teacher aide	Prepares instructional materials, helps students with classroom work, and supervises students when they are outside of the classroom.
Speech-language pathologist	Evaluates problems of speech and language. Consults with the classroom teacher about ways of coping with, compensating for, and overcoming a child's communication difficulties. Provides direct service to children with communication impairments.
School social worker	Provides a bridge of communication between the home and the school. Interviews parents and compiles a psychosocial history. May be responsible for handling problems of truancy. Frequently serves as case manager for the special education committee.
School physician	Evaluates a child's sight, hearing, physical development, medical needs, and physical factors that affect school progress.

Source: Adapted from Hopke (1990), New York State Education Department (1990), Reynolds and Fletcher-Janzen (1990), and Weinenstein and Pelz (1986).

of language continue to rise and learning must become an activity that is both self-initiated and self-corrected.

Metalinguistic Skills

The ability to think about and eventually talk about language is the most significant linguistic achievement of the school-aged child. Metalinguistic skill, as it is called, cuts across both spoken and written language and facilitates the child's acquisition of independent problem-solving abilities (van Kleeck, 1984).

In school, children's metalinguistic knowledge expands at all levels of language. As learners of semantics they must be able to discover and explain word definitions. They must deal comfortably with components of lexical organization: oppositions and similarities of meaning and subordinate and superordinate relationships. They must distinguish between literal and non-literal meanings and among various types of nonliteral meaning: word play, **irony**, humor, metaphor, and so on. As learners of grammar, children must be able to identify and manipulate **constituent** structures to clarify the meaning of what they read ("What does 'come what may' mean?"), to improve their writing ("Where should this paragraph go?"), or to learn foreign languages ("What's the imperfect form of 'poder'?"). To participate fully in social situations, children must also develop **metapragmatic** skills, that is, to communicate about situational differences in language use in order to function adequately in peer groups ("Don't talk that way in mixed company"), in school ("That kind of language belongs on the playground, not in here"), and at work ("Don't say that to the boss"). The social penalties for using inappropriate language in any of these settings can be severe.

Differences Between Spoken and Written Language

In chapter 1, some of the similarities and differences between listening and speaking and reading and writing were introduced. When we review these and other similarities and differences between these two language forms, it may be easier to understand why some children with learning disabilities find the demands of the two forms unequal.

Children learning to read and write face much stiffer demands for lexical understanding and use. When they speak, children can take advantage of physical context and listener knowledge to patch up deficiencies in vocabulary. Deictic words such as "these" and "here" work wonderfully in speech when they are accompanied by an appropriate gesture. But in writing they must function **anaphorically**, that is, the items or place to which they refer must have been explicitly mentioned earlier in the text. Thus, deictic words cannot be used to overcome a lack of vocabulary. In speech, generous allowance is made for the use of vague words. We all say "thing," "stuff," "guy," and "sort of" and allow others to do the same. In writing, however, more precise communication is expected.

Words must be carefully evaluated for subtle differences in meaning, using tools such as a dictionary or thesaurus if necessary. And since this is the expectation for writing, it follows that children will confront more sophisticated vocabulary when they read. Indeed, many words will be found only in the context of reading. To be successful readers, therefore, children must develop extensive recognition vocabularies that, for the most part, are triggered only by the visual stimulus of the word.

It is easy to observe that people do not write and talk the same way. Beyond the differences in vocabulary, however, it is not always simple to identify the formal differences between the two. First, we must ignore those instances of writing masquerading as speech, such as dramatic conversations (in plays, soap operas) or television news where the reporter reads from the teleprompter while looking into the camera. *Real* speech is characterized by a high rate of formulation breakdown—repetition, pauses, filled pauses, revision—while published writing is free of these disturbances. More important, though, are the differences in the *lexical density* and *redundancy* of written and spoken language (Perera, 1984). Following is an example of the same information presented in spoken and written form:

Spoken Language

The man came into the store and came up to the counter. He asked me for some change and I told him that we didn't make change, you know, because people are always asking us for change, but I told him that the laundromat next door had a change machine, so he could get some there.

Written Language

When the man came into the store, he came up to the counter and asked for some change. Because of all the requests we receive for change, I referred him to the change machine in the laundromat next door.

Whereas speech has a high frequency of repetition, rephrasing, and clausal coordination, the preference in writing is for conciseness characterized by single statements employing clausal embedding. These constructions, while elegant, cannot be comprehended as easily, especially by children with language impairment.

Differences Between Home and School Language

A child new to school soon discovers that life in a classroom is different from life at home. Most people would say that the child must learn to follow a new set of *routines*. Scholars have refined this concept and re-labeled it as an event script. A *script* is a generalized representation of the varied experiences that occur within an event (Creaghead, 1990). For example, as adults we have internalized a range of experiences about conducting transactions in banks. Consequently, we know what to expect when we enter an unfamiliar bank: There will be forms to fill out, a line to stand in, and tellers to serve us. We "know the routine," but we know it in a sufficiently general way that it can be adapted to any bank, not just the one we usually use.

To act appropriately in the classroom, normally achieving children must learn a number of scripts, which can be summarized as follows (Creaghead, 1990):

Arriving	Recess
Coming to class	Going home
Snack time	Getting objects, information, and help from the teacher
Following verbal directions	
Cleaning up	Answering the teacher's questions during lessons
Completing workbook pages	
Story time	Reading aloud
Getting homework	Following oral directions
"Show and tell"	Getting information and help from peers
Changing classes	
Group time	Chatting with peers
Reading group	Negotiating rules for games and play
Free play	
Reading for information	Planning and negotiating group projects
Making things	
Taking tests	Explaining and defending behavior
Field trips	
Group lessons	Relaying messages
Going outside	Giving reports
Lunch	Pretending, role playing
Going to the bathroom	Giving directions

Students with learning disabilities also must know the scripts because more than 90% of these children are taught in regular education classrooms for some part of their school day (12th Annual Report to Congress on the Implementation of the Education of the Handicapped Act, cited by National Joint Committee on Learning Disabilities, 1991b). Scripts serve to govern behavior in various classroom situations, but they also set the ground rules for communication. Children must know when they can speak freely and when they must request permission. They must know that the question "Can you tell us about . . . ?" is really a request for an elaborated reply and should not be answered with a simple "yes" or "no." They must know when it is appropriate to seek help from friends and when it is not.

Most of the language differences in school pertain to pragmatics; children learn to vary their use of language in different interpersonal and instructional contexts. We should not overlook, though, the changes in semantic and grammatical complexity that also accompany the school experience. Children are introduced to a host of new words in the classroom. Some of these words describe objects, people, and activities of the school itself ("assembly," "roll call," "principal," "report card," "grade"). Others are words that are crucial to instruction ("turn the page," "skip," "alike," "identical," "opposite"). There is also less fine tuning in the commands given in the classroom. Teachers typically must address an entire group of students and therefore cannot tailor instructions ("pick up the scissors—the ones right next to you—on the table"), as might a parent speaking to an individual child.

Differences in Developmental Expectations for Language Knowledge and Use

Another way of viewing the changes that can affect children's school performance is simply to reflect on what we expect them to know at different ages. Both the content and method of school instruction change from grade to grade, as we saw in chapter 1. In some cases, these changes can serve to trigger learning problems where none had existed previously. For example, children who struggle in learning to read might be diagnosed with dyslexia in Grades 1 and 2. They might continue to learn normally in other academic areas where the method of instruction is the lecture and visual demonstration. Beginning in Grade

3, however, these children would be asked to do more of their learning through reading and, consequently, they might begin to lag behind in several subjects.

COMMUNICATION PROBLEMS IN CHILDREN WITH LEARNING DISABILITIES

Characterizations of children with learning disabilities are based on research in which they have served as subjects. All conclusions from research should be regarded as tentative and subject to revision by future studies that replicate, refute, or reinterpret the earlier findings. Readers should be aware that at least three general criticisms have been made of research on children with learning disabilities:

1. Most studies have selected subjects who display a significant discrepancy between achievement and intelligence test scores, the standard required by most state laws. Such criteria do not exclude children whose learning problems are due to poor motivation, poor instruction, or inadequate opportunities for learning (Roth & Spekman, 1989). Thus many investigations may have been conducted with children who are not truly learning disabled, as it is properly defined.

2. Some studies have been conducted with students attending parochial schools, which do not have explicit criteria for identifying children with learning disabilities (e.g., Bryan, Donahue, & Pearl, 1981; Donahue, Pearl, & Bryan, 1980). Results from these studies may not be representative of the population of *system-identified* children with learning disabilities (Dudley-Marling, 1985). It should be noted, however, that quantitative comparison of these studies with ones that employed standard subject selection criteria showed no significant difference in outcome (Lapadat, 1991).

3. Studies that use samples of system-identified children with learning disabilities may produce different findings than studies where children are identified by means of research criteria. In particular, comparison of the two types of investigations suggests that system-identified samples tend to underestimate the abilities of females with learning disabilities (Vogel, 1990).

With these criticisms in mind, we can examine some of the major findings about the language skills of children with learning disabilities.

Semantics

Research on problems at the level of semantics falls into two broad categories: difficulty in organizing word meanings and difficulty in retrieving lexical items either during naming tasks or in spontaneous speech. Many professionals consider word meaning and word retrieval as separate clinical problems but, as we shall see, at least one interpretation of the research views them as different manifestations of an underlying semantic deficit.

Word Meanings   Both clinical observation and controlled experiments indicate that children with learning disabilities have underdeveloped lexical systems. This is reflected by their impoverished vocabularies and poor metalinguistic knowledge. For example, in comparison with their normal-achieving peers, first-grade children with learning disabilities showed significantly poorer performance on all sections of the *Boehm Test of Basic Concepts,* which requires them to identify words in the categories of quantity, space, time, and miscellaneous (Kavale, 1982). Another study indicates that this problem persists throughout the school years, as adolescents with learning disabilities showed poor scores on the comparative, passive, temporal, and familial subtests of the *Wiig-Semel Test of Linguistic Concepts* (Riedlinger-Ryan & Shewan, 1984)

Clinical reports on children with learning disabilities frequently cite their difficulty with more advanced assessments of literal word meaning. For example, they are commonly found to misunderstand words with multiple meanings such as "toast," "rear," or "catch" (Wiig & Semel, 1984). They are also much less proficient at recognizing and using words that are structurally related such as antonyms, synonyms, superordinates, and subordinates (Wiig & Semel, 1975). In a study that asked 4- to 9-year-old children with and without learning disabilities to relabel objects with a different word, the impaired children produced significantly more nonmeaningful responses such as word play ("paemp" for "lamp"), repetitions, or related but different word forms ("wrench" for "hammer") (Lewis & Kass, 1982). Poor lexical knowledge was also evidenced in a study of the definitions produced by adolescents with learning disabilities, which suggested that they understood only "limited, concrete aspects of the concept while abstract, general aspects were overlooked" (Wiig & Semel, 1975, p. 584). For example, "apple" might be defined as "something you eat" and "history" as "something you learn in school." Abstract words such as "material" or "opinion" were defined incorrectly by the majority of the students with learning disabilities.

An even more problematic lexical task for children with learning disabilities is the comprehension and use of nonliteral meanings. Even though these students often perform comparably to other students on standardized tests of literal comprehension, they are poorer at explaining sentences consisting of **metaphors**, involving atypical or nonliteral description or comparison (e.g., "Spring is a lady in a new coat") than their nondisabled peers (Nippold & Fey, 1983). They tend to err by giving literal responses. Children with learning disabilities apparently are better at understanding similes (e.g., "David was like a thirsty puppy finding water") than metaphors (e.g., "David was a thirsty puppy finding water"), though they improve on both kinds of comprehension tasks as they grow older (Seidenberg & Bernstein, 1986). This difference in comprehension has been interpreted as due to metacognitive factors, that is, a simile explicitly indicates with the word "like" that a comparison is being made. Children with learning disabilities apparently need this verbal cue in order to recognize that a nonliteral meaning is being expressed. Cues provided by story context or pictures have not been found effective in shifting these children from literal to nonliteral interpretations (Lee & Kamhi, 1990).

Word Retrieval   There is both agreement and dispute over the so-called word retrieval skills of children with learning disabilities. Clinicians and researchers are in accord that these children show differences in verbal behavior. In both **confrontation naming** and spontaneous speech, children with learning disabilities produce a range of behaviors that are either different from those of normally achieving children or occur with higher frequency (Blachman, 1984;

Denckla & Rudel, 1976a, 1976b; German, 1979, 1982; Rudel, Denckla, & Broman, 1981; Wiig & Semel, 1975):

1. Items are described without being directly named (**circumlocution**).
2. Another word is substituted for the target.
3. A previous response is repeated (**perseveration**).
4. Low-information words such as pronouns and indefinite adverbs ("somewhere," "sometime," etc.) are used excessively.
5. There is greater delay in producing the target word.
6. Extra verbalizations are produced (e.g., "oh, it's uh . . .").
7. Target words are preceded by initial-sound repetitions (e.g., "f, f, thumb").
8. There are greater difficulties in naming to description ("What do you call the end of your shirt sleeve?").

Different interpretations have been offered on the nature of the impairment that produces these behaviors. By analogy with the deficits seen in adults with brain injuries, some have described the impairment as one of word retrieval (German, 1982; Wiig & Semel, 1984). In this view, the children are presumed to have adequately *learned* certain vocabulary but to have trouble retrieving and using that vocabulary productively. In contrast to this account are the findings and explanations of a series of experiments by Kail and Leonard (1986). Drawing on their study of children 6 to 14 years of age with specific language impairment, they suggest that these children do not show a specific retrieval deficit. Instead, it is argued, they are slower and less efficient at word retrieval tasks because of their less elaborated word knowledge, which renders them less effective at using common retrieval strategies based on semantic and phonological linkages. That is, children with language impairment retrieve words in the same way as nonimpaired children, but they are less successful because the words have been learned less completely. This explanation collapses the clinical categories of word meaning and word retrieval into one problem area, which might be termed a *generalized semantic deficit*.

Grammar

For many years, the general impression has been that children with learning disabilities perform at lower levels on most measures of language form. For example, between the ages of 7:8 and 12:5 years, students with learning disabilities show a very gradual linear increase in utterance length (Andolina, 1980). Over the same period, normally achieving children are consistently higher in average utterance length. Even more interesting, the normal children exhibit periods of rapid growth, whereas the children with learning disabilities maintain a constant slow rate of growth.

There is other evidence of grammatical impairment from studies employing structured communication tasks. For example, when asked to describe unfamiliar objects to listeners who could not see them, children with learning disabilities at Grades 2, 4, 6, and 8 produced fewer words per T-unit (one main clause with all the subordinate clauses attached to it) and per main clause than normally achieving students at the same grade levels (Donahue, Pearl, & Bryan, 1982). At the level of morphology, 7- and 8-year-old children with learning disabilities showed poorer command of past tense inflections than a normally achieving control group (Moran & Byrne, 1977). Most errors occurred with irregular forms. There was evidence of adaptation to the problem in the disabled children's frequent use of the **obligatory form** "do" or the **catenative** "finished + verb" to signal past events. Another study of children with learning disabilities at the same age showed significantly lower scores on the *Berry-Talbott Test of Comprehension of Grammar* but the same order of difficulty as their nondisabled peers (Vogel, 1983). These findings have led many professionals to characterize all children with learning disabilities as slow learners of grammatical form.

Recent research, however, indicates that there is a subgroup of students with learning disabilities who do not display grammatical disability, as judged by the type and accuracy of structures produced in spontaneous story telling (Roth & Spekman, 1989). The students examined ranged in age from 8:0 to 13:11 years. They attended a private school for students with learning disabilities and had IQ scores that were approximately 15–20 points higher than those typically found in research samples of children with learning disabilities. Judging from this study, we should be careful not to assume that a child with learning disabilities will have impairments of language form, especially if the IQ is higher than the mean score of 100.

Narratives

An important area of assessment in children of school age is the comprehension and production of language units larger than the sentence. *Discourse analysis* is relevant to both spoken and written language. The analysis of spoken discourse is often conducted by asking children to produce or listen to and answer questions about narratives (stories). A body of research using these techniques has now developed, and it paints a fairly clear picture of the problems exhibited by children with learning disabilities:

▷ Their spontaneous narratives are shorter and contain fewer complete episodes (Garnett, 1986; Roth & Spekman, 1986).

▷ Their character descriptions are shallow, with few references to internal states such as fear, anger, revenge, or surprise (Montague, Maddux, & Dereshiwsky, 1990; Ripich & Griffith, 1988; Roth & Spekman, 1986).

▷ They are less successful in judging the comparative importance of information in a story (Garnett, 1986).

▷ They give the impression of being egocentric narrators who do not consider the needs of the audience. This may be due to inadequate mastery of discourse cohesion devices such as anaphoric reference (Garnett, 1986).

▷ They may have less knowledge of the world to help them interpret events and motivations in stories (Garnett, 1986).

▷ In retelling stories, they reduce the amount of information contained in the original narrative (Montague et al., 1990; Ripich & Griffith, 1988).

▷ They show a greater rate of communication breakdowns (stalls, repairs, and abandoned utterances) in narration than in conversation, which is not true of nondisabled children (MacLachlan & Chapman, 1988).

▷ They are immature in their ability to answer **inferential** questions about stories read to them. These questions require them to reason with the facts presented in the narrative rather than simply recall the verbatim content of the story. Problems with inferential reasoning are especially acute for children with lower receptive vocabularies (Crais & Chapman, 1987).

Pragmatics

Many studies of children with learning disabilities have examined their ability to use language effectively in various kinds of communicative situations. In dyadic or group conversations, researchers have been interested in how well these children maintain a topic, how well they repair breakdowns in the conversation, and how well they adjust to different listeners and different levels of shared information. Readers should be aware that much of this research has been heavily criticized for problems in design. For example, there are many studies suggesting that the types of utterances produced by children with learning disabilities are somehow different. There are indications that they produce more requests and make more negative or competitive statements. However, each of these studies has tended to use its own set of pragmatic categories to analyze the behavior of the children. Consequently, there is little corroboration of findings across studies, and it can be questioned whether they indeed show a consistent result (Dudley-Marling, 1985).

Allowing that at least some of the research is flawed, there is a consensus that differences exist in the pragmatic language behaviors of children with and without learning disabilities. Lapadat (1991) used a metaanalytic statistical procedure[1] to compare the results of 33 studies in six pragmatic categories: vocabulary selection and use, topic management, use of different speech acts, paralinguistic and nonverbal behaviors, conversational turn taking, and stylistic variation. She found that there were differences in all six categories between children with language disorders or learning disabilities and typically developing children. The differences were significantly greater in the categories of lexical selection and use and speech acts than in turn taking and stylistic variation. This result suggests that so-called pragmatic deficiencies are more likely due to linguistic than to social deficits.

Topic Management   Children with learning disabilities are likely to behave differently in verbal interactions with their peers. For example, when asked to work with a group in making a choice, children with learning disabilities are less likely to take the lead, keep the group on task, and persuade their peers to agree with their opinions (Bryan, Donahue, & Pearl, 1981). They are similarly passive in situations where they are asked to act as an interviewer. They ask fewer questions overall, and those they do ask tend to be ones that require only simple responses (Bryan, Donahue, Pearl, & Sturm, 1981).

An interesting analysis has been performed on transcripts of conversation between 9- to 13-year-old children with learning disabilities and nondisabled children of the same age and gender. Both the impaired and nonimpaired children were found to produce utterances at several levels of responsiveness (the degree to which an utterance is on task and relates to what the partner has said) and informativeness (the degree to which an utterance seeks information from the partner). The children with learning disabilities, however, produced higher-level types less frequently (Mathinos, 1991). Responsiveness was found to be correlated with the children's self-perception of social acceptance and self-worth. It was also correlated with how well the children knew their conversational partner. Thus the conversational engagement of children with learning disabilities appears to be a function of the goals they set for conversation, namely, to avoid excessive demands and the possibility of peer rejection.

Referential Communication   The ability to establish reference with a conversational partner is necessary to avoid miscommunication. It is frequently studied, however, using contrived activities such as a

---

[1]*Metaanalysis* is a statistical procedure that allows researchers to compare the results from multiple studies and reach conclusions about common findings. Comparison is made between *treatment effects,* a measure of the difference between the subject groups in each study.

Inappropriate use of social language may isolate children with learning disabilities from their peer group.

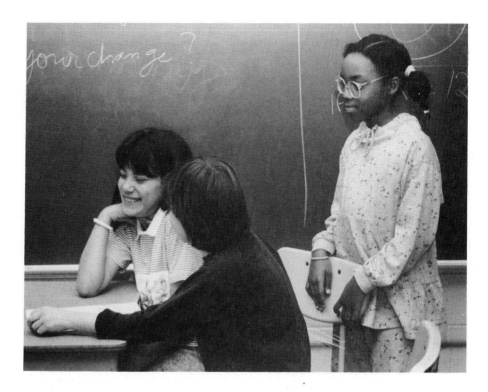

barrier task, in which two children sit on opposite sides of a screen that allows them to hear but not see each other. Recall from chapter 6 that in a barrier task, both children are given identical pictures or unusual geometric forms. One child will be asked to select a picture and then describe it so that the partner can select the same picture from his or her set. Nearly all studies of referential communication in children with learning disabilities have been of this type (Dudley-Marling, 1985). We should therefore be careful not to assume that the referential problems that have been identified in this research will also be found in the natural conversational behavior of these children.

In general, most experiments using referential communication tasks have found that children with learning disabilities provide descriptions that are less useful to their listeners (Noel, 1980; Spekman, 1981). However, at least one study used a similar experimental task and found no difference between children diagnosed as both language impaired and learning disabled and their nondisabled peers. The study did

find a significant difference between these groups and a group of younger nondisabled children, suggesting that age is the most potent factor in causing referencing problems (Meline, 1986). Presumably the inconsistency in research findings is due to variation in the subjects selected and the referential communication task employed.

Register Variation   Competent language users are able to modify their language in different contexts and with different conversational partners (**register** variation), thereby ensuring that their message will be understood and will not offend. Research that has studied the ability of children with learning disabilities to vary language in this way has not yielded a clear conclusion. For example, Bryan and Pflaum (1978) asked fourth- and fifth-grade children with and without learning disabilities to teach a game to a classmate of the same age and to a kindergarten child. They found that boys with learning disabilities did not modify the syntactic complexity of their language in the two situations. But girls with learning disabilities and normally achieving boys did modify their language, using less complex language when interacting with the younger children. To further complicate the picture, they found that normally achieving girls used *more* complex language with the kindergartners

Another investigation of language variation examined the MLUs of four children talking to an adult examiner (Soenksen, Flagg, & Schmits, 1981). The normally achieving students had significantly higher MLUs in conversation with the adult, whereas students with learning disabilities did not. There were, however, no consistent differences in pragmatic functions between the disabled and nondisabled children. With so few children in the study, we must not overinterpret these findings. There is stronger evidence to suggest that children with language-learning disabilities or reading disabilities do not differ greatly from typically developing children in how they respond to changes in situational variables. The grammatical complexity of all the children's utterances varies in similar ways when they speak with or without contextual support (for example, having the objects they are talking about present or absent) or are asked to describe a picture, explain an event, or tell a story (Masterson & Kamhi, 1991).

Conversational Repair   All conversations break down at some point, and the ability to detect and repair these disruptions is an important language competency, especially when the function of the conversation is to inform. Children with learning disabilities appear to be less effective, both as speakers and as listeners, in effecting conversational repairs. For example, one study asked teenage boys with learning disabilities to explain a game to a naive listener and then examined their responses to requests for clarification that were made during their explanations (Knight-Arest, 1984). Compared to normally achieving peers, the boys with learning disabilities were found to produce more language but with lower informational content. They relied more often on nonverbal demonstrations and gestures and often just repeated rather than reformulating their messages. When roles are reversed and children with learning disabilities are listeners rather than speakers, they are less likely to

request clarification of ambiguous messages (Donahue et al., 1980).

Reading

To read and understand a page of text requires a number of psycholinguistic processes to operate in sequence (Glass & Perna, 1986):

1. The letters on the page must be decoded to form an accurate phonological image of each word.
2. The definitions of the individual words must be retrieved from memory.
3. The syntactic and semantic information contained in these definitions must be combined to form a representation of the entire sentence.
4. The representations of the individual sentences must be combined to create an understanding of the entire passage.
5. If an individual is reading aloud, then speech production skills must also be brought to bear.

A disruption of any stage of the process will ultimately produce an impairment in reading.

Children with reading disabilities show a lack of phonological awareness in comparison with good readers and are, therefore, likely to struggle at the stage of phonological decoding. They perform inferiorly on segmentation tasks that require them, for example, to divide words into syllables or syllables into phonemes (Bryant & Bradley, 1981; Kamhi & Catts, 1986; Liberman, Shankweiler, Fischer, & Carter, 1974; Treiman & Baron, 1981). In one study it was found that poor readers in second and fourth grades were less accurate at distinguishing sentences from prosodic cues of pitch, stress, and pause. The poor readers in the fourth grade performed at levels comparable to those of good second-grade readers. Thus, they also appeared to lag developmentally in the acquisition of these nonsegmental phonological skills (Mann, Cowin, & Schoenheimer, 1989). Memory experiments indicate that children with reading disorders are impaired in their short-term recall of linguistic stimuli but not of nonlinguistic stimuli, suggesting that they have difficulty in encoding verbal stimuli phonologically (Cohen, 1982; Torgesen, 1985).

Semantic representations also may be difficult for children with reading disabilities to generate. Along with other types of children with learning disabilities, poor readers exhibit word-finding deficits (Blachman, 1984). They also have trouble identifying sentences that are grammatically ill-formed, which suggests that syntactic cues to meaning are probably not well represented (Kamhi & Koenig, 1985). On the other hand, a comparison of good readers and poor readers in the fourth grade found that although the poor readers had lower scores on a test of syntactic comprehension, there was no significant correlation between syntactic comprehension and reading comprehension when vocabulary was controlled. This suggests that "the acquisition of vocabulary drives all other aspects of language development, including syntactic competence, auditory comprehension and reading comprehension" (Glass & Perna, 1986, p. 358). Thus, it is not clear whether breakdowns in forming semantic representations during reading should be attributed primarily to lexical or syntactic factors, or to other influences such as discourse referencing. A study of 10th- and 11th-grade students with and without learning disabilities showed that the impaired children had significantly more difficulty in comprehending the referent of anaphoric pronouns that appeared in reading passages (Fayne, 1981).

Oral reading can be impaired by breakdowns at any of the previous stages and can also be affected by subtle speech production problems that may appear infrequently in conversation. Adolescents with reading disorders have been found to make significantly more errors in naming and repeating multisyllabic words and repeating phonologically complex phrases. Their performance on these speech production tasks correlates significantly with their measured reading ability (Catts, 1986). Furthermore, when asked to speak as rapidly as possible, college students with dyslexia repeated complex phrases more slowly and had a higher rate of "slips of the tongue," that is, substitutions of sounds for phonetically similar segments that occur in similar syllable positions (e.g., "she shells" for "seashells") (Catts, 1989). This finding suggests that students with dyslexia are deficient in their ability to plan phonetic sequences and may explain many of the disruptions commonly seen in their oral reading.

What reason can be offered for the apparent speech impairments of children who are poor readers? In a study aimed at this question, Kamhi, Catts, and Mauer (1990) asked second- and third-grade children with reading disorders and their nondisabled peers to produce four multisyllabic nonsense words. The children with reading disorders needed significantly more trials to master the task. They were also significantly poorer in recognizing the correct response when they produced an error. This suggests that their problems are the result of phonological encoding deficits and not speech production difficulties.

Writing

Without adequate skills in spoken language and reading, a student is destined to struggle with writing as well. The foundation abilities in writing—knowledge of vocabulary, syntax, and discourse structure—are derived from these same abilities in speech. Hence, certain writing problems are predictable from and will be consistent with these same problems in spoken language production.

There is also a very close and important relationship between reading and writing. Perera (1984) notes three aspects to this relationship:

1. Reading teaches the characteristic structures of written language.
2. Children must be able to read their own writing in order to evaluate and edit it to suit its intended audience.
3. Children must be able to proofread their own writing to correct superficial errors of spelling, grammatical form, and others.

The problems students meet in learning to write are varied, as would be expected for a complex activity that depends on many subskills. Scott (1991) has reviewed studies of children and adults who are low-achieving students or who have been diagnosed with learning or reading disabilities. She summarizes the findings under six headings:

1. *Productivity.* In controlled writing tasks, such as creating a story to match a picture, poor writers produce fewer words and sentences.
2. *Text structure.* There is an overall lack of coher-

ence and text organization. Topics are not well introduced, and conclusions are not logical. Errors occur in the use of cohesion devices such as pronouns and temporal adverbs.

3. *Sentence structure.* Sentences are grammatically less complex and contain errors of omission, substitution, and form agreement. The connective "and" is overused, and subordinating conjunctions ("if," "because," "since") are often used incorrectly.

4. *Spelling.* Poor writers have a higher frequency of spelling errors and tend to produce more *nonphonetic* errors, that is, errors that are inconsistent with the pronunciation of the target word (e.g., "skool/school" is phonetic, "sookl/school" is nonphonetic).

5. *Lexicon.* The type:token ratio obtained from samples of poor writing is lower, indicating that words tend to be used repetitively.

6. *Handwriting.* Letters are poorly formed, unevenly spaced, and may contain a mix of lower- and uppercase, printing and cursive writing.

IMPLICATIONS FOR INTERVENTION

In recent years, there has been a shift in the practices of many professionals providing services to children with learning disabilities. The previously dominant model for delivering service to these children was to separate them from their normally achieving peers and conduct special teaching sessions away from the classroom. This model has now been replaced in some educational settings by one in which children with learning disabilities remain in their classrooms for most instruction and educators from different disciplines collaborate in a comprehensive program of intervention. Consequently, professionals today must be aware of the issues relevant to both traditional individual instruction and approaches that emphasize collaboration across disciplines.

The chief concern of all practitioners must be the efficacy of their intervention strategies. How effective are our methods for treating the problems of children with learning disabilities? The answer to this question depends, to some degree, on the way in which we measure success. As noted earlier in this chapter,

research indicates that learning disabilities persist throughout the school years. Most children with learning disabilities emerge from school with poorer preparation for work and, as a result, tend to have lower-paying jobs (Shapiro & Lentz, 1991). There is evidence to suggest, then, that these children are not able to compete with their normally achieving peers when their secondary education is complete.

Other research indicates that children with learning disabilities do improve, but perhaps not as much as other children with language impairments. Analyzed as a group, language intervention studies show that the amount of improvement is larger for children classified as language disordered or language-learning disabled (38 percentile gain) than for those classified as learning disabled (22 percentile gain) or reading disordered (13 percentile gain) (Nye, Foster, & Seaman, 1987). These differences probably reflect a common practice in diagnostic classification. That is, younger children with language impairments are usually described as language disordered, whereas language-impaired children of school age are labeled as learning disabled. The population of children labeled as learning disabled is, therefore, likely to be older and to receive language intervention in a school setting.

What does this indicate about the efficacy of language intervention for children with learning disabilities? At least three interpretations are possible:

1. Intervention is less effective with school-age children because of the increased complexity of the language system.
2. Intervention is less effective with older children because of neurological or social changes.
3. Intervention is less effective because our methods of treating this population are less effective.

At this point, we lack research information that favors one interpretation over another. For that matter, it may be that all the interpretations are correct to some extent. An additional factor may be the amount of language intervention children receive. Children with language impairments identified before school age may receive intervention prior to entering school, and intervention may continue during the school years. In contrast, children identified as learning disabled may not be identified until the school years, when intervention may first commence. We can do nothing to change the complexity of language and the fact that it increases with age. We can, however, begin to work as early as possible with language-impaired children and perhaps forestall or lessen certain types of learning disabilities. We can also improve our methods of intervention with school-age children by investigating instructional, motivational, professional, and other variables that affect the success of our efforts.

Issues in Regular Education

Professionals should be sensitive to the fact that learning disabilities interact with both developmental changes in children and shifts in the organization of the classroom. Language problems may be manifested at different grade levels as new competencies are required (Bashir, 1989). For example, word-finding difficulties may first be discovered as children attempt to join in class discussions or produce extended oral narratives. They may be treated for the problem and develop greater oral language competence. Later in school, however, they will be required to produce written texts that demand even greater precision of expression. Word-finding difficulties are then likely to reappear. As children move from grade to grade, the structure of their formal education changes: The amount of play time decreases, and the number of different subjects and teachers increases. Children with learning disabilities will require special attention as they make major grade transitions, such as between kindergarten and first grade, third and fourth grades, and elementary and junior high school (Bashir & Scavuzzo, 1992). These are times when professionals should be especially alert to referrals from classroom teachers, and they may want to assist in observing and identifying children who reveal new learning problems.

The move toward mainstreaming of students with handicaps was based on the perception that regular classrooms would provide better educational and social models. This change in practice, though generally well reviewed, has produced certain problems that must be addressed in the years ahead. The National Joint Committee on Learning Disabilities (1991b) has identified a number of problems related to the education of students with learning disabilities in regular education classrooms. These are listed in Table 7.4, along with the Committee's proposed recommendations for corrective actions.

Psychological Problems and Reactions

An important piece of the puzzle presented by children with learning disabilities may be their psychological state. One would expect most of these children to show some frustration as they work to overcome their handicaps. However, the manner in which this frustration is exhibited can be socially acceptable (stamping feet, crying, avoidance, periods of depression) or unacceptable (screaming, fighting). There is evidence that boys with learning disabilities react with more frustration and antisocial behavior than girls with similar impairments. One explanation offered for this finding is that girls with learning disabilities are more likely to seek social approval by being nice, whereas boys so impaired seek to be group leaders or to excel in athletics. The opportunity to be nice exists for all of the girls, but leadership roles or athletic prowess are possible for only a few of the boys. Therefore, girls with learning disabilities are better able to seek and receive social approval than their male counterparts (Caplan & Kinsbourne, 1974).

One of the touted benefits of mainstreaming is that it will improve the self-image of children with disabilities by not isolating them from their nondisabled peers. However, in a comparison of third-grade children with learning disabilities to their nondisabled peers in an integrated classroom, it was found that the children with learning disabilities scored lower on measures of scholastic competence, behavioral conduct, and global self-worth (Bear, Clever, & Proctor, 1991). On the other hand, the nondisabled boys in the integrated classroom scored consistently higher than the nondisabled boys in a nonintegrated classroom. Thus, it was the *nondisabled* children whose attitudes appeared to benefit from mainstreaming.

In one segment of the population with learning disabilities, psychological problems extend beyond frustration. One group of investigators performed psychiatric evaluations on children seen for treatment in

TABLE 7.4   Problems and Recommended Solutions for the Education of Students with
Learning Disabilities in Regular Education Classrooms

Problem	Recommended Solution
Teachers often are required to adhere rigidly to a prescribed curriculum and materials and, therefore, may not have the flexibility to address the unique needs of students with learning disabilities.	Establish instructional conditions and environments that allow teachers to capitalize on the strengths and remediate or compensate for the weaknesses of students with learning disabilities. These should include: ▷Appropriate materials and technology. ▷Flexibility in determining the array of skills necessary for attainment of overall curricular objectives.
Adequate support services, materials, and technology often are not available for either the teacher or the student with learning disabilities.	Ensure the availability of services needed to support the education of students with learning disabilities in the regular education classroom, including: ▷Appropriate related services for students. ▷Consultation services for teachers. ▷Direct services for students from teachers certified in the area of learning disabilities and other qualified professionals such as school psychologists, counselors, speech-language pathologists, reading teachers, audiologists, and social workers. ▷Teaching assistants or aides trained to work with students who have learning disabilities.
Time and support for the ongoing planning and assessment that are needed to make adjustments in students' programs and services often are inadequate.	Provide sufficient time for collaborative planning among and between professionals and parents.
Communication concerning students with learning disabilities among administrators, teachers, specialists, parents, and students is often insufficient for the development and implementation of effective programs.	

a communication disorders clinic (Baker & Cantwell, 1982). They found that of the children who presented with speech and language disorders (mean age, 4.9 years), 45% also exhibited psychiatric disorders. Of the children who presented with pure language disorders (mean age, 9.3 years), 95% exhibited psychiatric disorders ranging from hyperactivity to schizophrenia. Studies of juvenile delinquency point to a relationship among learning disability, negative self-image, and delinquency (Prizant et al., 1990). Many teachers and other professionals are not aware of these relationships and may need to be educated regarding the prevalence of communication problems in behavior-disordered or emotionally disturbed individuals.

The Collaborative Service Delivery Model

The traditional model for service delivery in the public schools was for professionals to pull individual children or small groups of children out of the classroom. Instruction was then provided in a setting remote from the classroom. Professionals were often unaware of children's school curriculum or of the academic problems they were having (Magnotta, 1991). This model began to change with implementation of

PL 94-142, which required the development of an Individualized Education Program (IEP) for each student and an interdisciplinary approach. Because an IEP has to be approved by all the educators working with a particular child, for example, the classroom teacher, school psychologist, speech-language pathologist, and reading specialist, educators began to work as part of an instructional team, reviewing and endorsing one another's efforts. In most cases, however, they also continued to work independently of the other team members. That is, they carried out their assessments and intervention without the direct assistance or consultation of the rest of the team.

The continuing problem of professional isolationism in service delivery has prompted at least one professional group to respond. Earlier in this chapter, we noted that the ASHA Committee on Language Learning Disorders (American Speech-Language-Hearing Association, 1991) has recommended that speech-language pathologists consider the merits of a *collaborative* service delivery model. There are several differences in practice under this model:

▷ Speech-language pathologists work as part of a transdisciplinary team consisting of educators, parents, and the student.
▷ All treatment goals, assessment methods, intervention procedures, and documentation systems are mutually planned by members of the team.
▷ Team members share responsibility for implementation of the educational plan.
▷ Special education as well as regular instruction take place in the classroom. An example of a typical classroom schedule is shown in Table 7.5.

A number of advantages accrue from the collaborative model:

▷ Treatment occurs within genuine communicative contexts.
▷ Intervention is not limited by a service schedule but can take place throughout the school day.
▷ Intervention can be provided by agents other than the speech-language pathologist.
▷ The setting is more appropriate for the use of procedures such as modeling, role playing, and group problem solving.

TABLE 7.5   Example of Primary Level Classroom Schedule for Transdisciplinary Teaching Program

Time	Activity
9:00–9:30	Journal writing and overview of day
9:30–10:30	Reading and learning centers
10:30–11:00	Recess and washroom
11:00–11:25	Storytelling
11:25–12:00	Mathematics
1:00–1:15	Free reading and writing centers
1:15–1:30	Weekly reader
1:30–1:45	Handwriting
1:45–2:15	Metalinguistic word search activity related to current unit
2:15–2:45	Think and draw activity related to current unit
2:45–3:05	Social studies, science, or health
3:05–3:20	Reward activity for behavior system
3:20	Ready for home

Source: Adapted from Hoffman (1990).

▷ There can be joint review and modification of texts and curriculum by all members of the educational team.
▷ Treatment time can be shared by team members.
▷ Self-esteem is promoted by allowing children to demonstrate to teachers their successes as well as their failures. In a traditional pull-out model, all time is spent focusing on a child's disabilities.
▷ Peer tutoring can take place, and the strengths of one student can be used to help the weaknesses of another.

The Traditional Service Delivery Model

Though support for the collaborative service delivery model is growing, there will continue to be settings and circumstances in which traditional pull-out service is provided and is appropriate. This does not mean, however, that specialists cannot or should not seek to improve lines of communication between themselves and other educators engaged in teaching children with learning disabilities. Specialists in communication should be active in suggesting ways to promote more effective language learning in the classroom. At a minimum, teachers should be advised to avoid lengthy or grammatically complex instructions that rely on prosodic cues for their proper interpretation (Mann, Cowin, & Schoenheimer, 1989). Following is a list of other general recommendations that could be made to a classroom teacher (Dudley-Marling & Searle, 1988):

1. Create a physical setting that promotes talk by providing work stations for collaborative learning and maintaining a set of regularly changing classroom displays that serve as the focus of conversation.

2. Promote verbal interaction in the process of learning by leading group discussions, asking children to verbalize as they problem-solve, and using cross-age and -ability groupings so that children explain concepts and processes to audiences other than their teachers.

3. Provide opportunities to use language for a variety of purposes other than the traditional ones of conveying information or checking on procedures. For example, children might be encouraged to persuade the teacher or their classmates to make a particular decision, to tell jokes, to discuss feelings, or to explain something they know to an unfamiliar listener. Guests invited to the classroom can serve an important role as confederates.

4. Encourage children to talk by avoiding evaluative responses ("Don't say bestest") or overly directive comments ("Now tell us how you felt when that happened") and by giving children ample time to respond to questions and prompts.

A common problem of the traditional service delivery model is that skills learned outside the classroom do not always generalize back to that setting. Hence, professionals must plan in advance to promote generalization of learning. Hughes (1989) suggests five strategies:

1. Select targets that meet specific classroom needs or that draw upon classroom information as material for teaching specific language behaviors. For example, select vocabulary that has already been presented as part of a child's science or history lessons, or work on inferential comprehension using materials from social studies. This strategy requires professionals to be familiar with the curricular content of their students.

2. Watch in the classroom for evidence of generalization. Observations can be done by assistants, but professionals retain responsibility to ensure that the observers are given clear "recognition rules" and a simple means for recording data (Dollaghan & Miller, 1986).

3. Reduce the differences between the therapeutic and classroom environments. For the most part, this means simulating the classroom situation. By role-playing the interactions and linguistic demands that occur in the classroom, children are better prepared to use their newly learned behaviors when they leave the therapy setting.

4. Program the classroom environment to provide children with challenges, prompts, and rewards that will facilitate generalization. Teachers, assistants, and peers can be recruited to assist in different ways.

5. Teach children to monitor their own language behavior in the classroom. Helpful techniques

Intervention Strategies

Regardless of the service model they use, professionals teaching children with learning disabilities must possess a repertoire of instructional methods. Students with learning disabilities are identified by their failure to achieve academically when provided with conventional instruction. Therefore, the focus of most work with these children is to find alternative ways for them to learn. Sometimes this means getting them to *do* something that normally achieving children do not need to do in order to learn. Sometimes it means getting them to *stop* doing something that is impeding them from learning.

Cognitive Training   Comparison of children with learning disabilities to normally achieving children shows that the former exhibit a less mature cognitive style. This has been described in several studies in which different kinds of learning tasks were presented:

▷ Children with learning disabilities responded with more **impulsivity** and used less mature strategies in problem-solving tasks (Copeland & Weissbrod, 1983).

▷ They tended to mislabel items during naming tasks. This is due to poor semantic organization but has also been interpreted as the result of *hyperexcitability,* an impairment in the ability to inhibit the selection of inappropriate or irrelevant labels from the memory store (Kail & Leonard, 1986; Lewis & Kass, 1982).

▷ Children 8 to 14 years of age with learning disabilities have been found to show less mature strategies for organizing and rehearsing words for recall. They showed no improvement with age unless the words were presented to them in a preorganized set. They also rehearsed single words, in contrast to their normal peers, who, as they grew older, began to rehearse several words at a time (Cermak, 1983).

▷ Seventh-grade children with learning disabilities did not detect logical inconsistencies in stories they read unless they were previously cued to look for them. However, once cuing was provided, their performance approached that of the nondisabled children (Bos & Filip, 1984).

These findings suggest that a simple approach to improving learning performance is to identify instances of impulsive responding. A child may then be prompted ("Take your time") and reinforced for acting reflectively. A more in-depth analysis is needed to uncover immature rehearsal or problem-solving strategies. Once a learning task has been identified that is difficult for a child, the cognitive and linguistic requirements of that task must be analyzed, usually through introspection. Professionals must ask themselves, How do I perform this task? What steps do I follow? Then the same information must be obtained from the child, either by observing while the task is performed or by asking direct questions. (Children may or may not be able to describe what they do.) If a child's strategies are different from those of the professional, then intervention may focus on introducing the new strategies through prompts and cues, which are then gradually removed to promote spontaneous use. If the child's strategies are the same as the clinician's, then alternative methods of rehearsal (e.g., visualization) or problem solving (e.g., verbalization of each step) must be explored.

When the language behaviors giving trouble are more complex, they require more intricate methods of instruction. Pehrsson and Denner (1988) describe an approach to reading and writing instruction that makes use of *semantic organizers.* As shown in Figure 7.1, students are taught to identify and use either cluster patterns, which show superordinate-subordinate relationships, or episodic patterns, which show a change or sequence of events. The clusters are drawn with circles and connecting lines either while reading or as a preliminary organization before writing. The professional models both the thought process and the mechanical process of constructing the clusters, and then gradually turns over the responsibility for doing them to the student.

Lexical Semantics   Not surprisingly, recommendations for the treatment of word retrieval difficulties vary according to the manner in which the problem is analyzed. Based on their finding that word-retrieval problems are the result of less elaborated lexical storage, Kail and Leonard (1986) recommend the following activities to strengthen a word's paradigmatic and syntagmatic associations:

Paradigmatic

1. Teach diverse functions of a word's referent, for example, "ball" (object in a game, shape formed with modeling clay).
2. Illustrate the referent of a word with nonidentical exemplars, for example, "capsule" (a form of medicine, a conveyance for space travel, an infant car seat).
3. Compare and contrast referents from similar categories, for example, clothing (shirt, blouse, blazer, jacket).
4. Teach superordinate categories (reptiles, senses, forms of government).

FIGURE 7.1 Examples of Semantic Organizers. (After Pehrsson & Denner, 1988.)

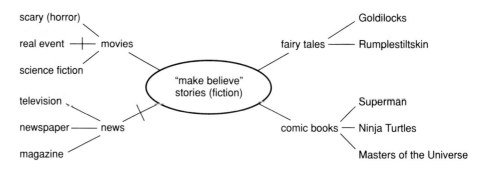

Cluster organizer for writing about "make believe" stories

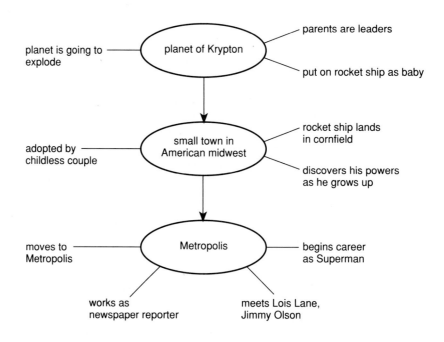

Episodic organizer for retelling the story of Superman

Syntagmatic

1. Illustrate attribute, agent, and locative terms commonly used with the word, for example, "handcuffs" (pair of, police, wrist).

2. Illustrate the word's syntactic privileges of occurrence; for example, "desperate" precedes a noun or follows a copular verb.

3. Explain the phonetic and morphological characteristics of the word; for example, "prejudice" has three syllables, begins with a consonant cluster, and contains a prefix.

In contrast, German (1982) recommends that treatment procedures be based on an analysis of substitution types. Children who produce visually similar substitutions might be asked to concentrate on visualizing the target word. Conversely, they might be given a cue that complements the visual information that seemingly is already available to them, for example, an auditory cue such as the initial sound of the word.

Fawcett and Nicolson (1991) reported on the results of a vocabulary training program administered by parents to teenage children with dyslexia. They found that both traditional and enriched methods of instruction produced short-term improvements in both word knowledge and lexical access speed. Traditional methods consisted of worksheets, crosswords, word bingo, and missing letter exercises, all of which aimed to help students link words with their definitions. The enriched training, shown in Table 7.6, led to slightly better long-term effects. The authors recommend that for children with age-appropriate receptive vocabulary, either training approach could be used to improve lexical access speed. For children with poor receptive vocabulary, enriched training should be used with target words matched to the child's current vocabulary level.

A specific approach to word retrieval improvement that has been comparatively well studied is the *keyword mnemonic strategy*. Target words are recoded as other *keywords* that are familiar and picturable. The target and keyword are then related by means of a visual image. For example, to learn the word "celibate," it might be related to the word "cell." The visual image could then be a priest (who is celibate) sitting in a small room with bars on the windows (cell). Keyword instruction has been found to be substantially more effective than direct instruction in teaching new word definitions to junior high school students with learning disabilities (Mastropieri, Scruggs, Levin, Gaffney, & McLoone, 1985). The effectiveness of the technique was maintained when students were required to form their own mnemonic images. In a study of comparative effectiveness, the keyword and other techniques were applied in a classroom with 12-year-old students who were poor readers. The keyword technique proved to be the most effective and to produce the highest levels of retention in a 10-week follow-up test (Condus, Marshall, & Miller, 1986).

The techniques reviewed previously are mostly suited for the teaching of literal word meanings. In order to understand metaphors, children must possess a set of skills:

▷ They must be able to remember the stimulus; for example, upon hearing of a legal verdict, a speaker might say, "That's a hard pill to swallow."

▷ They must have knowledge of the features being compared; that is, they must understand how legal decisions are rendered and enforced, and they must understand that pills come in varying shapes and sizes.

▷ They must be able to pick out the shared features of the elements being compared; that is, both the legal decision and the pill must be somehow taken in and accepted.

▷ They must consider the topic of conversation and the **extralinguistic** context; that is, the conversation up to this point has *not* been concerned with drugs or vitamins, and there is no literal interpretation of the speaker's utterance that is relevant to the topic of jurisprudence.

Therefore, a teaching program for metaphors must evaluate and be able to remediate deficits in any or all of these areas (Nippold & Fey, 1983).

Narratives   Several suggestions can be made to students to improve their narrative skills. Because of the finding that more communication breakdowns occur as utterance length increases, children with language-learning disabilities should be encouraged to produce narratives with linguistically simple structures (MacLachlan & Chapman, 1988). As they listen to or produce narratives, they should be asked to pay particular attention to the goals, motives, thoughts, and feelings of the characters (Montague, Maddux, & Dereshiwsky, 1990). These children should be engaged frequently in reading or listening to and discussing stories. They can be supported in their narratives by helping them to identify explicitly the topic of their story, as well as the specific structural components. Following are

TABLE 7.6 Examples of Worksheets for Enriched Vocabulary Training

Day 5 Answer these questions

(Please read the question and three possible answers aloud and ring the answers your child chooses)

Words: rogue   hermit   sleuth   urge   berate   baffle.

What would a rogue do? Why?
(1) Steal apples from a tree   (2) Help an old lady across the road   (3) Climb a mountain

What would a hermit do? Why?
(1) Live alone in a cave   (2) Live in a high rise flat   (3) Live in a commune

What would a sleuth do? Why?
(1) Visit a prisoner   (2) Solve a murder   (3) Makes cakes for tea

Think of one more thing for each word

Day 8 Finish the sentences

(Please read the sentences aloud and write in the words for your child—encourage him if he has difficulty)

Words: urge   berate   baffle   rogue   hermit   accomplice

Things people can do to others

Urge
(1) The children were urged to try harder to . . .   (2) At the winning line the boy was urged to . . .

Berate
(1) Katy is often berated for . . .   (2) The duchess berated Alice, shouting . . .

Baffle
(1) The police were baffled by . . .   (2) The magician baffled . . .

Day 10 Feelings and word overlap

How do you feel about a rogue? If you saw one at a pantomine would you cheer or boo?

What about a hermit? Are they goodies or baddies?

What about an accomplice? Are they honest or dishonest?

How would you feel if someone urged you, berated you, baffled you? Why?

Could a rogue be an accomplice? Why? Could a hermit be a rogue? Why?

Could an accomplice be a hermit? Why? Could a hermit berate you? Why?

Could an accomplice baffle you? Why? Could a rogue urge you? Why?

Source: From "Vocabulary Training for Children with Dyslexia," by A. J. Fawcett and R. I. Nicolson, 1991, *Journal of Learning Disabilities,* 24, p. 381. Copyright 1991 by PRO-ED, Inc. Reprinted by permission.

some questions that can be asked in preparation for producing a narrative (Garnett, 1986):

Setting:	Who? Where? When?
Event:	What happened to the main characters?
Goal:	What are the main characters trying to do?
Attempts:	What happens when they try to do it?
Reactions:	What are the feelings? What are the plans?
End:	How does it turn out?

Intuitively, one might think that visual aids would assist children in maintaining the sequence and organization of a narrative. It has been found, however, that using line drawings to assist narrative production by children with learning disabilities actually caused them to provide less information (Ripich & Griffith, 1988). It appears that having shared visual information with the listener reduces the demand on the children to supply that information orally. Thus, if the goal of treatment is to enhance the production of oral narratives, clinicians should not use visual aids to facilitate the child's recall. Auditory cues should be supplied instead.

Reading and Writing Historically, the treatment of reading disabilities in children has been the responsibility of learning disabilities specialists. The approach favored by most of these specialists has been one of teaching component reading skills: word attack, word recognition, oral reading, sentence comprehension, and others (Cirrin, 1991). This contrasts with the developmental language perspective that has been taken by many speech-language pathologists who work with reading-impaired children (Kamhi & Catts, 1991). Therefore, the expertise of the two professionals may be complementary, and either or both may be asked to provide intervention to a particular child.

Earlier in this text and in this chapter, it was noted that spoken language, reading, and writing exist in a relationship that is both sequential and reciprocal. Basic language skills are learned in spoken form and must be present in order for reading skills to take root. Reading skills, in turn, are crucial for the development of writing. As children grow older, the mutual influence of all three skills becomes greater and greater.

Professionals must ensure that children with learning disabilities possess adequate basic language skills to support their first efforts at learning to read. Most important, children must have attained adequate levels of phonological awareness to enable them to decode letter–sound relationships (Catts, 1991). Children who have not developed such awareness can be helped through activities that emphasize word rhyming, phoneme segmentation (such as sound blending), and sound–letter relationships (such as categorizing words by letter and then noting common sounds) (Blachman, 1991).

Reading skills must be supported by a variety of linguistic and metalinguistic abilities. Awareness and recognition of grammatical function words may be a critical element of some children's reading failure (Blank, 1990). In that case, metalinguistic instruction about the purpose of function words and drill to promote visual recognition of them may facilitate the child's reading efforts. Semantic skills, both literal and nonliteral, can also be key to children's ability to predict and decipher words and phrases they encounter on the page (Roth & Spekman, 1991). Finally, children's familiarity with common schemas, as well as their understanding of narrative structure, can help them to unravel more complex texts (Westby, 1991). *Self-summarization* training (students asking themselves "Who or what is the paragraph about?" and "What is happening to them?") has been shown to lead to significant improvement in reading comprehension by students with learning disabilities in Grades 6 to 8 (Malone & Mastropieri, 1992). The addition of self-monitoring—using a card to prompt the self-summarization strategy—resulted in better transfer of improvement.

Intervention for writing problems should be contingent on students having attained sufficient spoken language and reading skills to support their efforts at writing. Once that is assured, a hierarchy of instruction, such as that proposed by Dagenais and Beadle (1984) might be used:

1. Improve students' motivation and attitudes toward writing.
2. Improve content skills.
3. Improve linguistic craftsmanship, including spelling.

Curricula developed for normally achieving students can be used in modified form with children who are learning disabled. Extra time must be provided and directions must be translated to each student's level of comprehension. Verbal discussion before and during writing exercises is helpful in organizing the task and encouraging self-monitoring. Dictation of text can be used to develop content skills while reducing the demands for linguistic craftsmanship. Correction should focus only on the target behavior and should ignore all other errors.

SUMMARY

In this chapter we have seen that:

▶ Learning disabilities emerged as a diagnostic category in the 1960s, and the term has since been redefined several times. Definitions written by USOE and the NJCLD are currently the most influential.

▶ Children with learning disabilities have been divided into subtypes by researchers, but there is no agreed-upon scheme for diagnostic classification.

▶ The category learning disabilities includes and overlaps with several other diagnostic categories: dyslexia, underachievement, attention deficit-hyperactivity disorder (ADHD), specific language impairment (SLI), phonological processing disorder, developmental apraxia of speech, central auditory processing disorder (CAPD), and minimal brain dysfunction (MBD). Professionals should be aware of the relationships among these terms.

▶ Diagnostic criteria for learning disabilities are set by every state. In some instances, these criteria depart from the USOE and NJCLD definitions. A common criterion is that a child must exhibit a discrepancy between intelligence and achievement scores.

▶ About 2 million American children are diagnosed with learning disabilities. More boys than girls are identified. There is evidence to suggest an hereditary factor.

▶ Language disorders and learning disabilities may be different manifestations of a single impairment. The problems tend to persist throughout the school years and beyond.

▶ Many learning disabilities can be understood as resulting from the demands of formal education. Children must become more sophisticated in their metalinguistic knowledge. They must learn a new set of rules and requirements for written language, which differ in many ways from those for spoken language. They must understand the scripts for language use at school.

▶ Lexical difficulties are common in children with learning disabilities. These children appear to be generally deficient in their lexical knowledge and organization, which leads to problems in word retrieval and word usage. Nonliteral meanings, expressed in metaphors and other figurative language, are especially problematic.

▶ Most children with learning disabilities exhibit problems with at least some aspects of grammar, though there appears to be a subgroup that shows no such impairment.

▶ Both comprehension and production of narratives may be impaired.

▶ Pragmatically, children with learning disabilities tend to be unassertive, and they have limited ability to modify their language to suit different situations or to repair conversational breakdowns.

▶ Reading and writing are complex behaviors requiring a number of subskills. Consequently, difficulties occur at many different levels of processing, and children with learning disabilities present a variety of impairment profiles.

▶ The model for the treatment of learning disabilities is slowly changing from the traditional practice of working individually with students away from the classroom. Educational planning by a professional team is mandated in most schools, and there is a trend toward collaborative intervention and teaching.

▶ Cognitive training, by focusing on general deficiencies such as impulsiveness and poor task analysis, offers an approach to the treatment of many different learning problems. More specific intervention strategies have been applied successfully to improve lexical organization and retrieval, narrative production, and reading and writing skills.

Theories of learning disabilities are still being formed and undergo frequent revision. In this situation, professionals are likely to find varying explanations of learning problems and disparate recommendations for intervention. This makes it especially important that we critically evaluate new information and, in working with individual children, remain willing to try innovative approaches when regular methods do not succeed.

REFERENCES

American Psychiatric Association. (1987). *Diagnostic and statistical manual of mental disorders* (third edition, revised). Washington, DC: American Psychiatric Association.

American Speech-Language-Hearing Association. (1991). A model for collaborative service delivery for students with language-learning disorders in the public schools. *Asha, 33* (Suppl. 5), 44–50.

Andolina, C. (1980). Syntactic maturity and vocabulary richness of learning disabled children at four age levels. *Journal of Learning Disabilities, 13,* 27–32.

Baker, L., & Cantwell, D. P. (1982). Psychiatric disorder in children with different types of communication disorders. *Journal of Communication Disorders, 15,* 113–126.

Bashir, A. S. (1989). Language intervention and the curriculum. *Seminars in Speech and Language, 10,* 181–191.

Bashir, A. S., & Scavuzzo, A. (1992). Children with language disorders: Natural history and academic success. *Journal of Learning Disabilities, 25,* 53–65.

Bear, G. C., Clever, A., & Proctor, W. A. (1991). Self-perceptions of nonhandicapped children and children with learning disabilities in integrated classes. *The Journal of Special Education, 24,* 409–426.

Beitchman, J. H., Nair, R., Clegg, M., & Patel, P. G. (1986). Prevalence of speech and language disorders in 5-year-old kindergarten children in the Ottawa-Carlton Region. *Journal of Speech and Hearing Disorders, 51,* 98–110.

Bennett, F. S., Ruuska, S. H., & Sherman, R. (1980). Middle ear effusion in learning disabled children. *Pediatrics, 66,* 254–260.

Blachman, B. (1984). Relationship of rapid naming ability and language analysis skills in kindergarten and first-grade reading achievement. *Journal of Educational Psychology, 76,* 610–622.

Blachman, B. (1991). Phonological awareness and word recognition: Assessment and intervention. In A. G. Kamhi & H. W. Catts (Eds.), *Reading disabilities: A developmental language perspective* (pp. 133–158). Boston: Allyn and Bacon.

Blakeslee, S. (1991, September 15). Study ties dyslexia to brain flaw affecting vision and other senses. *New York Times,* pp. A1, A30.

Blalock, J. (1982). Persistent auditory language deficits in adults with learning disabilities. *Journal of Learning Disabilities, 15,* 604–609.

Blank, M. (1990). *Sentence master* (computer program). Winooski, VT: Laureate Learning.

Bos, C. S., & Filip, D. (1984). Comprehension monitoring in learning disabled and average students. *Journal of Learning Disabilities, 17,* 229–233.

Bryan, T., Donahue, M., & Pearl, R. (1981). Learning disabled children's peer interactions during a small-group problem-solving task. *Learning Disability Quarterly, 4,* 13–22.

Bryan, T., Donahue, M., Pearl, R., & Sturm, C. (1981). Learning disabled children's conversational skills: The "TV Talk-Show." *Learning Disability Quarterly, 4,* 250–259.

Bryan, T., & Pflaum, S. (1978). Linguistic, cognitive and social analysis of learning disabled children's social interactions. *Learning Disability Quarterly, 1,* 70–79.

Bryant, P., & Bradley, L. (1981). Visual memory and phonological skills in reading and spelling backwardness. *Psychological Research, 43,* 193–199.

Bunch, G. W., & Melnyk, T. (1989). A review of the evidence for a learning-disabled, hearing-impaired sub-group. *American Annals of the Deaf, 134,* 297–300.

Caplan, P. J., & Kinsbourne, M. (1974). Sex differences in response to school failure. *Journal of Learning Disabilities, 7,* 232–235.

Catts, H. W. (1986). Speech production/phonological deficits in reading-disordered children. *Journal of Learning Disabilities, 19,* 504–508.

Catts, H. W. (1989). Speech production deficits in developmental dyslexia. *Journal of Speech and Hearing Disorders, 54,* 422–428.

Catts, H. W. (1991). Phonological processing deficits and reading disabilities. In A. G. Kamhi & H. W. Catts (Eds.), *Reading disabilities: A developmental language perspective.* Boston: Allyn and Bacon.

Cermak, L. S. (1983). Information processing deficits in children with learning disabilities. *Journal of Learning Disabilities, 16,* 599–605.

Cirrin, F. M. (1991). Issues in determining eligibility for service: Who does what to whom? In A. G. Kamhi & H. W. Catts (Eds.), *Reading disabilities: A developmental language perspective* (pp. 345–368). Boston: Allyn and Bacon.

Clements, S. D. (1966). *Minimal brain dysfunction in children. Terminology and identification* (NINDS Monograph No. 3, U.S. Public Health Service Publication No. 1415). Washington, DC: U.S. Department of Health, Education, and Welfare.

Cohen, R. (1982). Individual differences in short-term memory. *International Review of Research in Mental Retardation, 11,* 43–77.

Condus, M. M., Marshall, K. J., & Miller, S. R. (1986). Effects of the keyword mnemonic strategy on vocabulary acquisition and maintenance by learning disabled children. *Journal of Learning Disabilities, 19,* 609–613.

Copeland, A. P., & Weissbrod, C. S. (1983). Cognitive strategies used by learning disabled children: Does hyperactivity always make things worse? *Journal of Learning Disabilities, 16,* 473–477.

Crais, E., & Chapman, R. (1987). Story recall and inferencing skills in language/learning-disabled children. *Journal of Speech and Hearing Disorders, 52,* 50–55.

Crary, M. (1984). Phonological characteristics of developmental verbal dyspraxia. *Seminars in Speech and Language, 5,* 71–83.

Creaghead, N. A. (1990). Mutual empowerment through collaboration: A new script for an old problem. *Best Practices in School Speech-Language Pathology, 1,* 109–116.

Crystal, D. (1984). *Linguistic encounters with language handicap.* New York: Basil Blackwell.

Dagenais, D. J., & Beadle, K. R. (1984). Written language: When and where to begin. *Topics in Language Disorders, 4,* 59–85.

Decker, S., & DeFries, J. (1980). Cognitive abilities in families with reading disabled children. *Journal of Learning Disabilities, 13,* 53–58.

Denckla, M., & Rudel, R. (1976a). Naming of object-drawings by dyslexical and other learning disabled children. *Brain and Language, 3,* 1–15.

Denckla, M., & Rudel, R. (1976b). Rapid "automatized" naming (R.A.N.): Dyslexia differentiated from other learning disabilities. *Neuropsychologia, 14,* 471–479.

Dollaghan, C., & Miller, J. (1986). Observational methods in the study of communicative competence. In R. Schiefelbusch (Ed.), *Language competence: Assessment and intervention.* San Diego: College-Hill Press.

Donahue, M. (1986). Linguistic and communicative development in learning-disabled children. In C. Ceci (Ed.), *Handbook of cognitive, social, and neuropsychological aspects of learning disabilities* (Vol. 1). New York: Erlbaum.

Donahue, M., Pearl, R., & Bryan, T. (1980). Learning disabled children's conversational competence: Responses to inadequate messages. *Applied Psycholinguistics, 1,* 387–404.

Donahue, M., Pearl, R., & Bryan, T. (1982). Learning disabled children's syntactic proficiency on a communicative task. *Journal of Speech and Hearing Disorders, 47,* 397–403.

Dudley-Marling, C. (1985). The pragmatic skills of learning disabled children: A review. *Journal of Learning Disabilities, 18,* 193–199.

Dudley-Marling, C., & Searle, D. (1988). Enriching language learning environments for students with learning disabilities. *Journal of Learning Disabilities, 21,* 140–143.

Esterly, D. L., & Griffin, H. C. (1987). Preschool programs for children with learning disabilities. *Journal of Learning Disabilities, 20,* 571–573.

Fawcett, A. J., & Nicolson, R. I. (1991). Vocabulary training for children with dyslexia. *Journal of Learning Disabilities, 24,* 379–383.

Fayne, H. (1981). A comparison of learning disabled adolescents with normal learners on an anaphoric pronominal reference task. *Journal of Learning Disabilities, 14,* 597–599.

Finucci, J. M., & Childs, B. (1981). Are there really more dyslexic girls than boys? In A. Ansara, N. Geschwind, A. Galaburda, M. Albert, & N. Gartrell (Eds.), *Sex differences in dyslexia* (pp. 1–10). Baltimore: Orton Dyslexia Society.

Frankenberger, W., & Fronzaglio, K. (1991). A review of states' criteria and procedures for identifying children with learning disabilities. *Journal of Learning Disabilities, 24,* 495–500.

Freeman, B., & Parkins, C. (1979). The prevalence of middle ear disease among learning impaired children. *Clinical Pediatrics, 18,* 205–212.

Garnett, K. (1986). Telling tales: Narratives and learning-disabled children. *Topics in Language Disorders, 6,* 44–56.

German, D. (1979). Word-finding skills in children with learning disabilities. *Journal of Learning Disabilities, 12,* 176–181.

German, D. (1982). Word-finding substitutions in children with learning disabilities. *Language, Speech, and Hearing Services in Schools, 13,* 223–230.

Gersten, J., & Gersten, R. (1978). Proportion of boys and girls in a program for children with learning disabilities. *Archives of Physical and Medical Rehabilitation, 59,* 72–75.

Gibbs, D. P., & Cooper, E. B. (1989). Prevalence of communication disorders in students with learning disabilities. *Journal of Learning Disabilities, 22,* 60–63.

Glass, A. L., & Perna, J. (1986). The role of syntax in reading disability. *Journal of Learning Disabilities, 19,* 354–359.

Guyette, T. W., & Diedrich, W. M. (1981). A critical review of developmental apraxia of speech. In N. J. Lass (Ed.), *Speech and language advances in basic research and practice* (Vol. 5). New York: Academic Press.

Hammill, D. D. (1990). On defining learning disabilities: An emerging consensus. *Journal of Learning Disabilities, 23,* 74–84.

Hoffman, L. T. (1990). The development of literacy in a school-based program. *Topics in Language Disorders, 10,* 81–92.

Hopke, W. E. (Ed.) (1990). *The encyclopedia of careers and vocational guidance* (8th ed.). Chicago: J. G. Ferguson.

Hughes, D. L. (1989). Generalization from language therapy to classroom academics. *Seminars in Speech and Language, 10,* 218–229.

Kail, R., & Leonard, L. (1986). Word-finding abilities in language-impaired children. *ASHA Monographs* (No. 25). Rockville, MD: American Speech-Language-Hearing Association.

Kamhi, A. G., & Catts, H. (1986). Toward an understanding of developmental language and reading disorders. *Journal of Speech and Hearing Disorders, 51,* 337–347.

Kamhi, A. G., & Catts, H. W. (1991). *Reading disabilities: A developmental language perspective.* Boston: Allyn and Bacon.

Kamhi, A. G., Catts, H. W., & Mauer, D. (1990). Explaining speech production deficits in poor readers. *Journal of Learning Disabilities, 23,* 632–636.

Kamhi, A. G., & Koenig, L. (1985). Metalinguistic awareness in normal and language-disordered children. *Language, Speech, and Hearing Services in Schools, 16,* 199–210.

Kamphaus, R. W., Frick, P. J., & Lahey, B. B. (1991). Methodological issues and learning disabilities diagnosis in clinical populations. *Journal of Learning Disabilities, 24,* 613–618.

Kavale, K. (1982). A comparison of learning disabled and normal children on the Boehm Test of Basic Concepts. *Journal of Learning Disabilities, 15,* 160–161.

Kavale, K. A., & Forness, S. (1985). *The science of learning disabilities.* Boston: College-Hill Press.

Keith, R. W. (1984). Central auditory dysfunction: A language disorder? *Topics in Language Disorders, 4,* 48–56.

Knight-Arest, I. (1984). Communicative effectiveness of learning disabled and normally achieving 10- to 13-year-old boys. *Learning Disability Quarterly, 7,* 237–245.

Lahey, M. (1990). Who shall be called language disordered? Some reflections and one perspective. *Journal of Speech and Hearing Disorders, 55,* 612–620.

Lapadat, J. C. (1991). Pragmatic language skills of students with language and/or learning disabilities: A quantitative synthesis. *Journal of Learning Disabilities, 24,* 147–158.

Lee, R. F., & Kamhi, A. G. (1990). Metaphoric competence in children with learning disabilities. *Journal of Learning Disabilities, 23,* 476–482.

Lewis, R. B., & Kass, C. E. (1982). Labelling and recall in learning disabled students. *Journal of Learning Disabilities, 15,* 238–241.

Liberman, I., Shankweiler, D., Fischer, F., & Carter, B. (1974).

Reading and the awareness of linguistic segments. *Journal of Experimental Child Psychology, 18,* 201–212.

Livingstone, M. S., Rosen, G. D., Drislane, F. W., & Galaburda, A. M. (1991). Physiological and anatomical evidence for a magnocellular defect in developmental dyslexia. *Proceedings of the National Academy of Sciences, 88,* 7943–7947.

Lyon, G. R. (1985). Neuropsychology and learning disabilities. *Neurology and Neurosurgery, 5,* 1–8.

Lyon, G. R., & Risucci, D. (1988). Classification of learning disabilities. In K. A. Kavale (Ed.), *Learning disabilities: State of the art and practice* (pp. 44–70). Boston: College-Hill Press.

MacLachlan, B. G., & Chapman, R. S. (1988). Communication breakdowns in normal and language learning-disabled children's conversation and narration. *Journal of Speech and Hearing Disorders, 53,* 2–7.

Magnotta, O. H. (1991). Looking beyond tradition. *Language, Speech, and Hearing Services in Schools, 22,* 150–151.

Malone, L. D., & Mastropieri, M. A. (1992). Reading comprehension instruction: Summarization and self-monitoring training for students with learning disabilities. *Exceptional Children, 58,* 270–279.

Mann, V. A., Cowin, E., & Schoenheimer, J. (1989). Phonological processing, language comprehension, and reading ability. *Journal of Learning Disabilities, 22,* 76–89.

Masters, L., & March, G. (1978). Middle ear pathology as a factor in learning disabilities. *Journal of Learning Disabilities, 11,* 103–106.

Masterson, J. J., & Kamhi, A. G. (1991). The effects of sampling conditions on sentence production in normal, reading-disabled, and language-learning-disabled children. *Journal of Speech and Hearing Research, 34,* 549–558.

Mastropieri, M. A., Scruggs, T. E., Levin, J. R., Gaffney, J., & McLoone, B. (1985). Mnemonic vocabulary instruction for learning disabled students. *Learning Disabilities Quarterly, 8,* 57–65.

Mathinos, D. A. (1991). Conversational engagement of children with learning disabilities. *Journal of Learning Disabilities, 24,* 439–446.

Mattis, S., French, J., & Rapin, I. (1975). Dyslexia in children and young adults: Three independent neuropsychological syndromes. *Developmental Medicine and Child Neurology, 17,* 150–163.

Meline, T. J. (1986). Referential communication skills of learning disabled/language impaired children. *Applied Psycholinguistics, 7,* 129–140.

Mercer, C. D., Hughes, C., & Mercer, A. R. (1985). Learning

disabilities definitions used by state education departments. *Learning Disability Quarterly, 8,* 45–55.

Merrell, K. W. (1990). Differentiating low achieving students and students with learning disabilities: An examination of performance on the Woodcock-Johnson Psycho-Educational Battery. *The Journal of Special Education, 24,* 296–305.

Montague, M., Maddux, C. D., & Dereshiwsky, M. I. (1990). Story grammar and comprehension and production of narrative prose by students with learning disabilities. *Journal of Learning Disabilities, 23,* 190–197.

Moran, M., & Byrne, M. (1977). Mastery of verb tense markers by normal and learning-disabled children. *Journal of Speech and Hearing Research, 20,* 529–542.

Murphy, V., & Hicks-Stewart, K. (1991). Learning disabilities and attention deficit-hyperactivity disorder: An interactional perspective. *Journal of Learning Disabilities, 24,* 386–388.

National Joint Committee on Learning Disabilities. (1985). Learning disabilities: Issues in the preparation of professional personnel. *Asha, 27,* 49–51.

National Joint Committee on Learning Disabilities. (1989). Issues in learning disabilities: Assessment and diagnosis. *Asha, 31,* 111–112.

National Joint Committee on Learning Disabilities. (1991a). Learning disabilities: Issues on definition. *Asha, 33* (Suppl. 5), 18–20.

National Joint Committee on Learning Disabilities. (1991b). Providing appropriate education for students with learning disabilities in regular education classrooms. *Asha, 33* (Suppl. 5), 15–17.

New York State Education Department. (1990). *A parent's guide to special education.* Albany, NY: The State Education Department.

Nippold, M., & Fey, S. H. (1983). Metaphoric understanding in preadolescents having a history of language acquisition difficulties. *Language, Speech, and Hearing Services in Schools, 14,* 171–180.

Noel, M. (1980). Referential communication abilities of learning disabled children. *Learning Disability Quarterly, 3,* 70–75.

Nye, C., Foster, S. H., & Seaman, D. (1987). Effectiveness of language intervention with the language/learning disabled. *Journal of Speech and Hearing Disorders, 52,* 348–357.

Pehrsson, R. S., & Denner, P. R. (1988). Semantic organizers: Implications for reading and writing. *Topics in Language Disorders, 8,* 24–37.

Perera, K. (1984). *Children's writing and reading: Analysing classroom language.* London: Basil Blackwell.

Prizant, B. M., Audet, L. R., Burke, G. M., Hummel, L. J., Maher, S. R., & Theadore, G. (1990). Communication disorders and emotional/behavioral disorders in children and adolescents. *Journal of Speech and Hearing Disorders, 55,* 179–192.

Reichman, J., & Healey, W. (1983). Learning disabilities and conductive hearing loss involving otitis media. *Journal of Learning Disabilities, 16,* 272–278.

Reynolds, C. R., & Fletcher-Janzen, E. (Eds.). (1990). *Concise encyclopedia of special education.* New York: Wiley.

Riedlinger-Ryan, K., & Shewan, C. (1984). Comparison of auditory language comprehension skills in learning-disabled and academically achieving adolescents. *Language, Speech, and Hearing Services in Schools, 15,* 127–136.

Ripich, D. N., & Griffith, P. L. (1988). Narrative abilities of children with learning disabilities and nondisabled children: Story structure, cohesion, and propositions. *Journal of Learning Disabilities, 21,* 165–173.

Roth, F. P., & Spekman, N. J. (1986). Narrative discourse: Spontaneously generated stories of learning-disabled and normally achieving students. *Journal of Speech and Hearing Disorders, 51,* 8–23.

Roth, F. P., & Spekman, N. J. (1989). The oral syntactic proficiency of learning disabled students: A spontaneous story sampling analysis. *Journal of Speech and Hearing Research, 32,* 67–77.

Roth, F. P., & Spekman, N. J. (1991). Higher-order language processes and reading disabilities. In A. G. Kamhi & H. W. Catts (Eds.), *Reading disabilities: A developmental language perspective* (pp. 159–198). Boston: Allyn and Bacon.

Rudel, R., Denckla, M., & Broman, M. (1981). The effect of varying stimulus context on word-finding ability: Dyslexia further differentiated from other learning disabilities. *Brain and Language, 13,* 130–144.

Satz, P., & Morris, R. (1981). Learning disability subtypes: A review. In F. J. Priozzolo & M. C. Wittrock (Eds.), *Neuropsychological and cognitive processes in reading* (pp. 104–141). New York: Academic Press.

Scarborough, H. S., & Dobrich, W. (1990). Development of children with early language delay. *Journal of Speech and Hearing Research, 33,* 70–83.

Scott, C. M. (1991). Problem writers: Nature, assessment, and intervention. In A. G. Kamhi & H. W. Catts (Eds.), *Reading disabilities: A developmental language perspective* (pp. 303–344). Boston: Allyn and Bacon.

Seidenberg, P. L., & Bernstein, D. K. (1986). The comprehension of similes and metaphors by learning-disabled and nonlearning-disabled children. *Language, Speech, and Hearing Services in Schools, 17,* 219–229.

Shapiro, E. S., & Lentz, F. E., Jr. (1991). Vocational-technical programs: Follow-up of students with learning disabilities. *Exceptional Children, 58,* 47–59.

Shaywitz, S. E., Escobar, M. D., Shaywitz, B. A., Fletcher, J. M., & Makuch, R. (1992). Evidence that dyslexia may represent the lower tail of a normal distribution of reading ability. *New England Journal of Medicine, 326,* 145–150.

Shaywitz, S. E., & Shaywitz, B. A. (1988). Attention deficit disorder: Current perspectives. In J. F. Kavanagh & T. J. Truss, Jr. (Eds.), *Learning disabilities: Proceedings of the national conference* (pp. 369–567). Parkton, MD: York Press.

Shaywitz, S. E., & Shaywitz, B. A. (1991). Introduction to the special series on attention deficit disorder. *Journal of Learning Disabilities, 24,* 68–71.

Siegel, L. S. (1989). IQ is irrelevant to the definition of learning disabilities. *Journal of Learning Disabilities, 22,* 469–478.

Smoski, W. J., Brunt, M. A., & Tannahill, J. C. (1992). Listening characteristics of children with central auditory processing disorders. *Language, Speech, and Hearing Services in Schools, 23,* 145–152.

Soenksen, P. A., Flagg, C. L., & Schmits, D. W. (1981). Social communication in learning disabled students: A pragmatic analysis. *Journal of Learning Disabilities, 14,* 283–286.

Spekman, N. (1981). A study of the dyadic verbal communication abilities of learning disabled and normally achieving 4th and 5th grade boys. *Learning Disability Quarterly, 4,* 139–151.

Strauss, A. A., & Kephart, N. C. (1955). *Psychopathology and education of the brain-injured child; Vol. II. Progress in theory and clinic.* New York: Grune & Stratton.

Strauss, A. A., & Lehtinen, L. E. (1947). *Psychopathology and education of the brain-injured child.* New York: Grune & Stratton.

Torgesen, J. (1985). Memory processes in reading disabled children. *Journal of Learning Disabilities, 18,* 350–357.

Treiman, R., & Baron, J. (1981). Segmental analysis ability: Development and relation to reading ability. In T. Waller & G. MacKinnon (Eds.), *Reading research: Advances in theory and practice* (Vol. 3). New York: Academic Press.

U.S. Department of Education. (1990). *To assure the free appropriate public education of all handicapped children: Twelfth annual report to Congress on the implementation of The Education of the Handicapped Act.* Washington, D.C.: Author.

van Kleeck, A. (1984). Metalinguistic skills: Cutting across spoken and written language and problem-solving abilities. In G. P. Wallach & K. G. Butler (Eds.), *Language learning disabilities in school-age children* (pp. 128–153). Baltimore: Williams & Wilkins.

Vogel, S. A. (1983). A qualitative analysis of morphological ability in learning disabled and achieving children. *Journal of Learning Disabilities, 16,* 416–420.

Vogel, S. A. (1990). Gender differences in intelligence, language, visual-motor abilities, and academic achievement in students with learning disabilities: A review of the literature. *Journal of Learning Disabilities, 23,* 44–52.

Wallach, G. P., & Liebergott, J. W. (1984). Who shall be called "learning disabled": Some new directions. In G. P. Wallach & K. G. Butler (Eds.), *Language learning disabilities in school-age children* (pp. 1–14). Baltimore: Williams & Wilkins.

Weisenstein, G. R., & Pelz, R. (1986). *Administrator's desk reference on special education.* Gaithersburg, MD: Aspen Publishers.

Wender, P. (1971). *Minimal brain dysfunction in children.* New York: Wiley-Interscience.

Westby, C. E. (1991). Assessing and remediating comprehension problems. In A. G. Kamhi & H. W. Catts (Eds.), *Reading disabilities: A developmental language perspective* (pp. 199–260). Boston: Allyn and Bacon.

Wiig, E. (1986). Language disabilities in school-age children and youth. In G. Shames & E. Wiig (Eds.), *Human communication disorders: An introduction* (2nd ed.) (pp. 331–379). New York: Merrill/Macmillan.

Wiig, E., & Fleischmann, N. (1980). Knowledge of pronominalization, reflexivization, and relativization by learning disabled college students. *Journal of Learning Disabilities, 13,* 571–576.

Wiig, E., & Semel, E. (1975). Productive language abilities in learning disabled adolescents. *Journal of Learning Disabilities, 8,* 578–586.

Wiig, E., & Semel, E. (1984). *Language assessment and intervention for the learning disabled* (2nd ed.). New York: Merrill/Macmillan.

Willeford, J. A., & Burleigh, J. M. (1985). *Handbook of central auditory processing disorders in children.* Orlando, FL: Grune & Stratton.

Yoss, K. A., & Darley, F. L. (1974). Developmental apraxia of speech in children with defective articulation. *Journal of Speech and Hearing Research, 17,* 399–416.

· Chapter 8 ·

Language and Children with Autism

Steven H. Long

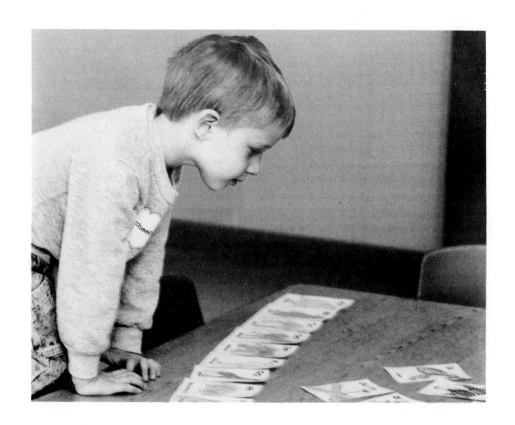

OBJECTIVES

Upon completion of this chapter, the reader should be able to:

▶ Define autism and other etiological categories with which it overlaps.

▶ Discuss the therapeutic technique known as facilitated communication and the challenge it poses to traditional thinking about what autism is and how it should be treated.

▶ Describe how research on children with autism is conducted.

▶ Identify and describe general characteristics of the language of children with autism.

▶ Discuss principles of language intervention for children with autism.

Professionals who serve children with language disorders are prone to change their minds. Usually these changes are relatively small: A theory might be updated to take account of new research information, or a new intervention tactic might be adopted that refines previous practice. The disorder of autism, however, has been associated with wide swings in thinking. Such large changes cause many reactions among professionals. There is fascination with the enigmatic nature of autism, frustration that many previous beliefs about it are eventually proven wrong, and optimism that the new ideas will improve the efficacy of treatment.

AN OVERVIEW OF CHILDREN WITH AUTISM

Autism was first described as a syndrome, or unique collection of behaviors, by Kanner in 1943. The patients he studied were children of normal or near-normal intelligence. Therefore, the focus of his description was on their unusual social and communicative impairments. He characterized the children as aloof and withdrawn, able to communicate only in repetitive utterances, fascinated by inanimate objects, and intolerant of changes in routine (Kanner, 1943). The cause of autism was and still is unknown, but for the next three decades following Kanner's published observations it was generally considered to be a type of emotional disturbance. As such, it was sometimes interpreted as resulting from environmental influences during the early years of life (e.g., Bettelheim, 1967). Because of this belief, the parents of children with autism were often—and, we now know, un-

fairly—held responsible for the condition. Treatment efforts were as likely to be concerned with changing the family as with changing the child.

Since the 1970s two major shifts in thinking about autism have occurred, and there are indications that a third shift is currently underway. One change has been in the conception of the disorder. Autism is now clearly viewed as a *developmental* rather than an *emotional* or *psychiatric* disorder (American Psychiatric Association, 1987). Hence, it is more closely aligned with mental retardation and other forms of developmental disability than with childhood schizophrenia and other types of psychotic disorders. The second change has been in our beliefs about the origin of the disorder. Though much about autism is still not understood, it is now generally accepted that the condition is present from birth. Therefore, autism does not stem from the actions of the parents in rearing their children but, in all likelihood, results from the genes they contributed in making them.

The third shift in thinking cannot be fully evaluated at present. It is resulting from an innovative approach to intervention known as *facilitated communication*. This approach will be described more fully later in this chapter, but it must be mentioned at the outset because of the challenge it presents to traditional views about the disabilities and the potential of children with autism. Briefly, facilitated communication combines elements of physical support and positive expectation to allow individuals with autism to communicate by typing messages (Biklen, 1992; Crossley, 1991). It has revealed that many of these individuals are literate and possess linguistic, cognitive, and even social abilities never imagined by their families or by the professionals who work with them. To anyone who observes a child with autism communicating with the help of a facilitator, it is obvious that, at least for some individuals, our assumptions and our methods of evaluation have been inadequate. What is currently unknown is the extent to which we have been blind to these underlying abilities. Facilitated communication may eventually reveal that we have been wrong about nearly all children with autism, or it may show that these startling abilities exist in only a small subpopulation. Further research on facilitated communication is an important priority and will determine how great our shift in thinking about autism must be.

Diagnostic Criteria

Despite the relatively short history of autism as a clinical category, it has become one of the most complicated areas of medical and educational diagnosis. The number of terms used to describe children with autism and related disorders has grown quickly, especially in recent years. A group of these terms is listed and defined in Table 8.1. The proliferation of labels has resulted from research on what constitutes the core of autism and distinguishes it from other similar disorders. To many professionals, the distinctions among these terms are subtle and may even seem irrelevant in matters of clinical practice. After all, if several children are labeled differently but receive the same treatment, what purpose does the label serve? This is a fair question, and the framers of diagnostic categories may in the future need to consider "response to treatment" as one of the characteristics that define subgroups of children with autism and related disorders.

Nevertheless, professionals rely on diagnostic categories to do their work, so we must address the issue of how syndromes are defined and distinguished. To begin with, we should note a simple linguistic and clinical distinction. The word *autism,* a noun, should refer always to a clinical syndrome that is defined by a unique set of behavioral criteria. Those criteria have changed at various points over the last half century, but the notion of autism as a syndrome has remained unchanged (Wetherby, 1989). In contrast, the word *autistic,* an adjective, has frequently been used by clinicians to describe individual behaviors in children who may or may not meet the criteria for the syndrome of autism. For example, many children with profound mental retardation exhibit self-injurious (head banging, biting) or stereotypic (arm flapping, grimacing) behaviors that are also observed in children with autism. Perhaps because these actions are so dramatically bizarre and are associated with autism, they are often called *autistic* or **autisticlike** behaviors. This practice is regrettable for two reasons. First, it gives a sloppy description of the behaviors themselves. To say that a child has "autisticlike behaviors" is akin to saying that someone "acts depressed." Second, the term *autisticlike* suggests to the uninformed listener or reader that a child has been diagnosed with autism, when this may not be the case.

As noted previously, the category of autism has been revised over the years. Several well-recognized scholars have had substantial influence in shaping professional opinion about the diagnostic boundaries of the disorder (e.g., Rutter, 1978; Wing, 1981). Since 1980, however, the major arbiter in the matter of definition has been a group of professionals assembled by the American Psychiatric Association, whose work is published in the *Diagnostic and Statistical Manual of Mental Disorders.* The third edition of this manual (DSM-III) was published in 1980; a revision (DSM-III-R) was published in 1987. The definition of Autistic Disorder contained in DSM-III-R is cited in Table 8.2. This definition now serves as the standard for scholars in the field and for many professionals involved in the diagnosis of autism. Although the DSM-III-R definition carries the weight of scholarly authority, the legal definition of autism is determined by each state. A survey conducted in 1985 indicated that the two state agencies most commonly providing diagnostic services for autism—the Departments of Mental Health and Public Instruction—often utilize different diagnostic criteria and permit different professionals (e.g., psychiatrist, school psychologist, special education teacher) to make the diagnosis (Vicker & Monahan, 1988). Without some investigation of a child's individual case history, therefore, the criteria that were applied in a diagnosis of autism will not be clearly known.

The DSM-III-R diagnostic criteria for autism are designed to deal with the inherent heterogeneity of the

TABLE 8.1 Terminology Used to Describe Children with Autism and Related
Psychotic and Developmental Disorders

Term	Description/Comment
Autistic disorder	The most severe form of pervasive development disorder and hence the only form recognized in DSM-III-R (American Psychiatric Association, 1987) as a unique diagnostic category. See Table 8.2 for a description of diagnostic criteria.
Infantile autism	Diagnostic category used in DSM-III (American Psychiatric Association, 1980). Criteria were similar to those used in DSM-III-R except that (1) a specific contrast was made with childhood schizophrenia and (2) the modifier *infantile* was included to specify that the condition existed only if onset occurred before 30 months of age. This age-of-onset requirement was deleted in DSM-III-R.
Kanner's syndrome or "classic" autism	A term used by some professionals to designate children with autism who resemble the patients originally described by Kanner (1943). Specifically, these are children who show the social, communication, and behavioral aberrations associated with autism but do not show intellectual impairment.
Rett syndrome	A progressive neurological disorder occurring in girls. It is associated with worsening dementia, loss of facial expression and purposeful hand use, ataxia, diminished interpersonal contact, and stereotyped movements (Rutter & Schopler, 1987).
Asperger syndrome	A diagnostic label not appearing in DSM-III-R but often used in the literature on pervasive developmental disorders. Individuals with this condition exhibit social and communicative deficits, but typically at a higher level than individuals with autism. For example, an individual with Asperger syndrome may interact socially but display numerous behavioral oddities such as social unawareness, lack of common sense, repetitive interests, and pedantic speech (Gillberg, 1991). The condition overlaps with mild forms of autism but has a better prognosis (Bishop, 1989).
Schizoid and schizotypal personality disorder	Two types of personality disorders, in contrast to developmental disorders, are described in DSM-III-R. The chief feature of schizoid personality disorder is "indifference to social relationships and a restricted range of emotional experience and expression" (American Psychiatric Association, 1987, p. 340). Individuals with these characteristics might by diagnosed by some professionals as having Asperger syndrome (Rutter & Schopler, 1987). Schizotypal personality disorder is associated with social deficits but also shows "oddities of behavior, thinking, perception, and speech" (American Psychiatric Association, 1987, p. 341).
Pervasive development disorder not otherwise specified (PDDNOS)	A diagnostic category introduced in DSM-III-R that is used for children who meet some but not all of the criteria for autistic disorder, schizophrenia, schizotypal, or schizoid personality disorder (American Psychiatric Association, 1987). Clinically, these children typically appear to be less impaired than children diagnosed with autistic disorder.
Residual autism	A term used to describe individuals who once met the criteria for autistic disorder but, because of developmental changes and improvements, no longer do.
Heller syndrome/ disintegrative psychosis	A condition in which a child's social, communicative, and cognitive development is normal during the first 3 or 4 years of life but then suddenly disintegrates, and behaviors characteristic of pervasive development disorder emerge (Rutter & Schopler, 1987). This syndrome is extremely rare and, according to DSM-III-R, a child following this pattern is better diagnosed with autistic disorder or PDDNOS (American Psychiatric Association, 1987).
Schizophrenia	A condition in which social and communicative behaviors are affected in ways similar to those seen in autism. Schizophrenia, however, is classified as a *psychosis*, in contrast to a *pervasive developmental disorder*. It contrasts with autism in several ways (see Table 8.4).

TABLE 8.2   DSM-III-R Diagnostic Criteria for Autistic Disorder

The Child Must Show at Least...	Example Typical of a Younger or More Handicapped Child	Example Typical of an Older or Less Handicapped Child
Two behaviors that demonstrate qualitative impairment in *reciprocal social interaction:*		
1. Marked lack of awareness of the existence or feelings of others	Treats a person as if he or she were a piece of furniture	Has no concept of the need of others for privacy
2. No or abnormal seeking of comfort at times of distress	Does not seek comfort even when ill, hurt, or tired	Seeks comfort in a stereotyped way; for example, says "cheese, cheese, cheese" whenever hurt
3. No or impaired imitation	Does not wave good-bye	Mechanically imitates others' actions out of context
4. No or abnormal play	Does not actively participate in simple games	Involves other children in play only as "mechanical aids"
5. Gross impairment in ability to make peer friendships	No interest in making peer friendships	Shows interest in friendship but does not understand conventions of social interaction, for example, reads phone book to uninterested peer

One behavior that demonstrates qualitative impairment in *verbal and nonverbal communication* and in *imaginative activity:* (Behaviors listed first are typical of younger or more handicapped children. Behaviors listed later are typical of older or less disabled children.)

1. No mode of communication, such as communicative babbling, facial expression, gesture, mime, or spoken language	No communicative babbling, facial expression, gesture, mime, or spoken language
2. Markedly abnormal nonverbal communication	Stiffens when held, does not make eye contact when making social approach, maintains fixed stare in social situations
3. Absence of imaginative activity	No playacting of adult roles, fantasy characters, or animals
4. Abnormal speech production	Monotonous or questionlike intonation, high pitch
5. Abnormal language form or content	Immediate echolalia, use of "you" for "I," idiosyncratic language, irrelevant remarks
6. Inability to initiate or sustain conversation	Monologues are produced without allowing others opportunity to speak

One behavior indicative of a *restricted repertoire of activities and interests:*

1. Stereotyped body movements	Hand flicking or twisting, spinning, head banging, complex whole-body movements
2. Persistent preoccupation with parts of objects	Sniffs objects, repetitive feeling of texture of materials, attachment to unusual objects (e.g., example, carrying around piece of string)
3. Distress over changes in trivial aspects of environment	Gets upset when a vase is moved from its usual position
4. Unreasonable insistence that routines be followed	Insists that the same route be followed when shopping
5. Restricted range of interests and preoccupation with one narrow interest	Interested only in lining up objects, amassing facts about meteorology, or pretending to be a fantasy character

Source: Adapted from American Psychiatric Association (1987).

disorder. That is, they recognize that children with autism present a wide range of aberrant behaviors. Stereotyped descriptions of children with autism nearly always include behaviors such as echolalia, idiosyncratic language (e.g, repeating television commercials), fascination with mechanical objects, and unusual motor behavior (e.g., toe walking). But these behaviors, though they may be common, are not found in all cases of autism.

Is there a behavior or behaviors that unambiguously identify autism in a child? If the question is asked this way, the answer has to be no. However, researchers have asked another related question: Do certain behaviors found in autism more reliably distinguish it from other disorders? Two studies have examined the records of children with autism and similar disorders and have used statistical analyses to determine the distinctive characteristics of autism (Dahl, Cohen, & Provence, 1986; Siegel, Vukicevic, Elliott, & Kraemer, 1989). The studies agree that social impairment is the hallmark characteristic. Specifically, Siegel et al. (1989) found that, of the behaviors cited in the DSM-III-R definition, the most predictive characteristic was a marked lack of awareness of the existence or feelings of others followed by a persistent preoccupation with parts of objects.

It must be noted again that our current working definitions of autism are based on traditional interactions with these children. Clinical experiences with facilitated communication challenge many traditional notions about the performance of individuals with autism. In particular, written messages from individuals with autism, including children as young as 3 years, suggest much greater social awareness and interaction ability than their behavioral profiles would lead us to expect (Biklen, 1990a, 1992; Biklen & Schubert, 1991). Some of these reported messages are as follows:

I AI DONT WANT TO BE AUTISTIC. NOBODY REALLY ZUNDERSTANDS WHAT IT FEELS LIKE. (Adult: How does it feel?) IT IS VERY LONELY AND I OFTEN FEEL LOUSY. MY MOOD IS BAD A LOT. I FEEL LESS LONELI WHEN I AM WITH KIDS. (Biklen, 1992, p. 15)

IM NOT RETARDED. MY MOTHER FEELS IM STUPID BECAUSE I CANT USE MY VOICE PROPERLY. (Biklen, 1990, p. 296)

ARE YOU MARRIED?
(Adult: I am.)

WHAT'S YOUR WIFE'S NAME?
(Adult: Sari)
FUNNY NAME (Biklen, 1990, p. 308)

I FEEL LONELY WHJEN I HAVE NO KIDS AT MY HOUSE. I WANT MY MOM TO KNUOW THAT I LIKE TO BE WITGH KIDS. (Biklen & Schubert, 1991, p. 47)

Prevalence

Estimates of the prevalence of autistic disorder have fluctuated slightly in accordance with shifts in the criteria used to diagnose the disorder. Current estimates based on the DSM-III-R criteria are that autism occurs in approximately 4 to 5 children in every 10,000. An additional 5 to 10 children in every 10,000 are affected by pervasive developmental disorder not otherwise specified (see Table 8.1) (American Psychiatric Association, 1987).

All forms of pervasive developmental disorder occur more frequently in males than in females, with different studies suggesting ratios ranging from 2:1 to 5:1 (American Psychiatric Association, 1987). The ratio for autistic disorder, in particular, has been estimated at 3:1 or 4:1. The more frequent impairment of males has no ready explanation, but it is one of the features of autism that distinguish it from mental retardation (Rutter & Schopler, 1987). Although females with autism are diagnosed less frequently, several studies have found them to have lower measured IQs than males with autism (Lord & Schopler, 1985, 1989; Lord, Schopler, & Revicki, 1982). Inasmuch as IQ is the best known predictor of outcome in individuals with autism, it can be inferred that females tend to present as more difficult clinical cases (Gillberg, 1991). Females have also been found to develop seizure disorders in higher proportions than males, which may contribute further to their poorer observed outcomes (Volkmar & Nelson, 1990).

Associated Problems

The core features of autism, which are outlined in the DSM-III-R diagnostic criteria, are social impairment, communicative impairment, and repetitive or highly restricted (**stereotyped**) behavior that replaces more imaginative forms of action. These features most accurately distinguish autism from other developmental disabilities, but they do not describe all the aberrant behaviors one is likely to find in children with autism. Table 8.3 summarizes some of the other significant conditions associated with autism.

What Causes Autism?

The short answer to this question is, simply, that we do not know. There are a number of methodological problems that make the search for the cause more difficult:

1. Autism is not a discrete disorder but represents the most severe form of pervasive developmental disorder. Therefore, the cause of autism must also account for the problems of children who have related disorders.

2. There is significant variation in the types and severity of problems manifested by children with autism. Whatever is causing the disorder must be interacting with other developmental factors to produce such a diverse array of behavioral profiles.

3. In most children with autism, the disorder is first manifested as an impairment in social skills observed at around 18 months (Johnson, Siddons, Frith, & Morton, 1992). Even then, however, it may not be possible to make a confident diagnosis. Consequently, researchers are unable to study the disorder until the children have become toddlers or preschoolers. This serves to keep certain information about the origins of the problem hidden from investigators.

4. The social and communicative impairments of children with autism have always made developmental testing extremely difficult, especially when the children are young (Lord & Schopler, 1989). In addition, the information gained from experience with facilitated communication has highlighted individual cases where past assessments have failed to reveal a child's abilities (Biklen, 1990a). When the accuracy of measurements is doubted, it is hard to find support for causal theories. After all, the data they are based upon may be wrong.

In spite of these obstacles, research on autism has assembled an impressive amount of information and has brought many issues into focus. For many years,

there has been a consensus that the underlying problem in autism is neurophysiological rather than environmental (Menyuk & Wilbur, 1981). Acknowledgment of this fact has led researchers to compare autism with other childhood disorders known to have a neurophysiological cause such as mental retardation and schizophrenia. The reasoning is that if autism can be linked to any of these other disorders, then it may be possible to develop an explanation of autism based on what is known about the other disorders. The evidence has indicated, however, that autism is distinctive. Table 8.4 summarizes some of the findings that differentiate autism from other neurophysiological disorders of childhood.

Some scientists have taken the position that the behaviors evidenced in autism can be traced to specific neurophysiological mechanisms and that these mechanisms must, therefore, be dysfunctional. Thus, it has been suggested that the primary deficit is in

1. Areas of the limbic system that are responsible for arousal, attention, and motor responsiveness (Maurer & Damasio, 1982) *or*

2. Areas of the cerebellum that facilitate arousal and attention (Courchesne, 1987) *or*

3. A combination of cortical and subcortical areas that are responsible for attachment and social behavior (Fein, Pennington, Markowitz, Braverman, & Waterhouse, 1986) *or*

4. Neuromotor systems underlying voluntary or intentional movement (Biklen, 1990a). This last suggestion is linked with the therapeutic approach of facilitated communication that will be considered later in this chapter.

Heredity

As with all serious developmental disorders, investigators have been intrigued with the role of heredity in causing autism. Although research in this area is ongoing, the current body of opinion may be summarized as follows:

▷ There is a slight tendency for autism to **aggregate** (occur more than once) in the same family. This occurs in approximately 1–3% of families who have one child with autism. Although this is a small percentage, it is 50 to 100 times greater

TABLE 8.3 Associated Problems in Children with Autism

Mental retardation	Over three quarters of all children with autism are mentally retarded, based on IQ test scores. In most cases the tests indicate a moderate level of retardation (IQ 35–49) (American Psychiatric Association, 1987; Rutter & Schopler, 1987).
Motor behavior deficits	Along with their propensity for repetitive movements (see Table 8.1), many children with autism are poorly coordinated and display odd hand and body postures (American Psychiatric Association, 1987). Their performance on copying tasks suggests that deficits in visual monitoring of motor performance are responsible for some of their motor difficulties (Fulkerson & Freeman, 1980). Proponents of facilitated communication have suggested that one of the primary impairments of autism is an inability to *initiate* voluntary movements, a motor apraxia (Biklen, 1990).
Unusual sensory behavior	Children with autism may show either hyposensitivity or hypersensitivity to certain stimuli. They may be oblivious to heat, cold, or pain but show extreme distress when they hear certain sounds or are touched unexpectedly.
Hearing loss	Fluctuating, negative middle-ear pressure is more common in children with autism than in unimpaired children. This results in more frequent middle ear infections (Konstantareas & Homatidis, 1987), though it is not necessary for an infection to develop in order for a child's hearing to be affected. When compared to children with learning disabilities—another group with a higher than normal prevalence of middle ear pathology—children with autism show greater negative pressure and a marked tendency toward bilateral involvement (Smith, Miller, Stewart, Walter, & McConnell, 1988).
Seizures	Approximately one third of all patients develop epilepsy during early childhood or adolescence (Gillberg, 1991; Volkmar & Nelson, 1990). The onset of seizures tends not to occur during *middle* childhood, for reasons that are not understood (Volkmar & Nelson, 1990).
Fragile X syndrome	Children with autism show a higher than normal prevalence of Fragile X syndrome, a genetic condition associated with mental retardation and certain behavioral abnormalities. Fragile X syndrome has been found at rates varying from 0% to 20%, depending on the identification criteria employed. When stringent criteria were followed, it appeared in only 2.7% of cases (Piven, Gayle, Landa, Wzorek, & Folstein, 1991). The reason for the association, even though it may be small, is unknown.

than the chance probability (Folstein & Rutter, 1988).

▷ There is a greater tendency for autism to aggregate with other disorders such as mental retardation or language impairment. This has been estimated to occur in 10–15% of families that

also have a child with autism (Folstein & Rutter, 1988). Research also suggests that the *parents* of children with autism may have subtle communication problems of their own (Landa, Folstein, & Isaacs, 1991).

▷ Preliminary studies indicate that autism may also

TABLE 8.4 Evidence Distinguishing Autism from Other Neurophysiological Disorders

Autism versus . . .	Mental Retardation
Onset of seizures (in about 25% of children) occurs during adolescence	Onset of seizures occurs during early childhood
Very rarely occurs in Down syndrome or cerebral palsy	Usually occurs in Down syndrome and cerebral palsy
Occurs much more frequently in males (approximately a 4:1 ratio)	Occurs only slightly more frequently in males
Children have difficulty discriminating socioemotional cues (e.g., facial expressions)	Children can read such cues at a level commensurate with MA

Autism versus . . .	Schizophrenia
Onset typically occurs before 30 months of age	Onset typically occurs during adolescence
Family history of schizophrenia is rare	Family history of schizophrenia is greater than chance
Delusions and hallucinations are rare	Delusions and hallucinations are hallmark behaviors
Abnormal behaviors are persistent	Abnormal behaviors are episodic
Seizures occur in about 25% of cases	Seizures are rare

Autism versus . . .	Developmental Disorder of Receptive Language
Occurs much more frequently in males (approximately a 4:1 ratio)	Approximately equal in sex distribution (males are predominant in *expressive* language disorder)
Prognosis for improvement is generally poor	Prognosis is generally good
Wider and more severe cognitive handicaps	Milder cognitive handicaps
Persisting socioemotional and behavioral problems	Emotional and behavioral problems appear secondary to language impairment and tend to improve as language does

Source: Adapted from Folstein and Rutter (1988) and Rutter and Schopler (1987).

aggregate with certain social or psychological problems in other family members. Compared to the parents of children with Down syndrome, the parents of children with autism show a significantly greater prevalence of anxiety disorder and a rate of manic-depressive disorder that probably exceeds that in the general population (Piven et al., 1991). It is important to note that these findings do not support the earlier—and now discredited—theory that autism results from insensitive parenting practices.

▷ Most cases of autism are *idiopathic,* that is, they result from unknown factors, and the probability that the condition will recur in other children cannot be well estimated. A small number of cases, however, can be linked to specific genetic disorders such as Fragile X syndrome (Folstein & Rutter, 1988). In these instances, the role of heredity is better understood and more accurate genetic predictions can be made.

▷ It is not even clear that autism itself is inherited. Instead, children may inherit a language or social impairment of some kind. This impairment may then interact with certain factors in the environment (illness, emotional trauma, exposure to toxins) to produce autism (Folstein & Rutter, 1988).

Natural History of Autism

One of the many mysteries about autism is that the condition is not generally recognizable until around 18 months. At that age, some but not all children who will eventually be diagnosed show a noticeable difference in social behaviors such as smiling or responding to people (Johnson, Siddons, Frith, & Morton, 1992). In most cases, the onset of autism occurs between 18 and 36 months of age. Children who later present more severe symptoms tend to have an earlier age of onset. This probably reflects the behavior of the parents more than that of the child: Severe symptoms are more likely to be recognized at an early age than mild ones. The term *age of onset,* as it is commonly used, is more accurately described as *age of recognition* (Short & Schopler, 1988).

Many of the early signs of autism are deficiencies in a child's communicative behaviors prior to the emergence of speech. Whereas both typically developing children and nonautistic children with mental retardation show a strong attraction to the sound of their mother's voice, children with autism show no such interest or even prefer to listen to environmental sounds such as restaurant noise (Klin, 1991).

When they are engaged in interactions with other people, children with autism show deficiencies in gestural joint attention skills (Mundy, Sigman, Ungerer, & Sherman, 1987; Wetherby & Prutting, 1984). That is, they rarely point to or show objects to their partners. These behaviors are frequent among preverbal typically developing children, as is the use of eye contact to attract and then direct a partner's attention. Yet compared to MA- and LA-matched groups of children with mental retardation, children with autism rarely show these behaviors (Mundy, Sigman, & Kasari, 1990).

In later childhood, children with autism begin to display the wide range of impairments in social interaction, communication, and imaginative play that characterize the disorder (see Table 8.2 for a summary). Recently a number of scholars have suggested that these diverse problems may have a single underlying cause, namely, an inability to attribute mental states to themselves or to others (Baron-Cohen, 1991; Frith, 1989; Tager-Flusberg, 1992; Yirmiya, Sigman, Kasari, & Mundy, 1992). This inability to engage in **metarepresentational** thinking means that children do not understand or relate to the thought processes of people with whom they interact. Obviously this problem would significantly limit their capacity to initiate and sustain social relationships, which rely on the ability to "read" the mood, desires, and intentions of social partners. Similarly, communication requires an ability to evaluate messages according to the context in which they are produced. Part of that context is the thinking and emotional state of the speaker. We routinely relate the two in statements such as "Mommy is sad because she thought you were lost." Children with metarepresentational problems are likely to be confused by this kind of sentence because they cannot imagine the emotions of the mother that would result in sadness. A further consequence of a metarepresentational problem is that children do not observe the subtle cues issued by their conversational partners that signal when they are expected to talk, when they should yield their turn, when they should clarify a statement they have made, and so on. Hence, the marked deficiencies in the pragmatics of communication they may exhibit may result from metarepresentational problems.

Most imaginative activity also depends on representations of what others are thinking. This is apparent in role-playing games, which demand that children be able to think like the individuals they are impersonating, whether it is a parent, a policeman, a store owner, or a doctor.

The social and communicative impairments observed in young children with autism often improve in later childhood. Treatment, of course, is one of the factors influencing this improvement. Long-term studies of individuals with autism have indicated, however, that many of them suffer an aggravation of symptoms during adolescence. Most commonly there is an increase in hyperactivity, aggressiveness, self-destructiveness, and insistence on routine. The reason for this deterioration, and the reason it strikes some individuals but not others, are unknown. Some of the causes that have been suggested are the adolescent onset of epilepsy in some individuals, the hormonal changes of puberty and their influence on the nervous system, and the physical growth of the child, which exacerbates the effect of any behavioral problems (Gillberg, 1991).

COMMUNICATION IN CHILDREN WITH AUTISM

Recall from chapter 6 that many studies of language impairment in children with mental retardation have relied on the technique of matching subjects by CA, MA, or LA. A similar procedure has been used to study language impairments of children with autism. In principle, this method should yield comparisons between groups of children (e.g., children with autism, children with mental retardation, and children who are developing typically) that are unconfounded by differences in age, intelligence, or general language level. However, children with autism are frequently difficult to match with others. Because of their tendencies to echo speech addressed to them and to produce stereotyped phrases and sentences, MLU counts are likely to be less stable and less representative than for other children (Wetherby & Prutting, 1984). Similarly, IQ matching is difficult for children with autism because their performances are highly variable at different ages and with different types of intelligence tests (Lord & Schopler, 1989). As noted earlier, some of the performances that have emerged from facilitated communication cast doubt on the adequacy of our methods for assessing intelligence in children with autism (Biklen, 1990a). Consequently, in the future there may be reason to challenge some of the findings to be reviewed here and to recommend that research be conducted using different techniques.

The verbal abilities of children with autism range from the total absence of speech to communication that is fully adequate in phonological and grammatical form but is remarkable for its semantic or pragmatic

irregularities. At both ends of this severity continuum, the behaviors evidenced by children with autism overlap with those shown by children with other developmental disorders. Obviously, a child with no speech may have one of several disorders: autism, mental retardation, psychogenic mutism, hearing impairment, and others. On the other hand, a child whose problems are exclusively semantic and pragmatic may have a history of autism, learning disability, mental retardation, or head injury. Thus, neither the degree of severity nor the level(s) of language impairment will unambiguously identify a child with autism. Nevertheless, various studies have suggested a profile of language skills that is generally characteristic of the disorder. In this profile certain abilities are relatively *preserved,* that is, they appear to be commensurate or nearly commensurate with a child's intellectual level. It is important to note that these components of the child's language typically will not be age appropriate and, therefore, may be a focus of clinical intervention. It is generally believed, however, that these language difficulties are secondary to intellectual impairment and, therefore, can be expected to improve as general developmental gains are made. In contrast is a set of abilities that appear to be relatively *impaired* in children with autism. These are the communication behaviors that are most distinctive of autism and are frequently cited as diagnostic criteria (see Table 8.2).

Preserved Abilities

Segmental Phonology and Syntax   One of the most important generalizations that can be made about the language abilities of children with autism is that they do not show specific developmental impairment at the levels of segmental phonology (consonant and vowel production) or syntax (Bartolucci, Pierce, Streiner, & Eppel, 1976; Boucher, 1976; Tager-Flusberg, 1981). Thus, one can expect the following:

1. The speech they produce will be generally intelligible, in the same way that the speech of a typically developing child can be understood at any age, even though it is not yet adultlike.
2. Utterances will be free of glaring syntactic problems and will show a balance in structural

growth, meaning that they will not have a **telegraphic** quality caused by limited development of phrase structures and bound morphemes.

The presence of these abilities is a major linguistic difference between children with autism and children with language handicaps due to other causes such as mental retardation, deafness, or specific language impairment.

Lexical and Syntactic Comprehension   Many factors influence a child's understanding of language, among them the familiarity of the grammar and vocabulary, the familiarity of the topic, and the familiarity of the interactants. Under controlled conditions, it appears that children with autism are able to comprehend the linguistic code at a level consistent with their MA. That is, they can decode word meanings and semantic contrasts signified by changes in word order or by inflectional morphemes (Beisler, Tsai, & Vonk, 1987; Eskes, Bryson, & McCormick, 1990). This does not mean that a child with autism will understand language as would a typically developing child of the same age. For instance, a 5-year-old child with autism who has an MA of 2 years will doubtless present with comprehension difficulties because of limited vocabulary and immature cognitive development. Moreover, the child is very likely to exhibit abnormal pragmatic behaviors such as poor eye contact, interruptions of the other speaker, and poor observance of the rules for referencing old and new information (Baron-Cohen, 1988). Such deficits give the appearance of a comprehension problem, whether or not one really exists.

Imitation   Imitation is often considered an area of impairment for children with autism because of their tendency to imitate excessively and inappropriately, which we will discuss later. However, we should also observe that, unlike many children with other forms of language impairment, children with autism *can* imitate verbal stimuli. Thus, the ability to decode, store, and encode verbal messages is present, even though there may be very little depth to the language processing that occurs.

Impaired Abilities

Nonsegmental Phonology   In contrast to their ability to master individual sound segments (consonants and vowels), children with autism commonly display significant impairment in nonsegmental speech production, also referred to as *prosody*. Problems of this type take many forms and can vary considerably among children. Some of the most frequently reported aberrations are as follows (Baltaxe & Simmons, 1985; Goldfarb, Braunstein, & Lorge, 1956):

1. A stereotyped rhythmic pattern, described as "singsong," that is characterized by excessive sound prolongation.
2. Overly frequent and contextually inappropriate whispering.
3. Unusual fluctuations in vocal intensity.
4. Limited pitch range, resulting in monotonous speech.
5. Tonal contrasts that are inconsistent with the meanings expressed verbally, for example, sentences produced with rising intonation that clearly are not requests.

Difficulty with prosody cannot easily be explained as a developmental lag, as most nonsegmental functions are learned early in life by typically developing children (Crystal, 1981). The most straightforward account of the problem is that it is perceptual. Children with autism simply do not hear the contrasts in rhythm, rate, and intonation that are used in normal discourse. However, most studies that have used perceptual tasks to evaluate prosodic ability have found that children with autism perform comparably to typically developing children or to other groups of language-impaired children who do not present with difficulties of expressive prosody (Baltaxe & Guthrie, 1987; Frankel, Simmons, & Richey, 1987).

Idiosyncratic Language   Children with autism display several unusual verbal behaviors that, as a group, are referred to as idiosyncratic language. This term draws attention to the fact that, although there are similarities in how idiosyncratic language is learned or used, each child is unique in the specific words or phrases that are produced and in the contexts in which they occur.

All forms of idiosyncratic language appear to reflect either peculiarities of **semantic processing** or deficits in pragmatic competence. Children with autism have a proclivity to recall certain words or phrases only in the context in which they were first learned (Fay, 1980). Thus, a child may learn a word initially (e.g., "shoe") as a result of experiences with a particular object (sneaker) but will never generalize use of the word to other stimuli (other shoes, other people's shoes, pictures of shoes). Similarly, a word or phrase may seem to be triggered by the recurrence of the original conditions of learning, as in this example:

> Alex, when he was about 3 years old, was riding home at dusk with his mother, who told him that for supper they would have "sea scallops to eat." Just as she said this, the car ahead (Mercury-Comet, 1960 vintage) with peculiar slanting tail lights stopped and the tail lights lit up. For three or four years afterward, Alex would recite "sea scallops to eat" whenever he saw this type of tail-light on a car. (Simon, 1975, p. 1442)

A distinction is sometimes made between idiosyncratic language, where conventional words or phrases are used with unconventional meanings, and **neolo-gisms**, where a new word or words are coined. Examples of the two behaviors are given in Table 8.5. Children with autism produce both forms, though neologisms are far less frequent and usually consist of incorrect combinations of morphemes (e.g., "glass-able" for "breakable") rather than wholly invented strings of phonemes (e.g., "glufer"). Neither idiosyncratic language nor neologisms are unique to children with autism. They are found less frequently in the spontaneous speech of children with mental retardation, as well as that of young children who are developing typically. In children with autism, however, they are more likely to draw attention. This is because they are more frequent and because they occur in older children who are no longer given license to "play" with language in these ways (Volden & Lord, 1991).

Idiosyncratic language varies in frequency and character among different children with autism. In some children the process is highly creative, so that idiosyncratic forms will appear at one time and may not reappear in other conversations. In contrast, other children make repeated use of the same word or phrase, often in contexts where it seems meaningless. It appears unlikely that this behavior has the same

TABLE 8.5 Examples of Neologisms and Idiosyncratic Language in Children with Autism

Utterance	Interpretation
Idiosyncratic Language	
"It makes me want to as deep as *economical* with it"	"withdraw as much as possible"
"They're having a meal and then they're finishing and *siding* the table"	"clearing the table"
"And *wave* their things on the floor in the bathroom"	"leave their things"
"If they even take it *true* enough"	"If they take it seriously enough"
"*But in the car, it's some*"	"But in the car, there's something different"
"*In Thames, with about 8 years ago*"	"In the Thames, about 8 years ago"
Neologisms	
"And he's seriously wounded like *cutes and bloosers*"	"cuts and bruises"
"She's bawcet"	"She's bossy"

Source: Adapted from Volden and Lord (1991), p. 118.

function for all children that produce it. The suggestion has been made, however, that highly repetitive utterances are used primarily to deal with comprehension difficulties and to structure conversation so that it is more predictable. Coggins and Frederickson (1988) studied a 9-year-old boy with autism who frequently repeated the phrase "can I talk." By analyzing where the utterance occurred in conversational sequences, they were able to determine that it did not occur randomly but nearly always was directed to the conversational partner, the child's father. Furthermore, the utterance tended to occur in the middle of speaking exchanges and often followed adult attempts to direct activities or introduce new topics. The conclusion was that the utterance was used to force a change in speaker turn and thereby help the child to cope with overwhelming conversational demands.

Pronoun Difficulties   Confusion and substitution of pronominal forms frequently occur in the speech of children with autism. Some of their errors, such as confusion of gender ("he" for "she" or "it") or case substitution ("him" for "he"), are also commonly found in young typically developing children and in children with other forms of language impairment. To some extent, therefore, the pronoun difficulties observed in autism are merely a predictable component of their total language impairment. The problem that appears distinct to autism is the persistent confusion of the first- and second-person singular forms. Children with autism often use "you" to refer to themselves and "I" or "me" to refer to others. A number of explanations for this phenomenon have been proposed. In years past the problem was viewed as a failure of ego differentiation, but this idea has been abandoned, along with other psychopathological accounts of autism. Among the current explanations are the following:

1. Children with autism are specifically impaired in their ability to understand and use certain deictic forms, that is, words whose meaning is determined by the communicative context. Because the interpretation of "I," "you," and "me" changes along with the speaker, they find it difficult to grasp the underlying meaning of these words.

2. The problem with pronominal reference is another aspect of the difficulty children with autism have with metarepresentation. That is, they do not clearly differentiate between their own and others' mental states and, therefore, struggle with the language forms that explicitly mark this difference (Frith, 1989). If this explanation is correct, one would expect pronoun use to improve as gains are made in nonverbal behaviors that direct others' attention (e.g., eye contact and gesturing).

3. Children with autism may have attention deficits that interfere with their ability to observe pronoun use in speech between other individuals (Oshima-Takane & Benaroya, 1989). Because they do not attend to conversation when others are speaking, they do not witness the normal shift in pronoun use. This means that they will not master pronouns as a result of incidental exposure to conversational models. Additional focused exposure to pronoun shifting, as might be provided in a language intervention program, should be helpful, according to this explanation.

Echolalia   One of the most salient characteristics of children with autism is the frequency with which they repeat utterances addressed to them. This behavior is described as **echolalia** when it appears to occur in an automatic and unthinking way, that is, when the listener believes the speech was repeated without communicative intent (Howlin, 1982; Prizant & Rydell, 1984). Descriptions of echolalia frequently distinguish between two types: *immediate* echolalia, the exact repetition of a word or words directly after they are spoken, and *delayed* echolalia, which occurs some time after the original utterance is produced. A third type sometimes mentioned, *mitigated* echolalia, refers to immediate repetitions that contain some change to the utterance. In both research and clinical practice, the distinctions among these types of echolalia are often difficult to make. For example, there is no standard for judging how much of a time delay must occur before echolalia is considered delayed rather than immediate (5 seconds? 1 minute? half an hour?). Similarly, there is no agreement on the quantity or quality of changes that must be present in a mitigated echolalic response (one word changed? one inflection?

change in intonation?). All in all, one must be careful not to assume that these terms are used with identical meanings by all professionals.

In the past, it was often assumed that the repetitions of children with autism were without intention and, therefore, should be regarded as pathological signs of their language disorder. At the same time, however, it has always been recognized that echolalia is not limited to children with autism but that it also occurs in children with mental retardation, as well as in typically developing children. A distinction between normal and pathological echolalia has been maintained on the basis of three pieces of evidence. First, the frequency of echolalia is higher in children with autism than in those who have mental retardation or who are developing typically (Cantwell, Howlin, & Rutter, 1977). Second, echolalia continues to occur at later ages in children with autism, while it usually disappears by the age of 2½ to 3 years in typically developing children (Howlin, 1982). Third, some research has suggested that imitation serves a role in facilitating the grammatical development of typically developing children (Tager-Flusberg & Calkins, 1990). It is also sometimes said that the repetitions of children with autism are qualitatively different, being almost exact copies of what is said to them, whereas those of other children more frequently contain changes in certain words or inflections or in the prosodic features of the utterance. Support for this belief comes largely from published clinical observations rather than experimental measurements and comparisons.

In recent years, echolalia has come to be viewed as less of a pathological behavior in individuals with autism, mostly because of research demonstrating that this repetition does have communicative intent. That intent is not found in the words themselves—these are borrowed from the conversational partner—but rather in the combined effect of the repetition, its prosody, any simultaneous nonverbal cues, and the context in which it is produced. Studies have confirmed that not all echolalia is interactive, that is, intended to be communicative (Prizant & Duchan, 1981; Prizant & Rydell, 1984). However, careful videotape analysis has revealed that echolalia can serve a range of interactive communicative functions. For example, echolalia might begin when the listener's attention is diverted

and persist until attention is gained; in this instance it appears to serve a "calling" function. In another case, echolalia might be used merely to fill a conversational turn. The child is facing the listener and it is the child's turn to talk, but there is no overt indication of communicative intent, such as heightened prosody, in the echolalic utterance.

It also has been speculated that the poor comprehension skills of children with autism may be a primary variable in causing echolalia (Fay, 1969). There is limited empirical support for this position. One study of 10 children with autism found a striking relationship between the frequency of echolalia in speech samples and scores on a standardized comprehension test (Roberts, 1989). It is possible, then, that echolalia is an adaptive response to breakdowns in comprehension. As understanding improves and other means become available for solving specific comprehension problems (e.g., requests for repetition or clarification), echolalia will no longer be needed and should, therefore, decrease in frequency.

Interestingly, as evidence has accumulated showing that echolalia serves various pragmatic purposes for children with autism, other research indicates that it does not seem to help in the acquisition of grammar. Studies comparing the spontaneous and immediately imitated utterances of children with autism have found that their echolalic utterances are less grammatically complex, with the possible exception of the early stages of acquisition (Howlin, 1982; Tager-Flusberg & Calkins, 1990). Thus, imitation does not appear to be the primary means by which new grammatical forms are learned, though it may play a more significant role in phonological or lexical acquisition.

Communicative Functions   Even though echolalia is frequent in many individuals with autism, it does not make up their total communication system. If echolalia is put to one side, what sorts of speech acts are most commonly performed by these children? Results from different studies on this question are not easily compared because of differences in the way verbal and nonverbal behaviors are classified. However, it appears reasonably clear that children with autism are most competent in performing instrumental communicative acts. These acts serve either to regulate the behavior of a conversational partner (e.g., by asking for an action to be performed or an object to be retrieved) or to comply with requests (e.g., by giving the partner a requested object). Children with autism are much less competent at gaining and directing the attention of the conversational partner, as might be achieved by making eye contact, pointing, or showing objects (Loveland, Landry, Hughes, Hall, & McEvoy, 1988; Mundy, Sigman, & Kasari, 1990; Mundy, Sigman, Ungerer, & Sherman, 1987; Stone & Caro-Martinez, 1990; Wetherby & Prutting, 1984). Compared to children with developmental language delay and typically developing children matched for language level, children with autism initiate communicative acts much less frequently (Loveland et al., 1988). They prefer, as a rule, to follow rather than lead in a conversation and to engage their partners at a level that requires little sharing of interest and attention (Frith, 1989).

The Concept of Asynchronous Development

Studies of the communicative functions used by children with autism have indicated that the frequency of those functions across categories is significantly different from that of other children. Those studies do not show, however, that the functions themselves are aberrant. Children with autism display the same communicative behaviors as typically developing children, but the profile of pragmatic functions they use is likely to be significantly different. It has been suggested that the essential problem is one of timing and sequence. Normal communicative functions are acquired in an abnormal order, so that at any one time, a child with autism may exhibit a set of behaviors that is developmentally scattered (Wetherby, 1986; Wetherby & Prutting, 1984; Wetherby, Yonclas, & Bryan, 1989). For example, children with autism commonly lack many of the joint attention functions seen in preverbal typically developing children, but they may possess other, more developmentally advanced functions such as requests for information. It has been suggested that this **asynchrony** in the emergence of pragmatic communication functions may be the result of underlying social and cognitive deficits in autism (Wetherby & Prutting, 1984). As with typically developing children,

the emergence of more advanced pragmatic behaviors appears to be correlated with the use of more symbolically advanced forms of communication (Stone & Caro-Martinez, 1990). As higher-level functions increase, so does the frequency of speech and gesture, replacing motoric acts and vocalization as the primary means of communication.

Facilitated Communication

No discussion of the communication abilities of children with autism is complete without considering the dramatic results being gained through facilitated communication. Yet, it is a remarkably simple procedure, as shown in Table 8.6. **Facilitated communication** is accomplished by means of various devices that have keyboard input and some type of readable output. This may be a computer, a specialized augmentative communication device, or just an electric typewriter.

It is not excessive to say that facilitated communication has burst on the clinical scene and defied the expectations of many professionals. As recently as 1983, for example, Schuler and Goetz wrote as follows about the potential of individuals with autism to communicate without speech:

> Overall conclusions, guidelines or recommendations regarding the use of nonspeech modes with the autistic population as a whole may never emerge or be substantiated. But what should be realized is that autistic individuals as a rule do not excel in nonverbal forms of communication, nor do they spontaneously make up signs or gestures. Because of their deficiencies of symbolic and communicative abilities, it would be unrealistic to expect dramatic breakthroughs. (p. 86)

Yet, what appears to occur for at least some individuals with autism who use facilitated communication *is* a dramatic breakthrough. Many of the impairments observed in spoken language, such as pronoun confusions and echolalia, are not present in the language they type on a keyboard (Biklen, 1992). Moreover, there have been stirring reports of changes in both the semantics and pragmatics of communication (Biklen, 1990a). Individuals with minimal ability to interact verbally have revealed in their facilitated messages a much higher than expected level of vocabulary, a greater attention span, a sense of humor, and an

TABLE 8.6   Elements of Facilitated Communication

Physical support	Adult supports the forearm or hand of the student, thereby helping to isolate the index finger and to slow movement toward the target on the keyboard or picture. Assistance is provided in *starting* movement toward the target, but the student is *not guided* to the target.
Initial training	Student is helped to gain accuracy in pointing by practicing with pictures, then advancing to letters, and finally to the keyboard.
Maintain focus	Adult reminds the student to keep watching the keyboard, to maintain a comfortable position for pointing, to keep the index finger isolated and extended, and to reduce extraneous actions such as hand flicking, screeching, or slapping objects. When echolalia occurs, the student is asked to type what he or she wants to say.
Avoid testing for competence	Adult encourages natural communication, providing appropriate amounts of encouragement. Students are *not* tested to determine their skill at communicating information.
Set-work	Initially students are given structured communication tasks in which their answers are fully or partly predictable, for example, math problems or sentence completion exercises. Communication is then gradually made more open-ended.
Fading physical support over time	The amount of support is gradually reduced over a period of months or years. For example, at first the adult may grasp the student's wrist, then merely support the wrist from below, then touch the sleeve, then stand adjacent but make no contact.

Source: Adapted from Biklen (1992) and Biklen and Schubert (1991).

awareness of and responsiveness to the mental state of their conversational partner. Judging from the anecdotal evidence, the number of topic initiations is considerably greater than those occurring in spoken conversations.

Taken as a whole, the much higher level of language abilities witnessed with facilitated communication may mean that "we must rethink the notion of autism as a social cognitive disability" (Biklen, 1992, p. 17). Most of the early writings on facilitated communication, however, have consisted of clinical descriptions of individuals who have benefited from the treatment. Often few details are provided about the social, educational, or communication histories of the subjects, so that it is unclear for whom the method is successful (Calculator, 1992; McLean, 1992). It has

not been claimed that facilitated communication will work effectively for all children with autism (Biklen & Schubert, 1991). Beyond the denial that it is a panacea, though, it is difficult to predict how many children can be helped. In the Australian clinic where the approach was pioneered, an assessment of 431 individuals over 5 years of age found that 70% of them were able to type a comprehensible sentence without a model (Crossley, 1992). Although not all the clients in this sample had been diagnosed with autism (all were intellectually impaired), the reported statistic does suggest that the number of candidates for facilitated communication is potentially large. However, some critics of the approach have raised the question: How much may the facilitator be influencing the child's communication and how much actually represents the child's own communication? What are needed now are more carefully controlled research studies to evaluate the approach.

IMPLICATIONS FOR INTERVENTION

All language disorders are complex and require careful assessment to sort out different levels of impairment. In children with autism, this complexity is raised one or more notches because of the intricate interactions between language, cognition, and social behavior, all of which are impaired at the same time. Faced with the enormity of the problems in this population, professionals have struggled to find effective intervention approaches. The lack of success many have experienced has resulted in an understandable tendency to abandon older methods whenever a recognizably new treatment comes along (McLean, 1992). Consequently, the swings in clinical practice have been wider in the area of autism than with other types of childhood language impairment. The current enthusiasm for facilitated communication is readily understandable when viewed in this historical context.

Regardless of the specific treatment approach a professional employs, it is important to understand and observe certain general principles of clinical practice. These principles should be consistent with the core information about autism reviewed to this point in the chapter.

Assessment

Assessment of children with autism is difficult and may not be appropriately done by the nonspecialist. Depending on the type of population they serve most frequently, many professionals may routinely use some norm-referenced tests to evaluate their clients. But the nature of the social impairment in children with autism makes most standardized testing unreliable. Many of these children lack the ability to attend to stimuli presented in a fixed manner; they may have no consistent verbal or nonverbal means of responding; and the responses they produce may be contaminated by the intrusion of echolalia or idiosyncratic language. The best results may therefore be obtained from a standardized observation protocol such as the *Au-tism Diagnostic Observation Schedule,* summarized in Table 8.7. In this procedure eight different tasks are presented to a child. Each task is intended to tap a different communicative behavior, with the aim of assessing the child's pragmatic abilities under a range of social and cognitive demands. The order of the tasks and the materials used can be varied to suit the age of the child and the flow of the interaction. The flexibility of the tasks and the technique of subtly "pressing" the child to produce certain kinds of communicative behaviors are well designed to meet the challenges presented by individuals with autism.

Service Model

As we have seen elsewhere in this text, the traditional model for providing intervention in the schools has been to remove a child from the classroom and provide brief therapy sessions at another location. This pull-out model makes several assumptions about the entry-level skills and motivation of the child that are not tenable for children with autism (Peck & Schuler, 1983). It is designed to supplement, not replace, an

TABLE 8.7 Components of the Autism Diagnostic Observation Schedule

Task	Target Behavior(s)
Construction task	Asking for help
Unstructured presentation of toys	Symbolic play
	Reciprocal play
	Giving help to interviewer
Drawing game	Taking turns in a structured task
Demonstration task	Descriptive gesture and mime
Poster task	Description of agents and actions
Book task	Telling a sequential story
Conversation	Reciprocal communication
Socioemotional questions	Ability to use language to discuss socioemotional topics

Source: Adapted from Lord et al. (1989), p. 189.

academic curriculum and, therefore, presupposes a minimum level of language development, an ability to learn and generalize, and a motivation to acquire language that may not be present in a child with autism. When the traditional model fails, creative approaches must be tried that balance structure and flexibility. As we have seen, many children with autism insist that routines be observed and will become highly distressed if they are not. It is therefore important that intervention approaches cater adequately to this need. On the other hand, programs that are too structured may not allow children to develop skills in the use of natural language (Prizant, 1982). The result may be language that appears unnatural to others and does not generalize well outside of the school setting. Efforts at developing a collaborative service model to address the needs of all handicapped children in school are especially important for individuals with autism.

The timing of services is another issue pertinent to intervention with autism. As noted earlier in this chapter, autism is rarely identified by infant screenings conducted during the first 18 months but is recognized in nearly all cases before 36 months of age. The implication, of course, is that one does not find infant stimulation programs for children with autism of the type that exist for other conditions (e.g., Down syndrome). On the other hand, it is not necessary—and indeed, would be ill-advised—to wait until a child with autism is of school age before initiating services. Evaluation of one early intervention program for high-functioning preschool children with autism found that they made significant developmental gains, as measured by IQ scores and standardized language test scores (Harris, Handleman, Gordon, Kristoff, & Fuentes, 1991). Some of the children were mainstreamed with typically developing preschoolers, while others were enrolled in a class consisting solely of individuals with autism. Interestingly, both groups showed equivalent gains in language ability (Harris, Handleman, Kristoff, Bass, & Gordon, 1990).

Special Considerations

Children with autism are known to have a number of associated problems (see Table 8.3) that may require special management during intervention. It is plain that all children must be evaluated and, if appropriate, treated for hearing loss and seizure, two conditions where there appears to be elevated risk in autism. The hypersensitivity of certain children may also dictate a change in teaching methods. Touch can be used to guide or reinforce—it is, for example, used systematically in facilitated communication—but a period of adjustment may be needed. Because of the auditory sensitivity of many children with autism, behavioral problems may be reduced if visual and physical prompts are used instead of verbal explanations (Schuler & Goetz, 1983).

As we have seen, studies of the communicative functions used by children with autism indicate that they emerge in a different sequence than in typically developing children (Loveland, Landry, Hughes, Hall, & McEvoy, 1988; Wetherby & Prutting, 1984). One may argue, therefore, that language intervention should be structured to reflect this different order of acquisition (Wetherby, 1986). Specifically, it should be expected that a child with autism will establish instrumental functions before ones that attract or direct attention. This means that in the first stage of intervention the goal may be to facilitate requests or protests. Procedures that often induce a communicative need for requests and protests, such as placing objects out of reach, withholding an important part of a toy, or sabotaging a play activity, are described in chapter 15 and in other therapy texts (e.g., Fey, 1986). It is not certain, however, whether such techniques are effective for children with autism. One study has found that neither adult direction (e.g., looking at and tapping an object) nor procedures designed to motivate communication (e.g., not sharing a desired food) increased joint attention behaviors (Landry & Loveland, 1989).

At the second stage of intervention, children with autism can be encouraged to use communications that attract attention to themselves. The inherent tendency toward ritualistic behavior might be used to establish behaviors such as greeting or requesting a social routine (e.g., playing pattycake or peekaboo). At the third stage, children may be taught functions that direct another person's attention. The earliest of these are labeling an object and commenting on an environmental event. The behaviors themselves can be introduced through various modeling approaches, discussed in chapters 6 and 15. Clinicians should be mindful, however, that children with autism often begin to direct others' attention by means of echolalia (Prizant & Duchan, 1981; Prizant & Rydell, 1984). Hence, it is important to monitor the child's contextual use of echolalia and evaluate whether changes in that behavior indicate the emergence of more sophisticated communicative functions.

Intervention Models

Duchan (1984) identified behaviorism, psycholinguistic theory, and social interaction theory as the intellectual sources for different methods used in the treatment of autism. Though many current intervention approaches borrow elements from all of these models, the distinction remains useful for sorting among various methods.

Behaviorism   In the 1960s and 1970s the elements of behavior modification were applied with great enthusiasm to the treatment of autism (Lovaas, 1977). Behavioral methods begin by analyzing language behaviors into a detailed series of steps. For example, to teach a child to name might require training the following behaviors in sequence: sitting, attending to the trainer's face, nonverbal imitation, verbal imitation, labeling in response to questions, and labeling in response to other stimuli. Behavior modification was also used to decrease self-injurious behavior and promote social interaction.

During this early period of investigation, both rewarding and **aversive** stimuli were employed to establish operant control over a behavior. In one notorious experiment, electric shock was used as a negative reinforcer (Lovaas, Schaeffer, & Simmons, 1965). Most recent behaviorist proposals, however, are strictly nonaversive. Desirable behaviors, such as the acquisition of specific signing skills, have been taught through a sequence of prompting, fading, stimulus rotation (the systematic introduction of new targets), and reinforcement (Carr, Kologinsky, & Leff-Simon, 1987). Undesirable behaviors have also been reduced by teaching a replacement behavior. For example, autistic leading—a request made by grasping an adult's wrist and leading him or her to the desired object—was diminished by teaching children to point to what they wanted (Carr & Kemp, 1989). Delayed echolalia was reduced in one child by observing the behavior and discovering that it served the communicative function of requesting help. The child was then taught an appropriate substitute behavior, the request "Help me" (Durand & Crimmins, 1987).

Psycholinguistic Theory   Early behavior modification programs to teach language were characterized by massed practice, a specialized treatment setting, and instructional episodes initiated by an adult (Carr et al., 1987). These techniques were effective in training new forms, but they often failed to produce results that generalized outside of the training sessions and yielded true communication. To meet this problem, many current intervention programs now emphasize *incidental teaching,* a technique in which teaching interactions occur in a child's typical environment (home or classroom) and are allowed to arise naturally out of the situation that transpires (see chapter 6). Comparisons of incidental teaching with traditional behaviorist methods have indicated that the more natural method is just as efficient in establishing new language behaviors in individuals with autism and is more effective in promoting generalization to everyday settings (Elliott, Hall, & Soper, 1991; Koegel, O'Dell, & Koegel, 1987). The method lends itself to classroom use and can be taught effectively to classroom teachers (Dyer, Williams, & Luce, 1991).

Social Interaction Theory   In contrast to the methods that grow out of behavioral and psycholinguistic theory, *social interaction theory* does not recommend a specific intervention strategy (Duchan, 1984). Instead, it offers a perspective on communicative interactions and suggests that some of the pragmatic deficits associated with autism may arise when adults do not make good conversational adjustments. For example, one study of four children with autism talking to their mothers and teachers found that the children produced more adequate responses when adults asked yes/no questions, questions that were conceptually simple, and questions that were related to the child's topic (Curcio & Paccia, 1987). Duchan

(1983) analyzed the interaction among a 9-year-old child with autism, his speech-language pathologist, and his mother. She discovered that the adults rarely departed from a teaching mode of conversation. They consistently set the topic and used directive communication acts to elicit specific responses from the child. This, in turn, led the child to produce a very narrow range of communicative behaviors. There is no simple solution to this problem. Duchan points out that attempts to be nurturing are generally ineffective with children with autism because they tend to remain socially withdrawn. When a child does not act spontaneously, adults are thwarted from using nurturing behaviors such as utterance expansions and responses related to the child's topic. The solution Duchan suggests is to (1) modify directive behaviors so that they allow more flexibility of response, for example, asking questions that have several correct answers, and (2) show nurturance by construing abnormal behaviors as normal, for example, responding to the intent of an echolalic utterance rather than its content.

The insights from social interaction theory can be applied to intervention in three areas:

1. Professionals can observe or record conversations between children and their parents or teachers. By coding the types of utterances produced by the adult(s) and the adequacy of the child's responses, it is possible to determine any relationships between the two. This may lead to recommendations to the adults that they increase certain behaviors and decrease others to promote more adequate language use by the child.

2. Professionals should observe themselves and carry out the same type of analysis on their own interaction with the child. Many clinical conversations contain stimuli that are intended to be facilitating (e.g., requests for repetition or clarification) but that may have undesirable effects on a child with autism.

3. If a child with autism is enrolled in a classroom with typically developing children, then social interaction analysis can be used to improve the effectiveness of peer-mediated intervention. In *peer-mediated programs,* typically developing children are shown how to initiate social interactions with children with

autism, for example, by commenting on what an impaired child is doing or by offering to share a toy. Once the typically developing children have been shown how to make initiations, they are verbally prompted to do so. Then, gradually, prompts are eliminated so that the behavior becomes spontaneous (Odom & Watts, 1991). Early analysis of how children with autism interact with adults or with their unimpaired peers may indicate what types of gambits are most successful at stimulating social interactions. These gambits would then become the ones taught to all of the typically developing children involved in the intervention program.

Nonspeech Options

Communication training for children with autism is not limited to spoken language. As in children with mental retardation, the decision on whether to teach speech is a fundamental one that will have an impact on all subsequent intervention efforts. The case for teaching nonverbal communication to children with autism has always been stronger than the case for teaching it to children with mental retardation. At least three arguments can be advanced in its favor:

1. Most children with autism appear to have mental retardation as well as the unique social and communicative impairments characteristic of autism. They therefore appear to be doubly (or triply) thwarted in their ability to acquire speech.
2. There is evidence that the auditory systems of children with autism are somehow different from those of typically developing children (Konstantareas, 1985). Whether these differences are responsible for their difficulty in oral communication is unknown, but they do provide a rationale for teaching language through visual and tactile-kinesthetic stimulation.
3. Certain attributes of children with autism, such as their poor eye contact, insistence on routines, and interest in mechanical devices, suggest that they might be well matched with alternative/augmentative communication systems.

Sign Language It is apparent from a number of published studies that sign language alone or simul-

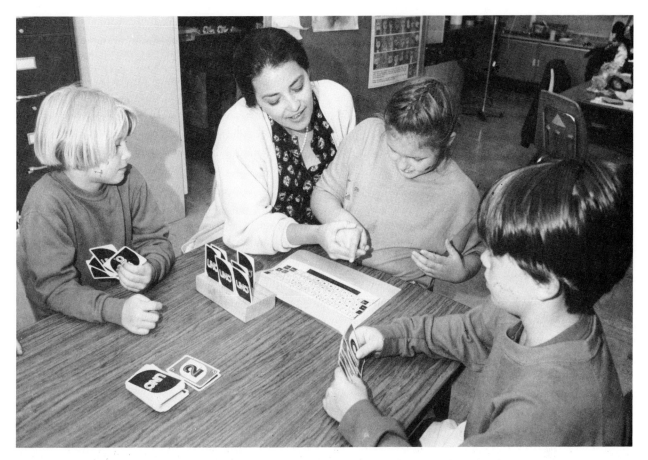

Alternative forms of communication may help children with autism interact socially with others.

taneous communication (sign and speech) training can produce effective communication skills in children with autism (Konstantareas, 1985). These methods seem particularly effective during the beginning stages of language learning. Research has not yet settled the issue of whether sign language training interferes with the learning or use of speech. Some investigators maintain that sign language has either no effect or a facilitating effect on speech acquisition (Konstantareas, 1985). Other findings support the view that at least some children with autism—those who are poor at verbal imitation—are visually "overselective" and tune out speech in favor of visual stimuli (Yoder & Layton, 1988). At this point, the general conclusion must be that sign language training may be effective but may not be equally so for all children

with autism. Future studies may help clinicians to determine which children are the best candidates for this type of intervention.

Facilitated Communication   As mentioned earlier, facilitated communication has produced some spectacular successes and has provoked considerable debate among professionals. In reexamining Table 8.6, a critical element in this method is *support,* both physical and social-emotional. It is a basic tenet of facilitated communication that individuals with autism should be treated no differently from other competent communicators (Biklen, 1990a). Pains are taken to avoid condescending practices such as speaking in a caretaker register (with a slower rate and exaggerated intonation), simplifying messages, or providing unnaturally high rates of reinforcement. The skill required for facilitated communication is for the adult facilitator to straddle the line between adequate and excessive support. If too little physical support is provided, a child with autism will be unable to overcome what is believed to be an impairment in the initiation of voluntary movement (Biklen, 1990a). If too much physical support is given, then it may not be possible to sense the child's hand movement and the adult may begin unwittingly to guide the movement. Similarly, if emotional support is not present in the form of encouragement, praise, and responsiveness to the child's messages, then motivation may lag. But too much encouragement may appear insincere and may cause the child to lose confidence in the adult. Experience with facilitated communication has demonstrated that confidence is an essential ingredient in success. When children are asked to communicate with new partners,

they commonly appear to regress in ability and require more support (Crossley, 1991).

Beyond the basic elements of facilitated communication, it is occasionally necessary to troubleshoot specific motoric problems (e.g., abnormal muscle tone, difficulty in extending the index finger, tremor) or abnormal patterns of response (e.g., perseveration on the same selection, impulsive movement). Specific procedures have been recommended to deal with these complications (Crossley, 1991). Communication can also be problematic when an individual with autism has echolalic or idiosyncratic language that interferes with attempts to communicate through typed messages. This difficulty is overcome by showing understanding of the condition, asking the impaired individual to try not to speak, and ignoring inappropriate speech when it occurs. If necessary, the adult may stop speaking and join with the child in typing messages (Biklen, 1990b).

SUMMARY

In this chapter we have seen that:

▶ Autism is a developmental rather than an emotional or psychiatric disorder. Evidence suggests that it has a genetic basis, though a single cause has yet to be identified.

▶ Autism is the most severe of a range of pervasive developmental disorders, all of which are characterized by social, communicative, and cognitive deficits.

▶ Children with autism are heterogeneous. Consequently, the diagnostic criteria established in DSM-III-R specify a wide range of behaviors as signs of the disorder. All children diagnosed with autism must exhibit some impairment in each of the categories of social interaction, communication and imagination, and a repertoire of activities and interests.

▶ Autism is associated with a number of sensory and motor handicaps. These handicaps are not found in all individuals with autism, however, and they are not included among the diagnostic criteria for the disorder.

▶ Autism is identified in nearly all children between 18 and 36 months of age, with more severe cases tending to be identified earlier.

▶ Certain language abilities tend to be relatively preserved in autism; that is, they are commensurate with the MA of the child. Segmental phonology and syntax, lexical and syntactic comprehension, and imitation are the abilities in this category.

▶ Language abilities that appear to be specifically impaired in children with autism are nonsegmental phonology and pronominal use. These children produce language that is frequently idiosyncratic or echolalic. Pragmatically, they are delayed in their use of language to share or direct attention, and they infrequently produce communicative acts considered to be initiating.

▶ An underlying cognitive deficit in children with autism may be their inability to think about and compare their own and others' mental states.

▶ Experiences with facilitated communication have challenged many of the prevailing notions about autism. Children communicating by means of typed messages, aided by the physical and emotional support of an adult, have sometimes demonstrated linguistic, cognitive, and social abilities previously unrecognized and unexpected.

▶ Intervention for children with autism requires special skills in assessment and a nontraditional service delivery model. Treatment methods based on principles of behaviorism, psycholinguistic theory, and social interaction theory have all been used successfully to promote verbal language learning and reduce aberrant communication behaviors.

▶ Communication by means other than speech is an increasingly popular intervention option. Both sign language and facilitated communication appear to be effective options. Facilitated communication, in particular, appears to offer the potential for achieving dramatic gains for at least some individuals.

Autism is often described as an enigmatic disorder because of its mysterious origin and the unusual behaviors that characterize it. Recent research has added to our understanding of autism but, at the same time, has raised new questions about the abilities of children with the disorder. Our views of what autism is and how it can be remediated seem destined to change—perhaps fundamentally—over the next few years. Stay tuned.

REFERENCES

American Psychiatric Association. (1980). *Diagnostic and statistical manual of mental disorders* (third edition). Washington, DC: American Psychiatric Association.

American Psychiatric Association. (1987). *Diagnostic and statistical manual of mental disorders* (third edition, revised). Washington, DC: American Psychiatric Association.

Baltaxe, C., & Guthrie, D. (1987). The use of primary sentence stress by normal, aphasic, and autistic children. *Journal of Autism and Developmental Disorders, 17,* 255–271.

Baltaxe, C., & Simmons, J. Q. (1985). Prosodic development in normal and autistic children. In E. Schopler & G. Mesibov (Eds.), *Communication problems in autism.* New York: Plenum Press.

Baron-Cohen, S. (1988). Social and pragmatic deficits in autism: Cognitive or affective? *Journal of Autism and Developmental Disorders, 18,* 379–402.

Baron-Cohen, S. (1991). Do people with autism understand what causes emotion? *Child Development, 62,* 385–395.

Bartolucci, G., Pierce, S., Streiner, D., & Eppel, P. (1976). Phonological investigation of verbal autistic and mentally retarded subjects. *Journal of Autism and Childhood Schizophrenia, 6,* 303–316.

Beisler, J. M., Tsai, L. Y., & Vonk, D. (1987). Comparisons between autistic and nonautistic children on the Test for Auditory Comprehension of Language. *Journal of Autism and Developmental Disorders, 17,* 95–102.

Bettelheim, B. (1967). *The empty fortress: Infantile autism and the birth of the self.* New York: Free Press.

Biklen, D. (1990a). Communication unbound: Autism and praxis. *Harvard Educational Review, 60,* 291–314.

Biklen, D. (1990b). *Facilitated communication with people who have speech.* Unpublished manuscript.

Biklen, D. (1992). Typing to talk: Facilitated communication. *American Journal of Speech-Language Pathology, 1(2),* 15–17, 21–22.

Biklen, D., & Schubert, A. (1991). New words: The communication of students with autism. *Remedial and Special Education, 12,* 46–57.

Bishop, D. V. M. (1989). Autism, Asperger's syndrome and semantic-pragmatic disorder: Where are the boundaries? *British Journal of Disorders of Communication, 24,* 107–121.

Boucher, J. (1976). Articulation in early childhood autism. *Journal of Autism and Childhood Schizophrenia, 6,* 297–302.

Calculator, S. N. (1992). Perhaps the emperor has clothes after all: A response to Biklen. *American Journal of Speech-Language Pathology, 1,* 18–20, 23–24.

Cantwell, D. P., Howlin, P., & Rutter, M. L. (1977). The analysis of language level and language function. *British Journal of Disorders of Communication, 12,* 119–135.

Carr, E. G., & Kemp, D. C. (1989). Functional equivalence of autistic leading and communicative pointing: Analysis and treatment. *Journal of Autism and Developmental Disorders, 19,* 561–578.

Carr, E. G., Kologinsky, E., & Leff-Simon, S. (1987). Acquisition of sign language by autistic children. III: Generalized descriptive phrases. *Journal of Autism and Developmental Disorders, 17,* 217–229.

Coggins, T. E., & Frederickson, R. (1988). Brief report: The communicative role of a highly frequent repeated utterance in the conversations of an autistic boy. *Journal of Autism and Developmental Disorders, 18,* 687–694.

Courchesne, E. (1987). A neurophysiological view of autism. In E. Schopler & G. B. Mesibov (Eds.), *Neurobiological issues in autism* (pp. 285–324). New York: Plenum Press.

Crossley, R. (1991). Communication training involving facilitated communication. *Communicating Together, 9,* 19 22.

Crossley, R. (1992). Lending a hand: A personal account of the development of facilitated communication training. *American Journal of Speech-Language Pathology, 1,* 15–18.

Crystal, D. (1981) *Clinical linguistics.* New York: Springer-Verlag.

Curcio, F., & Paccia, J. (1987). Conversations with autistic children: Contingent relationships between features of adult input and children's response adequacy. *Journal of Autism and Developmental Disorders, 17,* 81–93.

Dahl, E. K., Cohen, D. J., & Provence, S. (1986). Clinical and multivariate approaches to the nosology of pervasive developmental disorders. *Journal of the American Academy of Child Psychiatry, 25,* 170–180.

Duchan, J. F. (1983). Autistic children are noninteractive: Or so we say. *Seminars in Speech and Language, 4,* 53–61.

Duchan, J. F. (1984). Clinical interactions with autistic children: The role of theory. *Topics in Language Disorders, 4,* 62–71.

Durand, V. M., & Crimmins, D. B. (1987). Assessment and treatment of psychotic speech in an autistic child. *Journal of Autism and Developmental Disorders, 17,* 17–28.

Dyer, K., Williams, L., & Luce, S. C. (1991). Training teachers to use naturalistic communication strategies in classrooms for students with autism and other severe handicaps. *Language, Speech, and Hearing Services in Schools, 22,* 313–321.

Elliott, R. O., Hall, K., & Soper, H. V. (1991). Analog language teaching versus natural language teaching: Generalization and retention of language learning for adults with autism and mental retardation. *Journal of Autism and Developmental Disorders, 21,* 433–447.

Eskes, G. A., Bryson, S. E., & McCormick, T. A. (1990). Comprehension of concrete and abstract words in autistic children. *Journal of Autism and Developmental Disorders, 20,* 61–73.

Fay, W. H. (1969). On the basis of autistic echolalia. *Journal of Communication Disorders, 2,* 38–49.

Fay, W. H. (1980). Aspects of language. In W. H. Fay & A. Schuler (Eds.), *Emerging language in autistic children.* Baltimore: University Park Press.

Fein, D., Pennington, B., Markowitz, P., Braverman, M., & Waterhouse, L. (1986). Toward a neuropsychological model of infantile autism: Are the social deficits primary? *Journal of the American Academy of Child Psychiatry, 25,* 198–212.

Fey, M. E. (1986). *Language intervention with young children.* Boston: College-Hill Press.

Folstein, S. E., & Rutter, M. L. (1988). Autism: Familial aggregation and genetic implications. *Journal of Autism and Developmental Disorders, 18,* 3–30.

Frankel, F., Simmons, J. Q., & Richey, V. E. (1987). Reward value of prosodic features of language for autistic, mentally retarded, and normal children. *Journal of Autism and Developmental Disorders, 17,* 103–113.

Frith, U. (1989). A new look at language and communication in autism. *British Journal of Disorders of Communication, 24,* 123–150.

Fulkerson, S. C., & Freeman, W. H. (1980). Perceptual-motor deficiency in autistic children. *Perceptual and Motor Skills, 50,* 331–336.

Gillberg, C. (1991). Outcome in autism and autistic-like conditions. *Journal of the American Academy of Child and Adolescent Psychiatry, 30,* 375–382.

Goldfarb, W., Braunstein, P., & Lorge, I. (1956) A study of speech patterns in a group of schizophrenic children. *American Journal of Orthopsychiatry, 26,* 544–555.

Harris, S. L., Handleman, J. S., Gordon, R., Kristoff, B., & Fuentes, F. (1991). Changes in cognitive and language functioning of preschool children with autism. *Journal of Autism and Developmental Disorders, 21,* 281–290.

Harris, S. L., Handleman, J. S., Kristoff, B., Bass, L., & Gordon, R. (1990). Changes in language development among autistic and peer children in segregated and integrated preschool settings. *Journal of Autism and Developmental Disorders, 20,* 23–31.

Howlin, P. (1982). Echolalic and spontaneous phrase speech in autistic children. *Journal of Child Psychology and Psychiatry, 23,* 281–293.

Johnson, M. H., Siddons, F., Frith, U., & Morton, J. (1992). Can autism be predicted on the basis of infant screening tests? *Developmental Medicine and Child Neurology, 34,* 316–320.

Kanner, L. (1943). Autistic disturbances of affective contact. *Nervous Child, 2,* 217–250.

Klin, A. (1991). Young autistic children's listening preferences in regard to speech: A possible characterization of the symptom of social withdrawal. *Journal of Autism and Developmental Disorders, 21,* 29–42.

Koegel, R. L., O'Dell, M. C., & Koegel, L. K. (1987). A natural language teaching paradigm for nonverbal autistic children. *Journal of Autism and Developmental Disorders, 17,* 187–200.

Konstantareas, M. M. (1985). Review of evidence on the relevance of sign language in early communication training of autistic children. *Australian Journal of Human Communication Disorders, 13,* 81–101.

Konstantareas, M. M., & Homatidis, S. (1987). Brief report: Ear infections in autistic and normal children. *Journal of Autism and Developmental Disorders, 17,* 585–593.

Landa, R., Folstein, S. E., & Isaacs, C. (1991). Spontaneous narrative-discourse performance of parents of autistic individuals. *Journal of Speech and Hearing Research, 34,* 1339–1345.

Landry, S. H., & Loveland, K. A. (1989). The effect of social context on the functional communication skills of autistic children. *Journal of Autism and Developmental Disorders, 19,* 283–299.

Lord, C., Rutter, M. L., Goode, S., Heemsbergen, J., Jordan, H., Mawhood, L., & Schopler, E. (1989). Autism diagnostic observation schedule: A standardized observation of communicative and social behavior. *Journal of Autism and Developmental Disorders, 19,* 185–212.

Lord, C., & Schopler, E. (1985). Differences in sex ratios in autism as a function of measured intelligence. *Journal of Autism and Developmental Disorders, 15,* 185–193.

Lord, C., & Schopler, E. (1989). The role of age at assessment, developmental level, and test in the stability of intelligence scores in young autistic children. *Journal of Autism and Developmental Disorders, 19,* 483–499.

Lord, C., Schopler, E., & Revicki, D. (1982). Sex differences in autism. *Journal of Autism and Developmental Disorders, 12,* 317–330.

Lovaas, O. I. (1977). *The autistic child: Language development through behavior modification.* New York: Irvington.

Lovaas, O. I., Schaeffer, B., & Simmons, J. Q. (1965). Building social behavior in autistic children by use of electric shock. *Journal of Experimental Research in Personality, 1,* 99–109.

Loveland, K. A., Landry, S. H., Hughes, S. O., Hall, S. K., & McEvoy, R. E. (1988). Speech acts and the pragmatic deficits of autism. *Journal of Speech and Hearing Research, 31,* 593–604.

Maurer, R. G., & Damasio, A. R. (1982). Childhood autism from the point of view of behavioral neurology. *Journal of Autism and Developmental Disorders, 12,* 195–205.

McLean, J. (1992). Facilitated communication: Some thoughts on Biklen's and Calculator's interaction. *American Journal of Speech-Language Pathology, 1,* 25–27.

Menyuk, P., & Wilbur, R. (1981). Preface to special issue on language disorders. *Journal of Autism and Developmental Disorders, 11,* 1–13.

Mundy, P., Sigman, M. D., & Kasari, C. (1990). A longitudinal study of joint attention and language development in autistic children. *Journal of Autism and Developmental Disorders, 20,* 115–128.

Mundy, P., Sigman, M. D., Ungerer, J. A., & Sherman, T. (1987). Nonverbal communication and play correlates of language development in autistic children. *Journal of Autism and Developmental Disorders, 17,* 349–364.

Odom, S. L., & Watts, E. (1991). Reducing teacher prompts in peer-mediated interventions for young children with autism. *Journal of Special Education, 25,* 26–33.

Oshima-Takane, Y., & Benaroya, S. (1989). An alternative view of pronominal errors in autistic children. *Journal of Autism and Developmental Disorders, 19,* 73–85.

Peck, C. A., & Schuler, A. L. (1983). Classroom-based language intervention for children with autism: Theoretical and practical considerations for the speech and language specialist. *Seminars in Speech and Language, 4,* 93–103.

Piven, J., Chase, G. A., Landa, R., Wzorek, M., Gayle, J., Cloud, D., & Folstein, S. E. (1991). Psychiatric disorders in the parents of autistic individuals. *Journal of the American Academy of Child and Adolescent Psychiatry, 30,* 471–478.

Piven, J., Gayle, J., Landa, R., Wzorek, M., & Folstein, S. E. (1991). The prevalence of Fragile X in a sample of autistic individuals diagnosed using a standardized interview. *Journal of the American Academy of Child and Adolescent Psychiatry, 30,* 825–830.

Prizant, B. M. (1982). Speech-language pathologists and autistic children: What is our role? *Asha, 24,* 531–539.

Prizant, B. M., & Duchan, J. F. (1981). The functions of immediate echolalia in autistic children. *Journal of Speech and Hearing Disorders, 46,* 241–249.

Prizant, B. M., & Rydell, P. J. (1984). Analysis of functions of delayed echolalia in autistic children. *Journal of Speech and Hearing Research, 27,* 183–192.

Roberts, J. M. A. (1989). Echolalia and comprehension in autistic children. *Journal of Autism and Developmental Disorders, 19,* 271–281.

Rutter, M. L. (1978). Diagnosis and definition of childhood autism. *Journal of Autism and Childhood Schizophrenia, 8,* 139–161.

Rutter, M. L., & Schopler, E. (1987). Autism and pervasive developmental disorders: Concepts and diagnostic issues. *Journal of Autism and Developmental Disorders, 17,* 159–186.

Schuler, A. L., & Goetz, L. (1983). Toward communicative competence: Matters of method, content, and mode of instruction. *Seminars in Speech and Language, 4,* 79–91.

Short, A. B., & Schopler, E. (1988). Factors relating to age of onset in autism. *Journal of Autism and Developmental Disorders, 18,* 207–216.

Siegel, B., Vukicevic, J., Elliott, G. R., & Kraemer, H. C. (1989). The use of signal detection theory to assess DSM-III-R criteria for autistic disorder. *Journal of the American Academy of Child and Adolescent Psychiatry, 28,* 542–548.

Simon, N. (1975). Echolalic speech in childhood autism. *Archives of General Psychiatry, 32,* 1439–1446.

Smith, D. E. P., Miller, S. D., Stewart, M., Walter, T. L., & McConnell, J. V. (1988). Conductive hearing loss in autistic, learning-disabled, and normal children. *Journal of Autism and Developmental Disorders, 18,* 53–65.

Stone, W. L., & Caro-Martinez, L. M. (1990). Naturalistic observations of spontaneous communication in autistic children. *Journal of Autism and Developmental Disorders, 20,* 437–453.

Tager-Flusberg, H. (1981). On the nature of linguistic functioning in early infantile autism. *Journal of Autism and Developmental Disorders, 11,* 45–56.

Tager-Flusberg, H. (1992). Autistic children's talk about psychological states: Deficits in the early acquisition of a theory of mind. *Child Development, 63,* 161–172.

Tager-Flusberg, H., & Calkins, S. (1990). Does imitation facilitate the acquisition of grammar? Evidence from a study of autistic, Down's syndrome and normal children. *Journal of Child Language, 17,* 591–606.

Vicker, B., & Monahan, M. (1988). The diagnosis of autism by state agencies. *Journal of Autism and Developmental Disorders, 18,* 231–240.

Volden, J., & Lord, C. (1991). Neologisms and idiosyncratic language in autistic speakers. *Journal of Autism and Developmental Disorders, 21,* 109–130.

Volkmar, F. R., & Nelson, D. S. (1990). Seizure disorders in autism. *Journal of the American Academy of Child and Adolescent Psychiatry, 29,* 127–129.

Wetherby, A. M. (1986). Ontogeny of communicative functions in autism. *Journal of Autism and Developmental Disorders, 16,* 295–316.

Wetherby, A. M. (1989). Language intervention for autistic children: A look at where we have come in the past 25 years. *Journal of Speech Language Pathology and Audiology, 13,* 15–28.

Wetherby, A. M., & Prutting, C. A. (1984). Profiles of communicative and cognitive-social abilities in autistic children. *Journal of Speech and Hearing Research, 27,* 364–377.

Wetherby, A. M., Yonclas, D. G., & Bryan, A. A. (1989). Communicative profiles of preschool children with handicaps: Implications for early identification. *Journal of Speech and Hearing Disorders, 54,* 148–158.

Wing, L. (1981). Language, social, and cognitive impairments in autism and severe mental retardation. *Journal of Autism and Developmental Disorders, 11,* 31–44.

Yirmiya, N., Sigman, M. D., Kasari, C., & Mundy, P. (1992). Empathy and cognition in high-functioning children with autism. *Child Development, 63,* 150–160.

Yoder, P. J., & Layton, T. L. (1988). Speech following sign language training in autistic children with minimal verbal language. *Journal of Autism and Developmental Disorders, 18,* 217–229.

Chapter 9

Language and Hearing-Impaired Children

Stephanie D. Shaw

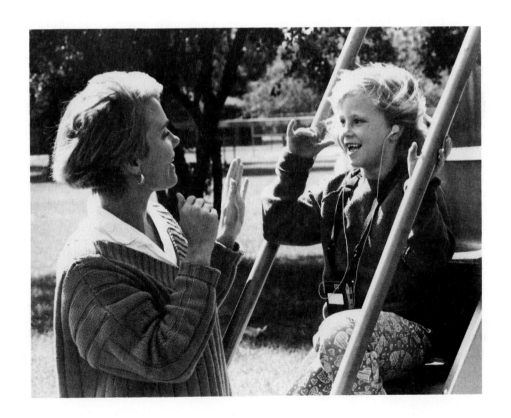

OBJECTIVES

Upon completion of this chapter, the reader should be able to:

- ▶ Define and describe mild to profound hearing impairments and their etiologies, and the impact of various degrees of loss on communication skills.

- ▶ Understand additional factors contributing to the performance of the child.

- ▶ Understand the complex interplay of speech acoustics and background noise in affecting speech perception.

- ▶ Describe the impact that hearing impairment has on oral language in terms of syntax, morphology, semantics, pragmatics, segmental and suprasegmental speech aspects, and intelligibility.

- ▶ Relate language skills to academic achievement and communication choices.

- ▶ Understand the essential aspects of intervention, including early identification, sound amplification systems, and educational management.

There is no question that hearing losses in children interfere with their acquisition of oral language, and the degree of disability from a hearing impairment is often measured in terms of its effects on communication. In this chapter, we review aspects of hearing loss as they relate to speech and language performance. We also discuss academic achievement as it relates to children with hearing impairments. Although hearing loss can occur in association with other disabling conditions, such as mental retardation, loss of vision, or cerebral palsy, this chapter focuses on children for whom hearing loss is the primary or sole problem.

AN OVERVIEW OF HEARING-IMPAIRED CHILDREN AND HEARING IMPAIRMENT

Hearing impairment, also called *hearing loss,* is a general term. It refers to difficulty in hearing at the same levels and with the same discriminative powers as other people. It produces a deficit in the sensitivity of the ear that can affect both loudness and clarity.

Hearing impairments are described in a number of ways. For example, they can be described with reference to etiology or the site of the lesion. Most commonly, they are described in terms of degree of loss, whereby the hearing deficit is quantified to give a **decibel** level. This is an average taken across some of the frequencies used in testing hearing. The hearing level obtained is then compared to a decibel range of normal hearing. Typically, what is known as the *three frequency average* is used, which is the average across 500, 1,000, and 2,000 Hertz (Hz) in the better ear.

A number of classification systems are available, most of which carry a functional descriptor with the degree of loss. The classification system that will be used here is that of Boothroyd (1982), which is based on extensive work on the speech perception capabilities of hearing-impaired children. Table 9.1 shows this classification system.

Decibel notation needs some explanation. Measures in decibels hearing level (dB HL) are those obtained when a hearing test is performed in the conventional way, using an audiometer and pure tone signals. These (dB HL) are weighted with a correction factor to make reporting of pure tone audiogram results easier, as the human ear is not equally sensitive at all frequencies. Decibels sound pressure level (dB SPL) is used to measure levels of speech and classroom background noise and the output of hearing aids. Measures in dB SPL do not have the correction factor to take account of the sensitivity of the ear. The

TABLE 9.1 Hearing Levels and Descriptions

Group	Hearing Level (dB HL)	Description
I	− 0–14	Normal hearing
II	15–30	Mild impairment
III	31–60	Moderate impairment
IV	61–90	Severe impairment
V	91–120	Profound impairment
VI	121 +	Total impairment

Source: Adapted from Boothroyd (1982).

differences in the two measures are not great, but information in texts on hearing impairment is presented both in dB HL and in dB SPL.

The term *hearing impairment* includes all forms of disability, ranging from mild to severe and profound. Depending on the effects of the hearing impairment, children are also described as hard of hearing or deaf. *Audition* is the primary means by which *hard-of-hearing* children acquire speech and language. It remains the modality for speech perception, despite the fact that amplification is usually required. Supplementary information comes from the visual channel, as it does for normally hearing individuals. In contrast, a *deaf* or *profoundly hearing-impaired* child is one who is unable to use the auditory channel as the primary means of acquiring speech and language or of maintaining communication. Deaf children rely much more on the visual and tactile channels as the primary input modalities for speech and language acquisition and maintenance (Boothroyd, 1982; Brill, MacNeil, & Newman, 1986).

From the point of view of intervention, the two groups of hearing-impaired children often have very different needs, as they have different primary input modalities. Attempts have been made to use an average hearing level in decibels to delineate deaf from hard-of-hearing children, and a number of different levels have been suggested. Children with hearing losses below 90 dB HL are regarded as deaf or profoundly impaired by Boothroyd (1982), whereas Ross (1982) puts the dividing line at around 95 dB HL, and Moores (1987) and Northern and Downs (1991) put the line at around 70 dB HL. The major problem with using an average hearing level is that the ability to understand speech cannot be predicted from a pure tone audiogram. Therefore, it may be unwise to attempt to define a cutoff point. Generally, the greater the degree of hearing loss, the more difficulty will be experienced with speech perception, or the understanding of speech. However, a child with a severe hearing loss (61–90 dB HL) may experience more difficulty in understanding speech, and may function more as a deaf child, than one with a loss of more than 90 dB HL. Erber (1979) demonstrated that it was extremely difficult to predict speech perception abilities for children with hearing losses of 85–100 dB HL. It is noteworthy that Brill and his colleagues, in providing a framework for the educational needs of the hearing impaired, leave out decibel dividers for the categories of deaf and hard of hearing. They prefer the use of functional descriptors (Brill et al., 1986).

Demographic studies demonstrate that far more children are hard of hearing than profoundly impaired. Ross, Brackett, and Maxon (1991) estimate that there are at least 16 to 30 times as many hard-of-hearing children as there are deaf children. Although 16 per 1,000 school children are considered hard of hearing, it may be that this figure is too low because of the levels used to define normal hearing (Ross et al., 1991). The majority of hearing-impaired children are mainstreamed.

Of importance is the change in ethnic background of the pupils making up the hearing-impaired school population. Between 1977 and 1984 the percentage of minority group children in the hearing-impaired school population increased, with the greatest increase occurring in the Hispanic population (Schildroth, 1986). This increase has implications for the programs serving these children.

Degree of Hearing Loss and Its Effects

Generally, the greater the hearing loss, the more difficulty the child will have in perceiving and understanding speech. In this section, degrees of impairment and their associated common characteristics will be presented. However, these must be interpreted as guidelines only because the speech and language deficits experienced by a hearing-impaired child result from a complex interaction of many different variables. Current literature testifies to the heterogeneous nature of the hearing-impaired population.

Important in understanding how hearing loss affects speech and oral language perception is some knowledge of the **frequency** (pitch) and **intensity** (loudness) of speech sounds. Therefore, prior to discussing the effects on language and speech that varying degrees of sound loss can have, an overview of speech acoustics is presented.

Acoustics of Speech   From chapter 2 we know that the different speech sounds are made up of different

FIGURE 9.1 Frequency Spectrum of Familiar Sounds Plotted on a Standard Audiogram. (From *Hearing in Children* [4th ed.] [p. 17] by J. Northern and M. Downs, 1991, Baltimore: Williams & Wilkins. Copyright 1991 by Williams & Wilkins. Reprinted by permission.)

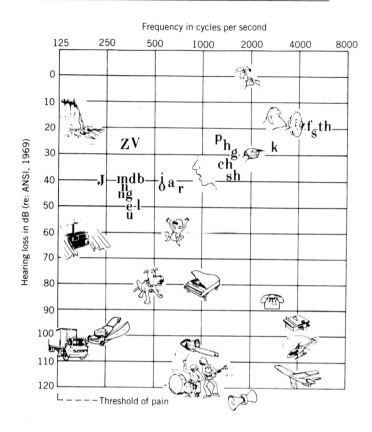

combinations of frequencies and intensities. Figure 9.1 gives the frequency spectrum of some speech sounds and some environmental sounds. The figure superimposes these sounds on an audiogram to provide a method of understanding hearing loss. The necessary adjustment from dB SPL to dB HL has been made. The frequencies are given along the top, and the relative intensities in dB HL are given down the left-hand side. Low frequencies are 250 and 500 Hz, middle frequencies are 1,000 to 2,000 Hz, and high frequencies are 3,000 Hz and above.

The average sound pressure level of conversational speech at 4 to 6 feet from the speaker is 60–65 dB SPL, and the sounds of speech contain energy between 100 and 8,000 Hz. The intensity of vowels is generally greater than that of consonants, with a 30-dB spread between the weakest and strongest speech elements at a given frequency location. If a speech signal is analyzed over time, considerable fluctuation is found, reflecting the relative strengths of the different sounds.

Some speech sounds are high in frequency or pitch, such as /s/, while others are low, such as /m/. Sounds that are voiced, such as /z/ and /m/, can have both high- and low-frequency information. In contrast, /s/ has no voicing and contains only high frequencies. Similarly, some speech sounds have high intensity, such as "or," as in "four," while others are low in intensity, such as "th," as in "think." Generally, vowels, such as /i/, /a/, and /u/, and voiced consonants, such as /m/, /b/, and /g/, are lower in frequency and more intense than the voiceless consonants, such as /p/, /t/, and /k/.

An important aspect of understanding speech perception relates to the properties of vowels and the acoustic information that vowels provide the listener. In chapter 2 we introduced concepts related to speech production and the acoustic characteristics that result. Recall that the passageway from the larynx consists of a series of coupled resonators—the pharynx, the mouth, and the nose. Recall also that the fundamental, or voicing, frequency is low (80–300 Hz for adult males and up to 500 Hz for adult females and children). The articulators modify the fundamental frequency by changing the shapes of the cavities or resonators, thus modifying the acoustic properties of the sound that emerges. The effect of these modifications results in the concentration of acoustic energy into clearly identifiable bands of energy at certain frequencies. These concentrations are called *formants* and are numbered from formant 1 (F1). It is primarily the first and second formants (F1 and F2) that are used in the perception of vowels, and they are differentiated largely on the basis of the ratio relationship between these formant frequencies. For example, for a female voice, for "ae" the average F1 is 860 Hz and the average F2 is 2,050 Hz. For "or" the average F1 is 590 Hz and the average F2 is 920 Hz. While the two vowels have similar F1 values, they have very different F2 values, making them easily distinguishable acoustically (Ross et al., 1991). Figure 9.2 superimposes the range

of values for fundamental frequency, the formant frequencies of the vowel sounds, and the consonants on to an audiogram. (The correction from dB SPL to dB HL has been made.)

In addition to the frequency information available from formants, the beginning and end of each vowel utterance reflect the transition or change in frequency from one sound to another. The F2 transition contains the most important cue for identification of neighboring consonants, particularly for identifying the place of articulation of the consonant. For example, the voiceless stops /p/, /t/, and /k/ show the same manner of articulation, but the F2 and F3 transitions from the consonant to the vowel differ, allowing the individual to distinguish between /pa/, /ta/, and /ka/ (Lieberman & Blumstein, 1988).

For hearing-impaired children, the nature of their impairment may prevent them from taking advantage of these acoustic cues. Imagine the child who has usable hearing only up to 1,000 Hz and turn again to

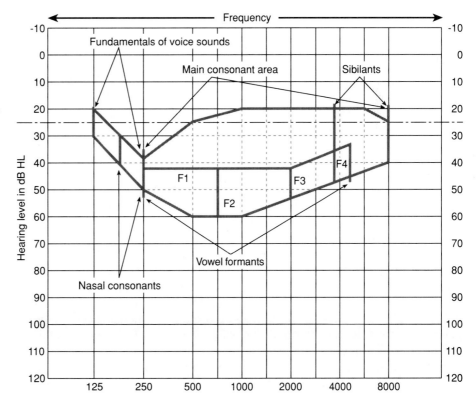

FIGURE 9.2 Acoustic Spectrum of the Speech Signal (HL Scale). (From *Assessment and Management of Mainstream Hearing-Impaired Children: Assessment and Principles* [p. 183] by M. Ross, D. Brackett, and A. Maxon, 1991, Austin, TX: PRO-ED. Copyright 1991 by PRO-ED. Reprinted by permission.)

Figure 9.2. This may make it difficult for the child to distinguish between, for example, /i/ and /I/ on the basis of frequency information and to recognize the difference in length of the vowels, but the child should have no difficulty distinguishing between /i/ and /u/ on the basis of frequency information. However, he or she will be unable to hear the voiceless consonant /s/, an important linguistic marker in English.

Erber and Alencewicz (1976) used speech materials to assess the functional hearing abilities of the severely and profoundly hearing impaired in an effort to establish which children could discriminate between segmental features or individual sounds and which children could discriminate only between the supra segmental features of loudness, duration, and pitch. They used a closed response set whereby the children were forced to choose a response to a stimulus from a finite set of possible responses. The majority of the children tested were able to categorize words accurately on the basis of suprasegmental features, for example, to identify a word as having one or two syllables. However, not all of these children were able to discriminate words within the same category, for example, "car"/"dog," demonstrating a deficit in perceiving the segmental features that are so closely related to the acoustic patterns received by the listener.

Further work has expanded this area. In a study using 120 children with hearing losses ranging from 55–123 dB HL, Boothroyd (1984) investigated how much of the acoustical information in the speech signal was used by children who wore hearing aids. He required the children to distinguish between phonemic contrasts and found the hearing levels beyond which there was only chance performance. These levels were (1) 75 dB for consonant place of articulation, (2) 85 dB for initial consonant voicing, (3) 90 dB for initial consonant continuance, (4) 100 dB for vowel place, (5) 105 dB for syllabic pattern, and (6) above 115 dB for vowel height. The variable that most affected performance was the ability to discriminate monosyllabic words such as "pen," "cat," and "shoe." Note that in these words, suprasegmental cues cannot be used to differentiate them. Rather, discrimination of frequency differences is required.

As we discuss the effects of varying degrees of hearing loss in the next sections, it may be helpful to refer regularly to Figures 9.1 and 9.2. As a simple example, use these figures and draw a horizontal line across the 30-dB level. A child with a flat hearing loss across the frequencies at this level would not hear the sounds for the entries above this line. Most hearing losses, however, are not the same in all frequencies, which needs to be remembered as we look at the effects of varying degrees of loss. We also need to keep in mind the different frequency characteristics of speech sounds from the preceding discussion of the acoustics of speech and relate this information to the degree of loss.

Mild Hearing Loss (15–30 dB HL) Children with this degree of hearing loss should develop speech and language spontaneously. Such losses have traditionally been considered to cause only minimal difficulty for the child, with the main problem involving hearing faint speech. However, because these children are not always in advantageous listening conditions, they often miss essential auditory information. The last few decades have produced research findings that have considerably increased our awareness of the effects of mild impairments on speech and language development and academic achievement. Professionals no longer tend to discount the negative impact that mild hearing losses can have on children. *Minimal* intervention for children with mild permanent hearing losses consists of fitting them with hearing aids, encouraging the use of visual as well as auditory cues, and providing preferential seating. With early and appropriate intervention, any language delay these children may experience should be successfully remediated. The problems faced by children with fluctuating and/or temporary hearing losses, as opposed to mild permanent losses, will be discussed further in a later section.

Moderate Hearing Loss (31–60 dB HL) Children with this degree of hearing loss definitely benefit from the fitting of hearing aids as soon as possible following diagnosis, as without amplification, conversational speech is not completely audible. Children at the lower end of this range often rely on a visual supplement to the auditory signal. Many of these children have delayed language skills and speech problems, particularly with consonants. Generally, voice can be monitored adequately, and voice quality is normal. Without appropriate intervention, these children will not develop to their full capacity in speech, language, or academics. They may remain at an educational disadvantage throughout the school period. With appropriate amplification and intervention, they have good audibility and speech perception, as well as reasonable potential to develop normal or nearly normal speech and language. These children are generally placed in normal classes, with preferential seating.

Severe Hearing Loss (61–90 dB HL)   Children with this degree of hearing loss have considerable difficulty hearing conversational speech sufficiently well for discrimination unless they wear amplification. Those with the most severe impairments respond only to sounds that are high in intensity and at close range, even with amplification. Some may have poor auditory discrimination skills. Even with amplification, there is frequently a delay in developing language. Speech will also be delayed, with consonant, vowel, and diphthong errors. Some children in this group may show abnormal voice quality. Other factors also play a significant part, and the range of spoken language abilities is wide. The outcome for these children depends largely on how early the hearing loss is detected and intervention begun. Audition should be the main input modality for these children, but with increased reliance on visual cues, particularly in poor acoustic conditions and for those children at the bottom of the hearing range. Good results can be achieved with early fitting of hearing aids and appropriate speech, language, and educational intervention. Some of these children may function in a regular classroom, but many will need special educational assistance and perhaps even special placement.

Profound Hearing Loss (91–120 dB HL)   Children with this degree of hearing loss are the ones least likely to benefit from auditory input, and many of them will rely heavily on tactile and visual cues. Amplified auditory input will give them information about environmental sounds and the suprasegmental features of speech. However, in most cases, it will not provide them with sufficient information to discriminate speech. Accordingly, the development of ade-

quate oral language is difficult for these children, and many need to use total communication or manual communication (discussed later in the chapter) in order to communicate. A very small number of children in this group may actually have no measurable hearing levels. They are generally reported as having "hearing levels" of about 120 dB, probably because they feel the test stimuli in the lower frequencies. Such children have speech and language skills below those of their peers who have only slightly better hearing. This is a powerful demonstration of what can be achieved with just a small amount of residual hearing (Levitt, McGarr, & Geffner, 1987).

Total Hearing Loss (121 + dB HL)   Children with this degree of hearing loss do not hear even with auditory amplification. It appears that they feel rather than hear sounds. Vision is the primary modality through which they acquire language. Some of these children may benefit from inputs from cochlear implants or tactile devices.

Age of Onset of Hearing Loss and Its Effects

Hearing loss is often described in terms of the age at which it occurred. It has been the custom to divide losses into congenital loss, which is present at birth or occurs in the immediate postnatal period, and **acquired** loss, which occurs after birth, when the child has had some exposure to language through audition. As the age of onset of loss is an important factor in determining the linguistic outcome, there has been a recent trend to refer to congenital losses and those that occur shortly after birth as *prelingual hearing losses* and those that occur after the child has been exposed to a considerable amount of conversational language as *postlingual hearing impairments*. There is no agreed-upon age level that is used to divide these two groups, and some would argue that, as language development begins at birth, the distinction is meaningless (Osberger & Hesketh, 1988). However, there are differences in linguistic performance between the two groups, and 2 years of age is generally used as the dividing line. The earlier a hearing impairment occurs, the more likely it is to have a deleterious effect on speech and language development. In addition, the more severe the loss, generally the more severe the linguistic impairment.

Congenital, or prelingual, losses have many different causes. According to a recent survey, genetic factors (heredity) and meningitis (inflammation of the membranes covering the brain and/or spinal cord) in the immediate postnatal period are the two most common causes (Schildroth, 1986). Other causes are prematurity and maternal rubella, with the latter declining as a cause. Acquired losses also have many different causes, and again, the most common causes are meningitis and genetic factors. Other causes are severe viral infections such as influenza and mumps, trauma that results in injury to the skull, and blood clots in the vessels supplying the inner ear (Schildroth, 1986). Another important cause of postlingual hearing loss is that due to middle ear infections or otitis media (Northern & Downs, 1991). The loss sustained is usually temporary, but it can be permanent. It is important to distinguish between congenital and genetic losses. As is obvious from the preceding discussion, not all congenital losses are genetic in origin and not all genetic losses are congenital. Genetic losses can develop in the prelingual period, but they may not develop until early adulthood.

Site of Lesion and Types of Hearing Loss

The site of the lesion, that is, the location of the damage to the hearing mechanism that causes the hearing loss, will have an impact on the hearing status of the child. Hearing losses are generally divided into two types, depending on the site of the lesion. The type caused by damage in the external ear canal, the eardrum, or the middle ear is referred to as conductive hearing loss. Damage to these parts of the ear generally affects the mechanical aspects of hearing, that is, how sound waves are transferred to the inner part of the ear. The hearing deficit consists of a loss of intensity. Sounds do not sound loud enough. However, there is no loss in discriminative ability. Thus, clarity is not impaired. Therefore, the child with a conductive hearing loss is able to be (re)habilitated effectively and should be able to use oral language to communicate. Conductive losses fit into the mild or moderate cate-gories described earlier. In the majority of cases, the hearing loss can be treated medically or surgically.

Sensorineural hearing loss is caused by damage to the inner ear, in the cochlea and/or the eighth (or acoustic) nerve. The hearing deficit typically causes both a loss of intensity and a loss of clarity, so that the child has difficulty discriminating speech. Sounds can be intensified through the use of appropriate amplification, but they are not necessarily made any clearer. Another problem for many sensorineurally impaired children is abnormal sensitivity to loud sounds, or **recruitment**. With this deficit, the point at which a sound is just heard compared to where it becomes uncomfortably or even painfully loud is reduced. This means that the child may have a very restricted range of usable hearing (reduced *dynamic range*), with soft sounds unable to be heard and loud sounds unable to be tolerated. As a result, the successful fitting of hearing aids and the perception of speech are severely compromised in some children. It is important to bear in mind that for all people, whether hearing impaired or not, whether suffering from recruitment or not, there is a maximum loudness limit above which sound becomes uncomfortable and then painful. The degree of sensorineural impairment varies across all categories, from mild to profound.

Sensorineural hearing loss generally is not amenable to medical intervention. Recently, however, some surgical intervention has become possible with the development of cochlear implants. An electrode is surgically implanted into the cochlea to stimulate the eighth nerve directly. However, this intervention is available only to a small number of profoundly impaired individuals who meet strict selection criteria.

Some children experience what is called a **mixed hearing loss**, that is, a loss that has both a conductive and a sensorineural element. The loss may have one or more causes, and the particular difficulties experienced will depend on the configuration of the loss. By *configuration,* we mean the particular frequencies affected by the loss and the extent to which each frequency is affected.

A small number of children present with what is termed *central auditory dysfunction.* There is not necessarily a decrease in auditory sensitivity, but there are varying degrees of difficulty with auditory comprehension. The topic is both a complicated and controversial one, as we have seen in previous chapters.

Stability of Hearing Loss

Some hearing losses are not stable over time. Boothroyd (1982) classified losses according to a stability factor as stable, progressive, and fluctuating. In a *stable* hearing loss, the child has access to the same quality of auditory signals across time. This consistency of auditory signals permits the child to incorporate sounds into perceptual development. In a *progressive* hearing loss, the hearing deteriorates over time, requiring the child to adapt to poorer and poorer auditory information. In a *fluctuating* hearing loss, as the loss varies the child experiences inconsistency in the auditory signal received. This can cause difficulties particularly when the child responds to sounds on some occasions and not on others. The variation in attending to auditory stimuli is sometimes viewed as willfully inconsistent behavior. It may also be that sound is not integrated into the child's perceptual development and is not given priority as a means of learning. The effects of fluctuating losses, particularly in the language development period, may be far-reaching and may lead to problems with auditory attention even after hearing has returned to normal. Children with otitis media, or middle ear disease, frequently experience fluctuating hearing loss (Northern & Downs, 1991).

Other Contributing Factors and Their Effects

Many factors in addition to age of onset and degree, type, and stability of loss may influence the performance of hearing-impaired children. It is frequently difficult to assess the precise impact that these factors may have on an individual child's performance. However, as they can significantly influence performance, it is imperative that they be considered.

One important factor is the hearing status of the parents. It has been suggested that normally hearing parents of hearing-impaired children are frequently so devastated by learning of their child's impairment that they undergo periods of psychological and emotional stress that can reduce their ability to relate to their child. This has a bearing on the way they relate to their child through the use of language and auditory stimulation. Normally hearing parents of hearing-impaired children have been shown to be more physically manipulative, more verbally dominant, and less likely to allow the child-directed discourse that usually occurs with young normally hearing children. In addition, there is sometimes a decrease of verbal input to the child in the initial period after the diagnosis (Cross, Johnson-Morris, & Nienhuys, 1980). The child, therefore, does not receive the necessary verbal input for language development. Through counseling and support, parents are usually able to increase the amount and type of auditory input to their child, thereby returning to a more dyadic interaction similar to what the normal hearing child experiences (Kenworthy, 1986).

Deaf parents, on the other hand, may view their child's hearing impairment with less distress and are able to communicate effectively, either through the use of audition or through the use of manual communication. In their early years, the children of deaf parents are more likely to have relatively good receptive and expressive language skills but poor speech skills. In contrast, the children of hearing parents are more likely to have superior speech skills (White & White, 1987).

The ability to attribute the results just presented to the hearing status of the parents is complicated by another important factor—child's age at intervention. The benefits of early intervention have long been supported by professionals. Early intervention may lead to emotional stability of the parents and child, more advanced linguistic skills, better communication abilities, and better educational development and achievement. A recent longitudinal study on the linguistic skills of a large number of hearing-impaired children reaffirmed this belief. Early intervention alone may not achieve superior skills, but children who have not received intervention at an early age have been found to perform well below the level of other children who have (Levitt et al., 1987).

A third factor that may affect performance is the presence of other handicapping conditions, such as developmental delay, cerebral palsy, visual deficit, or behavioral disturbance. The impact that other condi tions may have on the child's perceptual and linguistic performances will vary considerably, but these conditions need to be taken into account both during the intervention process and when assessing the outcome of intervention (Boothroyd, 1982; Levitt et al., 1987).

Background Noise

An important problem among hearing-impaired children is background noise. Background noise is affected by the level of noise in a room, the acoustics of the room, and the distance between the talker and the listener. The first two variables produce what is known as *room reverberation*. A room with highly reverberant surfaces, such as glass and wood, will produce a relatively high level of background noise and will hamper the listener in perceiving a speech signal.

Normally hearing people have difficulty understanding speech if the background noise is too high; hearing-impaired individuals have even more difficulty. A number of studies demonstrate the difficulty that hearing-impaired children have in classrooms with high levels of background noise (Berg, 1987). Profoundly impaired children, in particular, have severely hampered speech perception with even low levels of background noise (Erber, 1971, 1979).

Signal-to-noise ratio is used to describe the relationship of the signal that the child needs to hear (usually speech) to the level of background noise that is present. A signal-to-noise ratio of 0 dB means that the signal and noise are at the same level. A signal-to-noise ratio of +20 dB (where the signal is 20 dB greater than the noise) is generally suitable for normally hearing children. Hard-of-hearing and deaf children need a signal-to-noise ratio of +30 dB (Berg, 1987).

Unfortunately, many classrooms do not have favorable signal-to-noise ratios, particularly those with highly reflective surfaces, such as hardwood or vinyl floors and windows without coverings. In fact, some classrooms have a negative signal-to-noise ratio at times, such that the signal is less intense than the background noise. In a recent survey of 45 classrooms where hearing-impaired children were mainstreamed, a third of the rooms recorded background noise levels in excess of 70 dB SPL (Ross et al., 1991).

ORAL LANGUAGE AND SPEECH CHARACTERISTICS

This section examines the speech and language characteristics of the hearing-impaired child. It is a rather difficult subject, as a wide range of speech and language behaviors are exhibited by these children. Children with mild hearing loss have linguistic behaviors closer to those of children with normal hearing than to those of children with a profound or even severe loss.

Professionals have considered the nature of the deficit, that is, whether it is quantitatively different, and therefore delayed, or qualitatively different, and therefore, deviant. The majority have concluded that *delayed* is the more appropriate descriptor and that the linguistic development of the hearing impaired follows normal development, but at a much slower rate. This issue was recently addressed in a report of a comprehensive study of the linguistic behaviors of a large group of hearing-impaired children. Delay was seen across all the children studied. However, deviant forms were observed both in older children who were attempting to use more complex linguistic structures and in older children who had the poorest language skills and the poorest hearing levels. It is likely that deviance is a result of many years of delayed development and that the two processes are interdependent (Levitt et al., 1987).

Irrespective of the descriptors used, documentation and observation show that hearing-impaired children have speech and language problems that are the result of auditory deprivation. They do not learn language as efficiently as normally hearing children and must frequently be taught correct forms that appear naturally in the speech of the normally hearing. Language problems have been observed in children with mild and moderate hearing losses (Davis, Elfenbein, Schum, & Bentler, 1986). However, the linguistic skills of the severely and profoundly impaired have received much more study. This may, in part, be because these children have traditionally been placed in schools and classes for the hearing impaired and thus represent a more accessible population. Generally, the more severe the auditory deficit, the more severe the verbal deficit. Levitt et al. (1987) show that speech and communication skills are generally related to hearing level. Language skills decrease with hearing level to about 80 dB. Between 80 and 115 dB, decreasing hearing level is not necessarily a predictor for language level. Beyond 115 dB, language and speech levels are very poor.

Syntax and Morphology

Longitudinal and cross-sectional studies on the hearing impaired have determined that there is considerable delay in the development of syntax and morphology. The extent of the delay varies widely and is generally related to the severity of the hearing loss (Davis & Hardick, 1981; Engen & Engen, 1983). Much of the research on syntax has focused on older children and has used written test materials, sometimes making comparisons difficult with the data on normally hearing children (Levitt, 1987; Quigley, 1978). Of particular concern is that many children tested on a longitudinal basis never reach the levels of their normally hearing peers. This has enormous implications for professionals in their choice of language instruction, textbooks, and presentation of all language materials.

Studies of moderate and severely hearing-impaired children show acquisition of verb forms with age, but at a much slower rate than in normally hearing children. Particular difficulty has been noted with accurate use of main verb forms (Presnell, 1973; Wilcox & Tobin, 1974). Not surprisingly, most difficulty was found with those forms that are difficult for normally hearing children. The present perfect, such as "have spoken," and the negative passive, such as "The candy was not found by the girls," are consistently reported as being the most difficult to master. In examining comprehension of medially embedded clauses, such as "The man who has the limp caught the bus," Levitt (1987) found that only about one third of the children were able to perform adequately. A similar finding was reported by Davis and Blasdell (1975). They found that children misunderstood embedding 49% of the time. These findings raise academic concerns, as Ross (1982) has noted that relative clauses are present in second-level reading primers. Hearing-impaired children, when required to interpret sentences, tend to do so on the basis of word order, imposing the simple subject-verb-object rule on complex sentences. Although this pattern is seen in young, normally hearing children, hearing-impaired children tend to persevere longer with its use and some never acquire other interpretation strategies.

Function words tend to be omitted in the expressive language of the hearing impaired. *Function words,* such as the articles "a," "the," and "an" and the prepositions "to" and "of," are normally unstressed in spoken language, thus making them lower in intensity and less visible in a lipreading pattern. They are often the words masked by the background noise present in classrooms. Incorrect patterns that the children produce verbally may be modeled by an adult with emphasis on the content words, thus compounding the problem. Hearing-impaired children's speech, therefore, consists predominantly of nouns and, to a lesser degree, verbs, which gives it a telegraphic quality (Davis & Hardick, 1981).

Limited research has been done on the morphological characteristics of the hearing-impaired. In parallel with the work on syntactic characteristics, marked delays have been found in morphological development for children with severe and profound losses (Russell, Power, & Quigley, 1976). The limited research on children with mild to moderate hearing losses shows delays of about 5½ years (Brown, 1984). This significant delay has implications for the educational achievement of such children, many of whom are in normal classes with high levels of background noise.

In hearing-impaired children, the sequence of morphological development appears to pattern that of normally hearing children. The areas that have received most attention are verb endings and noun forms. Noun forms are reported to be easier to learn than verb forms (Taylor, 1969). The easiest verb forms are the present progressive, such as the "ing" marker in "running." There is more difficulty with past tense markers, and the third-person singular present tense ("runs") presents the most problems. This hierarchy corresponds to the information on the language development of the normally hearing presented in chapter 3. The possessive marker on nouns, such as "the girl's ball," appears to be the easiest noun form mastered. More difficulty is encountered with plural markers, such as "two pig" for "two pigs." Hearing-impaired children also tend to apply regular rules to irregular plural nouns ("mices") and to collective nouns ("sheeps"), and they use irregular plural forms as singular nouns ("The men was hot").

The problems seen in morphology may again be related to the fact that the word endings are usually unstressed, with consequent reduced visibility and intensity. An additional factor is that the marker /s/, a common one in English, is high in frequency and low in intensity, making its perception difficult, particularly in background noise. In many cases where it is to be used, there is built-in linguistic redundancy, such as in the sentence "The three cats are playing." In this example, plurality is denoted by "three" and "are." The information gained from the /s/ on cats is repetitive and may well be ignored by hearing-impaired children who focus on the higher content forms.

Semantics

A number of studies have focused on semantics. Patterns tend to follow other areas of study, with the most severe deficits found among the profoundly impaired. Davis et al. (1986) found that even mild hearing losses are likely to result in delays in vocabulary development ranging from 1 year to more than 3 years. Delays for profoundly impaired children may be as much as 4 to 5 years (Markides, 1970). Again, most research has centered on the profoundly hearing impaired, although children with all degrees of hearing loss show vocabulary deficits that are both quantitatively and qualitatively different from those of normally hearing children. There is evidence that hearing-impaired children experience developmental gaps in their word knowledge. They miss out on basic concepts at the preschool level and may never catch up (Moeller, McConkey, & Osberger, 1983; Osberger, 1986).

With receptive vocabulary, hearing-impaired children show difficulty in comprehending words and understanding word meanings. In addition to the delays noted earlier, there is evidence that the delay widens as these children grow older (Davis, 1974; Templin, 1966). Vocabulary size does not grow as quickly as it does in normally hearing children, and vocabulary growth may not show the systematic gains seen in normally hearing children.

The expressive vocabularies of the hearing impaired show similar problems. Their vocabulary use is closely tied to the present and literal and is used in limited ways, with few synonyms (Moeller et al., 1983). These children use fewer numbers of words and fewer types of words compared to their normally hearing peers (Brannon, 1968; Easterbrooks, 1987). Among the severely and profoundly impaired, there is a *lower type-token* ratio, the ratio used to express the number of different words a child uses in relation to the number of words in a language corpus (Easterbrooks, 1987). Expressive vocabulary samples of hearing-impaired children show a lack of function words such as demonstrative pronouns, auxiliary verbs, and connectives (Brannon, 1968). One of the reasons suggested for the vocabulary delay is that the hearing impaired have to rely on being taught new vocabulary, whereas the normally hearing learn it vicariously. The poor vocabularies of the hearing impaired reflect the dependence of many of them on the visual channel, where incidental language learning is less likely.

Semantic concept development is also delayed. It appears that concepts such as size and space, which are more easily perceived through vision, are learned earlier and more easily than other concepts, such as time. The *Boehm Test of Basic Concepts* (Boehm, 1970) has been administered to children with varying degrees of hearing loss; significant delays have been found, even with mild and moderate losses. The test was administered by Davis (1974) to a group of 24 children with mild to moderate hearing losses between the ages of 6 and 8 years. All of the childen were mainstreamed for part or all of their schooling. Time concepts were the most difficult, and space concepts were the least difficult. The children experienced marked difficulty with the test, with 75% of them scoring below the 10th percentile. Even greater difficulty with this test was experienced by a group of 13- and 14-year-old severely and profoundly impaired children (Brenza, Kricos, & Lasky, 1981). Of these children, 39% exhibited semantic or syntactic-semantic errors on the production task. On the comprehension task, 80% of them scored lower than the 10th percentile, and 66% scored below the 1st percentile. The results suggested that with increasing age, hearing-impaired children do not achieve age-appropriate language comprehension skills. The authors of this study examined the textbooks used by these children. Of particular concern was their finding that 80% of the textbooks assumed that the examined concepts were understood by the children.

Some authors have suggested that the difficulty hearing-impaired children have with vocabulary may reflect a deficit in the semantic notions that underlie oral language. However, the few applicable studies suggest that this is not generally the case. Bellugi and Klima (1972) showed that when deaf children of deaf parents learn language, the semantic relations they acquire are very similar to those acquired by normally hearing children, despite the fact that the communication modality is sign. In another investigation, Curtiss, Prutting, and Lowell (1979) studied semantic development in hearing-impaired preschool children and found that although they evidenced delay, these children demonstrated a number of semantic functions. The authors point out that the delay is not surprising given the difficulty of coding meaning nonlinguistically. They noted that there were differences in the frequency of use of some forms compared to their use by the normally hearing, and they attributed this difference to the ease with which some forms are coded visually compared to others. Although the hearing-impaired children were learning oral English, they relied on nonverbal forms of communication such as gestures.

An examination of hearing-impaired children's use of abstract language shows particular difficulties with the understanding of language that is not literal. Much English language usage is concrete, familiar, and geared to the present. However, English also uses idiom, slang, puns, and metaphors. The experiences of hearing-impaired children are more tied to the present, and this makes it difficult for them to learn abstract word usage (Moeller et al., 1983). Rather, they tend to attach literal meanings to many figurative forms. Forms such as "in one ear and out the other" and "I ran like the wind" may lead to confusion and misunderstanding.

Recent reports have suggested that these difficulties are educationally based rather than an outcome of the hearing loss per se. Easterbrooks (1987) reported on a study using two groups of hearing-impaired children, one age 7 to 8 years and the other age 11 to 12 years, and groups of normally hearing children. She required them to classify objects and pictures using adjectives with opposite meanings, for example, "happy" and "sad." Although the responses of the older hearing-impaired group were similar to those of the normally hearing 7- to 8-year-olds, even the younger children could use adjectives metaphorically. Easterbrooks suggests that it is lack of exposure and lack of expectation on the part of educators that play a part in how children function with semantic forms. This opinion is also expressed by Iran-Nejad, Ortony, and Rittenhouse (1981).

Earlier, it was pointed out that hearing-impaired children tend to know few synonyms. They may also know only one meaning for a word that may have more than one meaning, for example, "bear" the animal and "bear" meaning the ability to tolerate something. Their language often seems stilted, as they do not have a variety of words to denote shades of meaning. For example, a hearing-impaired child may use "happy" to convey a range of feelings, from mild contentment to extreme delight. Frequently, the words these children use can be conveyed accurately by visual means. As they grow older, they fail to show subtle changes in language use of the society.

In everyday situations, hearing-impaired children can rely on context and use familiar words. However, once outside familiar contexts and words, they have difficulty. From an academic standpoint, the effects of reduced vocabulary can be extremely detrimental, as these children are unable to understand the language used in specific academic disciplines and the language used in textbooks. As pointed out before, hearing-impaired children do not benefit from incidental language learning on television or radio and from conversing with others. They have particular difficulty retaining academic vocabularies (Ross, 1982), and because of their poor language skills, they are unable to figure out meanings from linguistic contexts.

Pragmatics

Many hearing-impaired children fail to learn such things as the rules that govern conversation. Behaviors such as turn taking, repair strategies, clarification, and topic negotiation are frequently not mastered. Some of these difficulties may be related to the children's lack of mastery of syntax. For example, failure to follow the rules for turn taking may be related to difficulties with question formation. These problems may also result from the way in which many hearing-impaired children learn language. For these children, linguistic principles and rules are taught as a series of exercises in the classroom or clinic. The children do not know how to incorporate the skills learned into everyday conversational settings, and frequently linguistic instruction does not provide the skills necessary to do this (Kretschmer & Kretschmer, 1980).

Normally hearing children master language competence through a series of developmental stages during which they are exposed to a wide variety of interactive auditory experiences. Kretschmer and Kretschmer (1980) assert that if communicative competence is to develop in the hearing impaired, the same developmental sequence needs to be followed.

Relatively few studies have concentrated on pragmatic development and function in the hearing impaired. The Curtiss et al. (1979) study on a group of profoundly impaired preschoolers who were in an auditory/oral program examined a variety of verbal and nonverbal pragmatic behaviors. The children used a range of pragmatic intentions, although expressed primarily through nonverbal means. In some cases, their pragmatic abilities exceeded their semantic abilities, presumably because the former could be expressed more readily in a nonverbal form. The most commonly used pragmatic functions were the earliest-developing ones in normally hearing children, such as labeling, naming, acknowledging, and demanding. McKirdy and Blank (1982) examined communicative intent in dyads of profoundly impaired and normally hearing preschoolers. They reported a delay in discourse, with the best response from the hearing impaired occurring when they initiated conversation. The hearing-impaired children encountered more difficulty when they were required to respond to their part-

ners, and they gave inappropriate and ambiguous responses to utterances of greater linguistic complexity.

In habilitative and rehabilitative management of the hearing impaired, one needs to do more than teach linguistic forms. These children need to see linguistic forms function as communication tools. They must be exposed to vocabulary describing basic concepts that are interesting to them. The use of language as a way to exchange information, to interact at an interpersonal level, and to enjoy such interaction needs to be emphasized if the subtleties of pragmatic functioning are to be developed (Kretschmer & Kretschmer, 1980).

A Language Disorder Masked by Hearing Loss?

The causes of hearing loss discussed earlier include some that are known to affect the peripheral hearing mechanism only, such as certain genetic causes, while others can also affect central nervous system functioning. It is possible that some children with sensorineural hearing loss have other problems that could reduce further their ability to develop language. In discussing hearing-impaired children with additional handicaps, Levitt (1987) notes that some children labeled minimally brain damaged in the absence of neurological data had scores among the lowest recorded for the entire group of children studied. Additionally, there may be a group of hearing-impaired children who have concomitant learning disabilities (Bunch & Melnyk, 1989), and we have discussed the relationship between language disorders and learning disabilities in previous chapters. It is possible that the language performances of some hearing-impaired children can be accounted for only in part by their hearing losses. The hearing impairment would add to an existing language problem or possibly mask a language disorder. There are, however, currently limited empirical data to support such conjectures, which therefore remain speculative. A cautionary note is sounded by Levitt (1987), who suggests that there is a danger in labeling children as possibly having other disabilities in the absence of supporting data. Such labels may lead educators to lower their expectations for the children so labeled.

Speech Production

Speech production in the hearing impaired is most affected by the degree of hearing impairment and the frequencies involved. Children with losses in high-frequency areas are unable to hear high-pitched sounds such as /s/, and some children also have difficulty with accurate perception of vowels. There are differences between the speech characteristics of the severely and profoundly impaired (Gold & Levitt, 1975). These differences are seen in both the number and the types of errors. Generally, the greater the hearing loss, the more likely the errors will extend from consonants and vowels to errors in stress, pitch, and voicing. Production errors affecting consonants and vowels are referred to as *segmental errors,* while those affecting timing, intonation, and stress are referred to as *suprasegmental errors* (Osberger & McGarr, 1982).

Segmental Errors   Consonants produced in the middle of the mouth are most likely to be deleted. Substitution of consonants also occurs, with voiced sounds often substituted for voiceless ones. Studies using both profoundly impaired and hard-of-hearing children have reported that sounds using tongue tip placement are more likely to be in error than other consonants. Such sounds are the stops /t/ and /d/, the fricatives /s/, /z/, "sh," and "th," and the affricatives "ch" and "j." The affricatives are ranked as most difficult for both the profoundly hearing impaired and the hard of hearing (Markides, 1970; Smith, 1975). In some instances, production of sound substitutions results in consonants that cannot be recognized as English or in consonants that are used in certain dialects of English, such as substituting a glottal stop for "g."

The difficulties of hearing-impaired children in producing vowels and consonants result from a combination of factors. Many of the consonants are low in intensity and high in frequency, making their accurate perception difficult. In addition, many hearing-impaired children have poor discriminative powers, even if the sounds are made intense enough for them. A number of sounds are able to be seen, such as /p/, /b/, and /m/, although it is difficult to tell the difference between them if only a lipreading pattern is used. In the absence of language competence, it is frequently difficult for the hearing-impaired child to use contextual cues to supplement lipreading. Similarly, it is difficult to discriminate vowels on the basis of lipreading. Many consonants, such as /k/, /g/, and "ng," cannot be seen. Poor auditory and visual input places the hearing-impaired child at a severe disadvantage for learning and monitoring speech. Intervention is necessary for these sounds to be recognized and produced.

Suprasegmental Errors   Most reports on the suprasegmental aspects of speech in the hearing impaired have centered on the errors produced by the profoundly impaired (Osberger & McGarr, 1982). The speech of hard-of-hearing children is less likely to contain such errors, as the nature of their hearing loss usually permits adequate monitoring of their voices (Markides, 1970). Numerous suprasegmental errors are possible, and they are sometimes difficult to separate. These errors also affect the listener's perception of segmental characteristics. A number of terms are used to describe the voice quality of the hearing impaired, among them *harsh, strident, nasal, strained, breathy, hoarse,* and *monotonous.*

Errors in timing can result in slow, labored speech that often distorts the transition between vowels and consonants. The rate of speech of the severely and profoundly hearing impaired has been reported to be 128 to 145 words per minute, in contrast to 134 to 210 words per minute for normally hearing speakers (John & Howarth, 1965). Breath control is frequently inadequate, resulting in either too much or too little air expenditure in utterances. Poor pharyngeal control can occur in conjunction with poor breath control, resulting in speech that is nasalized. Pitch can be either too high, too low, or monotonous, with little control over pitch change. Loudness is also reported to be a problem with some children (Davis & Hardick, 1981).

Intelligibility

Descriptions of speech and language errors do not always state whether the speaker can be understood by the listener. *Intelligibility* is a measure of the listener's response, and there are two common methods of expressing it. One is to rate a speech sample on a 5- or 7-point scale, with descriptors that vary from "completely intelligible" to "completely unintelligible." The other is to calculate the percentage of intelligibility based on the number of words understood in a corpus. Studies using different hearing-impaired populations and different methods have consistently reported that as hearing impairment increases, intelligibility decreases (Markides, 1983). Similarly, as the number of segmental and suprasegmental errors increases, intelligibility decreases. Intelligibility is also affected by the listener's experience, the listener's view of the speaker, context, and repetition (Monsen, 1983). Although, in general, the greater the hearing impairment, the less intelligible the speech, the relationship is less clear-cut with profound impairment. While many profoundly impaired children have unintelligible speech, many others can be understood by the majority of their listeners.

THE EFFECTS OF MILD HEARING IMPAIRMENT

Recently, there has been discussion of the need to redefine normal hearing. The normal hearing range of 0–14 dB HL given by Boothroyd earlier in this chapter reflects new definitions. In 1981 Downs suggested that the 25-dB cutoff point that was being used in many school screening programs was too lenient. Northern and Downs (1991) now use average hearing levels of 15–30 dB HL to define a mild hearing loss. To illustrate for normally hearing individuals the effects of a mild loss, Downs (1981) suggested that the individual block both ears with the finger tips, producing about a 25-dB loss. If you try this, you will notice difficulty understanding your favorite TV show, particularly if background noise is present.

Ear Infections

The most frequent etiology of mild hearing losses is otitis media with effusion (fluid), or middle ear infection. It is one of the most common childhood illnesses, and it causes hearing deficits of varying degree and for varying lengths of time (Teele, Klein, & Rosner, 1984). One of the notable aspects of otitis media is that although it may present with fever and pain, it may also be insidious, occurring with no easily observable symptoms of illness, yet causing hearing losses that are both fluctuating and recurrent. As a result, the child receives inconsistent auditory information (Downs, 1981). In this hearing impairment, the child will usually hear the more intense parts of the speech signal, such as voiced consonants and vowels, but will have difficulty with the voiceless fricatives (/s/, "sh," "th," and /f/) and the voiceless stops (/p/, /t/, and /k/). The unstressed parts of speech, such as function words and morphological endings, will be less audible.

The last two decades have produced many studies on the effects of episodic otitis media on speech, language, and academic development. Early studies demonstrated speech and language delays in children with a history of otitis media, as well as problems with sound blending, auditory discrimination, auditory memory, and auditory closure skills. It was suggested that these deficits remained long after the active ear disease and the accompanying hearing loss, and that poor listening strategies resulted in continued educational underachievement (Brandes & Ehinger, 1981; Lehmann, Charron, Kummer, & Keith, 1979; Zinkus, Gottlieb, & Schapiro, 1978). However, Ventry (1980) and Paradise (1981) questioned the possibility of overinterpretation of such results and the validity of the design of the studies. Both were careful to point out that they were not questioning the hypothesis that mild hearing impairments could lead to communicative and academic delay. However, they suggested that the results of the studies they reviewed were inconclusive.

Recent studies have attempted to resolve these questions. While it appears that the hearing deficit caused by otitis media is responsible for lowered language performance (Friel-Patti & Finitzo, 1990; Wallace, Gravel, McCarton, & Ruben, 1988), it also appears that once hearing has returned to normal, there are no measurable or obvious long-term effects on language performance (Gravel & Wallace, 1992; Roberts, Burchinal, Davis, Collier, & Henderson, 1991). However, there is some evidence that more subtle aspects of language and speech reception may be influenced for some time after the period of active ear disease, such as the ability to discriminate in noise or the ability to take advantage of some speech perception cues (Clarkson, Eimas, & Marean, 1989). Frequent bouts of otitis media, and thus frequent changes in hearing status, would be more likely to have long-term negative influences on the child's speech, language, and academic performance.

Irrespective of the nature of the long-term effects of intermittent, mild hearing loss resulting from otitis media, it is clear that a mild hearing loss, when present, has an impact on a child's auditory capabilities. Inability to hear clearly in a noisy preschool or elementary classroom can lead to misunderstanding, inability to participate appropriately, and behavioral problems. A child who is unable to follow the classroom activities easily quickly becomes distracted. Such a child often presents a confusing picture to parents and teachers. The child fails to respond appropriately to an auditory signal, with the result that the signal is increased, either by the adult's speaking louder or moving closer to the child, who then responds to what is now a more intense signal. The child in such a situation is perceived as "difficult." Unfortunately, hearing impairment is often not (initially at least) considered a possibility in such a scenario.

It is clear that early identification and intervention with children who have otitis media is important, especially as hearing status has been identified as the crucial factor in the language performance of these children. The American Academy of Pediatrics (1985) recognized the need to treat middle ear disease by issuing a policy statement urging prompt diagnosis and treatment in order to restore normal hearing as quickly as possible, thereby reducing the possible impact of the disease on language and academic skills.

In conclusion, it is important to note that otitis media also occurs in children with sensorineural hearing impairment. It can exacerbate the child's hearing loss, often severely compromising the effectiveness of amplification. One fifth of sensorineurally impaired students, mostly younger ones, had otitis media in a study on the language of the hearing impaired (Osberger, 1986). Unfortunately, the condition and its effects on an already hearing-impaired population often go undetected for months (Osberger & Danaher, 1974).

Unilateral Hearing Loss

Unilateral hearing loss has traditionally been regarded as posing no particular educational and communicative difficulties; in fact, it is rarely considered when the effects of hearing impairment are discussed (Bess, Klee, & Culbertson, 1986). A prevalence of 3 per 1,000 for losses of 45 dB HL or more among school-age children was reported by Bergman (1957); 75% of these cases are thought to be congenital. Because children with unilateral hearing loss frequently are able to hear and, therefore, respond to auditory signals and appear to develop language at a normal rate, they are often not identified as hearing impaired until they reach school age, when they may be identified through school hearing screening programs (Shepard, Davis, Gorga, & Stelmachowicz, 1981) or after other labels such as *inattentive* have been applied.

Most hearing screening procedures used with infants and young children are insensitive to unilateral hearing loss. The effects of unilateral impairment on the auditory experience include difficulty hearing when the affected ear is toward the sound source, difficulty localizing the source of sounds, and difficulty hearing in the presence of background noise. Given the generally high levels of background noise in classrooms, it is clear that there are many occasions when a unilaterally hearing-impaired child could be disadvantaged. For example, a child sitting in an area where the impaired ear is toward the teacher and at the back of the class, and therefore farther from the signal, with an average level of background noise, will likely experience an auditory signal that is severely reduced.

Recent reports address the subtle effects of unilateral hearing loss on language development and education. One report compared unilaterally impaired children with losses of 45 dB HL or more with normally hearing children. Few differences in performance were found between the groups on standardized language tests; however, 32% of the hearing-impaired group had failed a grade in school compared to none in the other group. The verbal IQs of the children who had failed were significantly lower than those of the children who had succeeded (Klee & Davis-Dansky, 1986). Further support for the difficulties of children with unilateral impairments compared to their normally hearing peers comes from a study reported by Culbertson and Gilbert (1986). In this study, more unilaterally impaired children had repeated a grade or needed special education or tutoring. There were no differences between the groups on cognitive or self-concept measures, but the unilateral group had lower scores on academic tests of word recognition, spelling, and language.

The majority of unilateral impairments are permanent. While these children may not require extensive special education services, an effort should be made to understand the nature of the auditory problems they experience. The use of FM wireless type of hearing aids for these children is recommended in many cases, as the auditory signal can be presented to the child with minimal background noise (Bess et al., 1986).

MANUAL COMMUNICATION

Several communication methods used with the hearing impaired rely exclusively or partly on conveying the speaker's message to the receiver by using the hands for arbitrarily agreed-upon signs and/or fingerspelling. Among these are American Sign Language (ASL), total communication, and cued speech. Cued speech, first proposed by Cornett (1967), is a supplement to help resolve the ambiguities arising from a lipreading pattern. Recall from chapter 1 that ASL uses hand signs and fingerspelling; it is regarded as a language because it has its own grammar and vocabulary (Osberger & Hesketh, 1988). **Total communication** (**TC**) uses sign, fingerspelling, and spoken language to convey meaning, thereby incorporating the use of the visual, manual, and auditory systems. It has developed out of SEE systems that, as we recall from chapter 1, use sign but preserve the word order of English. The use of TC has become widespread over the last two decades.

There has long been debate over the best communication methods to use in the education of the hearing impaired. Prior to the use of TC, education was either manual, using ASL, or auditory/oral, with the use of signing and fingerspelling prohibited and an

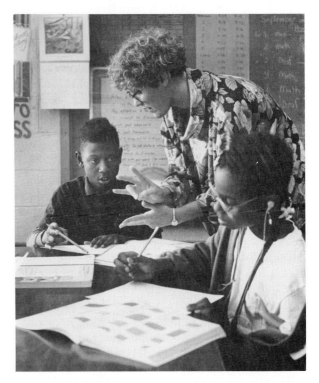

Total communication (TC) educational programs for hearing-impaired children use auditory, oral, and visual modes of communication.

emphasis on improving each child's auditory discrimination and lipreading. Disillusionment grew out of the results of auditory/oral education, where it was observed that many children had failed to develop the expected oral skills. In fact, many failed to become competent communicators, exhibiting unintelligible spoken language skills and such delayed levels of language development that their academic achievement was severely restricted. These discouraging results led, in part, to the popularity of TC.

Research into the outcome of different communication and educational methods remains controversial. Studies in the 1960s showed generally higher performances for deaf children of deaf parents who used ASL in areas such as educational achievement, lipreading, reading and writing skills, self-image, maturity, independence, sociability, and popularity (Denton, 1966; Meadow, 1968; Quigley & Frisina, 1961; Stevenson, 1964). For the most part, these children's performances were compared to those of deaf children of normally hearing parents, a factor that may have confounded the findings.

Subsequent studies attempted to examine directly the impact of different communication and educational methods on the development of hearing-impaired children. Brasel and Quigley (1977) examined the linguistic and academic skills of four groups of children. Two groups were orally trained, one of which had active parental involvement at all stages of the educational process. The other two groups were manually trained, one in ASL and the other in a form of manually coded English. There was no difference in the abilities of the two orally trained groups, but there were significant differences between them and the manually trained groups, with the latter achieving better on academic and language measures. However, different conclusions were reported by Geers, Moog, and Schick (1984), who examined the performances of deaf children from auditory/oral and TC programs on the *Grammatical Analysis of Elicited Language—Simple Sentence Level* (GAEL-S). These researchers concluded that the scores of the auditory/oral children were superior to those of the TC children. The results of other studies have also been inconsistent. Several authors either favored programs with a manual component or found no significant difference (Montgomery, 1966; Moores, Weiss, & Goodwin, 1978; Quigley, 1969; Seewald, Ross, Giolas, & Yonovitz, 1985). However, other authors obtained results that favor auditory/oral programs (Greenberg, 1980; Jensema & Trybus, 1978). What is clear is that the introduction of TC into programs for the hearing impaired has not resulted in the hoped-for improvement in language skills (Levitt et al., 1987; Osberger, 1986).

Jensema and Trybus (1978), reporting on a national study conducted through the Office of Demographic Studies, concluded that academic success or failure is based on a number of variables in addition to communication mode, such as the child's hearing level, the family's income, and the child's age at intervention. Two recent large longitudinal studies have reinforced

this finding. Levitt et al. (1987) suggest that competence in linguistic and academic areas cannot necessarily be predicted from the educational environment and that factors beyond our control, such as the etiology and degree of hearing impairment, may be more important. As a result of a 4-year study on preschool children, Musselman, Lindsay, and Wilson (1988) reported that age, degree of hearing loss, and intelligence are the most important correlates of development. Although these researchers did find that auditory/oral children scored higher on some measures of spoken language than did TC children, two important points should be noted. First, the selection methods for educational placement tended to put lower-achieving children into TC programs. Second, the language output of the preschoolers may have been related in part to the signing level of their parents, which in most cases was fairly limited. The parents had learned signing only after their children were diagnosed as hearing impaired.

It is argued that children who are exposed to sign from birth, such as children born to deaf, signing parents, develop language that follows essentially the same pattern that hearing childen demonstrate in their normal development (Bonvillan, Nelson, & Charrow, 1976). There is concern that deaf children of hearing parents who do not have such early exposure to language may be more delayed in their language learning. A study by White and White (1987) on the language performance of preschoolers found better language performance in the deaf children of deaf parents than in the deaf children of hearing parents. On the other hand, the speech of the children with hearing parents was superior to that of the children with deaf parents.

A discussion of the controversy surrounding manual versus auditory/oral communication needs to look at the social and emotional impact that each approach may have on the hearing-impaired children and their families. A frequent argument is that those who use manual communication isolate themselves from the rest of society, as they limit their interactions to those who can sign. Furthermore, they expose themselves to societal biases due to lack of knowledge and understanding. On the positive side, they can relate well to their hearing-impaired peers who also sign. This skill gives them an environment in which they can share thoughts and emotions, without the isolation and frustration that come from being unable to communicate.

The argument that the use of sign isolates the hearing-impaired person needs to be examined with reference to the skills of those who are educated in auditory/oral environments. In many instances, the speech intelligibility of these children is poor. Only a few individuals close to these children are able to understand their spoken language, so that the communicative interactions of the children are limited. If such children were lost, they might have difficulty supplying authorities with their names and addresses. Proponents of sign say that at least the hearing-impaired signer has a group with which to communicate, whereas the child who does not sign and has unintelligible speech is sometimes left even more isolated.

Cued speech consists of 12 hand signals used around the mouth to supplement simultaneously what is available through audition and lipreading. For example, the sounds /t/ and /d/, which look alike on the lips, have different hand signals. Ambiguity and, thus, frustration are reduced for both the speaker and the listener. The use of cued speech significantly improves the receiver's ability to interpret spoken language and to target a correct sound in speech production training. It may also be useful in promoting the acquisition of spoken language (Clarke & Ling, 1976; Ling & Clarke, 1975; Nicholls & Ling, 1982). Mohay (1983) found that in a group of prelinguistic, profoundly deaf children who used cued speech, there were slight increases in the lengths of their utterances and decreases in other forms of gestural communication. However, the overall amount and diversity of their linguistic utterances did not alter. It is possible that there is an ideal stage of development during which cued speech could be introduced, but at the moment the benefits of using cued speech with young, hearing-impaired children are inconclusive. There are no reports in the literature indicating that the use of cued speech is widespread.

We must view the hearing-impaired population as heterogeneous and their educational and linguistic achievements as confounded by a number of vari-

ables. It is clear that no one communication and educational approach will suit all hearing-impaired children (Levitt, 1987; Osberger & Hesketh, 1988; White, 1984; White & White, 1987).

ACADEMIC ACHIEVEMENT

Hearing-impaired children are consistently reported as performing on a par with their hearing peers on nonverbal tests of intellectual functioning but below their hearing peers on verbal tests of intellectual functioning (Davis et al., 1986). In addition, hearing-impaired children in a variety of educational settings perform well below their hearing peers on measures of academic achievement. These reports are disheartening in their consistency across age ranges and educational settings. But perhaps even more disturbing is the fact that the delay in academic areas tends to increase with time, so that the gap between the academic skills of the hearing impaired and those of their normally hearing peers increases with time (Davis, Shepard, Stelmachowicz, & Gorga, 1981; Paul & Young, 1975). In a study by Paul and Young (1975), one third of the children with moderate hearing losses increased their academic performance by less than 6 months over a 12-month period. This means that over a 3-year period of schooling, hearing-impaired children could experience a delay of 1½ years in academic skills.

The implications of such reports are disturbing and raise a number of questions. One important question is whether hearing-impaired children are receiving the services they need in school. Davis et al. (1981) reported that many of the children in their investigation had failed to receive complete assessments of language, speech perception, and academic and intellectual skills. Without adequate psychoeducational data on these children, it was not possible to plan the most effective intervention and educational placement. A study on the impact of PL 94-142 on the services handicapped children were receiving found that the law generally had a positive effect, although a number of issues needed attention. Large caseloads still existed, there were too few audiologists, and many children who had speech, language, and hearing

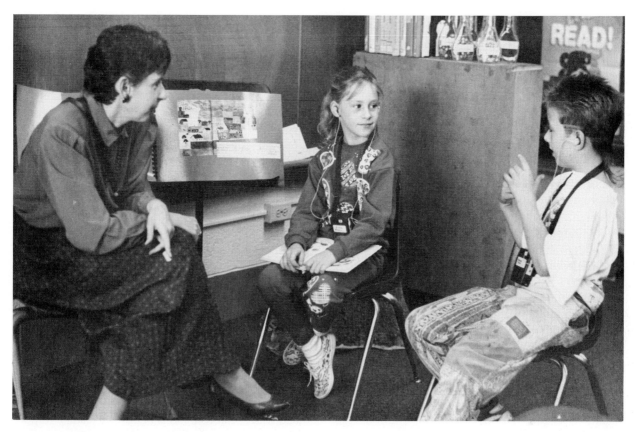

Hearing-impaired children may be at risk for learning to read.

needs were still not being adequately served (Mansour & Lingwall, 1985).

Learning to read is frequently regarded as an indicator of academic success (Osberger, 1986). For many hearing-impaired children, learning to read involves a two-step process: learning language and learning to read (Davis & Hardick, 1981). Many hearing-impaired children do not have an adequate base in auditory-oral language on which to build their reading skills. The reading perfomance of hearing-impaired children has consistently been reported as poor. A study by McClure (1966) revealed that 30% of hearing-impaired 16-year-olds were functionally illiterate and that 60% read at levels below the sixth grade. Only 5% were able to read at the 10th-grade level or better. Trybus and Karchmer (1977) demonstrated clearly the effect of the widening academic achievement gap as these children grow older. At the age of 14, hearing-impaired children read at more than five grades below normally hearing children, while at the age of 9 they were only one and one-half grades below. Severe delays in reading comprehension were also reported by Osberger (1986), who found the highest level of reading comprehension from 9 to 16 years to be comparable to that of a fourth grade child with normal hearing.

INTERVENTION AND MANAGEMENT

Early intervention is seen as important in the development of speech, language, and academic skills in the hearing impaired. Numerous studies have shown the benefits when intervention is begun at an early age (e.g., Levitt et al., 1987; White & White, 1987). Early intervention requires accurate and early diagnosis, fitting of appropriate amplification, early special education, and early speech and language intervention. Hearing-impaired children continue to need intervention throughout the school years.

Early Identification

Before successful intervention is achieved, the child's hearing status must be established. Throughout the United States in the last two decades, many hospitals and clinics have initiated programs to identify at-risk infants at birth or in the first year of life. These programs usually screen babies identified as at risk for hearing impairment and aim to identify moderate to severe hearing loss. Recent studies have demonstrated that reliable, cost-effective methods are available (Hyde, Riko, & Maliziz, 1990; Konkle & Jacobson, 1991).

The most recent statement of the Joint Committee on Infant Hearing Screening in 1990 (ASHA, 1991) lists several criteria that may be used to identify infants at risk for sensorineural hearing loss (Table 9.2). The statement departs substantially from previous risk statements in that two separate risk criteria are listed for different age groups.

The Joint Committee guidelines recommend when to screen and state that, wherever possible, the diagnostic process should be completed and habilitation begun by 6 months. Both electrophysiological and behavioral testing are recommended. Early testing may not identify children with mild hearing disorders, as infants require loud intensities to produce a response. It is also important to be aware that most programs for early identification are based on high-risk factors, and not all children with significant hearing loss will present with such factors. Of equal importance is that once a child is diagnosed as hearing impaired, intervention must begin. Current reports suggest that the delay between diagnosis and intervention is sometimes unacceptably long (Elssmann, Matkin, & Sabo, 1987; Jerger, 1990; Stein, Jabaley, Spitz, Stoakley, & McGee, 1990).

Otitis Media

The early identification guidelines just discussed are not designed to identify children who are at risk of hearing impairment and speech and language delay as a result of repeated or chronic middle ear infections. The prevalence of otitis media has long been associated with social conditions of poverty leading to poor living conditions, including poor nutrition, poor sanitation, and low levels of education. Native Americans,

TABLE 9.2 Risk Factors for the Identification of Hearing Loss in Infants and Toddlers	Group A Neonates (Birth–28 Days)	Group B Infants (29 Days–2 Years)
	Family history	Applicable factors from Group A
	Congenital infections	Parent/caregiver concern about communication development and developmental delay
	Craniofacial anomalies	Head trauma
	Low birth weight	Neurodegenerative disorders
	Hyperbilirubinemia	Diseases (e.g., mumps, measles) associated with sensorineural hearing loss
	Administration of ototoxic drugs	
	Bacterial meningitis	
	Severe depression at birth	
	Syndromes associated with hearing loss	

Source: Adapted from ASHA (1991).

including Eskimos, have been found to have high rates of otitis media (Northern & Downs, 1991). Additionally, any social group that lives in poverty, with its attendant problems, must be considered at risk for higher prevalence rates of otitis media.

Guidelines for screening hearing and middle ear function for children aged 3 years through Grade 3 have been prepared by the American Speech-Language-Hearing Association (ASHA, 1985, 1990). The emphasis is on screening on a regular basis (ideally, each year), thus preventing the long-term difficulties that can arise because of undetected mild to moderate hearing impairment.

Sound Amplification Systems

One of the key factors in intervention is the selection of appropriate amplification devices. With infants and young children, much time is required for the proper selection and fitting of a hearing aid by an audiologist. The procedure can be complicated by the fact that the audiologist often works with incomplete test data because of the difficulty of testing young children and because these children provide little or no feedback on the outcome of fitting.

Amplification systems are of two types—personal hearing aids (most common) and group amplification systems. The purpose of any type of hearing aid is to amplify sounds, making them louder, and to deliver them to the ear of the listener so that they are more easily detected. A personal hearing aid contains four basic components: a microphone, an amplifier, a receiver, and a battery. The microphone picks up sound waves and converts them into electrical energy. It is encased in the hearing aid itself and appears as either a small opening or a grid somewhere on the case. The amplifier then boosts the electrical signal. The receiver, which is built into the hearing aid in all but body-worn hearing aids, converts the amplified electrical energy back into sound waves, and the battery provides the power for all the other circuits. Each hearing aid has specifications for the type of battery needed, and it does not function if the battery is inserted incorrectly.

There are five types of personal hearing aids, their names reflecting where they are worn by the user: (1) body aids, (2) behind-the-ear (BTE) aids, (3) in-the-ear (ITE) aids, (4) in-the-canal (ITC) aids, and (5) eyeglass aids. The most common type of hearing aid for infants and children is the BTE. Also referred to as *ear-level aids,* these hearing aids have their components housed in a small, crescent-shaped case that fits behind the ear of the user. Figure 9.3 illustrates a typical BTE and its components. Body aids and eyeglass aids are seldom fitted today, and manufacturers are making few technical improvements for them. ITE and ITC aids are recommended by some manufacturers; they are small and inconspicuous, and the amplified signal they deliver is good. However, a number of factors, such as frequent need for repair and the requirement for safety, make them less durable and versatile for use with children (Beauchaine, Nelson Barlow, & Stelmachowicz, 1990).

With the exception of ITE and ITC aids, in which all the components are contained in the earpiece, personal hearing aids require the use of a separate earmold that fits into the user's ear. Earmolds are individually made for each ear from plastic-like materials. The earmold delivers the amplified sound into the ear canal. It is essential that the earmold fit snugly so that sound will not leak out around the sides. If this happens, the leaked sound is then fed back into the hearing aid microphone, causing a high-pitched squeal, known as *feedback,* that interferes with the listening of both the hearing aid's user and other people nearby. To avoid feedback, it is necessary to ensure a well-fitting mold by refitting it as the child grows. In older children this may be every 6 to 12 months, whereas in children under the age of 4, a refit may be needed every 3 to 6 months.

Use of group hearing aids for children has typically been associated with educational and/or (re)habilitative settings. Many different systems have been used, all of which enable the children to receive speech with a better signal-to-noise ratio. Some of these are hard-wired systems in which the speaker talks into a microphone and the children receive the amplified speech through headphones. Alternatively, a magnetic loop can be installed in a room, and the children can receive the amplified signal through their personal hearing aids.

In the past two decades, group amplification has been more commonly provided by frequency modulated (FM) radio hearing aids. With FM aids, the

FIGURE 9.3 An Example of a BTE Hearing Aid.

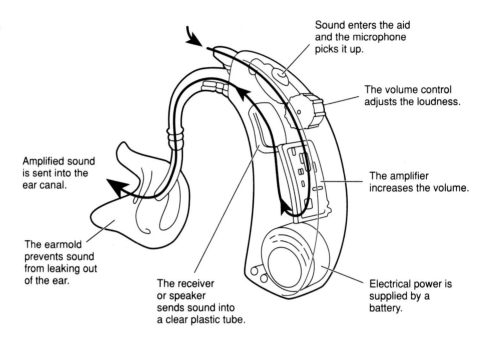

Sound enters the aid and the microphone picks it up.

The volume control adjusts the loudness.

The amplifier increases the volume.

Amplified sound is sent into the ear canal.

The earmold prevents sound from leaking out of the ear.

The receiver or speaker sends sound into a clear plastic tube.

Electrical power is supplied by a battery.

speaker wears a small radio transmitter and a microphone close to the mouth. The amplified signal can be directed into a sound field or, more often, the child wears a radio receiver and the signal can be directed to the ear, either through an earphone or through the child's personal BTE. The two major advantages of FM systems are that they provide an improved signal-to-noise ratio and at the same time permit movement of both the speaker and the child around the room. They are particularly beneficial where childen are mainstreamed in conditions with high levels of background noise.

If the child is to benefit from the hearing aid, the device must function properly. Daily monitoring should be performed by the child (if old enough) and by all adults in regular contact with the child. Either a personal earmold or a hearing aid stethoscope is needed. After inspection of the battery and tubing, the aid is turned on and turned to the "M" (microphone) setting so that the listener can evaluate the quality of the signal, listening for static or intermittent cutout (Flexer, 1990; Osberger & Hesketh, 1988; Reichman & Healey, 1989).

Recently, two methods of amplification have been offered to the profoundly hearing impaired. One is an implantable device, called a cochlear implant, and the other is vibrotactile and electrotactile devices. These devices supplement visual information and are designed for children whose hearing impairments are so profound that they are unable to benefit adequately from conventional hearing aids. The *cochlear implant* uses electrodes implanted into the cochlea to deliver electrical signals to the eighth (acoustic) nerve. A microphone is contained in a wearable speech processor, and acoustic signals are selectively amplified by the speech processor, using a processing system that highlights the speech signal. These signals are transmitted to a receiver implanted in the mastoid bone behind the ear, and the receiver then delivers an amplified signal to the electrodes. *Vibrotactile devices,* as their name implies, enable the wearer to feel vibration of sounds on the skin. The child wears something in contact with the skin that delivers an amplified, processed, tactile signal. Electrotactile devices deliver electrical pulses to the skin. They can be placed on the wrist, the fingers, the sternum (breast bone), and the abdomen.

Both cochlear implants and tactile devices have demonstrated benefits in clinical experiments over the past decade, although it is clear that neither device is able to give to the hearer a normal auditory signal. Speech perception, speech production, and language development benefits from cochlear implants vary widely, depending partly on whether the device fitted is single-channel or multichannel. Multichannel devices are able to provide more information to the user. Additional factors, such as the status of the individual hearing mechanism, age at which the device is acquired, age of onset of hearing loss, time since acquiring the device, amount of training with the device, and type of device, influence personal performance. The effects on learning can extend to beyond $1\frac{1}{2}$ years after receiving an implant (Osberger, 1990), and the best users are able to discriminate speech materials in conditions where a number of alternatives are possible. Tactile devices are generally more effective for increasing reception and production of suprasegmental aspects of speech. The skin is sensitive only to low-frequency sounds, with an optimal frequency range of 40–400 Hz; has a greatly reduced dynamic range; and cannot discriminate as finely between frequencies as can the ear. Some devices transpose high-frequency information, and the child learns to recognize, for example, high-frequency affrication from a position on the fingers. Evidence suggests that extensive training is vital if the wearer is to learn to do this (Osberger, 1990).

Language Intervention

Intervention with hearing-impaired children is multidisciplinary and involves parents, educators, audiologists, speech-language pathologists, counselors, and physicians. The parents and professionals use a team approach to plan and implement an intervention program for each child. Language intervention is a critical component, and progress is reflected not only in language performance but in cognitive, academic, and social developments as well. Equal importance should be placed on hearing management and language learning, as a consistent effort is needed to improve the generally poor language functioning reported for the hearing impaired. Language competence is the major determinant of academic achievement for the hearing impaired (Geers & Moog, 1989; Osberger, 1986).

Intervention needs to be tailored to the individual and the family, using the communication method that best suits each particular circumstance. In determining the most appropriate intervention strategy, two problems arise. The first centers on the sequences used in intervention and the second on the approaches employed. Intervention that begins early in a child's life follows a normal developmental pattern, with attempts to mirror for the child both the experiences of a normally hearing child and the normal development of language. Intervention that begins with an older child is frequently nonsequential, identifying and working on specific areas of weakness or need, a practice that receives support from some evidence of deviant versus delayed patterns in the language of some hearing-impaired children. Unfortunately, there are very little empirical data to support the use of either developmental or nondevelopmental sequencing in language intervention for the hearing impaired (Hasenstab, 1983; Osberger & Hesketh, 1988). Furthermore, many of the approaches used have not been designed specifically for the hearing impaired (Kretschmer & Kretschmer, 1978). The intervention strategies usually parallel those employed with other language-disordered children, modifying the input to accommodate the diminished auditory signal received by the children.

There are differing views on whether to emphasize the visual or the auditory modality. For children with more severe hearing losses, the visual modality may be emphasized. For those with less severe losses, the auditory modality may be emphasized. Finally, for those with profound hearing loss, the tactile modality may be emphasized. In very few cases is only one modality used exclusively. It is generally accepted that whatever approach works best to give the child a language base to ensure academic and social progress is the most appropriate one (Northern & Downs, 1991). Interpretation of this approach extends to whether or not manual communication is used in intervention for which the goal is oral language competence. The issues regarding the use of manual communication have already been discussed. However, it appears that the use of manual communication, in the context of TC, is conducive to the development of oral language.

For the preschool hearing-impaired child, there is ongoing debate over the best methodology, but professionals agree that the language learning should be an active process that includes experiences with people and objects—a necessary condition for learning. There is concern that if the child is placed in a structured, adult-directed learning situation, with repetition of important language structures, the child will not develop appropriate peer interaction and discourse. There is evidence that such skills are frequently deficient in the older hearing-impaired child (Easterbrooks, 1987; Moeller, Osberger, & Morford, 1987). On the other hand, there is concern that in the course of active learning, the child will concentrate on the materials or the visual/tangible environment and not the linguistic aspects of the activity. This has led to the use of many programs with a combination of activities, some child-directed and others teacher-directed. The teacher-directed activities may well involve materials that the child has selected, with the instructor modeling and expanding the linguistic aspects in the same way this is done for normally hearing children. In the majority of programs, parental involvement is essential, with the parents continuing to foster language through activities in both formal and informal situations away from a professional setting.

Studies have demonstrated that preschool hearing-impaired children are delayed in their conversational skills (Kretschmer & Kretschmer, 1978). This indicates the need for intervention programs to promote these skills, ensuring that the children are not just drilled on specific language structures. This can be difficult with hearing-impaired children. It is also possible that these children may sometimes receive an impoverished communication model, although recent experience suggests that a strong commitment to parental/caregiver education can reverse this trend (Luetke-Stahlman & Moeller, 1985).

In addition to making the language-learning process active, professionals need to select specific objectives for the child in the areas of form, content, and function. Unfortunately, little is known about how hearing-impaired children acquire form, content, and function skills (Moeller et al., 1987). In many programs, a sequence based on normal language development is used, as most evidence suggests that the hearing-impaired preschooler develops language in the same sequence as normally hearing peers. This teaching process initially concentrates on nouns and verbs and then progresses from words of location, such as "here" and "there," to spatial terms, temporal terms, and then to conditional and causal expressions.

Programs for the preschooler with a hearing impairment likely require a special focus on vocabulary development, as delay in this area is a serious problem in older hearing-impaired children (Osberger, 1986). Many programs use semantic classes of items such as "food," "transportation," or "family." This approach provides semantic information that can then be expanded to include syntactical aspects. A number of resources are available to help parents and professionals plan sequences and materials for use with the preschooler. One program developed for normally hearing children, which provides active learning tasks, is by Hohmann, Banet, and Weikart (1979).

For the school-age hearing-impaired child, speech and language intervention becomes extremely complex. Not only does the program need to be individualized for the child, but the demands of the educational process need to be considered. Educators and clinicians must work together to ensure that the child gets maximum benefit from intervention. An eight-step model has been presented by Reed and Bugen (1983). The model makes two assumptions: (1) the sequence of acquisition should follow that of the normally hearing child and (2) language learning should be interactive and involve both formal and informal experiences, with emphasis not only on the structures to be used but also on language as a means of communicating and interacting. The model includes planning grammatical targets, planning how to implement each target meaningfully, providing practice, reinforcing, and expanding the structures to higher levels of difficulty. Assessment is part of the model at all stages.

Using language and speech as an interactive communication process has been emphasized repeatedly (e.g., Kretschmer & Kretschmer, 1978). Children need to be involved with as many activities and as much material as possible to be encouraged to use language in an interactive manner.

There has always been considerable debate over the best methods of teaching language to this population. Certain approaches provide various systems for the children to follow. It is not possible to outline all of these approaches here. We will mention a few as examples. The *Fitzgerald Key* (Fitzgerald, 1949) provides a pattern for children to use in analyzing speech in a very structured fashion. Although now considered an artificial way of presenting language, it can be a useful guide for some children (Easterbrooks, 1987). The *Test of Syntactic Abilities* by Quigley and Power (1979) is a comprehensive assessment and instructional package for nine syntactic areas. A relatively recent proposal is to teach English as a second language (Hatfield, Caccamise, & Siple, 1978). Older children who have been reared in an ASL environment are later exposed to English as a second language, or younger children are exposed to both languages from the outset, effectively growing up bilingual. As with many approaches, empirical evidence of efficacy is lacking.

Educational Approaches

Over the last decade, the majority of hearing-impaired children have been educated in public schools. One of the key changes has been the provision of TC programs, whereby the child is exposed to both oral/aural and visual methods of presenting language (Moores, 1987). Prior to the introduction of TC, hearing-impaired children who were not mainstreamed were placed in either auditory/oral or manual programs. A frequent problem was the need for sufficiently sensitive diagnostic procedures to assist in choosing a program for a particular child. It was often recommended that a preschooler initially be enrolled in an auditory/oral program, assessed for progress, and either kept in the program or moved to a manual program. A common alternative now is for a hearing-impaired preschooler to be integrated into a hearing preschool, with speech-language and auditory intervention scheduled on an individual basis.

Assessment of suitability for a particular educational approach is a lengthy, complex process that focuses not only on auditory and communication skills but also on other areas, such as social development, educational ability, and family support. Schools for the hearing impaired frequently have a defined procedure to assess suitability for a particular program. An example is the program at the Clark School for the Deaf in Northhampton, Massachusetts (Gatty, Schneider, &

Gjerdingen, 1985). For children who are to be mainstreamed, particular school districts institute interdisciplinary assessment programs and incorporate input from many professionals, including audiologists, speech-language pathologists, regular and special educators, counselors, and parents. It is important that parental input be obtained and that the parents feel they are making informed choices about their child's future (Brill et al., 1986).

Scales are available to identify children who may need more emphasis on visual and tactile methods of communication. One such scale is the *Deafness Management Quotient* (DMQ) (Downs, 1974), which evaluates residual hearing, intelligence, family support, socioeconomic status, and central processing abilities. Another scale, the *Feasibility Scale for Language Acquisition Routing* (FSLAR), is reported by Rupp et al. (1977). A number of factors are considered, among them aided and unaided hearing, parental interaction, communication mode used by the child, age at first intervention, and behavior of the child during testing.

As we have seen throughout this chapter, there is a correlation between academic achievement and competent use of oral language. In turn, there is a correlation between language abilities and the degree to which hearing-impaired children use their auditory abilities. Over the past two decades an increasing number of assessment procedures, both formal and informal, has become available to assess the language and auditory abilities of the hearing impaired. A test battery approach is recommended to cover many aspects of language (Moeller et al., 1987; Nerbonne & Schow, 1989; Osberger & Hesketh, 1988). Examples of such batteries specifically for use with the hearing impaired are the *Grammatical Analysis of Elicited Language Tests,* designed for different age groups (GAEL-S, GAEL-P, and GAEL-C), published by the Central Institute for the Deaf, St. Louis, Missouri. These tests are complemented by the *Teacher Assessment of Grammatical Structure Tests* (TAGS), which consists of rating scales for the use of grammatical structures. The GAEL and TAGS suggest sequences for teaching grammatical structures.

Several tests are designed to assess auditory abilities, and an increasing number of useful tests designed specifically for the hearing impaired are available for this very important area. One example is the *Test of*

Auditory Comprehension (TAC), developed by Trammell (1979), which assesses discrimination, memory, sequencing, comprehension, and auditory figure-ground abilities. Another is the *Glendonald Auditory Screening Procedure* (GASP) developed by Erber (1982). It assesses phoneme detection, word identification, and sentence comprehension.

Whatever assessment procedures are used, it must be remembered that each child is an individual who brings to the assessment process a unique combination of abilities and needs. Decisions about educa-tional placement must be made with this fact in mind. Of equal importance is the need for ongoing appraisal of each child's development in academic and communication areas. Educational decisions may need to be changed as children develop and respond to their particular programs. Monitoring of intervention is essential so that the goals of language acquisition and educational achievement can be met for each child. These goals should remain foremost, irrespective of methodologies.

SUMMARY

In this chapter we have seen that:

▶ Children can have different types of hearing losses and a range of hearing levels. These factors combine to affect each hearing-impaired child's communicative functioning in a unique way.

▶ The degree of stability of hearing loss, the age of the child when the loss occurred, and the child's age when the loss is detected and intervention initiated also affect a hearing-impaired child's communicative functioning.

▶ The characteristics of a child's hearing loss combined with the acoustical characteristics of speech sounds, especially in connected speech, influence what parts of speech the child can and cannot detect. This, in turn, affects the child's speech and language performance.

▶ The amount of background noise is a significant factor in how well a hearing-impaired child can function in different listening environments.

▶ Hearing-impaired children can have problems with all aspects of language functioning, and these problems can be exacerbated in education because of the linguistic levels of the educational materials used. There is also evidence that the gap between hearing-impaired children's language level and that of their normally hearing peers widens as the hearing-impaired children grow older.

▶ Mild hearing losses caused by ear infections and unilateral hearing losses can negatively affect children's language and academic performances.

▶ The choice of communication and educational modes (manual, TC, auditory/oral) depends on the unique situation of each child. No one mode suits all children.

▶ Hearing-impaired children's academic achievements are frequently poor, and the gap between their achievements and those of their normally hearing peers increases with age. Reading levels are especially affected.

▶ Models of language intervention for hearing-impaired children generally follow normal developmental sequences, but there is little empirical evidence to support this practice. Little is known generally about how hearing-impaired children learn language, and even less is known about the efficacy of various intervention strategies.

Any degree of hearing loss puts a child at risk for language learning and academic achievement. There is no one documented correct method of intervention, but early identification, followed by early intervention that results from interdisciplinary cooperation and planning and that involves the parents from the beginning, gives the hearing-impaired child the best chance of succeeding.

REFERENCES

American Academy of Pediatrics. (1985). Pediatrics academy advises on language–otitis media link. *Asha, 27,* 12.

ASHA. (1985). Guidelines for identification audiometry. *Asha, 27,* 49–52.

ASHA. (1990). Guidelines for screening for hearing impairments and middle ear disorders. *Asha, 32*(Suppl. 2), 17–24.

ASHA. (1991). Joint Committee on Infant Hearing 1990 Position Statement. *Asha, 33*(Suppl. 5), 3–6.

Beauchaine, K. L., Nelson Barlow, N. L., & Stelmachowicz, P. G. (1990, June–July). Special considerations in amplification for young children. *Asha, 32,* 44–46.

Bellugi, U., & Klima, E. (1972). The roots of language in the sign talk of the deaf. *Psychology Today, 6,* 60–64.

Berg, F. S. (1987). *Facilitating classroom listening: A handbook for teachers of normal and hard of hearing students.* Boston: College-Hill Press/Little, Brown.

Bergman, M. (1957). Binaural hearing. *Archives of Otolaryngology, 66,* 572–578.

Bess, F., Klee, T., & Culbertson, J. (1986). Identification, assessment and management of children with unilateral sensorineural hearing loss. *Ear and Hearing, 7,* 43–51.

Boehm, A. (1970). *Boehm test of basic concepts.* New York: Psychological Corporation.

Bonvillian, J., Nelson, K., & Charrow, V. (1976). Language and language-related skills in deaf and hearing children. *Sign Language Studies, 12,* 211–250.

Boothroyd, A. (1982). *Hearing impairments in young children.* Englewood Cliffs, NJ: Prentice-Hall.

Boothroyd, A. (1984). Auditory perception of speech contrasts by subjects with sensorineural hearing loss. *Journal of Speech and Hearing Research, 27,* 134–144.

Brandes, P., & Ehinger, D. (1981). The effects of early middle ear pathology on auditory perception and academic achievement. *Journal of Speech and Hearing Disorders, 46,* 301–307.

Brannon, J. (1968). Linguistic word classes in the spoken language of normal, hard of hearing, and deaf children. *Journal of Speech and Hearing Research, 11,* 279–287.

Brasel, K., & Quigley, S. (1977). The influence of certain language and communication environments in early childhood on the development of language in deaf individuals. *Journal of Speech and Hearing Research, 20,* 95–107.

Brenza, B., Kricos, P., & Lasky, E. (1981). Comprehension and production of basic semantic concepts by older hearing-impaired children. *Journal of Speech and Hearing Research, 24,* 414–419.

Brill, R. G., MacNeil, B., & Newman, L. R. (1986). Framework for appropriate programs for deaf children—Conference of educational administrators serving the deaf. *American Annals of the Deaf, 131,* 65–77.

Brown, J. (1984). Examination of grammatical morphemes in the language of hard-of-hearing children. *Volta Review, 86,* 229–238.

Bunch, G., & Melnyk, T. (1989). A review of the evidence for a learning-disabled, hearing-impaired sub-group. *American Annals of the Deaf, 134,* 297–300.

Clarke, B., & Ling, D. (1976). The effects of using cued speech: A follow-up study. *Volta Review, 78,* 23–34.

Clarkson, R., Eimas, P., & Marean, G. C. (1989). Speech perception in children with histories of recurrent otitis media. *Journal of the Acoustical Society of America, 85,* 926–933.

Cornett, O. (1967). Cued speech. *American Annals of the Deaf, 112,* 3–13.

Cross, T., Johnson-Morris, J., & Nienhuys, T. (1980). Linguistic feedback and maternal speech: Comparison of mothers addressing hearing and hearing-impaired children. *First Language, 1,* 163–189.

Culbertson, J., & Gilbert, L. (1986). Children with unilateral sensorineural hearing loss: Cognitive, academic and social development. *Ear and Hearing, 7,* 38–42.

Curtiss, S., Prutting, C., & Lowell, E. (1979). Pragmatic and semantic development in young children with impaired hearing. *Journal of Speech and Hearing Research, 22,* 534–552.

Davis, J. (1974). Performance of young hearing impaired children on a test of basic concepts. *Journal of Speech and Hearing Research, 17,* 342–351.

Davis, J., & Blasdell, R. (1975). Perceptual strategies employed by normal-hearing and hearing-impaired children in the comprehension of sentences containing relative clauses. *Journal of Speech and Hearing Research, 18,* 281–295.

Davis, J., Elfenbein, J., Schum, R., & Bentler, R. A. (1986). Effects of mild and moderate hearing impairments on language, educational, and psychosocial behavior of children. *Journal of Speech and Hearing Disorders, 51,* 53–62.

Davis, J., & Hardick, E. (1981). *Rehabilitative audiology for children and adults.* New York: Wiley.

Davis, J., Shepard, N., Stelmachowicz, P., & Gorga, M. (1981). Characteristics of hearing-impaired children in the public schools: Part II—Psychoeducational data. *Journal of Speech and Hearing Disorders, 46,* 130–137.

Denton, D. (1966). A study in the education achievement of deaf children. In *Report of the Proceedings of the 42nd Meeting of the Convention of American Instructors of the Deaf.* Washington, DC: U.S. Government Printing Office, pp. 428–433.

Downs, M. (1974, January-February). The deafness management quotient. *Hearing and Speech News.*

Downs, M. (1981). Contribution of mild hearing loss to auditory language learning problems. In R. Roeser & M. Downs (Eds.), *Auditory disorders in school children.* New York: Thieme Stratton.

Easterbrooks, S. R. (1987). Speech/language assessment and intervention with school-age hearing-impaired children. In J. Alpiner & P. McCarthy (Eds.), *Rehabilitative audiology: Children and adults* (pp. 188–240). Baltimore: Williams and Wilkins.

Elssmann, S., Matkin, N., & Sabo, M. (1987). Early identification of congenital sensorineural hearing impairment. *The Hearing Journal, 40,* 13–17.

Engen, E., & Engen, T. (1983). *Rhode Island test of language structure manual.* Baltimore: University Park Press.

Erber, N. (1971). Auditory and audiovisual reception of words in low-frequency noise by children with normal hearing and by children with impaired hearing. *Journal of Speech and Hearing Research, 14,* 496–512.

Erber, N. (1979). Speech perception by profoundly deaf children. *Journal of Speech and Hearing Disorders, 44,* 255–270.

Erber, N. (1982). *Auditory training.* Washington, DC: Alexander Graham Bell Association for the Deaf.

Erber, N., & Alencewicz, C. (1976). Audiologic evaluation of deaf children. *Journal of Speech and Hearing Disorders, 41,* 256–267.

Fitzgerald, E. (1949). *Straight language for the deaf.* Washington, DC: Alexander Graham Bell Association for the Deaf.

Flexer, C. (1990, April). Audiological rehabilitation in the schools. *Asha, 32,* 44–45.

Friel-Patti, S., & Finitzo, T. (1990). Language learning in a prospective study of otitis media with effusion in the first two years of life. *Journal of Speech and Hearing Research, 33,* 188–194.

Gatty, J., Schneider, M., & Gjerdingen, D. (1985). The Clarke School visiting infant and parent (V.I.P.) program: An approach to short-term audiological/educational intervention. In I. G. Taylor (Ed.), *The education of the deaf: Current perspectives* (Vol. II, pp. 726–734). London: Croom Helm.

Geers, A., & Moog, J. (1989). Factors predictive of the development of literacy in profoundly hearing-impaired adolescents. *Volta Review, 91,* 69–86.

Geers, A., Moog, J., & Schick, B. (1984). Acquisition of spoken and signed English by profoundly deaf children. *Journal of Speech and Hearing Disorders, 49,* 378–388.

Gold, T., & Levitt, H. (1975). *Comparison of articulatory errors in hard of hearing and deaf children.* New York: Communication Sciences Laboratory, Graduate School and University Center, City University of New York.

Gravel, J. S., & Wallace, I. F. (1992). Listening and learning at 4 years of age: Effects of early otitis media. *Journal of Speech and Hearing Research, 35,* 588–595.

Greenberg, M. (1980). Mode use in deaf children: The effects of communication method and communication competence. *Applied Psycholinguistics, 1,* 65–79.

Hasenstab, M. (1983). Child language studies: Impact on habilitation of hearing-impaired infants and preschool children. In R. Truax & J. Schultz (Eds.), *Learning to communicate: Implications for the hearing impaired.* Washington, DC: Alexander Graham Bell Association for the Deaf.

Hatfield, N., Caccamise, F., & Siple, P. (1978). Deaf students' language competency: A bilingual perspective. *American Annals of the Deaf, 123,* 847–851.

Hohmann, M., Banet, B., & Weikart, D. (1979). *Young children in action.* Ypsilanti, MI: High/Scope Press.

Hyde, M., Riko, K., & Maliziz, K. (1990). Audiometric accuracy of the click ABR in infants at risk for hearing loss. *Journal of the American Academy of Audiology, 1,* 59–66.

Iran-Nejad, A., Ortony, A., & Rittenhouse, R. (1981). The comprehension of metaphorical uses of English by deaf children. *Journal of Speech and Hearing Disorders, 42,* 143–147.

Jensema, C., & Trybus, R. (1978). *Communication patterns and educational achievement of hearing impaired students.* Series T, Number 2. Office of Demographic Studies, Gallaudet College, Washington, DC.

Jerger, J. (1990). Neonatal screening. *Journal of the American Academy of Audiology, 1,* 57.

John, J., & Howarth, J. (1965). The effect of time distortions on the intelligibility of deaf children's speech. *Language and Speech, 8,* 127–134.

Kenworthy, O. T. (1986). Caregiver–child interaction and language acquisition of hearing-impaired children. *Topics in Language Disorders, 6,* 1–11.

Klee, T., & Davis-Dansky, E. (1986). A comparison of unilaterally hearing-impaired children and normal-hearing children on a battery of standardized language tests. *Ear and Hearing, 7,* 27–37.

Konkle, D., & Jacobson, J. (1991). Hearing loss in newborns, infants and young children. In W. F. Rintelmann (Ed.), *Hearing assessment.* Austin, TX: PRO-ED.

Kretschmer, R., & Kretschmer, L. (1978). *Language development and intervention with the hearing impaired.* Baltimore: University Park Press.

Kretschmer, R., & Kretschmer, L. (1980). Pragmatics: Development in normal-hearing and hearing-impaired children. In J. Subtelny (Ed.), *Speech assessment and speech improvement for the hearing impaired.* Washington, DC: Alexander Graham Bell Association for the Deaf.

Lehmann, M., Charron, K., Kummer, A., & Keith, R. (1979). The effects of chronic middle ear effusion on speech and language development—a descriptive study. *International Journal of Pediatric Otorhinolaryngology, 1,* 137–144.

Levitt, H. (1987). Interrelationships among the speech and language levels. In H. Levitt, N. McGarr, & D. Geffner (Eds.), Development of language and communication skills in hearing-impaired children. *Asha Monographs, 26,* 123–139.

Levitt, H., McGarr, N., & Geffner, D. (1987). Concluding commentary. In H. Levitt, N. McGarr, & D. Geffner (Eds.), Development of language and communication skills in hearing-impaired children. *Asha Monographs, 26,* 140–145.

Lieberman, P., & Blumstein, S. E. (1988). *Speech physiology, speech perception, and acoustic phonetics.* Cambridge: Cambridge University Press.

Ling, D., & Clarke, B. (1975). Cued speech: An evaluative study. *American Annals of the Deaf, 120,* 480–488.

Luetke-Stahlman, B., & Moeller, M. P. (1985). *Are parents trained to sign proficiently to their deaf children?* Paper presented at the ASHA National Convention, Washington, DC.

Mansour, S. L., & Lingwall, J. B. (1985). ASHA omnibus survey. *Asha, 27,* 37–40.

Markides, A. (1970). The speech of deaf and partially-hearing children with special reference to factors affecting intelligibility. *British Journal of Disorders of Communication, 5,* 126–140.

Markides, A. (1983). *The speech of hearing-impaired children.* Manchester: Manchester University Press.

McClure, W. (1966). Current problems and trends in the education of the deaf. *The Deaf American, 18,* 8–14.

McKirdy, L., & Blank, M. (1982). Dialogue in deaf and hearing preschoolers. *Journal of Speech and Hearing Research, 25,* 487–499.

Meadow, K. (1968). Early manual communication in relation to the deaf child's intellectual, social, and communicative functioning. *American Annals of the Deaf, 113,* 29–41.

Moeller, M. P., McConkey, A. J., & Osberger, M. J. (1983). Evaluation of the communicative skills of hearing-impaired children. *Audiology, 8,* 113–128.

Moeller, M. P., Osberger, M. J., & Morford, J. A. (1987). Speech-language assessment and intervention with pre-school hearing impaired children. In J. G. Alpiner & P. A. McCarthy (Eds.), *Rehabilitative audiology: Children and adults* (pp. 163–187). Baltimore: Williams and Wilkins.

Mohay, H. (1983). The effects of cued speech on the language development of three deaf children. *Sign Language Studies, 38,* 25–49.

Monsen, R. B. (1983). The oral speech intelligibility of hearing-impaired talkers. *Journal of Speech and Hearing Disorders, 48,* 286–296.

Montgomery, G. (1966). The relationship of oral skills to manual communication in profoundly deaf adolescents. *American Annals of the Deaf, 111,* 557–565.

Moores, D. (1987). *Educating the deaf: Psychology, principles and practices* (3rd ed.). Boston: Houghton Mifflin.

Moores, D., Weiss, K., & Goodwin, M. (1978). Early education programs for hearing-impaired children: Major findings. *American Annals of the Deaf, 125,* 925–936.

Musselman, C. R., Lindsay, P. H., & Wilson, A. K. (1988). An evaluation of recent trends in pre-school programming for hearing-impaired children. *Journal of Speech and Hearing Disorders, 53,* 71–88.

Nerbonne, M. A., & Schow, R. L. (1989). Auditory stimuli in communication. In R. L. Schow & M. A. Nerbonne (Eds.). *Introduction to aural rehabilitation* (2nd ed.) (pp. 81–123). Austin, TX: PRO-ED.

Nicholls, G., & Ling, D. (1982). Cued speech and the reception of spoken language. *Journal of Speech and Hearing Research, 25,* 262–269.

Northern, J., & Downs, M. (1991). *Hearing in children* (4th ed.). Baltimore: Williams and Wilkins.

Osberger, M. J. (1986). Summary and implications for research and educational management. In M. J. Osberger (Ed.), Language and learning skills of hearing-impaired students. *Asha Monograph, 23,* 92–98.

Osberger, M. J. (1990, April). Audiological rehabilitation with cochlear implants and tactile aids. *Asha, 32,* 38–43.

Osberger, M. J., & Danaher, E. (1974). Temporary conductive hearing loss in students with sensorineural hearing loss. *Volta Review, 76,* 52–56.

Osberger, M. J., & Hesketh, L. J. (1988). Speech and language disorders related to hearing impairment. In N. J. Lass, L. V. McReynolds, J. L. Northern, & D. E. Yoder (Eds.), *Handbook of speech-language pathology and audiology* (pp. 858–886). Toronto: B. C. Decker.

Osberger, M. J., & McGarr, N. (1982). Speech production characteristics of the hearing impaired. In N. Lass (Ed.), *Speech and language: Advances in basic science and research*. New York: Academic Press.

Paradise, J. L. (1981). Otitis media during early life: How hazardous to development? A critical review of the evidence. *Pediatrics, 68,* 869–873.

Paul, R. L., & Young, B. (1975). *The child with a mild sensorineural hearing loss: The failure syndrome*. Paper presented at the International Congress on Education of the Deaf, Tokyo.

Presnell, L. (1973). Hearing-impaired children's comprehension and production of syntax in oral language. *Journal of Speech and Hearing Research, 16,* 12–21.

Quigley, S. (1969). *The influence of fingerspelling on the development of language, communication and educational achievement in deaf children*. Champaign: Department of Special Education, University of Illinois.

Quigley, S. (1978). Effects of hearing impairment on normal language development. In F. Martin (Ed.), *Pediatric audiology*. Englewood Cliffs, NJ: Prentice-Hall.

Quigley, S., & Frisina, D. (1961). *Institutionalization and psycho-educational development of deaf children*. Washington, DC: CEC Research Monograph.

Quigley, S., & Power, D. (1979). *TSA syntax program*. Beaverton, OR: Dormac.

Reed, R., & Bugen, C. (1983). *A process approach to developing language with hearing impaired children*. Silver Springs, MD: National Association for the Deaf.

Reichman, J., & Healey, W. (1989). Amplification monitoring and maintenance in schools. *Asha, 31,* 43–45.

Roberts, J. E., Burchinal, M. R., Davis, B. P., Collier, A. M., & Henderson, F. W. (1991). Otitis media in early childhood and later language. *Journal of Speech and Hearing Research, 34,* 1158–1168.

Ross, M. (1982). *Hard of hearing children in regular schools*. Englewood Cliffs, NJ: Prentice-Hall.

Ross, M., Brackett, D., & Maxon, A. (1991). *Assessment and management of mainstreamed hearing-impaired children: Assessment and principles*. Austin, TX: PRO-ED.

Rupp, R., Smith, M. H., Briggs, P., Litvin, K., Banachowski, S., & Williams, R. H. (1977). A feasibility scale for language acquisition routing for young hearing-impaired children. *Language, Speech, and Hearing Services in the Schools, 8,* 222–233.

Russell, W., Power, D., & Quigley, S. (1976). *Linguistics and deaf children*. Washington, DC: Alexander Graham Bell Association for the Deaf.

Schildroth, A. (1986). Hearing-impaired children under age 6: 1977 and 1984. *American Annals of the Deaf, 131,* 85–89.

Seewald, R. C., Ross, M., Giolas, T. G., & Yonovitz, A. (1985). Primary modality for speech perception in children with normal and impaired hearing. *Journal of Speech and Hearing Research, 28,* 38–46.

Shepard, N., Davis, J., Gorga, M., & Stelmachowicz, P. (1981). Characterisitics of hearing-impaired children in the public schools: Part I—Demographic data. *Journal of Speech and Hearing Disorders, 46,* 123–129.

Smith, C. R. (1975). Residual hearing and speech production in deaf children. *Journal of Speech and Hearing Research, 18,* 795–811.

Stein, L. K., Jabaley, T., Spitz, R., Stoakley, D., & McGee, T. (1990). The hearing-impaired infant: Patterns of identification and habilitation revisited. *Ear and Hearing, 11,* 201–205.

Stevenson, E. (1964). A study of the educational achievement of deaf children of deaf parents. *California News*. Berkeley: California School for the Deaf.

Taylor, L. (1969). *A language analysis of the writing of deaf children*. Unpublished doctoral dissertation, Florida State University, Tallahassee.

Teele, D., Klein, J., & Rosner, B. (1984). Otitis media with effusion during the first three years of life and development of speech and language. *Pediatrics, 74,* 282–287.

Templin, M. (1966). Vocabulary problems of the deaf child. *International Audiology, 5,* 349–354.

Trammell, J. (1979). *Test of auditory comprehension*. North Hollywood, CA: Foreworks.

Trybus, R., & Karchmer, M. (1977). School achievement scores of hearing impaired children: National data on achievement patterns and growth patterns. *American Annals of the Deaf Directory of Programs and Service, 122,* 62–69.

Ventry, I. (1980). Effects of conductive hearing loss: Fact or fiction. *Journal of Speech and Hearing Disorders, 45,* 143–156.

Wallace, I. F., Gravel, J. S., McCarton, C. M., & Ruben, R. J. (1988). Otitis media and language development at 1 year of age. *Journal of Speech and Hearing Disorders, 53,* 245–251.

White, S. (1984). Antecedents of language functioning in the deaf: Implications for early intervention. ERIC Reports (ED 243–297, EC 162–425). Washington, DC: ERIC Clearing House.

White, S., & White, R. (1987). The effects of hearing status of the family and age of intervention on receptive and expressive oral language skills in hearing-impaired infants. In H. Levitt, N. McGarr, & D. Geffner (Eds.), Development of language and communication skills in hearing-impaired children. *Asha Monographs, 26,* 9–24.

Wilcox, J., & Tobin, H. (1974). Linguistic performance of hard of hearing and normal hearing children. *Journal of Speech and Hearing Research, 17,* 286–293.

Zinkus, P., Gottlieb, M., & Schapiro, M. (1978). Developmental and psycho-educational sequelae of chronic otitis media. *American Journal of Disorders of Childhood, 132,* 1100–1104.

· Chapter 10 ·

Language and
Bilingual-Bicultural Children

Steven H. Long

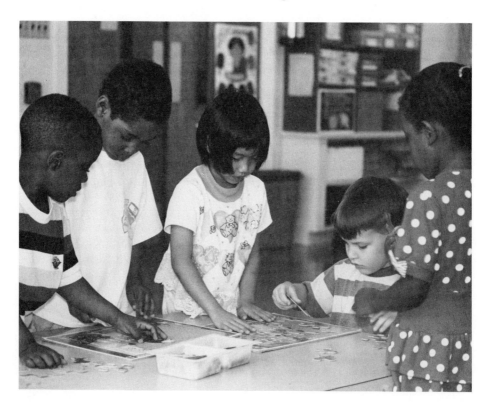

OBJECTIVES

Upon completion of this chapter, the reader should be able to:

▶ Discuss concepts of multiculturalism, linguistic variation, and second-language learning and their relevance to the classification, assessment, and treatment of language disorders in children.

▶ Describe general linguistic characteristics of the language of bilingual-bicultural children.

▶ Discuss principles of language assessment and intervention for bilingual-bicultural children.

The linguistic and cultural character of the United States is rapidly changing. Projections based upon current rates of immigration and new births indicate that by the end of the century, whites will be a minority of the population and one quarter of all children will come from homes at or below the poverty level. Thus it is likely that certain social, economic, and linguistic trends evident now will continue into the future. Many nonwhite children are raised in homes where languages other than English are spoken at least some of the time (McArthur, 1984). Other children, both nonwhite and white, learn a form of spoken English that differs from the form favored in most of America's schools and workplaces. As a result, many students are at risk for educational failure due to their language background and not because of a language impairment. At the same time, children who grow up in households that are ethnic, bilingual, or both are not immune from specific deficiencies in language learning. Consequently, professionals must be able to distinguish between language differences, which are the result of a child's linguistic environment, and language disorders, which are due to an impairment of language learning mechanisms.

CONCEPTS OF MULTICULTURALISM

Multiculturalism is a cover term for the racial, linguistic, and cultural variations in our society. Although there is much overlapping and interaction among the factors of race, language, and culture, they are in principle separate concepts:

▷ *Race* is a statement about an individual's biological attributes. By itself, race is of little importance to discussions of language acquisition and language disorders. The few exceptions occur when there are physical differences among races, which in turn can be related to variations in learning. For example, African-American children have a lower incidence of middle ear infection because the size and angle of their eustachian tubes permit better drainage. Insofar as otitis media may be a source of language difficulties in children, this racial difference may be of some significance.

▷ Most broadly, *language* refers to all the behaviors by which individuals communicate with one another. In the context of multiculturalism, however, we attend primarily to the differences in form (phonology, grammar, and vocabulary) that distinguish one language (English, Spanish, Japanese, etc.) from another and one variety of the same language (standard, nonstandard, American English, New Zealand English) from another variety. Differences in pragmatics are viewed as an aspect of culture rather than language. For example, Hispanic-American speakers tend to have a small distance between them during conversation (Taylor, in press). This appears to be true whether the speakers are **monolingual** (having only one language) or **bilingual** (sharing aspects of two languages) and, if they are bilingual, whether they are speaking Spanish, English, or a mixture of the two. Thus, the language behavior (Spanish) and the cultural behavior (standing close during conversation) are separable components of the communication of many but not all Hispanic-Americans. When we speak of language as a multicultural variable, the meaning should be restricted to those formal elements that will be learned and used by speakers.

▷ *Culture* is a statement about behaviors that are shared by a group of individuals. Members of an ethnic group will share many cultural elements as a result of ancestral links. Three large ethnic groups in the United States—African-Americans, Hispanic-Americans, and Asian-Americans—are commonly contrasted with one another and with white Americans of mostly European descent. As shown in Table 10.1, this comparison of behaviors across cultural groups reveals several differences with the potential to cause miscommunication. It is important to recognize that even though ethnicity cannot be changed, it does not compel an individual to follow certain cultural standards. To expect that all members of an ethnic group will behave in the same way is prejudicial. On the other hand, to be unaware of cultural differences and their potential effect on communication is unprofessional. There must be "a delicate balance between recognition of cultural orientations and stereotyping" (Cole, 1989, p. 68).

CONCEPTS OF LINGUISTIC VARIATION

Around the world, no two individuals communicate in exactly the same manner. The differences among people can be described in several ways. At the broadest level, we can identify nearly 1,000 different languages, each produced by 10,000 or more speakers (Crystal, 1987). Many of these languages are produced in several different forms or **dialects**, which vary from one another in grammar, vocabulary, and phonology. A language is distinguished from a dialect in two ways:

▷ A dialect is assumed to be a subset of a language and therefore should share a common core of grammatical and other characteristics with all other dialects of that language; and
▷ Speakers of different dialects should be able to understand one another whereas speakers of different languages should not.

The common core of a language is more evident in its written form than in its spoken form. Thus, an individual who knows English will be able to read a news-

TABLE 10.1   Some Differences in Communicative Behavior Across American Cultural Groups

White Americans	African-Americans	Hispanic-Americans	Asian-Americans
▷ Touching of hair is considered a sign of affection, especially between adults and children ▷ Uninvited touching between men and women may be considered harassing ▷ Direct eye contact is maintained during listening but avoided during speaking ▷ Public behavior should be emotionally restrained	▷ Touching of hair may be considered offensive ▷ Direct eye contact is avoided during listening but maintained during speaking ▷ Public behavior may be emotionally intense and demonstrative ▷ Interruption of another speaker during conversation is acceptable	▷ Touching occurs commonly during conversation ▷ Direct eye contact may be considered disrespectful ▷ A small distance is maintained between speakers during conversation	▷ Touching is more acceptable between members of the same sex than between men and women ▷ Backslapping is considered offensive ▷ Men and women do not customarily shake hands

Source: Adapted from Taylor (in press).

paper published in Canada, the United States, Great Britain, Australia, or any other English-speaking nation. However, the same individual, if he or she is from Kansas, may be unable to understand the English spoken in some parts of Scotland, Jamaica, New Zealand, or even Los Angeles. This calls attention to the fact that differences in pronunciation, or **accent**, are conspicuous features of a dialect and cause difficulty in communication between two speakers of the same language.

There is nothing inherently better about one dialect than another. However, within a society, factors of history, economics, and education can combine to favor a particular dialect and establish it as the standard. **Standard American English (SAE)** has been defined as "the real spoken language of the educated middle class" (Wolfram & Fasold, 1974, p. 21). All English-speaking nations are considered to have their own standard dialects, so it is customary to use the terms *American English, South African English,* and so on to refer to various national standard dialects (Quirk & Greenbaum, 1973).

The concept of a standard dialect is strongly associated with the educational level of the speaker. Individuals with considerable formal education tend to speak the standard dialect of the nation in which they live. They may also speak other dialects, depending on their personal background and experiences. The most invariant feature of a standard dialect is grammar. Whereas differences in vocabulary and pronunciation are identifiable features of regional dialects, these dialects are not usually considered nonstandard unless they include grammatical variation. Thus, we would expect educated speakers in Mississippi, New Hampshire, and Minnesota to show discernible differences in their speech, but these differences are primarily at the levels of phonology and vocabulary.

Because the standard dialect of a nation is generally the dialect of its more educated inhabitants, it is usually preferred in the classroom. Historically, this has led many speakers to identify standard dialectal forms as correct and nonstandard dialectal forms as wrong or substandard. At one time it was believed that non-standard dialects were immature forms of Standard English and that speakers who produced them were

less developed in their linguistic abilities. However, research by sociolinguists has shown convincingly that nonstandard forms of English are equally complex and have the same intellectual and linguistic requirements as the standard dialect (Labov, 1970; Trudgill, 1974).

Table 10.2 summarizes four of the factors contributing to communication differences among speakers of English. Geography and membership in an ethnic group are often considered together as comprising an individual's **speech community**. For example, most speakers who are raised in Texas produce speech that has phonological, lexical, and grammatical characteristics distinctive of that region. Collectively, these features are often described as a *twang* or *drawl* (though some might restrict those terms to descriptions of the differences in pronunciation). The features of Texan speech are sufficiently distinctive to constitute a regional dialect of English. However, this regional dialect is altered to varying degrees by the ethnic background of each speaker. We are most likely to find the prototypical Texas dialect among white speakers. In contrast, many African-American speakers from that state will produce **Black English Vernacular (BEV)**, an **ethnic dialect** used across the United States. Regional and ethnic influences interact, so that the BEV spoken by African-Americans living in Dallas is likely to differ in some respects from the BEV produced by African-Americans living in Seattle or Cleveland.

The influence of an ethnic dialect is sometimes difficult to separate from the effect of a native language other than English. Many characteristics of the dialect spoken by Hispanic-Americans are the result of **linguistic borrowing** from Spanish. English words may be pronounced with a Spanish accent, Spanish vocabulary may be substituted for English words in some contexts, and English syntax may be modified in ways that make it consistent with Spanish syntax. Some individuals speak only English but nevertheless maintain an influence from Spanish in their dialect. Others will speak both English and Spanish, though their English will likely reveal characteristics of Spanish, and vice versa. All immigrant groups from non-English-speaking countries can be expected to show a similar pattern. However, we tend to focus on particular ethnic

TABLE 10.2   Factors Contributing to Communication Differences Among Speakers

Regional dialect	Ethnic dialect	Register	Idiolect
Examples: Southern, Brooklyn	Examples: Black English Vernacular, Spanish-influenced English	Examples: formal, informal, caretaker	Examples: every individual speaker
Produces variation in:	Produces variation in:	Produces variation in:	Produces variation in:
▷ Phonology (e.g., use of vocalic /r/) ▷ Rate of speech ▷ Syntax (e.g., use of "y'all") ▷ Use of gestures ▷ Use of specific words or idioms ▷ Vocal intensity ▷ Vocal quality (e.g., nasality)	▷ Distance between speaker and listener ▷ Morphology (e.g., use of plural marker) ▷ Phonology (e.g., use of theta) ▷ Rate of speech ▷ Stress and intonation ▷ Syntax (e.g., use of copula) ▷ Use of specific words or idioms	▷ Distance between speaker and listener ▷ Eye contact ▷ Lexical specificity ▷ Rate of speech ▷ Stress and intonation ▷ Syntax (e.g., simple/complex) ▷ Use of gestures ▷ Use of specific words or idioms (e.g., formal/informal, common/uncommon) ▷ Vocal intensity	▷ Rate of speech ▷ Stress and intonation ▷ Use of gestures ▷ Use of specific words or idioms ▷ Vocal quality

dialects for social and demographic reasons. When the number of immigrants from a particular country or region becomes large, the language differences of those individuals can become a social issue, especially in education. This has occurred in the United States with both Hispanic-Americans and Asian-Americans; consequently we tend to identify dialectal issues with these two groups. The massive Asian and Hispanic immigration to America has also resulted in the formation of ethnic enclaves, especially in the larger cities. The insulation of these subcommunities helps to maintain ethnic dialects by keeping native languages in use and by mitigating the influence of English-speaking culture.

Beyond the effects of geography and ethnic background, we all vary our speech to suit the requirements of specific social communicative events. As young children, we learn that certain language forms are appropriate or required in one context but not another. An example is the use of polite language, which may not always be necessary at home or with peers but is mandatory with unfamiliar adults and in public

places. In school we learn to vary language further, especially along the lines of formal and informal usage. By adulthood we have developed a set of registers, which we employ in different social situations. The ability to shift from one register to another, or from one dialect to another or one language to another, is known as **code switching**. We switch codes when we talk in one way to a child and talk in another way to the child's parents. Students are likely to shift from an informal register with their classmates to a more formal didactic register with their teachers. Speakers of nonstandard ethnic dialects who are also competent users of standard English often adjust their use of nonstandard features to meet the expectations of a conversational partner. In a work or educational setting, the standard dialect will be used; in an ethnic social setting, the nonstandard dialect.

Of course, not all the features of an individual's communication are determined by region, ethnicity, or social situation. If they were, then many of us would sound far more alike than we do. What keeps us different is our uniqueness as individuals. Variation in everything from vocal tract anatomy to personal experiences provides everyone with an **idiolect**, that is, a distinctive combination of language characteristics.

Each person's idiolect can be compared to those of other persons within a speech community. When we evaluate children for language disorders, this is what is done. Typically, a child's idiolect is first compared to the standard dialect of the nation in which the child lives. If the child's language is found to be different, then the following possibilities must be explored:

▷ The child is learning the standard dialect but is language disordered.

▷ The child is learning a nonstandard dialect.

▷ The child is learning a nonstandard dialect *and* is language disordered.

To evaluate either of the last two possibilities requires a knowledge of the child's nonstandard dialect. Every feature of the child's language that differs from the standard dialect must be evaluated to determine whether it is disordered or merely a dialectal variation.

CONCEPTS OF SECOND LANGUAGE LEARNING

In theory, the perfect bilingual speaker is one who can comprehend and use two languages with equal facility. However, apart from professional translators, such competence is rarely attained. Far more common are individuals who

▷ are fluent in both written and spoken forms of their first (native) language and have less proficiency with a second language; or

▷ have equivalent but different areas of competence in two languages and therefore prefer to use one or the other in particular circumstances (e.g., at school, during play) or while engaged in certain tasks (speaking, reading, writing).

Many factors affect the process, and the result of second-language learning. The model environment for children is to learn two languages from birth. They should hear the two languages being spoken by both of their parents, as well as by their peers, other adults,

and speakers on radio and television. The children should be able to speak, read, and write both languages at school and in all other social experiences such as church, sports teams, and clubs. Of course, such an environment does not exist, even in the most multilingual nations. Bilingual acquisition is influenced by every variation from the model situation we have described.

For example, a daughter is born to a German university professor. Although the father speaks English, he does not use it at home. When the girl is 4, the father accepts a position at an American university and the family moves. The daughter is exposed to English through her American friends and their families, through television, and through her father, who now begins to speak it to her at home. The mother has limited knowledge of English and, therefore, speaks mostly German with the girl and with her father. In this scenario, the girl's language learning is affected by (1) the ages at which she was first exposed to German and English; (2) the switch in the language used by her father; and (3) the difference in the languages used by her mother and father. Because she learned German and English in sequence rather than simultaneously, the girl is less likely to have mixed the two languages (Dulay, Hernandez-Chavez, & Burt, 1978). At age 4 and beyond, she will be aware of the difference in the language skills of her two parents. Not only will she expect her mother to speak German, she may object if her mother attempts to use English with her (Volterra & Taeschner, 1978). On the other hand, the girl and her father may develop an elaborate system for code switching between German and English. For instance, they may use German when speaking affectionately but switch to English for an instructional purpose. Discipline may be meted out in English unless the child resists or disobeys in some way. In that case, the father may switch to German to emphasize his determination (Crystal, 1987).

Children who learn two languages simultaneously appear to go through a sorting-out process during the preschool years (Volterra & Taeschner, 1978). At first, these children acquire vocabulary from both languages but have few equivalent words. That is, if the name for a food item or body part or article of clothing is learned in one language, the child is unlikely to learn the same name in the other language. Later, when the child begins to combine words to form sentences, there is some mixing of vocabulary from the two languages. Nearly all of this mixing disappears, however, by the end of the third year. Thereafter, the vocabularies of the two languages are kept distinct and equivalent words are learned in each language. For a time, simultaneously bilingual children may mix the grammatical systems of the two languages. For example, a child learning Spanish and English may vary the order of nouns and adjectives, thereby creating ungrammatical or unusual sentences in both languages (e.g., "It's a clown silly" or "Es un tonto payaso"). Eventually, the two grammars become separate and children are able to switch between the languages without confusion or error.

LANGUAGE CHARACTERISTICS OF BILINGUAL-BICULTURAL CHILDREN

Although it is convenient at times to consider bilingual-bicultural children as a group, there are important linguistic and cultural differences among various ethnic populations. Analysis of language and culture can be done along a continuum of detail. At a broad level, we can identify four major ethnic groups in the United States: African-Americans, Hispanic-Americans, Asian-Americans, and Native Americans. The first three of these groups are statistically dominant, comprising over 59 million individuals in the 1990 census (ASHA Office of Minority Concerns, 1991). At a fine level of analysis, every major ethnic group can be seen to consist of many subgroups, which often vary greatly from one another in language and culture. Thus we could distinguish between African-Americans living in southern and northern states; we could differentiate among Hispanic-Americans based on their country of origin (Cuba, Mexico, El Salvador, etc.); and we could discriminate among Asian-Americans who have immigrated from different nations (Korea, Cambodia, Vietnam, etc.). Detailed knowledge of such subgroups may be crucial in certain educational settings. For the purposes of this chapter, however, we will examine only those broad linguistic and cultural differences that exist among the three largest minority populations.

Hispanic-American Children

A major factor in the English produced by Hispanic-American bilingual-bicultural children is the Spanish language. A unique dialect is formed as a result of the influence of and borrowing from Spanish phonology, grammar, and vocabulary.

Varieties of Spanish-Influenced English   Spanish, like English, has many national standard forms as well as nonstandard forms. Mexicans, Puerto Ricans, and Cubans are the predominant groups in the Hispanic population of the United States. Consequently, those national varieties of Spanish are the most influential. During the 1980s, however, there was a significant increase in Central and South American immigration, so that groups such as Salvadorans, Guatemalans, Columbians, and Hondurans are now more numerous and will have a greater impact on dialectal learning (ASHA Office of Minority Concerns, 1991). Many immigrants are working-class individuals with limited formal education. They may speak, and their children may therefore learn, a nonstandard dialect of Spanish that is considerably different from the standard dialect of their native country. Clearly, there are many varieties of Spanish spoken in America, which means that a wide range of effects on children are possible.

Language Profiles of Hispanic-American Bilingual-Bicultural Children   Several variables interact to produce different language profiles among Hispanic-American children. First, and most important, children's relative proficiency in English and Spanish can vary greatly, depending on such factors as the following:

▷ The age at which they were introduced to English and its effect on simultaneous or sequential acquisition.
▷ The bilingual fluency of the parents and other significant language models.
▷ The bilingual requirements or opportunities of the environment in which the children live.

TABLE 10.3   Profiles of Language Mixing and Separation

Monolingual English	Comprehends and produces English only.
Low mixed English/other language	Comprehends and produces both languages imperfectly, though English is slightly stronger. Mixes the languages in speaking.
English dominant	Comprehends and produces English well. Uses other language when required but has less proficiency with it.
Bilingual	Comprehends and produces both languages equally well. Code-switches easily.
Other language dominant	Comprehends and produces other language well. Uses English when required but has less proficiency with it.
Low mixed other language/English	Comprehends and produces both languages imperfectly, though other language is slightly stronger. Mixes the languages in speaking.
Monolingual other language	Comprehends and produces other language only.

Table 10.3 shows the different ways in which two languages may be mixed or kept separate. Some Hispanic-American children may be truly bilingual, highly competent in both their comprehension and production of Spanish and English. Others may have a dominant language that they are able to speak and understand well. They naturally prefer to use this language in all situations that allow it. Another possibility is for children to know elements of both Spanish and English but lack competence and confidence in either one. These children may be able to communicate effectively only by switching back and forth between the languages and by mixing Spanish and English vocabularies. Children with such low mixed dominance are not necessarily language disordered. Those who are language impaired probably mix languages as a compensatory strategy, while those who are not mix languages as a result of environmental influences.

A final group of Hispanic-American children may be monolingual, communicating only in English or Spanish. Obviously, children who are ethnic Hispanics and may have Spanish surnames are not obligated to know the Spanish language. This situation will occur more frequently in second- and later-generation families. Because of cultural traditions the children may know a considerable number of Spanish words and idioms, but they are functionally monolingual. In contrast, children who have recently arrived in America or have been raised in tightly knit Hispanic-American communities may speak only Spanish. Like the other monolingual children, they may have acquired some vocabulary, but otherwise they are incompetent in English.

A second variable affecting Hispanic-American children's language profiles is the dialect or dialects to which they are exposed. As we have seen, both Spanish and English are spoken in many dialectal forms. One child might learn a Puerto Rican standard form of Spanish and a BEV nonstandard form of English. Another child might combine a nonstandard form of Mexican Spanish with SAE. The possible combinations are potentially as great as the number of varieties of Spanish and English. In actuality, however, common combinations will be determined by patterns of immigration and settlement in the United States.

Individual variation in Hispanic-American children's pragmatic language profiles will be largely influenced by variables such as family expectations, ethnic pride, and cultural beliefs (Williams, Hopper, & Natalicio, 1977). We have noted that the Hispanic community in America is now quite diverse, which makes it increasingly difficult to generalize about "Hispanic culture" or "Hispanic value systems." It remains fair to say, however, that Hispanic-American children often display pragmatic communicative behaviors that are different from those of white middle-class children. They may, for instance, show more reluctance to extend topics—providing more information than is requested—in conversations with adults. This behavior, which is valued as a sign of creativity and social skill

TABLE 10.4   Consonants of Spanish and English

1. Consonants pronounced alike: f, s, h, m, n, l, w, j, ng	
2. English consonants that do not exist in Spanish: z, sh, zh (except in Argentina), /ʤ/, th (except in central Spain)	
3. Consonants pronounced differently	Explanation of Spanish pronunciation
b, v	Pronounced the same way, as a voiced bilabial fricative, a sound that does not exist in English.
p, k, ch	Produced without the following aspiration.
t, d	Produced as dental rather than alveolar stops. In the intervocalic position, /d/ is produced as a voiced interdental fricative /ð/.
g	Produced as /g/ only when it follows /n/, e.g., in "tango." Otherwise, it is produced as a voiced velar fricative, a sound that does not exist in English.
r	Produced either as a flap or as an alveolar trill, depending on the phonetic context.

Source: Adapted from Butt and Benjamin (1988).

among most whites, may be considered disrespectful among certain Hispanic-American groups.

Phonological Differences   Of the major European languages, Spanish has been estimated to be the second closest (after Italian) in overall structure to English (James, 1979, cited by Crystal, 1987). The two languages have very similar alphabets, spelling, and vocabulary. They are somewhat more distant in pronunciation and grammar. Spanish has slightly fewer consonants than American English, about 18 versus about 24. Table 10.4 compares the two consonant systems in terms of three groups. First, there are several sounds that are produced identically or nearly so. The pronunciation of these sounds presents little difficulty to bilingual or second-language learners of English. Second, there is a smaller group of sounds that occur only in English. Native speakers of Spanish will typically substitute phonetically similar Spanish sounds. For example, /s/ or /t/ will be substituted for "th," /s/ for /z/, and "ch" for "sh." The third group of sounds are ones that are sometimes or always produced differently in Spanish than in English. To the ear of a native English speaker, these consonants sound slightly distorted when native speakers of Spanish pronounce English words.

The Spanish vowel system also contains fewer sounds than its English counterpart, 5 compared to 12. Table 10.5 summarizes the points of contrast. All the Spanish vowels and diphthongs also exist in English, but there are seven vowels unique to English. Native speakers of Spanish tend to substitute for these English vowels phonetically similar vowels, for example, /i/ for /I/ and /a/ for /ʌ/. Another major influence on vowel production in the two languages is the difference in prosodic features. In English, the duration of vowels varies, depending on whether they occur in stressed or unstressed syllables. Thus, in the word "elephant" the vowel in the first, stressed, syllable is /ɛ/; the vowel in the second, unstressed, syllable is /ə/. In Spanish, vowel length is constant. Therefore, in the

TABLE 10.5   Vowels and Diphthongs of Spanish and English

Vowels pronounced alike: a, e, i, o, u (though they are not lengthened, as in English)
Diphthongs pronounced alike: aI, aU, eI, iu, oI
English vowels and diphthongs that do not exist in Spanish: I, ɛ, æ, ʌ, ə, ɔ, U, oU

Source: Adapted from Butt and Benjamin (1988).

word "elefante" the vowels in the first, second, and fourth syllables are all /e/. There is a natural tendency for native speakers of Spanish to retain their habit of producing equal vowel duration when they speak English. This habit, along with the vowel substitutions mentioned earlier, yields pronunciations such as /presiden/ for "president," /telefon/ for "telephone," and /mekani/ for "mechanic."

The contrasts we have drawn thus far are between the phonetic features of English and Spanish, that is, differences in which sounds are produced and how they are produced. There are also a number of phonological differences that can affect the pronunciation of bilingual children. Some of the most important ones are as follows:

▷ The fricative /ð/ occurs only in the **intervocalic** position in Spanish. Thus, in speaking English, it is typically substituted for by /d/ in the **prevocalic** (e.g., "this") or **postvocalic** (e.g., "smooth") position.

▷ In many dialects of Spanish (e.g., Cuban) /s/ is omitted in the postvocalic position.

▷ Consonant clusters containing /s/ as the first sound, such as /sp/, /st/, and /sk/, do not occur in the word-initial position in Spanish. Consequently native speakers will often insert a vowel before the cluster so that it conforms to the Spanish phonological rule, for example, /eskul/ for "school."

▷ Consonant clusters containing /s/ as the last sound, such as /ps/, /ts/, and /ks/, do not occur in the word-final position in Spanish. These clusters are commonly reduced in English words, for example, /bak/ for "box" or /kot/ for "coats."

▷ The only word-final consonants in Spanish are /s, n, r, l, d/. All other words end in vowels. Therefore the tendency is to omit consonants (e.g., /kæn/ for "can't") or add vowels to the ends of words, especially when the English and Spanish words are **cognates** (e.g., /fruta/ for "fruit").

It is important to be aware of phonological differences such as these because they frequently contain the key to understanding what seem to be inconsistencies in pronunciation. For example, a Hispanic-American child may correctly pronounce the consonants in the words /feðo/ "feather," /soni/ "sunny," and /mostod/ "mustard" but have difficulty with some of the same sounds in the words /do/ "those," /leto/ "lettuce," and /estó/ "stove." The reason for the difference is the influence of Spanish phonological rules.

Grammatical Differences   Comparison of English and Spanish grammar is considerably more complex than comparison of phonology because of the number of features involved. Many differences are relevant only to the language of adults and need not concern us in our discussion of children's grammatical learning. Some of the distinctions that are most pertinent to children are these:

▷ The position of adjectives in the noun phrase is more flexible in Spanish. The rules determining which adjectives precede and which follow a noun are difficult to formulate (Butt & Benjamin, 1988). However, the fact that Spanish allows **postmodifying** adjectives makes it more likely that bilingual children will attempt to use this structure in English, for example, "car green" instead of "green car."

▷ Nearly all Spanish adjectives can function as nouns if preceded by an article or **demonstrative**. English requires an indefinite pronoun to express the same meaning; for example, "los rojos" (literally, "the reds") has the same meaning as "the red ones" in English.

▷ Indefinite articles are omitted following certain uses of the copula, certain common verbs ("have," "buy," "take," "look for," "wear"), and certain prepositions.

▷ In referring to parts of the body, clothing, or other personal belongings, the possessive pronoun is replaced by the definite article; for example, "me quité los calcetines" is translated literally as "I took off the (i.e., my) socks."

▷ Spanish does not require the auxiliary verb "do" to support the transformation of statements into questions ("He did it" → "Did he do it?") or statements into negative commands ("Do it!" → "Don't do it!"). Questions are instead marked by rising intonation and negative commands by the insertion of "no" at the beginning of the sentence.

▷ Plurality is marked more redundantly in Spanish than in English. For instance, in the sentence "Han llegado los dos niños colombianos"/"The Columbian boys have arrived," plurality is marked five times: on the auxiliary verb, the article, the **quantifier**, the noun, and the adjective. Such redundancy permits Spanish speakers to omit some of the markers without loss of information. Omission of plural markers is especially common in dialects that delete the postvocalic /s/ (Iglesias & Anderson, 1993).

▷ Negation is marked on all constituents of a negative sentence; for example "Nunca veía a nadie en ninguna de las habitaciones" translates literally as "I never saw nobody in none of the rooms."

▷ "No" is used for all negation in the verb phrase, for example, "No puedo" ("I can't") or "No está aquí" ("He isn't here"). There is no equivalent to the English negative "not."

Characteristics of Spanish-Influenced English

The basic framework for identifying and understanding characteristics of Spanish-influenced English is knowledge of the two languages and the differences between them. We should recall, however, that the interaction between the languages is influenced by dialectal variation within Spanish and English. Moreover, it is not clear that interference from Spanish is the major cause of errors in Hispanic-American children's learning of English. One study of 145 Spanish-speaking children age 5 to 8 found that only 3% of their errors resulted from interference such as direct translation of Spanish grammar to English. A much larger percentage of errors appeared to be similar to immature forms produced by children learning English as their native language (Dulay & Burt, 1973).

Interference effects appear to be more potent in explaining the phonological characteristics of Spanish-influenced English. Table 10.6 provides examples of both grammatical and phonological interference errors that may be observed in Hispanic-American children. The frequency and consistency of such errors are likely to vary, depending on when and how the

children begin to learn English, as well as the degree of balance in their competence with the two languages.

African-American Children

Many African-American children learn a nonstandard dialect of American English. At one time this dialect was commonly described as *Black English*. However, that term implied that the dialect is used by all African-Americans, which is not the case. Consequently, it has been replaced by the description Black English *Vernacular* (BEV) to emphasize that it is the dialect of a particular speech community and not of an entire race. Sociolinguistic studies suggest that BEV is used to some extent by most African-Americans, but that the degree of usage varies by socioeconomic group. African-Americans of the lower working class are likely to use a high percentage of BEV linguistic features, whereas those of the upper middle class tend to use only a few features (Wolfram, 1986).

In 1977, a case was brought against the school district of Ann Arbor, Michigan, by African-American children attending elementary school there (*Martin Luther King Jr. Elementary School children v. Ann Arbor School District Board,* 1977). The argument put forward was that these children were faring poorly in school because they were speakers of BEV, which put them at a disadvantage in a school that required the use of SAE. To provide the African-American children with an equal educational opportunity, the court ruled, the school district must provide instruction that takes into account their linguistic differences. The Ann Arbor trial has played a major role in heightening American educators' awareness of linguistic differences and in forcing them to modify curricula so that these differences do not handicap the progress of African-American children.

Historical Issues The origin of BEV has been a disputed and controversial subject. Language is a major source of ethnic identity, and the origin of a language can become an issue of ethnic pride as well as a topic of academic study. One early view of BEV was that it was merely a *restricted code,* that is, a variety of language used by lower social classes that is character-

TABLE 10.6   Phonological and Grammatical Interference Errors
Found in Spanish-Influenced English

Example	Errors	Explanation
"She /tʃi/ no can help"	▷ Substitution of "ch" for "sh" ▷ Incorrect negative in the verb phrase	▷ "ch" not used in Spanish; "sh" is the closest form ▷ "no" is the only negative form in the verb phrase and always precedes the verb it modifies
"I want /wan/ the /di/ big"	▷ Reduction of cluster /nt/ → /n/ ▷ Substitution of /d/ for /ð/ ▷ Omission of indefinite pronoun "one"	▷ Spanish words do not end in /t/; cluster is reduced to conform to this rule ▷ /ð/ not used in word-initial position; /d/ is the closest form ▷ Article + adjective is the Spanish equivalent of the English phrase article + adjective + "one"
"He wearing /weɾin/ shirt /tʃut/, no?"	▷ Substitution of flap for /r/; substitution of /n/ for "ng"; substitution of "ch" for "sh" ▷ Omission of auxiliary verb "is" ▷ Omission of indefinite article "a" ▷ Use of "no" and rising intonation to form tag question	▷ Sounds do not exist in Spanish or are not allowed in certain phonetic contexts; closest forms are substituted ▷ Immature verb form (*not* an interference error) ▷ Indefinite articles not used following verb "wear" ▷ "No" + rising intonation is Spanish tag form when seeking agreement from listener

ized by, among other things, reduced syntax and a reliance on context for the interpretation of meaning (Crystal, 1987). This opinion of BEV has been largely abandoned, though the issue of a restricted code among lower social classes continues to be argued.

Scholars agree that BEV had its origins in the slave communities of the American South and then spread to northern urban centers as African-Americans migrated to those regions. There has been disagreement, however, about how the dialect first became established among the slaves. One position has been that BEV was derived from other dialects spoken by whites in the southern United States. It is clear, for example, that some of the linguistic features of BEV are also found in British dialects that were spoken in early American southern history (Trudgill, 1974). However, the best-supported and most widely accepted view is that BEV began in Africa as a **pidgin**, or very limited trade language, used to facilitate commerce between

Europeans and Africans. When a slave trade developed during the 1600s, this pidgin language came with the Africans to southeastern America. There it gradually merged with English to form a language of its own, known as a **creole** language, which has a systematic and elaborated grammar and vocabulary (Iglesias & Anderson, 1993). This creole language gradually evolved into what we recognize today as BEV. What is apparent from historical study is that BEV is a systematic and rule-governed variety of English that has evolved through processes that are well known to linguists. It should be viewed, therefore, as an independent linguistic system that is closely related to SAE but that has many of its own formal and functional characteristics.

Characteristics of BEV   BEV may be contrasted with SAE at each level of linguistic structure: pragmatics, semantics, phonology, and grammar. To a speaker of SAE, the interaction of BEV speakers may appear to be highly assertive and perhaps even excessively demonstrative. Loud talking, heated public arguments, and frequent interruptions of one's conversational partners are considered acceptable pragmatic behaviors in BEV. On the other hand, certain behaviors that SAE speakers may consider acceptable or only mildly rude are intolerable to BEV speakers, for example, asking personal questions of a new acquaintance or trying to break in on a conversation (Taylor, in press). Thus, neither dialect should be considered more polite than the other.

BEV has been a fertile ground for the development of slang, especially among inner-city populations. This is hardly surprising, because slang's most consistent function is to mark social or linguistic identity (Crystal, 1987). Some of the slang generated by BEV, such as the adjectives "cool" and "hip," has crossed over and become part of SAE. Other words and idiomatic phrases have remained unique to BEV and are unintelligible to individuals who do not know the dialect.

The major phonological features of BEV are summarized in Table 10.7. As indicated earlier, these features are characteristic of the dialect as a whole but are found to varying degrees in individual speakers.

When a standard articulation test was given to African-American and white children at 4 to 5 years of age, the BEV speakers were found to produce more of the phonological features characteristic of that dialect. However, the white children produced the same features (e.g., **reduction** of word-final consonant clusters) less frequently (Seymour & Seymour, 1981). It appears, therefore, that the phonological systems of BEV and SAE speakers do not become fully differentiated until later in childhood.

Table 10.8 shows some of the principal features of BEV grammar. Some grammatical markers that are obligatory in SAE are deleted in BEV in contexts where they are redundant. For example, the possessive noun marker is absent in the sentence "That be Rhonda purse" but present in the sentence "That be Rhonda's." Interactions can occur between phonological and grammatical features of BEV. For instance, the singular form of "desk" would be pronounced in BEV as /dɛs/ "des." To form the plural and yet still avoid a consonant cluster, BEV speakers produce /dɛsəz/ "desses" unless the word follows a numerical quantifier. In that case, the plural marker will be omitted: "My school got a hundred desk /dɛs/." Thus, the dialect's variations from SAE are both consistent and logical.

TABLE 10.7 Phonological Features of BEV

Phonological Variation	Example
Deletion of nasal at the end of a word and nasalization of the preceding vowel	comb → co /ko/ (with vowel nasalized) man → ma /mæ/ (with vowel nasalized)
Deletion of semivowels /r/ and /l/	store → sto /sto/ fool → foo /fu/ help → hep /hɛp/
Devoicing and weakening of final stops	hat → ha /hæ/ mad → mat /mæt/ or ma /mæ/ cake → ca /ke/ big → bid /bɪd/ or bi /bɪ/
Simplification of consonant cluster at the end of a word	last → lass /læs/ soft → sof /sɔf/
Substitution of f/th in the middle and at the end of a word; substitution of v/ð in the middle of a word	tooth → toof /tuf/ brother → brover /brʌvɚ/
Substitution of stop for interdental fricative at the beginning of a word	that → dat /dæt/ thin → tin /tɪn/

Sources: Adapted from Iglesias and Anderson (1993) and Labov (1970).

TABLE 10.8 Grammatical Features of BEV

Grammatical Variation	Example
Deletion of possessive marker with adjacent nouns	That Bobby bike (= Bobby's bike)
Deletion of plural marker when a numerical quantifier is used	I got two card
Different formation of indirect questions	I asked him did he know her name
No final -s in the third-person singular present tense	That dog bark all the time
Use of double negatives involving the auxiliary verb at the beginning of a sentence	Can't nobody fix that thing
Use of "be" to mark habitual action	I be goin' to school every day
Use of the copula is not obligatory	He mad My brother real big

Sources: Adapted from Baratz (1969) and Trudgill (1974).

Asian-American Children

Asian-Americans are the most culturally and linguistically diverse of the three major ethnic groups in the United States. There is no agreement on which nationalities should be included in the category of *Asian,* as it is not clear whether this term refers to a racial subtype, a geographical area, or a linguistic grouping. For our purposes, it will refer to a particular group of languages. Some languages, such as those spoken in India and the Philippines, will be excluded from our discussion, even though these might also be considered Asian.

Varieties of Asian Languages   The classification of languages raises some problems for which there are no clear solutions. Languages are usually compared in terms of their structural characteristics (grammar, vocabulary, and phonology) and historical origins. However, the weighting given to different structural levels is purely arbitrary. Thus, two languages that are grammatically distinct might be placed in different families, even though they share many phonological features. Historical information can assist in resolving some structural issues, but there are problems even here. Two languages that are historically distinct may be used by ethnic groups that, through migration and resettlement, come to live in the same area. Over time

the two languages that were once distinct will begin to influence and borrow from one another.

Asian languages that are widely spoken by immigrants to the United states are listed in Table 10.9, along with some of the phonological features of those languages that contrast with English. As can be seen, the phonological structure of Asian languages is markedly different from that of English. They tend to have a simpler segmental structure, with fewer vowels and consonants, and with word shapes that are largely monosyllabic and contain few consonant clusters. However, the suprasegmental structure of Asian languages is generally richer, with variation in tone and vowel length used to signal differences in word meaning.

Characteristics of Asian-Influenced English
The English spoken by Asian-American children may show the effect of interference from their native Asian language. The extent of this interference depends on the bilingual profile of each child. Recall that Table 10.3 shows a range of profiles that may be demonstrated by different children learning two languages. The precise nature of the interference will depend on the cultural and linguistic experiences of each child. For example, the language and behavior of a Hmong child may show little resemblance to those of a Korean

TABLE 10.9 Languages Widely Spoken Among Asian Immigrant Populations
and Their Contrasting Phonological Features

Language	Where Spoken	Contrasting Phonological Features
Japanese	Japan	No word final consonants, only five vowels, contrastive vowel length
Korean	North and South Korea, parts of China, Japan, and Russia	Contrastive vowel length
Mon-Khmer family		
Khmer	Kampuchea (Cambodia)	Large repertoire of consonant clusters
Vietnamese	Kampuchea (Cambodia), Laos, Vietnam	Tone language, no consonant clusters, essentially monosyllabic, only six final consonants
Sino-Tibetan family		
Chinese (Cantonese and Mandarin)	China	Tone language, no consonant clusters, essentially monosyllabic, few final consonants
Hmong	Northern Laos, Thailand, Vietnam	Tone language, only word-initial consonant clusters, only one final consonant
Tai family		
Lao (Laotian)	Laos, Thailand	Tone language, essentially monosyllabic

Sources: Adapted from Cheng (1987a,b) and Crystal (1987).

child. Table 10.10 summarizes some of the phonological and grammatical interference errors that are likely to occur in native speakers of Chinese or Vietnamese. Similar errors may be found among speakers of other Asian languages.

Besides their differences in language form, Asian-American children may vary in their pragmatic behavior. Because Asian cultural mores generally discourage children from interrupting or asserting themselves with adults, they may appear passive when observed alongside other American children. They may seem to avoid eye contact in dyadic conversation and yet stare openly in other situations (Cheng, 1987b). While pragmatic differences of this kind are subtle and may not interfere at all with peer interaction, they can interfere with assessment efforts and might be wrongly taken as an indication of limited language competence.

THE INFLUENCE OF POVERTY

To this point, we have examined the language development and language differences of ethnic American children from a purely cultural and linguistic perspec-

tive. In an ideal world, this would be the only viewpoint we would need to consider. It is apparent, however, that in a disproportionate number of cases, ethnic children are also children of poverty. While one white child in seven is poor, four out of nine African-American children and three out of eight Hispanic-American children are poor (National Center for Children in Poverty, 1990). The effects of poverty on the general health and development of children are well known:

> Children of poverty lack food, clothing, housing, medicine, and early learning assistance. These children face sickness, psychological stress, malnutrition, and underdevelopment. . . . As poor children progress through the school system, they face school failure, pregnancy, substance abuse, and economic stress. Illiteracy in the poor is endemic and cyclic as poor children become poor parents of more poor children. (Work, 1991, p. 61)

Each of the problems identified in the preceding paragraph can increase the risk of handicapping conditions, including language disorders. Poor mothers often receive no prenatal care during their pregnancies, and malnutrition and substance abuse can lead to

TABLE 10.10   Phonological and Grammatical Interference Errors
Found in the English of Native Chinese and Vietnamese Speakers

Example	Errors
"We go you house /haU/ yesterday /jɛtu'de/" (= "We went to your house yesterday")	▷ Omission of word-final /s/ (house) ▷ Reduction of cluster /st/ → /t/ (yesterday) ▷ Incorrect syllable stress (yesterday) ▷ Use of unmarked verb form (go) for irregular past tense form (sent) ▷ Substitution of pronominal forms (you/your) ▷ Omission of preposition "to"
"Him no buy book /bU/?" (= "Didn't he buy the book?")	▷ Omission of word-final /k/ (book) ▷ Omission of article "the" ▷ Simplified interrogative: auxiliary verb "did" omitted; question marked only by rising intonation ▷ Use of unmarked verb form (buy) for expanded verb phrase (did buy) ▷ Substitution of pronominal forms (him/he) ▷ Simplified negation: marked only by use of "no"
"That /dæ/ man two dollar /daral/ me" (= "That man gave me two dollars" or "That man gave two dollars to me")	▷ Omission of word-final /t/ (that) ▷ Substitution of /ð/ → /d/ (that) ▷ Substitution of liquid consonants /r/ and /l/ (dollar) ▷ Omission of plural marker when preceded by numerical quantifier (two dollar) ▷ Reversed ordering of direct and indirect objects (two dollar me) or omission of preposition "to"

Sources: Adapted from Cheng (1987a, 1987b).

premature delivery of babies with low birth weight. These babies have a substantially greater risk of incurring developmental problems. Even when poor children are born healthy, they can be raised in an environment that can be less stimulating and more dangerous than that of other children. As a result, they are likely to be delayed in certain areas of language learning compared to middle class children.

All professionals should differentiate between environmental conditions that result from cultural differences and those that are due to poverty. Nutritional choices, methods of discipline, and styles of verbal interaction all vary across cultural groups. Though differences in these behaviors may have short-term effects on language learning, they are not associated with a greater prevalence of language disorders. In contrast, the consequences of poverty can harm a child's nervous system, either from birth or during the early formative years. Such damage can lead to long-term language deficits from which a child is unlikely to recover.

ISSUES IN ASSESSMENT

It is estimated that 10% of the members of all racial/ethnic minority groups have disorders of speech, language, or hearing, the same percentage as the U.S. population as a whole (ASHA Office of Minority Concerns, 1991). The unique issue in the case of bilingual-bicultural children is that their language can be evaluated and categorized in any of four different ways:

1. Typically developing and speaking SAE.
2. Typically developing and speaking a nonstandard dialect.

3. Atypically developing and speaking SAE.
4. Atypically developing and speaking a nonstandard dialect.

The key to fair assessment is to determine each child's dialectal status and not allow a nonstandard dialect to interfere with the judgments made about language learning ability. This requires an awareness of the structural differences found in nonstandard dialects and a critical attitude toward assessment instruments, which may ignore the possibility of dialectal variation.

Testing Bias

Standardized testing is based on the premise of peer comparison. Stimuli are presented in an invariant manner to children of the same age so that their responses can be compared and each child's performance ranked. In order to determine a valid ranking, no child can be put at a disadvantage in responding to the test items. Thus, a child who is ill will not be tested, and special assistance must be provided if tests are to be used with children who have sensory or motor handicaps. It is sometimes more difficult to recognize the disadvantages faced by bilingual-bicultural children who undergo standardized testing. There are obstacles to be overcome in nearly every aspect of the evaluation process (Flaugher, 1978; Sattler, 1982). Some of the most common are as follows:

1. Cultural bias. Many standardized tests reflect white, middle-class backgrounds. This is typically seen in the choice of tasks and stimulus items. For example, it is routinely assumed that children will enjoy the activities of listening to stories, pointing to pictures, and answering requests for information. Such activities are common in middle-class households, and children from these homes have usually been reinforced extensively for taking part. But children from African-American, Hispanic-American, or Asian-American families may lack these experiences. Poverty and parental illiteracy may have stood in the way of book reading and other sorts of storytelling. Different cultural values may not have favored the type of question asking and answering that encourages middle-class children to display their knowledge for adults. Hence, bilingual-bicultural children may arrive at a testing session un-

prepared and unmotivated for the kinds of activities that will be presented to them.

2. Examiner sensitivity bias. Professionals who administer standardized tests may not be familiar with the linguistic and cultural characteristics of the bilingual-bicultural children they are asked to evaluate. This condition opens up the possibility of several types of misinterpretation. The speech of the bilingual-bicultural children may be only marginally intelligible to the examiner, who then must frequently ask for repetition or clarification. Such frequent requests can be interpreted by the children as an indication that they are performing poorly, which may make them reluctant to participate in the assessment. Another source of misinterpretation may be the pragmatic behavior of a child. As we have seen, bilingual-bicultural children may differ in their pattern of eye contact and in their willingness to respond to requests for information. An examiner who is unaware of these differences may construe these behaviors as nervousness, uncertainty, ignorance, or even defiance.

3. Examiner expectations bias. The experiences of certain examiners may lead them to anticipate a particular pattern of behavior from bilingual-bicultural children. Although standardized tests try to reduce variation in examiner's procedures, some discretion is always allowed. For example, most tests do not specify how long an examiner must wait for a child to respond to an item. Most examiners rely on their intuition in deciding whether a child is still thinking or does not know an answer. This intuition is formed from previous experiences with children similar to the one being tested. If those experiences suggest that a child will perform poorly, then the examiner is less likely to believe that additional time will enable a correct response.

4. Overinterpretation bias. A danger attached to all standardized assessments is that the examiner will draw broad conclusions from limited test data. For instance, it is inappropriate to conclude that a child's language comprehension is generally impaired when the only data to support this statement is a low score on a test of receptive vocabulary. With monolingual, middle-class children, such bias is avoided by administering more than one test and by combining information from standardized and nonstandardized assessment procedures. The same practice should be followed with bilingual-bicultural children. However, fewer tests are available that have been standardized on this population, and nonstandardized assessment can be difficult without the assistance of someone knowledgeable about a child's linguistic and cultural background.

5. *Linguistic bias.* Some tests may contain English words or idioms that are unfamiliar to bilingual-bicultural children. This may reduce the number of items to which a child responds or may change the demands of a task. For example, a bilingual child may not know some of the English words for common household items, which are frequently used in tests because they are assumed to be familiar. Language bias may also occur inadvertently in the idiomatic prompts and reinforcers used by the examiner, such as "Don't take your eyes off it" or "That's the way."

The problem of bias is not limited to the test or the examiner. Bilingual-bicultural children are likely to vary their performance, depending on how they perceive a communicative situation. For example, African-American children may not use BEV in settings that are perceived as formal (Seymour & Seymour, 1977). If children try to communicate in SAE and they do not know this dialect as well as BEV, the results of the assessment will be misleadingly low. On the other hand, children who are able to code-switch effectively from BEV to SAE may leave the impression that they speak only the standard dialect.

The concern over test bias applies to all instruments used to evaluate children's developmental abilities. Standardized intelligence tests have long been criticized for underestimating the competence of bilingual-bicultural children (Bransford, 1974; Hilliard, 1975; Reynolds, 1975; Rudman, 1977; Williams, 1974). Certain intelligence tests appear to yield higher or more reliable scores than others when administered to particular ethnic minority populations. Thus, the *Wechsler Intelligence Scale for Children-Revised* (WISC-R) (Wechsler, 1974) has been found to yield reliable scores when administered to Mexican-American

children (Raymond, 1979, 1980; Reschly, 1978). When lower socioeconomic African-American children were tested, the *Wechsler Preschool and Primary Scale of Intelligence* (WPPSI) (Wechsler, 1967) yielded significantly higher scores than the *Stanford-Binet Intelligence Scale* (Terman & Merrill, 1973). To reduce the bias inherent in intelligence instruments, it has been proposed that they be administered to bilingual-bicultural children only in a translated form. In one study of Mexican-American children, this practice resulted in better test performance (Zirkel, 1973). Translation of test items is difficult, however, without affecting the sensitivity of the test. Moreover, translation of tests into BEV does not appear to be of significant benefit to African-American children (Quay, 1971).

Standardized language tests have also been analyzed for evidence of bias. Among the findings are the following:

▷ From kindergarten to fourth grade, African-American students obtained increasingly lower scores than white students on the Grammatic Closure subtest of the *Illinois Test of Psycholinguistic Abilities* (Kirk, McCarthy, & Kirk, 1968). This result appears to be due to the appearance of more BEV grammatical features in older African-American students (Arnold & Reed, 1976).

▷ Both white and African-American children from a rural area of northeastern Georgia obtained scores on the *Wepman Auditory Discrimination Test* (Wepman, 1958) that were lower than those predicted by the test's norms (Hirshoren & Ambrose, 1976).

▷ African-American children matched for age and grade level with white children obtained statistically lower scores on the *Peabody Picture Vocabulary Test* (Dunn, 1965) (Kreschek & Nicolosi, 1973).

▷ Hispanic-American and African-American preschool children were more successful at imitating sentences containing BEV features, while their white counterparts performed better with SAE stimuli (Stephens, 1976).

▷ The *Test of Language Development* (Newcomer & Hammill, 1977), when administered to young BEV-speaking children, yielded scores significantly lower than those reported in the norms (Wiener, Lewnau, & Erway, 1983).

▷ A wide range of scores has been obtained when the Spanish version of the *Test for Auditory Comprehension of Language* (Carrow, 1973) has been administered to different groups of Hispanic-American children (Linares-Orama & Sanders, 1977; Rueda & Perozzi, 1977; Wilcox & Aasby, 1988). This variation appears due to differences in the socioeconomic status and educational experiences of the different subject groups.

It is apparent, therefore, that many standardized language tests are significantly biased against bilingual-bicultural children. This issue is of enormous concern to professional organizations involved in debates over assessment practices. In the past, several organizations and task forces have called for a moratorium on the use of particular tests until they are revised in content to include nonstandard language forms and revised in standardization to include ethnic minority populations (Vaughn-Cooke, 1983). Such dramatic action, along with other efforts to increase professional awareness of multiculturalism, has prompted publishers to revise existing tests and develop new instruments that better meet the needs of bilingual-bicultural children. New tests and materials for multicultural assessment are regularly reviewed in *Asha,* the journal of the American Speech-Language-Hearing Association (Cole & Campbell-Calloway, 1983; Cole & Snope, 1981; Deal & Yan, 1985).

Differential Diagnosis of Communicative Behaviors

Professionals who work with bilingual-bicultural children face the challenge of distinguishing between language differences and language disorders. The principles and requirements of this task have been stated succinctly in one official position paper:

> It is the position of the American Speech-Language-Hearing Association (ASHA) that no dialectal variety of English is a disorder or a pathological form of speech or language. Each social dialect is adequate as a functional and effective variety of English.

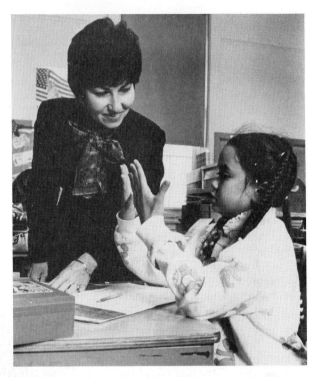

Some children who have language differences may also have language disorders, but not all do.

> ... It is indeed possible for dialect speakers to have linguistic disorders within the dialect. An essential step toward making accurate assessments of communicative disorders is to distinguish between those aspects of linguistic variation that represent the diversity of the English language from those that represent speech, language, and hearing disorders. The speech-language pathologist must have certain competencies to distinguish between dialectal differences and communicative disorders. These competencies include knowledge of the particular dialect as a rule-governed linguistic system, knowledge of the phonological and grammatical features of the dialect, and knowledge of nondiscriminatory testing procedures. (ASHA Committee on the Status of Racial Minorities, 1983, pp. 23–24)

The process of language evaluation for bilingual-bicultural children follows the usual steps of screening, diagnosis, and intervention. Screening should be conducted to identify children who are at risk for language disorders and who therefore ought to be evaluated in greater detail. Figure 10.1 illustrates the progression of a language evaluation for a child who is a member of a racial/ethnic minority group. Because not all minority children are bilingual or use a nonstandard dialect, Step 1 is to screen the child with an instrument that is based upon and standardized for SAE. If the child passes this screening, an optional second screening may be carried out to determine whether the child is also competent in a second language or in a nonstandard dialect. Children who fail the initial SAE screening should then be tested, if pos-

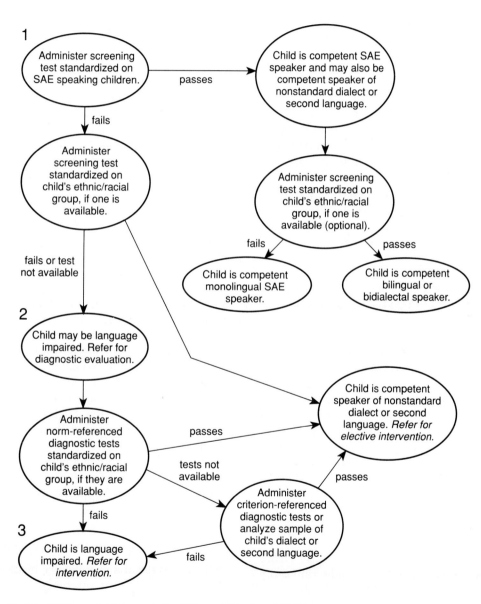

FIGURE 10.1   Model of Differential Diagnosis for Bilingual-Bicultural Children.

sible, in their native language or nonstandard dialect. A passing score on this screening would then establish that a child is not language impaired but rather language different.

Children who fail both language screenings arrive at Step 2, along with children who fail the SAE screening and cannot be tested in their native language or dialect. These children should now be evaluated more fully to determine whether they are actually language impaired. If nonbiased, norm-referenced tests are available, they should be administered. If a child receives passing scores on these tests, the result of the screenings would be discarded and the child would be assessed as a competent speaker of a second language or nonstandard dialect. If appropriate norm-referenced instruments do not exist to suit a particular child, then criterion-referenced tests or language sampling should be used to evaluate competence (Vaughn-Cooke, 1983). Pragmatic behaviors should receive particular attention in criterion-referenced appraisal. One study of bilingual Hispanic-American children found that pragmatic analysis was a better predictor of academic achievement than analysis of grammatical structure (Damico, Oller, & Storey, 1983). Language samples can be obtained by recording conversation that occurs during play. During this interaction, however, care should be taken to avoid the kinds of direct interrogation that are uncommon among members of certain racial/ethnic groups. The samples that are gathered should be evaluated using developmental criteria that have been well referenced for the speech community to which a child belongs. For example, Black English Sentence Scoring (BESS) (Nelson & Hyter, 1990), an adaptation of Developmental Sentence Scoring (DSS) (Lee, 1974), represents an attempt to honor the grammatical features of BEV, as well as to compare young African-American children to their linguistic peers. A child who fails either a norm-referenced or criterion-referenced assessment is diagnosed as language impaired (Step 3) and referred for language intervention.

The protocol just described and shown in Figure 10.1 is truly workable only if more nondiscriminatory assessment instruments become available. As a first step, some tests written in SAE and originally normed on mostly mainstream populations have been re-normed on minority populations. Such an approach is inadequate, however, because it only serves to verify that a child is incompetent as a speaker of SAE. What is needed are measures that can establish children's competencies in their native languages or nonstandard dialects. To serve this purpose, the tests must be conceived and developed specifically to evaluate a minority population. For example, in the case of BEV speakers, test tasks and stimulus items should be developed and field tested with African-American children to ensure that they are both motivating and familiar. Individual test items and appropriate responses must be based on a thorough knowledge of the BEV dialect (Vaughn-Cooke, 1983). The standardization population for the test must be representative of BEV speakers nationwide. At a minimum, it should be reflective of the social class distribution of African-Americans, as this is a variable known to affect BEV usage (Wolfram, 1986).

The problems of nonbiased assessment are equally great for children who speak languages other than English. Currently, more tests and other assessment materials exist in Spanish than in any other foreign language (Deal & Yan, 1985). However, these instruments are based upon different dialects of Spanish. What may be appropriate vocabulary and cultural assumptions for a Mexican-American child may not be suitable for a child from El Salvador. In all cases of assessment involving children who speak limited English, the assessment should be carried out in the child's native language. To do this, the examiner must possess "native or near native fluency in both the minority language and the English language" (ASHA Committee on the Status of Racial Minorities, 1985, p. 30). If the examiner is not trained in language assessment—for example, if a parent or relative serves this role—then time must be allowed for adequate instruction regarding the purposes, procedures, and goals of the assessment.

IMPLICATIONS FOR INTERVENTION

Language evaluation of bilingual-bicultural children can have three different outcomes:

1. Intervention is not recommended for children who are competent users of SAE and who may

also be competent users of another language or an English dialect.

2. *Prescribed language intervention* is recommended for children who fail to show competence in *any* language or dialect.

3. **Elective language intervention** is recommended for children who are not competent users of SAE but who are competent in a nonstandard dialect or a language other than English.

The distinction between prescribed and elective language intervention is based on the view that the traditional role of a language professional is to provide services to communicatively disordered individuals (ASHA Committee on the Status of Racial Minorities, 1983). Children who do not use SAE are not impaired in their ability to communicate; they merely communicate through another language form. Hence, following the traditional model, intervention should not be recommended for them. Nevertheless, professionals recognize that individuals who do not use SAE may be penalized educationally, socially, or vocationally (Terrell & Terrell, 1983). Many children, or their parents, may, therefore, request intervention to develop skills in the use of SAE.

Intervention for Language Differences and Language Disorders

Children recommended for prescribed language intervention need to develop competence with some language form, whether it is standard English, nonstandard English, or a language other than English. It is likely that many of the bilingual children in this category have a *low mixed* language dominance, that is, they combine elements of English and another language to form a mixture that is inadequate by the standards of both languages. Children whose language is influenced by a nonstandard dialect of English may also show signs of mixing. Among typically developing children, the acquisition of more than one language or dialect does not slow the rate of acquisition (Dulay et al., 1978). However, the commonsense assumption of most professionals is that a language-disordered child is hindered by bilingual instruction. The different rules for phonology and grammar, the greater vocabulary load, and the need to master the subtleties

of code switching all place demands on the child without necessarily improving the child's communicative effectiveness. The routine practice, therefore, is for professionals to begin by determining which language form will serve as the target of intervention.

There is no single formula by which to select the language form for instruction. Among the factors that must be weighed are the following:

▷ *Dominant language or dialect.* Although children receiving prescribed intervention are not competent in any language form, they may show greater strength in one form than another. For example, a 4-year-old Asian-American child from Korea may respond to simple commands in both Korean and English but display a larger receptive vocabulary in English. The child may speak in both languages but produce only minor or **formulaic** utterances in Korean, in contrast to two- and three-word combinations in English. In both languages, then, the competence is less than would be expected of a typically developing child of this age, yet English appears clearly to be the dominant language.

▷ *Availability of a service provider.* If intervention is to be provided in a language form other than SAE, it must be conducted by a professional or by a hired translator who is fully proficient in that other form (ASHA Committee on the Status of Racial Minorities, 1985). There are presently large discrepancies between the number of bilingual-bicultural children who qualify for prescriptive language intervention and the number of professionals able to work in language forms other than SAE. For example, as of 1992 only 1.5% of the membership of ASHA was African-American and only 1% was Hispanic-American (Cole, 1992). Only a handful of speech-language pathologists speak Asian languages (ASHA, 1990–1991). In many instances, therefore, professionals will need to rely on a hired translator or substantially improve their knowledge of a nonstandard dialect such as BEV. If these actions are deemed impractical, it may be a factor favoring the use of SAE in intervention.

▷ *Parental preference.* In all language intervention

the support and assistance of a child's parents should be recruited. This will obviously be difficult if (1) the parents are opposed to the language form selected for instruction or (2) they themselves are not proficient in that language form. Some parents want their children to become SAE speakers, even though they themselves may not be. An often overlooked fact of the Ann Arbor trial is that the parents of the African-American elementary students did not ask that their children be taught in BEV, only that their linguistic differences be considered in planning the curriculum for teaching them SAE (Bountress, 1987). Immigrant families frequently insist that their children learn SAE, as it is viewed as crucial to their economic improvement and cultural assimilation.

▷ *Speech community.* The most important insight that sociolinguistic study affords us is that language develops within a cultural context. We learn to speak and understand the variety of language used by those with whom we live and interact. For children, this means that peers and adult supervisors (parents, teachers, day-care providers, relatives, etc.) will be the most important linguistic influences. A child will have difficulty learning SAE when a nonstandard dialect is routinely heard at home, on the street, on the playground, and in the classroom. Conversely, it makes little sense to avoid SAE when that form dominates the child's environment.

Once a language form is chosen as the target for intervention, goals should be formulated that will increase the bilingual-bicultural child's language competence. In the main, the process of goal selection should observe the same principles as with mainstream language-impaired children (Fey, 1986). Some multicultural materials are available that may enhance a child's progress by providing stimuli that are more personally relevant (Cole & Campbell-Calloway, 1983; Deal & Yan, 1985). The major differences in the intervention procedure will be to (1) identify instances where a child's performance in the target language form appears to be influenced by the other language or dialect; (2) use assistants as models when neces-

sary; and (3) clearly identify what is an acceptable target behavior. An example of the first point is that Hispanic-American children being taught SAE syntax may be slow to learn interrogative reversals because of interference from Spanish syntax. This does not affect the manner in which the form is introduced (operant learning, modeling, etc.), but it does lead to a different expectation for how quickly the children will progress with that form. A case can be made for initially avoiding target forms where interference can be anticipated.

If instruction is provided in a language form other than SAE, professionals must be very careful to ensure that correct models are presented. This may require the use of an assistant who can present stimuli under the guidance of the professional. The intervention task and the stimuli to be presented should be worked out in advance so that the interaction with the child is as natural and uninterrupted as possible. Similarly, professionals must identify, perhaps with the assistant's help, what are acceptable responses to certain tasks. Once these are distinguished, the professional and the assistant may share the job of reinforcing the behaviors when they are produced by the child.

Intervention for Language Differences

Elective language intervention can occur under the following circumstances:

▷ A child is a proficient speaker of a nonstandard dialect or a language other than English.
▷ The child or his or her parents request intervention to facilitate the acquisition of SAE.
▷ Resources are available to support elective intervention for children with language differences, as well as prescribed intervention for children with language impairment.

The proficiency of these bilingual-bicultural children in a language form other than SAE means that they are competent language learners and should respond well to instruction. This conclusion, in turn, provides a rationale for working with the children in larger groups and using teacher aides and peer instructors to maximize resources. The role of the professional may vary from providing direct, individualized instruction to conducting inservice training and oversight of classroom activities.

The practice of elective language intervention is controversial and raises issues of ethnic identity, nationalism, economics, and professional training. To some extent, the issues are different for speakers of nonstandard dialects and speakers of languages other than English. In the Ann Arbor trial, for instance, the BEV-speaking children were described as "impaired by rejection by teachers who perceive dialectal variations as errors and indicative of an inferior linguistic system and intellectual inferiority" (Bountress, 1987, p. 55). The problem, then, was not the use of SAE in the classroom but the fact that teachers were insensitive to the African-American children's problems in learning that dialect. The solution devised by the Ann Arbor School Board, under court order, was to organize inservice programs to increase teachers' awareness of BEV and improve their ability to teach SAE to the African-American children.

The issue of ethnic sensitivity involves a different response in the case of children who speak little or no English. Politically, it is more difficult to make the case that these children should receive special instruction to help them make the transition to the use of SAE. As of 1988, 17 states had declared by statute, resolution, or constitutional amendment that English was the official language of the state. The effect of these laws has been mixed, and they have been challenged in court. However, they speak to the concern many citizens feel over the increasing linguistic diversity of America. They also reflect an apprehension that programs to accommodate non-English-speaking children will take resources away from other aspects of public education.

There is disagreement over which group of professionals should be responsible for elective language intervention. Some within the field of speech-language pathology are highly supportive of the practice and feel competent to serve as teachers. Others argue that elective intervention, especially with non-English speakers, requires skills not possessed by speech-language pathologists. They suggest that instruction is better offered by teachers of English as a second language (TESOL) or language arts teachers (Wiener, Bergen, & Bernstein, 1983).

At least three distinct purposes for elective language intervention can be identified. It may be that some but not all of these objectives are relevant to professionals in different settings:

1. Cultural assimilation. Especially in conditions where bilingual-bicultural children are a small minority, the mastery of SAE may help the development of peer relationships and facilitate interactions with adults at school and in the community.

2. Vocational opportunity. Difficulty in obtaining work is a problem that all children will face in the future if they do not speak SAE. It is futile to prepare children in other areas if they will be denied opportunities because of their language differences.

3. Literacy instruction. This was the basis of the Ann Arbor trial, and it remains a significant issue. The only form of English that is written—apart from creative works—is the standard dialect. To become literate, therefore, a child must learn that dialect. In the case of BEV, it remains unclear whether use of that dialect, as opposed to other socioeconomic factors, is the cause of reading difficulty (Harber & Bryen, 1976; Marwit & Neuman, 1974; Strickland, 1972). Interestingly, there was no follow-up investigation of the effectiveness of the changes made by the Ann Arbor School Board (Bountress, 1987). Experience with Hispanic-American children suggests that their reading success correlates with their oral language proficiency (Barnitz, 1980; Kaminsky, 1977). This appears to justify the recommendation of early elective intervention to improve oral SAE skills

If the decision is made to support elective language intervention for bilingual-bicultural children, instructional procedures should be tailored to match their age, environment, and language needs. Young children who speak languages other than English are often mainstreamed successfully in classes of predominantly SAE-speaking peers. They may require some initial support in making their needs known, and some of them will be silent for an extended period before they begin speaking in English (Saville-Troike, 1988). In circumstances where bilingual children form a sizable percentage of a class, mainstreaming may need to be supplemented with special programs to introduce English as a second language.

Children who use a nonstandard dialect should receive instruction targeted at contrasting structures in SAE. For example, speakers of BEV may benefit from SAE practice in the use of the copula, the formation of indirect questions, and the use of negation (see Table 10.8). It may assist children to practice switching from nonstandard to standard dialectal forms within the same communication task.

A child's age must be considered in relation to interference effects and to the amount of time available for instruction. In general, older nonnative speakers of English will have more difficulty with interference from their native languages. The same might be presumed to be true for speakers of nonstandard dialects. In both cases, however, a child's age may be offset by a high motivation to learn SAE (Cole, 1983). The linguistic needs of older children are more immediate, as they have fewer remaining years of school. In this case, professionals may opt for a more intense and selective approach to instruction, emphasizing those features of SAE that will most improve the intelligibility and public acceptability of an individual's communication.

SUMMARY

In this chapter we have seen that:

▶ Changes in the population of the United States are resulting in increased multiculturalism, that is, variation in race, language, and culture.

▶ Language variation exists on many levels: in different nations, in different regions of the same nation, among different ethnic groups, in different social situations, and among different individual speakers.

▶ Children learning more than one language can show varying degrees of competence with the different languages. Bilingual learning is affected by many factors. Patterns of acquisition appear to be different in children who learn the languages sequentially rather than simultaneously.

▶ A major influence on the English produced by Hispanic-American bilingual-bicultural children is the Spanish language. Most of the phonological variation and some of the grammatical differences they show from SAE can be explained as interference from a dialect of Spanish.

▶ Many African-American children learn a nonstandard dialect, known as Black English Vernacular, that evolved from the interaction of English and African languages. The dialect is systematic, with rule-governed features of phonology, grammar, semantics, and pragmatics.

▶ The English of Asian-American children may be influenced by the phonological and grammatical features of their native Asian languages. Some general contrasts exist between English and several Asian languages. However, there is considerable variation in the linguistic and cultural behaviors of Asian-American children.

▶ A high percentage of bilingual-bicultural children live in conditions of poverty. This may be responsible for a higher prevalence of certain language disorders in this population.

▶ Professionals who assess bilingual-bicultural children must distinguish between language differences and language disorders, either or both of which can occur in an individual.

▶ Many current tests of language and intelligence contain significant sources of bias when they are used with bilingual-bicultural children. They must be administered with caution. In the future, they should be replaced by new instruments developed for and standardized on racial/ethnic minority populations.

▶ Screening and diagnostic procedures for bilingual-bicultural children lead to a recommendation of no intervention, prescribed intervention, or elective intervention.

▶ Prescribed language intervention is for children who do not show proficiency in any language or dialect. Several factors must be considered by professionals in selecting the language or dialect for use in instruction. Assistance in interpreting a child's language or culture may be necessary.

▶ Elective language intervention is for children who are competent in a nonstandard dialect or another language but not in SAE. It may not be supported by all professionals or political factions. The form of intervention will vary, depending on the identified purposes of instruction, the number and ages of the children to be seen, and the resources that are provided.

The communication needs of bilingual-bicultural children have been highlighted by demographic changes, linguistic research, and legal action. Professionals are still in the process of responding to these needs, which require many changes in traditional methods of assessment and intervention. Much work remains to be done.

REFERENCES

American Speech-Language-Hearing Association. (1990–1991). *Directory of bilingual speech-language pathologists and audiologists, 1990–1991.* Rockville, MD: ASHA.

Arnold, K. S., & Reed, L. (1976). The Grammatic Closure Subtest of the ITPA: A comparative study of black and white children. *Journal of Speech and Hearing Disorders, 41,* 477–485.

ASHA Committee on the Status of Racial Minorities. (1983). Social dialects position paper. *Asha, 25,* 23–24.

ASHA Committee on the Status of Racial Minorities. (1985). Clinical management of communicatively handicapped minority language populations. *Asha, 27,* 29–32.

ASHA Office of Minority Concerns. (1991). 1990 census figures indicate increasing diversity. *Perspectives, 12,* 11.

Baratz, J. (1969). Language and cognitive assessments of Negro children: Assumptions and research needs. *Asha, 11,* 87–92.

Barnitz, J. (1980). Black English and other dialects: Sociolinguistic implications for reading instruction. *The Reading Teacher, 33,* 779–786.

Bountress, N. G. (1987). The Ann Arbor decision: In retrospect. *Asha, 29,* 55–57.

Bransford, L. (1974). Social issues in special education. *Phi Delta Kappan, 55,* 530–532.

Butt, J., & Benjamin, C. (1988). *A new reference grammar of modern Spanish.* London: Edward Arnold.

Carrow, E. (1973). *Test for auditory comprehension of language.* Austin, TX: Learning Concepts.

Cheng, L. L. (1987a). *Assessment and remediation of Asian language populations.* Rockville, MD: Aspen Publishers.

Cheng, L. L. (1987b). Cross-cultural and linguistic considerations in working with Asian populations. *Asha, 29,* 33–38.

Cole, L. (1983). Implications of the position on social dialects. *Asha, 25,* 25–27.

Cole, L. (1989). E pluribus pluribus: Multicultural imperatives for the 1990s and beyond. *Asha, 31,* 65–70.

Cole, L. (1992). We're serious. *Asha, 34,* 38–39.

Cole, L., & Campbell-Calloway, M. (1983). Resource guide to multicultural tests and materials, Supplement I. *Asha, 25,* 37–42.

Cole, L., & Snope, T. (1981). Resource guide to multicultural tests and materials. *Asha, 23,* 639–649.

Crystal, D. (1987). *The Cambridge encyclopedia of language.* New York: Cambridge University Press.

Damico, J. S., Oller, J. W., Jr., & Storey, M. E. (1983). The diagnosis of language disorders in bilingual children: Surface-oriented and pragmatic criteria. *Journal of Speech and Hearing Disorders, 48,* 385–394.

Deal, V. R., & Yan, M. A. (1985). Resource guide to multicultural tests and materials, Supplement II. *Asha, 27,* 43–49.

Dulay, H. C., & Burt, M. K. (1973). Should we teach children syntax? *Language Learning, 23,* 245–257.

Dulay, H. C., Hernandez-Chavez, E., & Burt, M. K. (1978). The process of becoming bilingual. In S. Singh & J. Lynch (Eds.), *Diagnostic procedures in hearing, language, and speech.* Baltimore: University Park Press.

Dunn, L. (1965). *Peabody picture vocabulary test.* Circle Pines, MN: American Guidance Service.

Fey, M. E. (1986). *Language intervention with young children.* Boston: College-Hill Press.

Flaugher, R. (1978). The many definitions of test bias. *American Psychologist, 33,* 671–679.

Harber, J., & Bryen, D. (1976). Black English and the task of reading. *Review of Educational Research, 46,* 387–405.

Hilliard, A. (1975). The strengths and weaknesses of cognitive tests for young children. In J. D. Andrews (Ed.), *One child indivisible.* Washington, DC: National Association for the Education of Young Children.

Hirshoren, A., & Ambrose, W. R. (1976). The Wepman Auditory Discrimination Test and Southern Piedmont Children. *Language, Speech and Hearing Services in Schools, 7,* 86–90.

Iglesias, A., & Anderson, N. (1993). Dialectal variations. In J.

E. Bernthal & N. W. Bankson (Eds.), *Articulation and phonological disorders* (3rd ed.). Englewood Cliffs, NJ: Prentice-Hall.

Kaminsky, S. (1977). *Language dominance, predicting oral language sequences and beginning reading acquisition: A study of first grade bilingual children.* Paper presented at the Annual Meeting of the American Educational Research Association, New York.

Kirk, S., McCarthy, J., & Kirk, W. (1968). *The Illinois test of psycholinguistic abilities* (rev. ed.). Urbana: University of Illinois Press.

Kreschek, J. P., & Nicolosi, L. (1973). A comparison of black and white children's scores on the Peabody Picture Vocabulary Test. *Language, Speech and Hearing Services in Schools, 4,* 37–40.

Labov, W. (1970). The logic of nonstandard English. In W. Frederick (Ed.), *Language and poverty: Perspectives on a theme.* Chicago: Rand McNally.

Lee, L. (1974). *Developmental sentence analysis: A grammatical assessment procedure for speech and language clinicians.* Evanston, IL: Northwestern University Press.

Linares-Orama, N., & Sanders, L. J. (1977). Evaluation of syntax in three-year-old Spanish-speaking Puerto Rican children. *Journal of Speech and Hearing Research, 20,* 350–357.

Martin Luther King Jr. Elementary School children v. Ann Arbor School District Board. (1977). 473 Federal Supplement 1371c Ed. Michigan.

Marwit, S., & Neuman, G. (1974). Black and white children's comprehension of standard and nonstandard English passages. *Journal of Educational Psychology, 66,* 329–332.

McArthur, E. (1984, October). What language do you speak? *American Demographics,* 32–33.

National Center for Children in Poverty. (1990). *Five million children: A statistical profile of our poorest young citizens.* New York: Columbia University Press.

Nelson, N., & Hyter, Y. (1990). *Black English sentence scoring: Development and use as a tool for non-biased assessment.* Short course presented at the Annual Convention of the American Speech-Language-Hearing Association, Seattle.

Newcomer, P., & Hammill, D. (1977). *Test of language development.* Allen, TX: Developmental Learning Materials.

Quay, L. (1971). Language, dialect, reinforcement and the intelligence test performance of Negro children. *Child Development Journal, 42,* 5–15.

Quirk, R., & Greenbaum, S. (1973). *A concise grammar of contemporary English.* New York: Harcourt Brace Jovanovich.

Raymond, D. (1979). Predictive validity of the WISC-R with Mexican-American children. *Journal of School Psychology, 17,* 55–66.

Raymond, D. (1980). Factor structure of the WISC-R with Anglos and Mexican-Americans. *Journal of School Psychology, 18,* 234–239.

Reschly, D. (1978). WISC-R factor structures among Anglos, Blacks, Chicanos, and native-American Papayas. *Journal of Consulting and Clinical Psychology, 46,* 417–422.

Reynolds, M. (1975). Implications for measurement. In W. Heuilly & M. Reynolds (Eds.), *Domain-referenced testing in special education.* Minneapolis: University of Minnesota Press.

Rudman, H. (1977). The standardized test flap. *Phi Delta Kappan, 59,* 179–185.

Rueda, R., & Perozzi, J. A. (1977). A comparison of two Spanish tests of receptive language. *Journal of Speech and Hearing Disorders, 42,* 210–215.

Sattler, J. (1982). *Assessment of children's intelligence and special abilities.* Boston: Allyn and Bacon.

Saville-Troike, M. (1988). Private speech: Evidence for second language learning strategies during the "silent" period. *Journal of Child Language, 15,* 567–590.

Seymour, H. N., & Seymour, C. M. (1977). A therapeutic model for communication disorders among children who speak Black English Vernacular. *Journal of Speech and Hearing Disorders, 42,* 247–256.

Seymour, H. N., & Seymour, C. M. (1981). Black English and Standard American English contrasts in consonantal development of four- and five-year-old children. *Journal of Speech and Hearing Disorders, 46,* 274–280.

Stephens, M. I. (1976). Elicited imitation of selected features of two American English dialects in Head Start children. *Journal of Speech and Hearing Research, 19,* 493–508.

Strickland, D. (1972). Black is beautiful or white is right. *Elementary English, 49,* 220–223.

Taylor, O. L. (in press). Clinical practice as a social occasion. In L. Cole & V. R. Deal (Eds.), *Communication disorders in multicultural populations.* Rockville, MD: American Speech-Language-Hearing Association.

Terman, L., & Merrill, M. (1973). *Stanford-Binet intelligence scale.* Boston: Houghton-Mifflin.

Terrell, S. L., & Terrell, F. (1983). Effects of speaking Black English upon employment opportunities. *Asha, 25,* 27–29.

Trudgill, P. (1974). *Sociolinguistics: An introduction.* New York: Penguin Books.

Vaughn-Cooke, F. B. (1983). Improving language assessment in minority children. *Asha, 25,* 29–34.

Volterra, V., & Taeschner, R. (1978). The acquisition and development of language by bilingual children. *Journal of Child Language, 5,* 311–326.

Wechsler, D. (1967). *Wechsler preschool and primary scale of intelligence.* New York: Psychological Corporation.

Wechsler, D. (1974). *Wechsler intelligence scale for children–Revised.* New York: Psychological Corporation.

Wepman, J. (1958). *Wepman auditory discrimination test.* Chicago: Language Research Association.

Wiener, F. D., Bergen, G., & Bernstein, D. K. (1983). Nonnative English speakers. *Asha, 25,* 18–22.

Wiener, F. D., Lewnau, L. E., & Erway, E. (1983). Measuring language competency in speakers of Black American English. *Journal of Speech and Hearing Disorders, 48,* 76–84.

Wilcox, K. A., & Aasby, S. G. (1988). The performance of monolingual and bilingual Mexican children on the TACL. *Language, Speech and Hearing Services in Schools, 19,* 34–40.

Williams, F., Hopper, R., & Natalicio, D. (1977). *The sounds of children.* Englewood Cliffs, NJ: Prentice-Hall.

Williams, R. L. (1974, May). Scientific racism and I.Q.: The silent mugging of the black community. *Psychology Today, 32,* 34, 38, 41, 101.

Wolfram, W. (1986). Language variation in the United States. In O. Taylor (Ed.), *Nature of communication disorders in culturally and linguistically diverse populations.* San Diego, CA: College-Hill Press.

Wolfram, W., & Fasold, W. (1974). *The study of social dialects in American English.* Englewood Cliffs, NJ: Prentice-Hall.

Work, R. S. (1991, November). Children of poverty: What is their future? *Asha, 33,* 61.

Zirkel, P. (1973). Spanish-speaking students and standardized tests. *Urban Review, 516,* 32–40.

· Chapter 11 ·

Language-Disordered Adolescents

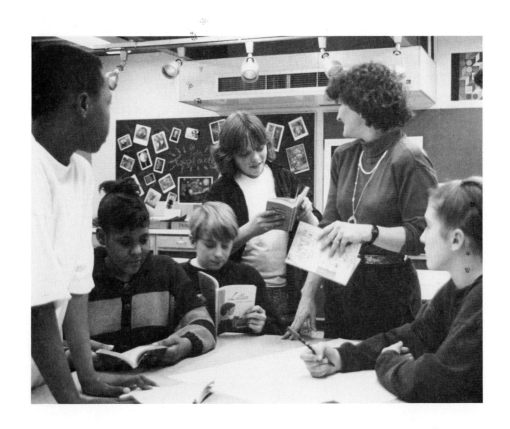

Upon completion of this chapter, the reader should be able to describe:

- Academic, social, and vocational implications of unresolved language disorders in adolescence.
- Reasons language-disordered adolescents remain a relatively neglected group professionally.
- Aspects of language development during adolescence.
- Characteristics of adolescents with language disorders.

- Various strategies used to identify adolescents with possible language disorders.
- Standardized and nonstandardized approaches for assessing adolescents' communicative performances.
- Principles guiding the development of intervention objectives and programs for language-disordered adolescents.

In sharp contrast to the abundant literature on children with language disorders, relatively little has been written about adolescents with these problems. At a practical level, this dearth of information limits professionals in providing valid and accountable assessment and intervention services for these adolescents. Despite the need for such services, many of these adolescents remain unidentified, unserved (Ehren & Lenz, 1989), or underserved, leading McKinley and Larson (1985) to use the phrase, "the neglected language disordered adolescent" (p. 2). In this chapter, we discuss problems related to language disorders in adolescence and reasons for the professional neglect in this area. Aspects of language development during adolescence and assessment procedures are reviewed, and current notions regarding intervention are examined. However, much remains either unknown or empirically unvalidated.

THE CONTINUING PROBLEM

When the first edition of this text was published in 1986, this section was entitled "The Problem" (Reed, 1986, p. 228). It was hoped that in this revised edition, published 8 years later, the section either could have been omitted or retitled something like "A Problem in Resolution." Unfortunately, the section needs to remain, and the title should most appropriately communicate the fact that adolescent language disorders have still received only marginal professional attention in the last several years. This is the situation despite convincing evidence that problems associated with

language disorders, in the absence of other conditions such as hearing loss, intellectual limitations, and physical disabilities, can persist into adolescence and even adulthood or can even emerge during adolescence (Aram, Ekelman, & Nation, 1984; Hall & Tomblin, 1978; Nippold & Fey, 1983; Tomblin, Freese, & Records, 1992; Weiner, 1974; Wiig & Fleischmann, 1980; Wiig & Semel, 1975, 1984). Weiner (1985) reviewed the studies that followed up the status of language-disordered children at a later point in their development, including individuals who were then adolescents or adults. Table 11.1 shows the results of the general group studies included in his review. In summarizing the findings, Weiner (1985) stated:

> In every one of the group studies reviewed here, a large number of the language disordered children were found on reevaluation to have remaining communication problems. In fact, in many of the studies a majority of the subjects continued to experience difficulties. This was true whether the interval between the original and follow-up evaluation was relatively brief or as long as 15 years. (p. 86)

Persisting language problems affect personal relationships, academic success during junior and senior high school, attainment of higher education, vocational and professional careers, and subsequent earning power (Ehren & Lenz, 1989). As one example, the 16-year-old boy described in Weiner's (1974) case study demonstrated problems with the semantic aspect of language, reading skills that only approximated a second-grade level, and syntactic and morphological

TABLE 11.1 General Group Follow-up Studies: Study Characteristics and Results

Study	Areas Covered	Nature of Evaluation	Major Results	Comments
de Ajuriaguerra et al., 1976	▷ Oral language ▷ Cognitive functioning ▷ Academic achievement ▷ Emotional and social development	Direct examination	▷ Each subject improved in most areas; development was generally proportionate to original level of functioning, with change usually not spectacular or even marked ▷ "Entire group retained aftereffects characteristic of dysphasia" (p. 355) ▷ Subjects tended to remain at same intellectual level on reexamination ▷ 4 of the 7 subjects in regular schools were 1 year delayed; 10 subjects were in special classes ▷ 7 subjects had "very unstable affective structures"; 4 were "seriously disturbed" (p. 363)	Wide range of measures used but not always adequately described; results often given in the form of interpretive statements rather than statistical results; emphasis in the report was on amount and nature of change rather than on final level of functioning
Griffiths, 1969	▷ Speech and language ▷ Academic achievement ▷ Social-emotional development	Direct examination; interview with parents, teachers, speech therapists	▷ 70% of subjects had speech and language within normal limits ▷ Subjects "without significant language disorders showed best overall results" (p. 50) ▷ Most subjects had problems with reading ▷ Most subjects had achieved a satisfactory level of "social development," but there was "evidence of considerable maladjustment" (p. 54)	Follow-up of children attending a school for defective children; 49 subjects had regular school placements, but few maintained satisfactory progress once removed from special school environment; apparently contradictory statements on social-emotional development
Beagley & Wrenn, 1970	▷ Speech	Questionnaire to parents	▷ 79.7% of subjects showed "a striking improvement in speech" (p. 1005) ▷ 53.2% of subjects still below expected level of speech development for age ▷ Those with average or above intelligence "showed considerable spontaneous improvement with or without speech therapy" (p. 1007) ▷ Those below average level of intelligence (IQ<80) who received therapy showed significantly greater improvement than did the untreated	The focus of the study was on the relationship between intelligence level and changes in speech

Study	Areas Covered	Nature of Evaluation	Major Results	Comments
Garvey & Gordon, 1973	▷ Speech and language ▷ Academic achievement ▷ Behavior problems	Speech and language directly examined in 51 subjects; simplified version of interview form sent in by 7; information obtained from medical officers, teachers, school therapists, parents, schools, hospital records	▷ 25 subjects in regular schools: 12 of these below expected level on language tests; 14 had reading and writing difficulties; 8 had behavior problems ▷ 9 subjects in schools for retarded: all below expected level on language tests; 8 had problems with academic subjects; 5 had behavior problems	Difficult report to follow: too much detail provided and not well organized; only the data on the children in regular schools and in schools for the retarded are reasonably reportable
Sheridan & Peckham, 1975	▷ Speech ▷ Academic achievement	Reports from parents, teachers, physicians	▷ 124 subjects (65.3%) in ordinary schools: of these, 69 (55.6%) had residual speech problems ▷ Scholastic attainment "remained notably depressed" when compared with the control group; those with residual speech problems and those without were "broadly similar" (p. 163) ▷ "Four times as many children with residual speech problems were considered 'maladjusted' at school compared with controls and three times as many children with satisfactory speech" (p. 163)	Part of a longitudinal study including 15,490 children born in a single week; original criterion for inclusion in the sample of children with marked speech defects was "appreciable unintelligibility of speech" at 7 years as noted by teachers and examining physicians
Wolpaw, Nation, & Aram, 1976	▷ Speech and language ▷ Academic problems	Direct examination for speech and language; source of information on academic problems not given	▷ Compared with original assessment, "all children's test scores improved" (p. 16) ▷ In general "original . . . language patterns were not identical to the follow-up . . . patterns" (p. 15) ▷ 7 subjects were in classes for the educably mentally retarded (EMR); 13 of 23 nonretarded had academic problems ▷ All EMR children still had language problems; apparently 16 of the non-EMR children also did	A brief report in which statistical results were not presented

Study	Areas Covered	Nature of Evaluation	Major Results	Comments
Strominger & Bashir, 1977	▷ Language ▷ Cognitive functioning ▷ Academic achievement	Direct examination	▷ Every child had remaining problems; most had problems in both spoken and written language ▷ 38 of the 40 children (95%) were below grade level on tests of oral reading, reading comprehension, and written language ▷ Considerable discrepancy found between Verbal and Performance IQs in most children; 26 of the 40 subjects (65%) scored higher in Performance IQ	Unpublished study reported by Maxwell and Wallach (1984)
Hall & Tomblin, 1978	▷ "Communication status" ▷ Academic achievement	Parent questionnaire; educational achievement test results from Testing Service files (not available for all subjects)	▷ 9 of 18 language impaired (LI) subjects and only 1 articulation impaired (AI) subject reported as still having communication problems ▷ All subjects had completed or were completing high school; 9 of the LI subjects were in the process of obtaining postsecondary education, as compared with 16 of the AI subjects ▷ On educational test scores "the LI group was consistently lower . . . than the AI comparison group" (p. 235), with differences significant at each grade level	Average scores of both groups fell within 1 SD of the mean; authors suggested that the groups were biased toward more "advantaged homes" (p. 237)
Kolvin, Fundudis, & Scanlon, 1979	▷ Speech and language ▷ Cognitive functioning ▷ Academic achievement ▷ Personality and behavior	Direct examination; teacher reports; parent inventory of behavior	▷ Retarded (delayed) speech group was significantly poorer than control group on articulation and language measures, on all cognitive measures, including Full Scale, Verbal and Performance IQs on the WISC, in reading, and on teacher reports ▷ Retarded speech group also had significantly more difficulties in personality and behavior	Part of a longitudinal study involving 3,300 children born in Newcastle-upon-Tyne in 1962; retardation of speech defined "as failure to use 'three or more words strung together to make some sort of sense' by the age of 36 months" (p. 3); carefully constructed study, unfortunately planned before more recent methods in psycholinguistics were available

Study	Areas Covered	Nature of Evaluation	Major Results	Comments
Aram & Nation, 1980	▷ Speech and language ▷ Academic achievement ▷ Special therapies and tutoring	Parent and teacher questionnaires	▷ "A good percentage" of the subjects had difficulties, ranging from 23.8% inability to understand single words to 49.2% inability to make speech sounds ▷ 40% were "below grade level in reading and math and almost 24% . . . in spelling" (p. 163) ▷ Approximately 40% were either in a special class or at least below expected age grade ▷ No significant correlation between length of preschool therapy and severity ratings in the initial or follow-up examinations; duration of speech therapy during the school years was significantly related to phonology at the examination and to "all areas of current speech, language and academic abilities rated" (p. 166)	Direction of the correlations was not given
King, Jones, & Lasky, 1982	▷ Communication problems ▷ Academic achievement ▷ Psychological development	Telephone interview with parent	▷ 42% "still had some type of communication problem" (p. 28), ranging from 80% of those who initially had no speech to 16% of those with articulation problems, to none of the children with articulation/fluency problems ▷ Academic problems were reported for 52% of subjects, particularly in reading; however, only 6% had grades below C ▷ 24% of the subjects were reported to have been in special education or ungraded programs at some point ▷ Only 8% were reported to have social and personal problems	The 15-year follow-up period must refer to the average length of the interval between examinations, because some of the children were less than 15 years of age at follow-up. The authors concluded that the overall low levels of academic achievement previously reported were not supported in this study; apparently this finding is based on the children's grades; however, it must be noted that a majority of the children were reported to have academic problems

TABLE 11.1, *continued*

Study	Areas Covered	Nature of Evaluation	Major Results	Comments
Aram, Ekelman, & Nation, 1984	▷ Speech and language ▷ Intelligence ▷ Academic achievement ▷ Social adjustment	Direct examination; parent questionnaire	▷ On the summary score of a language test, 14 of the 20 subjects (70%) fell below −2 SD ▷ 4 subjects had WISC-R Performance IQs in the borderline or defective range; 8 had Verbal IQs at the same level ▷ 8 subjects were in special classes; 7 more were in regular classes but required tutoring or had repeated a grade ▷ On the achievement test, over half of the subjects were below the 25th percentile ▷ The 14 male subjects were found to show more behavior difficulties than did the normative group on the scale used ▷ "The Leiter was found to be the single best predictor of intelligence . . . language proficiency . . . class placement and reading achievement" (p. 240)	

Source: Reprinted from Weiner, P., The value of follow-up studies, in *Topics in Language Disorders,* Vol. 5:3, pp. 81–83, with permission of Aspen Publishers, Inc., © 1985.

errors, even though his language problems were initially identified during his preschool years. Unfortunately, language intervention for this individual during his school years had been spasmodic. Although he was placed in a work-study special education program, his nonverbal IQ indicated that he had normal intelligence. This adolescent also experienced problems with peer relationships. Except for the other students in his work-study program, his peers either teased or ignored him.

As another example, Hall and Tomblin (1978) followed up 18 adults who as children had been diagnosed as having articulation problems and 18 adults who 13 to 20 years previously had been diagnosed as having language problems. Only 1 of the 18 in the articulation-disordered group continued to experience articulation problems as an adult. In contrast, over 50% of the adults in the language-disordered group had persisting language problems. Compared

to the adults in the articulation-disordered group, far fewer adults in the language-disordered group pursued higher education or received higher education degrees.

A further example of the continuing effects of language disorders in childhood comes from Aram et al. (1984), who reexamined the language, intellectual, behavioral, and academic characteristics of 20 adolescents, ages 13 to 16, who 10 years earlier had been identified as having language disorders. Fifteen of the 20 adolescents (75%) had required some form of special academic assistance, ranging from placement in classrooms for educable mentally retarded children to tutoring for specific subjects. On academic achievement tests, over half of the adolescents fell below the 25th percentile for spelling and reading. In social adjustment and school performance, they were less competent than their normally achieving peers. Behavioral problems were also greater for these students than for their normal counterparts. This last finding is consistent with those of Camarata, Hughes, and Ruhl (1988), who found that 71% of the children (aged 8 to 13 years) in a public school setting who had been identified as having mild/moderate behavioral disorders had language scores between one and two standard deviations below the means for the normative sample. (Unfortunately, none of these students had had language evaluations prior to the data collection for the research project.)

For the adolescents in the Aram et al. (1984) study, language skills continued to be deficient. All but 2 of the 20, or 90% of the students, obtained language test scores that placed them in the moderately to profoundly deficient range. These findings led Aram et al. (1984) to conclude that "language disorders recognized in the preschool years are only the beginning of long-standing language, academic, and often behavioral problems" (p. 240).

A language disorder in adolescence potentially limits opportunities for personal, vocational, and economic self-realization. The problem is not only the individual's, however; it is also society's. Because undereducation and underemployment are common results of a language disorder, potentially valuable human resources and contributions are wasted. In some instances, rather than contributing to society as a self-sufficient adult when the underlying potential to do so may have existed, an individual with residual language problems becomes a drain on society. In adolescence, juvenile delinquency, suicide, and drug and alcohol abuse have been linked to basic deficits in skills, including speaking and listening abilities (Berman & Siegal, 1975; Donahue & Bryan, 1984; Meltzer, Roditi, & Fenton, 1986; Prizant et al., 1990; Tarnopol, 1970). Asocial behavior and drug and alcohol dependency may continue into adulthood when underemployment, if not unemployment, also becomes a societal concern.

Several reasons account for the limited professional attention to adolescents' language disorders. One is the failure to realize the significant negative effects that persisting language problems have on all aspects of life. Another is the failure to understand that adolescents' academic, personal, or social difficulties may be related to language deficits (Comkowycz, Ehren, &

Hayes, 1987; Ehren & Lenz, 1989). As we have seen both here and in chapter 7, some language problems of children are not resolved by adolescence. In other instances, however, language problems may emerge when teenagers are confronted by the new social, vocational, and educational demands of secondary school (Bashir, Kuban, Kleinman, & Scavuzzo, 1983; Ehren & Lenz, 1989; Reed & Miles, 1989; Wiig & Semel, 1984). These students are at risk of having their language problems neglected because of inadequate identification or misdiagnosis. If academic problems are exhibited, the student is frequently relabeled as having a learning disability, and services, if any, are provided in a learning disabilities program (Damico, 1985; Ehren & Lenz, 1989). Chapter 7 discusses this topic in more detail.

The emphasis placed on preschoolers and elementary school children with language disorders has also led to the neglect of language-disordered adolescents. Early intervention to prevent, or at least lessen, academic and personal failures is the rationale behind this emphasis on young children. It is certainly a logical and worthwhile rationale, and often it works. However, the emphasis on young children has detracted attention from adolescents with language disorders. Ehren and Lenz (1989) even express the fear that the passage of PL 99-457, with its emphasis on the preschool population, "will provide another distraction from a commitment to improving adolescent services, as well as adding additional competition for resources" (p. 194).

Passage of PL 94-142 extended public school services for students to 21 years of age and mandated special services, including language intervention, for adolescents. However, services at the secondary level still are not fully implemented. In a 1992 article on the status of speech-language pathologists employed in the public schools, Blake (1992) reported that only 3.1% of these professionals worked in secondary schools. Unfortunately, this report went on to state that the given proportion was "consistent with data from the *Thirteenth Annual Report to Congress* (U.S. Department of Education, 1991), which indicate that the number of students identified as having speech-language impairments is quite high in the early elementary school years (ages 6–8) but decreases dramatically after age 9" (p. 82). An obvious issue is that if language disorders are not being identified in adolescents, then apparently there is no population needing the services of speech-language pathologists and, therefore, no need to employ them in secondary schools. The circular nature of this neglect continues when one then asks: If only a few speech-language pathologists are serving the secondary schools, who is available there to identify language-disordered adolescents in the first place?

In other instances, the historical lack of services at the secondary level may lead professionals serving language-disordered children who are progressing from elementary school to junior or middle school to dismiss these children in the belief that further services may not be available (Ehren & Lenz, 1989). Dismissal criteria from intervention, and the tools used to determine adequacy of language functioning, may further result in neglect of language-disordered adolescents (Damico, 1985; Ehren & Lenz, 1989; Larson & McKinley, 1987). As Larson and McKinley (1987) point out, "Many times formal tests seem to indicate that the student's language deficit has been cured, when in fact it has not" (p. 6). Some tests may not be sensitive to the language behaviors that can cause problems for students entering secondary schools. The problems surrounding dismissal criteria and procedures can be exacerbated by the erroneous perceptions that only minor language development changes normally occur beyond late childhood and that little more can be done after this developmental period to help (Ehren & Lenz, 1989; Larson & McKinley, 1987).

The very limited data on the prevalence of language disorders in adolescents add to their neglect. Again, we see that limited data may create the perception that there are no individuals with these problems. It would appear, however, that adolescents with language problems are more common than many professionals suspect. One of the few prevalence studies indicated that 7% of 1,028 secondary students in a regular education program failed an adolescent language screening test (Albritton, 1984). Of the students in remedial English classes for grades 9 to 12, 18% failed the screening test, a result that underscores the relationship between deficient oral language skills and poor academic achievement. When complete language assessments were conducted on the students who failed the screening, 35 of them were identified as language disordered and as needing intervention. This figure converts to an approximate prevalence rate of 3%, which is comparable to some prevalence data for learning disabilities (2.5 to 3%) or mental retardation (3%). Adolescents with language disorders may represent an equally large group needing intervention. Larson and McKinley (1987) suggest that this figure may, however, be closer to 5%. As another indication of prevalence, Ehren and Lenz (1989) summarized the results of a 1983 Florida Department of Education study, dealing with the identification of adolescent language problems. These authors reported that

> 73% of a high-risk population of middle school students, including students in compensatory education and special education, evidenced some degree of language disorder. This same study found a prevalence of language disorders of 80% for the group with learning disabilities. (p. 193)

As further documentation of prevalence, 45% of the students enrolled in special education programs in a junior high school in Arizona failed a screening test of language, as did 53% of the seventh-grade students (approximately 12–13 years of age) who had been placed in developmental reading classes because of reading problems (Despain & Simon, 1987). This latter finding once again points out the relationship between oral language ability and reading achievement. It is also disturbing because only about one half of the students in the developmental reading classes had been referred for special education services, including language intervention services, reflecting "the 'happenstance' nature of identification and composition of special education caseloads at the middle school level of education" (Despain & Simon, 1987, pp. 142–143).

At present there is no cohesive, integrated body of knowledge regarding normal language development during adolescence. There is also little knowledge about effective, efficient, and comprehensive assessment procedures for use with these teenagers; a limited number of standardized assessent tools; a paucity of information about what intervention strategies are most appropriate; and insufficient data regarding the objectives to emphasize in intervention. The lack of attention and research devoted to adolescents with language disorders led Prather (1984) to use the phrase "babes in the woods" (p. 159) to describe the state of the art in this area. In these circumstances, it may be no wonder that many professionals are not being adequately prepared to work with language-disordered adolescents and that they may feel somewhat "uncomfortable about their roles with adolescents" (Ehren & Lenz, 1989, p. 194), a feeling that could lead to a reluctance to pursue assertively implementation of services in the secondary schools.

Table 11.2 categorizes and summarizes various reasons language-disordered adolescents are a neglected population. These reasons are not mutually exclusive. They are interrelated, as we have seen in the previous discussion. Because of these interrelated reasons, Ehren and Lenz (1989) have used the phrase "self-perpetuating cycle" (p. 194) to describe the con-

TABLE 11.2   Reasons for the Neglect of Language-Disordered Adolescents

Lack of professional awareness	▷ Failure to realize the negative academic and personal effects of persisting language problems ▷ Failure to recognize that overt problems may stem from underlying language problems ▷ Perception that nothing can be done after childhood
Early intervention emphasis	▷ Emphasis on prevention detracting attention from adolescents
Federal public laws	▷ PL 99-457 emphasizing early intervention; detracting attention from adolescents; possible additional competition for resources for adolescent services ▷ PL 94-142 still not fully implemented at the secondary level
Misidentification/ misdiagnosis	▷ Academic problems as overt symptoms of underlying language problems lead to diagnosis of learning disabilities ▷ Problems associated with language problems that emerge in adolescence attributed to reasons other than language
Dismissal processes	▷ Tendency to dismiss students from services at the end of elementary grades ▷ Tests may not be sensitive to language problems that cause difficulty at the secondary level
Level of services in secondary schools	▷ Fewer services available at the secondary level ▷ Few speech-language pathologists employed in the secondary schools ▷ Historical belief among professionals in the elementary schools that secondary services do not exist ▷ Lack of information on the effectiveness of service delivery at the secondary level
Limited research on adolescent language	▷ Lessened professional awareness of the problem ▷ Limited prevalence data ▷ Unvalidated service delivery strategies ▷ Relatively few assessment and intervention tools ▷ Insufficient information on language development in adolescence
Level of professional preparation	▷ Professionals may feel uncomfortable about working with language-disordered adolescents ▷ Lack of assertiveness in pursuing services for adolescents

tinuing problem of providing services for language-disordered adolescents.

Despite the potentially significant number of adolescents with language disorders and despite the negative effects that language problems can have on an individual's life, the phrase "babes in the woods" is still an accurate description of what we know about these teenagers and their language difficulties. However, we must still provide for them the best services we can within the limits of our knowledge while we await the research results that will help guide the way to more informed and, hopefully, more effective assessment and intervention.

LANGUAGE DEVELOPMENT

The relatively few studies on adolescent language development have focused on isolated aspects of communication. In some instances, little or no differences in language performance have been found between students in early junior high school and those in later senior high school. Prather (1984) proposed two possible explanations for these apparent absences of language changes:

> First, current tests may be insensitive to the progress students make in language facility from fifth grade to high school. In other words, we may be testing the wrong factors. Second, there is the possibility that little changes in the student's ability to manipulate some aspects of language meaningfully beyond at least the fifth grade level. (p. 160)

To support her view that many tests may be insensitive to changes during these years, Prather reviewed the norms for the *Clinical Evaluation of Language Functions Advanced Level Screening Test* (Semel & Wiig, 1980) and the *Screening Test of Adolescent Language* (Prather, Breecher, Stafford, & Wallace, 1980) and pointed to the differences in the mean number of items passed by 5th and 12th graders. On the first screening instrument, 12th graders passed, on the average, only 4.4 more items (out of 52 possible items) than 5th graders. On the latter screening test, 12th graders tended to pass only 3.05 more items (out of 23 possible items) than 5th graders. According to

Prather, increases in test scores with advancing age in adolescence are only somewhat larger for more comprehensive language tests. Of the various tasks included in these tests, those focusing on syntax and morphology were less sensitive to language differences between grades or ages. In contrast, vocabulary tests and subtests showed more noticeable increases in scores during adolescence (Prather, 1984). It may be that the grammatical aspects of language are established by early adolescence and do not change substantially after that time, whereas semantic skills continue to increase. Alternatively, it may be that vocabulary tests are sensitive to language growth, whereas tests requiring grammatical manipulation are not, even though these skills continue to develop.

In the next sections, several aspects of language that appear to develop into adolescence are highlighted. Bloom's (1988) model, with its three components of language—form, content, and use—guides the discussion.

Form

As we recall from chapter 4, *form* refers to the structural aspects of language. Although length of utterance is one structural aspect used to estimate young children's level of language development, it has not generally been used with older children, adolescents, or adults. Children learn linguistic rules for embedding and deletion that can result in syntactically more complex utterances that are not necessarily longer. It is believed that control of these grammatical skills allows children to increase the density of ideas conveyed in a single utterance without a parallel increase in length.

In contrast to this view, there is evidence that length of utterance does continue to increase into and during adolescence (Klecan-Aker, 1985). For example, Chabon, Kent-Udolf, and Eglof (1982) found that length of utterance increased between 3 and 9 years of age. Other findings have shown that 14-year-olds use significantly longer utterances than 8-year-olds (Reed, 1990; Reed & Rasmussen, 1985). Ninth-grade students in Klecan-Aker and Hedrick's (1985) research also used longer utterances than sixth-grade students. Similarly, in their study of children in kindergarten and in first, second, third, fifth, and seventh grades, O'Donnell, Griffin, and Norris (1967) found that utterance length increased in successive grades.

The results of these investigations are consistent with those of Loban (1976), who examined longitudinally students' language development from kindergarten through 12th grade. There were three groups of students for whom Loban presented data. One group consisted of students whom teachers identified as having advanced language skills. The second group consisted of students whom teachers identified as having poor language skills. The third group was created by randomly selecting students from the advanced and poor language-proficient groups and pooling the results of their performances. Loban suggested that this last group represented average or typical language users.

His results revealed a relatively stable pattern of increasing utterance length throughout the grades for all three groups. Loban discounted interpreting these data as resulting from simple verbosity, that is, "an increased use of language without any significant increase in meaningful communication" (p. 25). In his study, utterance length was closely associated with overall syntactic complexity. Additionally, those students whom teachers rated as having advanced language skills consistently used longer statements than their less language-proficient counterparts. Table 11.3

summarizes the length data from these studies. Several cautions are, however, necessary in utilizing the information. The data are not directly comparable as not all of the studies used similar methods to separate language samples into utterances, the same definitions of utterances, and similar language sample tasks. The data should also not be viewed as normative, as none of the studies was designed as normative research. Table 11.3 does, however, illustrate the consistency with which various researchers have found that utterance length increases into and throughout the adolescent period.

We saw in chapter 3 that young children use complex sentences (which contain at least one dependent/subordinate clause) and that proficiency with this sentence type continues to grow into the adolescent years. In Hass and Wepman's (1974) study, the one clearly distinguishing developmental characteristic between the ages of 5 and 13 years was the increasing use of embedding (placing linguistic elements, such as a dependent clause, in the middle of utterances rather than at the end, as in "The man *who came to dinner* ate a lot" versus "The man ate a lot *when he came to dinner*"). In reviewing the results of her earlier work (Scott, 1984b), Scott (1988a) suggested that the use of multiply embedded utterances (those having three or more clauses) may be a "sensitive meas-

TABLE 11.3 Comparison of Adolescents' Lengths of Utterances

Grade*	Chabon et al. (1982)	Reed and Rasmussen (1985)	Loban[†] (1976)	Klecan-Aker and Hedrick (1985)	O'Donnell et al. (1967)
1	6.66		6.88		
2			7.56		
3		7.01	7.62		8.73
4	6.81		9.00		
5			8.82		8.90
6			9.82	9.03	
7			9.75		9.80
8			10.71		
9		7.99	10.96	10.15	
10			10.68		
11			11.17		
12			11.70		

*Grade = Age minus 5 years.
[†]Data presented for the average (random) group.

ure of linguistic growth" (p. 55). Her results indicated that the 10- and 12-year-old subjects in her study used more multiembedded utterances than the 6- and 8-year-old children.

Loban's (1976) results are basically similar. From kindergarten through 12th grade, students used more dependent clauses per statement with advancing age. Furthermore, the ratio of the number of words in these clauses to the total number of words in utterances increased throughout the grades. This finding is consistent with that of Klecan-Aker and Hedrick (1985), who reported that ninth graders used more words per clause than sixth graders. In Loban's study, students who represented average or typical language users in first grade devoted approximately 12% of the words in each of their utterances to dependent clauses. In contrast, these same students in 12th grade placed about 35% of their words per utterance in dependent clauses. As Loban states, "with increasing chronological age all subjects devote an increasing proportion of their spoken language to the dependent clause portion of their communication units" (p. 41). Consistent with the results regarding length, the more proficient language users employed a greater number of dependent clauses and devoted a greater proportion of each utterance to dependent clauses than average or poor language users. Reed's findings (Reed, 1990; Reed & Rasmussen, 1985) can be interpreted as supporting those of Loban, Scott, and Hass and Wepman. Fourteen-year-old students used more conjunctions, including those used to introduce dependent clauses, than 8-year-olds. More conjunctions mean more utterances containing dependent clauses and/or more sentences formed by conjoining two independent clauses. Increasing use and length of dependent clauses, especially dependent clauses embedded in utterances, appear to be characteristics of language development during adolescence.

Loban also investigated changes in the use of various types of dependent clauses with advancing age. For the average language users, the proportion of *noun clauses* (those functioning as nouns in utterances, as in "*What he wants* is a job") increased from 1st to 12th grade, while the proportion of *adverbial clauses* (those functioning as adverbs, as in "She will eat *when she comes home*") decreased in successive

TABLE 11.4   Proportions of Clause Types Used by Students Representing Those with "Average" Language Skills in Grades K–12

Grade	Noun Clauses	Adjectival Clauses	Adverbial Clauses
1	41.48	26.18	32.34
2	44.75	25.21	30.04
3	43.05	27.83	29.12
4	49.63	19.90	30.47
5	48.19	21.91	29.90
6	47.06	21.10	31.84
7	41.12	30.15	28.73
8	37.14	34.24	28.62
9	43.70	30.85	25.45
10	44.54	25.50	29.96
11	46.67	24.06	29.27
12	50.27	24.69	25.04

Source: Adapted from *Language Development: Kindergarten through Grade Twelve* by W. Loban, 1976, Urbana, IL: National Council of Teachers of English. Copyright 1976 by the National Council of Teachers of English. Adapted by permission.

grades (Table 11.4). With regard to *adjectival clauses*,[1] Table 11.4 shows that approximately 25% of the dependent clauses functioned as adjectives in both 1st and 12th graders' language, a finding suggesting little change in the frequency with which average language students use this clause type as they grow older. By 12th grade, about 50% of the clauses used were noun clauses, with adjectival and adverbial clauses each accounting for about 25% of dependent clause usage. A different pattern for adjectival clauses emerged for the group of students with advanced language skills. These students increased their use of adjectival clauses from 1st to 12th grade, in contrast to noun or adverbial dependent clauses. This increase clearly separated language-proficient children and adolescents from average and poor language users. As Loban (1976) concluded, "the evidence seems clear that an exceptional speaker . . . will use a progressively greater percentage

---

[1] An adjectival clause is one that is used to modify a noun. These are often relative clauses introduced by relative pronouns, although adjectival clauses can also be introduced with words such as "where," "why," and "when," as in "The meadow where we played was green."

of adjectival clauses in oral language, whereas the non-proficient speaker . . . or average speaker . . . will show no such percentage increases in the use of adjectival clauses" (p. 48). He pointed out that the greatest increase in the language-proficient students' uses of adjectival clauses occurred mainly in Grades 7, 8, and 9. It is interesting to note that these grades, with the corresponding ages of about 11 to 14, approximate the estimated ages at which children typically make the transition from Piaget's concrete operations stage to the formal thought stage.

Another potentially revealing finding concerns changes with advancing age in the use of adverbial clauses, in comparison to adjectival clauses, by proficient and nonproficient speakers. Whereas the proficient speakers' proportions of adverbial clauses declined as age and use of adjectival clauses increased, the nonproficient students' use of adverbial clauses remained higher than their use of adjectival clauses throughout the grades (Loban, 1976). In chapter 3 we saw that adverbial clauses are among the first types of dependent clauses young children acquire. It may be that poor language users retain this early-developing structure, whereas advanced language users shift to the more advanced adjectival clause as they grow older.

In summary, Loban's findings suggested that as students with average language ability progressed through elementary and secondary school, they used adverbial clauses less frequently and noun clauses more frequently, with the proportion of adjectival clauses remaining about the same in 1st and 12th grades. In contrast, proficient language students used more adjectival clauses with advancing age, particularly on entering adolescence, and fewer adverbial clauses. Their use of noun clauses remained basically the same throughout the grades. Finally, as the students with poor language skills grew older, the pattern of shift in their use of the three clause types was similar to that of the average language users. Table 11.5 shows the direction of change from Grade 1 to Grade 12 in clause type usage for these three groups of students. Although the average and poor language users demonstrated similar shifts, the poor language users used more adverbial clauses. This feature distinguished the poor language users not only from the

TABLE 11.5   Direction of Shift in Proportions of Clause Types Used from Grades 1–12 by Proficient, "Average," and Poor Language Users

Degree of Language Skill	Adjectival Clauses	Adverbial Clauses	Noun Clauses
Proficient	Increase	Decrease	No shift
Average	No shift	Decrease	Increase
Poor	No shift	Decrease	Increase

Source: Adapted from Loban (1976).

average students but from the language-proficient ones as well. This information may be useful in assessing the language skills of adolescents and in monitoring the progress of language-disordered adolescents during intervention.

In contrast to young children, the syntactic development of older children and adolescents is a much slower process and may sometimes be apparent only when linguistic structures that occur relatively infrequently in language are examined (Nippold, Schwarz, & Undlin, 1992; Scott, 1988b). Adverbial connectives are one category of low-frequency linguistic devices. *Adverbial conjuncts* (forms that indicate a logical relation between utterances, such as "*Nevertheless,* the burned cake was eaten") and *adverbial disjuncts* (forms that indicate an attitude or comment about the utterance, such as "There was, *of course,* some debate about the issue") are two types of these devices that connect utterances but do so outside of the internal syntactic structure of clauses. Scott (Scott, 1984a; Scott & Rush, 1985) investigated adverbial conjuncts and disjuncts in the language of students between 6 and 13 years of age. Compared to the younger students, the older ones used a greater variety of these forms, used them more frequently, and were more successful at metalinguistic tasks involving them. Compared to disjuncts, conjuncts occurred much more frequently. In fact, most disjunctive forms occurred in the language of the older students. While the young children used conjuncts rarely, they used disjuncts even more rarely. Although Scott (Scott, 1984a; Scott & Rush, 1985) identified a developmental trend for these structures up to 13 years of age, she indicated that teenagers used these forms far less often than adults (Crystal & Davy,

1975). This suggests that further development of these forms occurs during adolescence, a supposition supported, in part, by the findings of Nippold et al. (1992). In a study on adolescents' (ages 12 and 15 years) and young adults' (ages 19 and 23 years) use and understanding of adverbial conjuncts in reading and writing tasks, these authors found that performances on both tasks increased from early adolescence into early adulthood. Although the young adults demonstrated mastery of the adverbial conjuncts in the reading task, they did not demonstrate full mastery of this form in the writing task. Nippold et al., as well as Scott (1988b), caution, however, that care must be taken in considering possible expectations for normal adults. Nippold et al. (1992) write:

> In fact, many adults may never approach mastery of adverbial conjuncts or other types of literate words, particularly if their formal educational experiences ended with high school. As Scott (1988b) has emphasized, it is important to allow for several levels of adult competence when attempting to establish norms for advanced linguistic structures. (p. 113)

Content

We recall that *content* refers to the meaning of utterances, or the semantic aspect of language (Bloom, 1988). One measure of semantic growth is the number of words in an individual's vocabulary. Miller and Gildea (1987) estimate that at the time of high school graduation, the typical adolescent knows about 80,000 words. Adolescents' vocabularies also contain more words with abstract meanings than those of younger children. As both Nippold (1988b) and Prather (1984) point out, formal education combined with a greater variety of life experiences are major factors contributing to an adolescent's larger vocabulary. However, there are varying degrees to which the meanings of words are known and the number of contexts in which they can be used or understood correctly. Although young children might be able to use or understand a word in some contexts, the full meaning of the word, all the meanings for a word with several possible meanings, and/or the variety of its contextual uses may not be known (e.g., "hot," "imperial"). During adolescence, there is a continuing qualitative refinement in

lexical knowledge in addition to quantitative growth in the size of the lexicon.

Word definition skills are sometimes used as indices of semantic abilities. In discussing this aspect of semantic growth in adolescence, Prather (1984) provides an example from one of the verbal subtests of the *Wechsler Intelligence Scale for Children* (WISC) (Wechsler, 1949). She explains that scores on the vocabulary subtest increase substantially during the adolescent years. The task on this subtest requires definition of words, and in order to respond correctly, an adolescent must not only know the meanings of the words but also possess metalinguistic skills.

Children gradually increase their ability to define words. The definitions of 6-year-old children are primarily based on descriptions of concrete actions and functions. The definitions then evolve to those demonstrating knowledge of semantic relationships, similarities, and differences that are typical of children at about 8 years of age (Lund & Duchan, 1983; Werner & Kaplan, 1963). Lund and Duchan suggest that it may not be until about 12 years of age that definitions show features characteristic of adultlike definitions, and with "development . . . the tendency to produce a synonymous or categorical response steadily increases well into the adult years" (Nippold, 1988b, p. 44).

Another aspect of content is understanding relationships among the meanings of words, as in verbal analogies or the task on the similarities subtest of the WISC. According to Achenbach (1970), some students in Grades 5 to 8 (approximate ages, 10 to 13 years) complete verbal analogies as though they are responding to free association tasks. This may explain Prather's (1984) observation that although there is some increase in scores between 11 and 16 years of age on the similarities subtest of the WISC, the change is not as great as the increase noted on the vocabulary subtest. The ability to respond appropriately to verbal analogies may be a skill that is not fully acquired until late adolescence or even adulthood. And as Nippold (1988c) points out in her review of the research on verbal reasoning abilities of children and adults, the relationship between cognitive and semantic factors in these types of tasks is not clear.

Some statements are referred to as *ambiguous* because they can have more than one meaning. Without the support of context, the statements may not be interpreted accurately. Four types of ambiguity have been identified in the literature:

1. Phonological ambiguity, in which **homophones** are used, such as "He saw three pears (pairs)" (Shultz & Pilon, 1973, p. 730).
2. Lexical ambiguity that involves words with multiple meanings, such as "She wiped her glasses" (Wiig & Semel, 1984, p. 343).
3. Syntactic or surface structure ambiguity that results when words in a statement may be grouped in more than one way, depending on how they are said, such as "He told her baby//stories" and "He told her//baby stories" (Kessel, 1970, pp. 86–87). We see here that interpretation depends on the recognition of subtle differences in stress and juncture.
4. Deep structure ambiguity in which more than one set of linguistic relationships are possible between words of a statement, such as "The duck is ready to eat" (Shultz & Pilon, 1973, p. 728). In this statement, the duck can be interpreted as the subject or the actor of eating or as the object of another's action, that is, a main course about to be eaten.

A developmental sequence has been suggested in the ability to detect these types of ambiguities. Children apparently first learn to detect phonological ambiguities, with the greatest growth occurring between 6 and 9 years of age (Shultz & Pilon, 1973). Furthermore, children's skill in detecting phonological ambiguities remains superior to their ability to detect the other types through 10th grade, or about 15 years of age, the oldest group included in the Shultz and Pilon study. Detection of lexical ambiguities appears to develop next (Shultz & Pilon, 1973), although some children in the early elementary grades respond correctly to these ambiguities (Kessel, 1970). In contrast to syntactic and deep structure ambiguities, detection of lexical ambiguities is consistently better. Lexical ambiguities are detected at approximately 10 years of age (Shultz & Pilon, 1973; Wiig & Semel, 1984). The ability to detect syntactic and deep structure ambiguities is the last to develop. Correct response rates show marked improvement at age 12, with little or no skill

evidenced before this age (Shultz & Pilon, 1973; Wiig, Gilbert, & Christian, 1978). In separating syntactic from deep structure ambiguities, the ability to detect the first type may somewhat precede the ability to detect the second type. Accordingly, estimated ages of acquisition are 12 years for syntactic ambiguities and 12 to 15 years for deep structure ambiguities (Shultz & Pilon, 1973; Wiig et al., 1978; Wiig & Semel, 1984), although even some 15-year-olds may continue to have difficulties with both types. We see that the detection of alternative meanings inherent in ambiguities, especially the syntactic and deep structure types, requires relatively sophisticated semantic and metalinguistic skills.

The recognition of alternative meanings contained in ambiguities has also been related to the development of jokes and verbal humor in children's language (Spector, 1990). Several authors have noted that many jokes are based on linguistic ambiguity (Fowles & Glanz, 1977; Shultz & Horibe, 1974). It would not be surprising, therefore, to find a developmental pattern similar to that for ambiguities. This is generally the case. Before about 6 years of age, children may appreciate slapstick humor that is not directly tied to language, but they do not understand "humor created with language alone" (Lund & Duchan, 1988, p. 255). Gradually, children begin to appreciate jokes based on different types of linguistic manipulations. Jokes that involve phonological ambiguities are often the first to be recognized for their humor. Shultz and Horibe (1974) placed this skill at approximately 8 to 9 years of age. Next come the abilities, acquired sometime between 9 and 12 years of age, to recognize jokes based on lexical ambiguities and those involving syntactically based ambiguities. Jokes containing deep structure ambiguities are the last to be appreciated (Shultz & Horibe, 1974). Appreciation of humor in deep structure jokes is likely not acquired until sometime after age 12.

Nippold, Cuyler, and Braunbeck-Price (1988) extended the notion of adolescents' developing proficiency in understanding ambiguities to the comprehension of ambiguities that occur in advertising slogans. These authors asked students between the ages of 9 and 18 to explain the meanings of phrases in advertisements, such as the slogan for a picture of a new car running on a highway, "*Designed to move you*" (p. 473). As predicted, the ability to explain the ambiguities increased with age, with the greatest improvement occurring between the ages of 9 and 12 and improvement thereafter occurring at a more gradual rate. These authors suggested that the spurt in ability between 9 and 12 might be associated, in part, with a shift in Piagetian cognitive stages from concrete to formal operations that also occurs during this period. Although the 18-year-olds understood more of the ambiguities than the younger students, they did not understand all of the ambiguities, suggesting the possibility of further growth beyond late adolescence. Furthermore, all of the ambiguities in the slogans examined in this research were lexically based. Although we have indicated that the ability to detect lexical ambiguities may precede the ability to detect syntactic and deep structure ambiguities, the results of this study suggest that even the ability to understand lexical ambiguities continues to develop throughout adolescence and possibly into adulthood.

An aspect of figurative language associated with semantic growth in adolescence deals with comprehension and use of metaphors. A metaphor is a figurative use of language in which an attribute is employed to describe an entity or to compare entities not literally or typically associated with the attribute or each other. The semantic associations inherent in the use of metaphors require acknowledgment of similarities between domains usually seen as dissimilar. Many metaphors have become a common part of our language, such as "She is a hard person" or "He is soft." Others are less common, such as "The wind was an arrow looking for its bull's-eye." Common metaphors are referred to as *frozen forms,* whereas less common ones are termed *novel forms.* Similes are variations of metaphors. With **similes**, the inclusion of the word "like" or the phrase "as (adjective) as" makes the comparison or association explicit, such as "The wind was like an arrow looking for its bull's-eye." The development of the comprehension and use of metaphors and similes has been linked to age, cognitive growth, the syntactic forms of the similes and metaphors themselves, and schooling, as well as to semantic growth and exposure to such forms (Nippold, 1988a). Similes are sometimes thought to be easier than metaphors because of the explicit syntactic form similes employ in making comparisons. However, research has not fully supported this conclusion for older children and adolescents, although for younger children, comprehension of similes may be better than that of metaphors (Reynolds & Ortony, 1980).

Comprehension of metaphors has been shown to increase consistently with age (Billow, 1975; Dent, 1984; Nippold, Leonard, & Kail, 1984; Pollio & Pollio, 1979; Winner, Engel, & Gardner, 1980; Winner, Rosenstiel, & Gardner, 1976). Although children prior to attaining the concrete operations stage of cognitive development at about 7 years of age can understand some metaphors, this comprehension appears to be intuitively based. As children enter the concrete operations stage, skill in interpreting metaphors improves considerably and continues to improve into adolescence and the formal thought stage. Winner et al. (1976), in their study of 6- to 14-year-olds, found that only the adolescents were able to understand the metaphors accurately. The type of metaphor, whether frozen or novel, has also been shown to affect comprehension. Pollio and Pollio (1979) concluded that novel forms were more difficult to understand than frozen forms for all students from 9 through 13 years of age.

In contrast to comprehension of metaphors, use of metaphors appears to increase in a **U**-shaped pattern (Gardner, 1974; Gardner, Kircher, Winner, & Perkins, 1975; Winner, 1979). Although metaphors occur in young children's utterances, they are generally conventional, or frozen, forms. The novel forms that occasionally occur usually stem from inaccurate perceptions or limited cognitive and linguistic realizations. The use of metaphors tends to increase up to the elementary grades. However, during these elementary grades children seem to resist employing metaphoric language, possibly in attempts to conform to educational expectations (Gardner et al., 1975). Following this slump, metaphoric use increases again into adolescence, a period described as a peak in the development of metaphoric productions. As Lund and Duchan (1988) suggest, with "adolescence comes the cognitive and linguistic abilities needed to understand and produce metaphors based on a variety of links between domains" (p. 254). The use of frozen forms, in comparison to novel forms, continues to predominate, however, even in adolescence (Pollio & Pollio, 1979).

Idioms, such as "raining cats and dogs" and "slap in the face," are another form of figurative language. For the most part, **idioms** have both a figurative and a literal meaning. Similar to the developmental trends seen with metaphors and similes, comprehension of the figurative meaning of idioms seems to improve with age, with the majority of research findings suggesting a gradual growth in understanding into and throughout adolescence (Ackerman, 1982; Douglas & Peel, 1979; Lodge & Leach, 1975; Nippold & Martin, 1989; Prinz, 1983). Children in the early grades may well be able to understand the literal meanings of idioms (e.g., Ackerman, 1982; Lodge & Leach, 1975). Some of these children may also be able to comprehend some of the figurative interpretations. However, relative consistency in the ability to comprehend figurative meanings of idioms is not evidenced until adolescence, and some suggest that even older adolescents may not demonstrate complete mastery of idiomatic interpretation (Nippold & Martin, 1989; Prinz, 1983).

A number of factors may influence the degree of success in idiom comprehension. Among these are the frequency of exposure to specific idioms, the manner in which an individual is asked to indicate understanding, and the degree of supporting contextual information in interpreting the idioms (Abkarian, Jones, & West, 1992; Douglas & Peel, 1979; Gibbs, 1987; Lodge & Leach, 1975; Nippold & Martin, 1989). With regard to the influence of context, several authors have found that idioms presented in context, such as in short stories, are more easily understood than those presented in isolation, such as pointing to pictures that represent the meanings of idioms in response to the question "What does spilling the beans mean?" or explaining the meaning of idiomatic phrases. This pattern may be more applicable to younger students, who may be more contextually bound, than to adolescents and adults, who seem less dependent on context for comprehension (Ackerman, 1982; Gibbs, 1987; Nippold & Martin, 1989).

Statements, such as "A rolling stone gathers no moss" or "Don't put all your eggs in one basket" are proverbs. **Proverbs** are figurative expressions that ad-

vise, caution, comment, or encourage (Nippold, 1985, 1988a; Nippold, Martin, & Erskine, 1988). The ability to understand proverbs appears to develop later than the ability to understand similes, metaphors, and idioms (e.g., Billow, 1975; Douglas & Peel, 1979). That is, proverb comprehension is likely more difficult for children and adolescents than comprehension of these other types of figurative language. In fact, several authors have suggested that it is not until adolescence that proverb comprehension occurs at the figurative level rather than at the literal level (Billow, 1975; Douglas & Peel, 1979). However, studies employing different methods of investigating proverb comprehension—that is, in receptive tasks and/or those with supporting contexts rather than in tasks using proverb explanation—have suggested that children as young as 7, 8, and 9 years of age demonstrate rudimentary figurative comprehension of proverbs (Honeck, Sowry, & Voegtle, 1978; Nippold et al., 1988; Resnick, 1982). Despite the somewhat conflicting findings regarding the ages at which children begin to demonstrate an understanding of the figurative meanings of proverbs, most authors agree that comprehension of proverbs continues to improve during adolescence and, as with other types of figurative language, possibly into adulthood.

It may seem strange to see so much information about the development of figurative aspects of language included in this chapter. Competence in figurative language use is certainly not critical to everyday survival. It is, however, important to adolescents in their academic and social lives. They frequently encounter figurative language in their classrooms and textbooks (Lazar, Warr-Leeper, Nicholson, & Johnson, 1989; Nippold, 1991, 1993), especially in the language arts. Additionally, the use of slang and jargon, for which adolescents are renowned, is primarily based on figurative language. In fact, the ability to comprehend and use the slang and jargon of the peer group has been linked to peer acceptance and the ability to establish friendships during adolescence (Donahue & Bryan, 1984; Nippold, 1985, 1993). Nippold (1988a) even suggests that "gaining competence with figurative language during the 9-through-19 age range is an important part of becoming a literate person" (p. 179). It appears that an adolescent's ability to understand

and use figurative expressions *should not be sold short* (to use a figurative expression) as a measure of language development.

Use

In Bloom's (1988) model, *use* refers to the pragmatic aspect of language. Several studies provide indications of developing pragmatic skills in adolescents, although we have less information regarding this area of development than for the other aspects of adolescents' language. Our discussion here focuses on four components of language use: (1) the ability to adapt and modify language, depending on the status of the conversational partner; (2) the various speech acts and functions occurring in communication; (3) the paralinguistic features employed; (4) and the nonverbal communicative characteristics of adolescents.

According to Allen and Brown (1977), an adolescent who is a competent communicator effectively adapts language to suit the situation. That is, the adolescent uses code switching and different forms of communication based on the listener's characteristics. McKinley and Larson (1983, 1991) compared the characteristics of adolescent–adolescent conversations and adolescent–adult conversations of 13-, 14-, and 15-year-olds who were in the seventh, eighth, and ninth grades. In adolescent–adolescent conversations, the speakers used more questions, figurative language, and topic shifts than in adolescent–adult conversations. They especially used more abrupt topic shifts with their peers than with the adults. Positive verbal interruptions occurred more frequently in the adolescent–adult than in the adolescent–adolescent conversations, whereas the frequency of negative verbal interruptions did not differ in the two situations. These findings support Wiig's (1982a) observation that by 13 years of age, adolescents evidence the ability to change from *peer register* to *adult register* and from *formal register* to *informal register.* This adaptive communication skill is, however, apparently refined even more as adolescents grow older. By age 15, use of the formal register seems to be extended to include less familiar peers as well as adults (Wiig, 1982a). The informal register is apparently reserved for use with the adolescents' close friends. Differences in adolescents'

MLUs may also reflect the use of formal or informal register. Wiig (1982b) reports that teenagers' MLUs tend to be shorter with peers than with adults. She suggests that this difference stems from the use of more names and titles when adolescents converse with adults. The extra words in these forms of address, therefore, increase MLU.

Besides being able to adapt their messages according to the communicative situation, adolescents should have full use of all communicative functions and speech acts (Allen & Brown, 1977). However, the frequency with which adolescents employ different functions and acts appears to vary with the listener's age. When communicating with peers, 13-, 14-, and 15-year-olds use more functions designed to entertain than when conversing with adults (McKinley & Larson, 1983, 1991). Furthermore, the direction of information flow appears to be influenced by the age of the communicative partner. Teenagers use more receiving-of-information functions with peers but more giving-of-information functions with adults (McKinley & Larson, 1983, 1991).

As a factor by itself, age of the speaker also seems to affect which functions adolescents use more frequently, as well as the characteristics of conversational interactions. When the results of both conversational situations (adolescent–adolescent and adolescent–adult) were pooled, McKinley and Larson (1991) found that from 13 to 15 years of age, there was an increase in the number of positive verbal interruptions but no difference in the number of negative verbal interruptions. Additionally, from 13 to 15 years of age, there was a steady decline in the frequency of topic shifts in conversation. With regard to language functions, McKinley and Larson (1991) noted that these adolescents used the entertaining function less often and the communication readiness function more often. For the controlling function of language, Wiig (1982b) found that a significant increase in ability occurred between the 7/8 and 9/10 age groups. After 10 years of age, skill in using this function appeared to plateau. This developmental trend was similar for conversations with both peers and with adults.

When adolescents' ages are considered together with their conversational partners' ages, differing patterns may emerge. For example, in investigating the use of the ritualizing function with peers, Wiig (1982b) found no increase in children's ability between the ages of 7 and 14. In contrast, Wiig suggested that in communicating with adults, their skill in using the ritualizing function generally increased from 7 to 14 years. This pattern was also observed for the feeling function when peer interactions were examined. However, two developmental spurts were identified for the feeling function in adult interactions. One increase occurred between 7/8 and 9/10 years and the other between 11/12 and 13/14 years. A still different pattern emerged for the informing function when students interacted with adults. In this situation, no increase in skill was observed from 7 to 14 years. By contrast, in peer interactions, the skill increased between 7/8 and 9/10 years. From 10 to 14 years, Wiig found no further significant developmental changes for the informing function. Although Wiig's results regarding this function may appear to conflict with those of McKinley and Larson (1983, 1991), previously cited, no direct comparisons can be made. The two studies differed in the tasks used to examine this communicative function and the context in which the function was elicited. The results may, therefore, be artifacts of one or both of the research designs employed.

Gender of the adolescent speaker may also influence the frequency with which certain functions and speech acts are employed. McKinley and Larson (1991) reported that as a group, the 13-, 14-, and 15-year-old girls indicated a readiness for further communication more often than the boys. In contrast, the boys used the entertaining function more frequently. This latter result may be related to McKinley and Larson's additional finding that the boys incorporated more instances of figurative language in their communications than did the girls.

In chapter 3, Loban's (1976) findings regarding maze behavior in 1st through 12th-grade students were discussed. As we recall, the proportion of maze behavior—revisions, repetitions, hesitations, and false starts—was the same for both 12th graders and 1st graders. Nevertheless, Loban noted erratic increases and decreases in maze behavior in the fourth through ninth grades. In contrast, McKinley and Larson (1991) reported a decrease in maze behavior from seventh to ninth grade (13–15 years of age). However, care must

be taken in comparing the results of these two studies. Loban measured maze behavior as a proportion of overall length of utterance, whereas McKinley and Larson used absolute numbers of occurrences not tied to utterance length.

Nonverbal communication can enhance or detract from the meanings of utterances and the effectiveness with which messages are delivered. Adolescents' uses of nonverbal communication seem influenced by their communicative partners' ages and by their own genders and ages. In their report of their earlier work, which looked only at 13- and 14-year-olds, McKinley and Larson (1983) indicated that when conversing with adults, adolescent speakers used more supportive gestures and fewer neutral gestures than when talking with peers. In terms of the gender of the adolescent speaker and its effect on nonverbal communication, McKinley and Larson's results suggested that 13- and 14-year-old males employed more neutral gestures than females. However, male and female adolescents did not differ in their uses of supportive, nonsupportive, or mixed gestures. At 14 years, more neutral supportive gestures occurred than at 13 years. Again, we see that the age of the adolescent, as well as the adolescent's gender and the listener's status, affect an adolescent's overall communicative behaviors.

This discussion of language use seems to indicate that effective adolescent communicators are indeed adaptive to communicative situations. Often, this ability to adapt appears to change and improve with age during the adolescent years. However, to make these statements with certainty, much more research on the development of all aspects of adolescents' language skills is needed.

CHARACTERISTICS OF LANGUAGE-DISORDERED ADOLESCENTS

In chapter 7, the language characteristics of learning-disabled school-age children were discussed. Adolescents with language disorders may evidence language deficits similiar to those of younger school-age children with language disorders. That is, language-disordered adolescents may have difficulties with words with abstract or multiple meanings or figurative language expressions. Their syntactic structures may reflect simpler, less complex forms, or they may use dependent clause types or adverbial connectives less often than normal adolescents. Language-disordered adolescents also experience difficulties in relationships with both their peers and adults. These difficulties have been attributed, in part, to problems in their communicative interactions. They may not adapt their communications appropriately for their listeners or they may use inappropriate strategies, such as an aggressive or abrupt tone of voice, to deliver their messages. Their nonverbal behaviors may make their listeners uncomfortable, such as standing too close, or may communicate unintentionally hostile or negative messages. Problems may exist with both expression and comprehension. We might expect, however, that some language growth as a result of intervention, maturation, or both would have occurred between childhood and adolescence. Therefore, the language problems of adolescents may be more subtle and more difficult to identify than those of younger children. These factors can contribute to false negatives in identification (not identifying a problem when one actually exists) or misdiagnosis, as discussed previously.

The neglect of language-disordered adolescents means that less is known about their communicative characteristics than about those of younger children with language disorders. Larson and McKinley (1987) point out "that much of what is known about adolescents with communication disorders comes from related literature in learning disabilities and deaf education" (p. 8). Nevertheless, a few attempts have been made to consolidate what is known, or in some instances suspected, about the characteristics of some language-disordered adolescents. As can be seen in Figure 11.1, Simon's (1981b) model of expressive language competence compares competent and incompetent communicative behaviors in terms of three broad aspects: form, function, and style. Adolescents with language disorders may evidence a number of the communicative features listed as incompetent behaviors. Larson and McKinley (1987) developed an excellent summary of problems that may characterize the communication of adolescents with language disorders. Their summary, shown in Table 11.6, contrasts expected normal skills for adolescents with problematic behaviors in five areas: cognition, comprehension

and production of linguistic features, discourse, nonverbal communication, and survival language. These authors suggest that the expectations and problems listed in the table can provide a starting point in determining "where a given adolescent matches or mismatches with educators', parents' or peers' expectations"(p. 15). The determination of match and mismatch is an essential component of assessment and intervention for language-disordered adolescents (Larson & McKinley, 1988).

A recurring theme throughout this book has been that individuals with language disorders do not represent a homogeneous group, even individuals whose language difficulties stem from a disability given a common label, such as mental retardation. Adolescents with language disorders also do not represent a homogeneous group. Each language-disordered adolescent presents a unique profile of communicative strengths and weaknesses. An objective of the assessment process is to identify each adolescent's unique profile.

ASSESSMENT

Without a solid understanding of normal language development in adolescence, assessment is a difficult and demanding process. Simon's model, presented in Figure 11.1, provides a framework for assessing an adolescent's language functioning, as do the expected and problematic characteristics summarized by Larson and McKinley (1987), shown in Table 11.6. Several authors have also suggested that communicative competencies that school systems have developed for the secondary grades can serve as assessment guidelines (Boyce & Larson, 1983; Prather, 1984; Wiig & Semel, 1984).

Simon's (1981b) view that "language must 'work' for an individual" (p. 21) if it is to be functional may also provide a framework for the assessment of adolescents. For an adolescent, language must "work" in social, academic, and vocational contexts. This perspective implies, therefore, that in assessment, an adolescent's communicative performance in each of these contexts needs to be examined. If language is not working for the adolescent in any or all of these

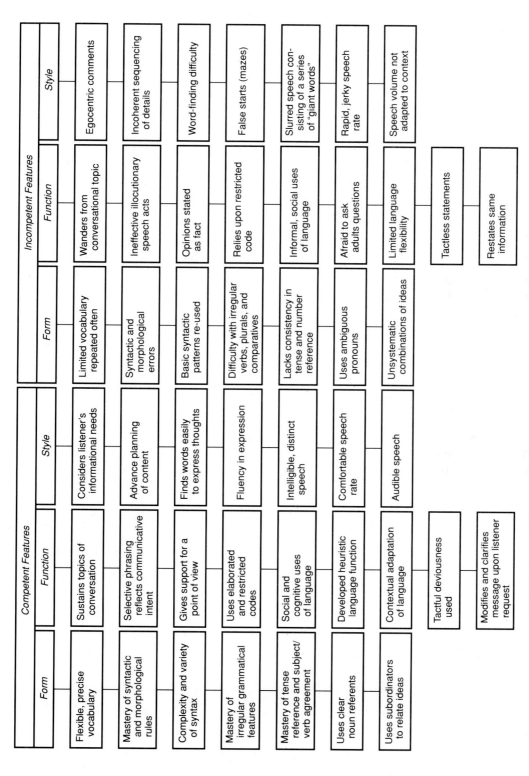

FIGURE 11.1 A Clinician's Model of Expressive Communicative Competence. (From *Communicative Competence: A Functional-Pragmatic Approach to Language Therapy* by C. S. Simon, 1981, Tucson, AZ: Communication Skill Builders. Copyright 1991 by C. S. Simon. Reprinted by permission.)

TABLE 11.6 Characteristic Problems of Adolescents with Communication Disorders

Expectations	Problems
A. Cognition	
1. To be at the formal operational level (Inhelder & Piaget, 1958).	They often remain concrete operational thinkers (Hains & Miller, 1980; Neimark, 1980).
2. To observe, organize, and categorize data from an experience (Feuerstein, 1980).	They make chaos out of order (Havertape & Kass, 1978).
3. To identify problems, suggest possible causes and solutions, and predict consequences (Alley & Deshler, 1979).	They may not recognize the problem when it exists; if they do, they do not know how to develop alternative solutions (Havertape & Kass, 1978).
4. To place concepts into hierarchial order (Feuerstein, 1980).	They often cannot place concepts in a hierarchy (Boyce & Larson, 1983, 1981).
5. To find, select, and utilize data on a given topic (Vermont, 1979).	They have limited strategies for finding, selecting, and utilizing data (Havertape & Kass, 1978).
B. Comprehension and Production of Linguistic Features	
1. To comprehend all linguistic features and structures (Duker, 1971).	They misunderstand advanced syntactical forms (Wiig & Semel, 1974, 1973).
2. To follow oral directions of three steps or more after listening to them one time (Vermont, 1977).	They do not always realize that they are being given directions (Boyce & Larson, 1983, 1981).
3. To use grammatically intact utterances (Simon, 1979).	They often use sentences that are fragmented and that do not convey their messages (Boyce & Larson, 1983, 1981).
4. To have a vocabulary capable of expressing ideas and experiences (Simon, 1979).	They have word-retrieval problems as well as a high frequency of low informational words (Wiig & Semel, 1975).
5. To give directions with clarity and accuracy (Vermont, 1977).	They often leave their listeners confused (Spekman, 1981).
6. To get information or assistance by asking questions and to respond appropriately to questions asked of them (Simon, 1979).	They may know what question or answer to give, but they do not know how to do so tactfully (Wiig, 1983).
7. To comprehend and produce the slang and jargon of the hour (Donahue & Bryan, 1984).	They do not comprehend or produce slang/jargon, thus they are ostracized from the group they most desire to be a member (Boyce & Larson, 1983, 1981).
C. Discourse	
1. To produce language that is organized, coherent, and intelligible to their listeners (Grice, 1975).	They use many false starts and verbal mazes (Simon, 1979).
2. To follow adult conversational rules for speakers (e.g., maintaining a topic, initiating conversation, turn taking) (Rees & Wollner, 1982).	They consistently violate the rules (Bryan, Donahue, & Pearl, 1981).
3. To be effective listeners during conversation without displaying incorrect listening habits (Nichols & Stevens, 1957).	They often have poor listening skills (Boyce & Larson, 1983, 1981).

Expectations	Problems
4. To make a report, tell or retell a story, and explain a process in detail (Vermont, 1977; Westby, 1985, 1984).	They often leave their listeners confused (Spekman, 1981).
5. To listen to lectures and to select main ideas and supporting details (Duker, 1971; Roeber, 1980).	They often do not grasp the essential message of a lecture (Blalock, 1981).
6. To analyze critically other speakers (Duker, 1971; Roeber, 1980).	Their judgements are arbitrary, illogical, and impulsive (Boyce & Larson, 1983, 1981).
7. To express their own attitudes, moods, and feelings and to disagree appropriately (Wiig, 1982a).	They have abrasive conversational speech (Wiig, 1983).
D. Nonverbal Communication	
1. To follow nonverbal rules for kinesics (Knapp, 1978).	They violate the rules and misinterpret body movements and facial expressions (Bryan, 1977; Wiig & Harris, 1974).
2. To follow nonverbal rules for proxemics (Knapp, 1978).	They violate the rules for social distance (Blalock, 1981).
E. Survival Language	
1. To comprehend and produce situational phrases and vocabulary required for survival in our society (Valletutti & Bender, 1982).	They do not have the necessary concepts and vocabulary needed in places such as banks, grocery stores, and employment agencies (Boyce & Larson, 1983, 1981).
2. To comprehend and produce concepts and vocabulary required across daily living situations (Valletutti & Bender, 1982).	They do not have the necessary concepts and vocabulary needed across daily living situations such as telling time, using money, and understanding warning signs (Boyce & Larson, 1983, 1981).

Source: From *Communication Assessment and Intervention Strategies for Adolescents* (pp. 16–18), by V. Lord Larson and N. McKinley, 1987, Eau Claire, WI: Thinking Publications. Copyright 1987 by Thinking Publications. Reprinted by permission.

settings, then a language disorder should be suspected and the adolescent should be more closely assessed.

The assessment of adolescents can be divided into two parts, each serving a different function. The first part consists of identifying adolescents who exhibit problematic language behaviors. The second part involves a more in-depth exploration of the adolescent's language functioning to either confirm or reject the initial identification and, if the identification is confirmed, to determine the targets for intervention. In the following sections, we discuss aspects of both parts of the assessment process. A few standardized tests are available to assist in this process. However, informal observation and nonstandardized assessment methods must also be employed.

Identification

Teacher referrals and language screening are two common methods of identifying language-disordered adolescents. These are not mutually exclusive methods. Both may, and probably should, be used.

Teacher Referrals   Referrals from regular education teachers, special educators, remedial teachers, and other specialists are effective ways of identifying adolescents with possible language problems. One critical factor in the success of this method is the degree to which these secondary school professionals understand and recognize the nature of language disorders in adolescents and know the potential sources of professional help for the adolescents. For this reason, information dissemination is important in providing services for language-disordered adolescents (Larson & McKinley, 1987, 1990; McKinley & Larson, 1985).

Information dissemination includes sharing with classroom teachers and support personnel (e.g., counselors, special educators, social workers, and principals) information about the characteristics of adolescents with language disorders, the ways in which language disorders can be manifested academically and socially, and the intervention services available. Imparting this information helps to ensure that those professionals who have daily contact with adolescents or who interact with them in a variety of situations make appropriate referrals for assessment (Larson & McKinley, 1987; McKinley & Larson, 1985). McKinley and Larson (1985) suggest that English and speech teachers are particularly important because they usually know the communicative skills of their students well. Appropriate referral through information dissemination is especially critical at the secondary level because the number of teacher referrals tends to decline with advancing grades (Damico & Oller, 1980).

Inservice presentations for secondary school professionals are one means of informing the school community about language disorders. To facilitate this process, Reed and Miles (1989) developed a set of eight videocassettes entitled *Adolescent Language Disorders: A Video Inservice for Educators.* The tapes cover such topics as oral language development in adolescence, characteristics of language-disordered adolescents, the academic and social impacts of language disorders in adolescence, and interdisciplinary intervention strategies. Each video is accompanied by a training guide that includes general inservice presentation guidelines, learning objectives, pre- and posttest questions, a glossary, discussion questions, additional resource information, and the script for the video. The series was designed to be used by all sec-

ondary educators, regardless of their specific areas of preparation in order to reduce the need for experts to present the inservices.

Asking informed educators to complete observational/behavioral ratings scales on their students is one way to obtain referrals. Several rating scales of language and language-related skills are available for use with adolescents (Cole & Wood, 1978; Loban, 1976; Larson & McKinley, 1987; Wood, 1982). Such ratings not only aid in identifying adolescents with possible language problems, they also direct assessment to areas of communication most highly suspect in an adolescent and indicate those aspects of an adolescent's language functioning that most concern others. This latter information is particularly useful because one critical function of language is to establish and maintain positive human relations. If an adolescent's communicative behavior is interfering with human interactions, the reasons for the ineffectual or negative uses of language need to be targeted for intervention.

Screening   Language screening tests are used to indicate in broad terms whether an individual's language skills are adequate or whether there is a discrepancy from normal expectations that is sufficient to warrant further assessment. Authors disagree about the benefits of mass screening of all students in secondary schools or even all students in specified grades in secondary schools, such as all 7th graders and all 10th graders (e.g., Comkowycz et al., 1987; Larson & McKinley, 1987; O'Connor & Eldredge, 1981; Tibbits, 1982). Some suggest that a more effective approach is selective screening of students who meet certain criteria, such as students in learning disabilities programs, those who received speech-language services in earlier grades, students receiving tutoring or remedial reading services, or adolescents at risk for dropping out of school (Comkowycz et al., 1987; Larson & McKinley, 1987).

Only a few standardized language screening tests for adolescents are commercially available. Four of these screening instruments are the *Clinical Evaluation of Language Fundamentals-Revised* (CELF-R): *Screening Test* (Semel, Wiig, & Secord, 1989), the *Screening Test of Adolescent Language* (STAL)

(Prather et al., 1980), the Mini-Screening Language Test for Adolescents (Prather, Brenner, & Hughes, 1981), and the *Adolescent Language Screening Test* (Morgan & Guilford, 1984). The first of these screening instruments, CELF-R, consists of six sections that examine various aspects of language expression and comprehension. It takes approximately 10 minutes to complete the test. The STAL, which contains 23 items spanning four areas that tap receptive and expressive language skills, takes about 7 minutes to administer. The miniscreening test is a shortened version of the STAL and includes only five items, one item each in sentence explanation, cause–effect explanation, and sentence repetition and two items in vocabulary. This miniscreening test requires about 90 seconds to complete. For the Adolescent Language Screening Test, 10 to 15 minutes are required to complete the seven subtests examining pragmatics, receptive vocabulary, concepts, sentence formulation, morphology, phonology, and expressive vocabulary, which include confrontation naming, naming to description, and use of lexical items.

Simon (1987) developed a group screening procedure, the *Classroom Communication Screening Procedure for Early Adolescents* (CCSPEA), to be used primarily with students in Grades 5 through 9. The procedure can be administered in the students' classrooms or in other group settings and takes about 50 minutes to complete. It is a paper-and-pencil task, although the writing is limited mostly to circling answers or writing single words, so that it can be used with students who have difficulty with written language. Areas of performance examined in this test include content, syntax, and metalinguistic comprehension, following oral and written directions, dealing with anaphoric reference and inferencing, and semantic skills involving synonyms and word definitions.

Language Assessment

Standardized Tests   Some of the more complete language tests for which norms include adolescent years are listed in Table 11.7. Most of these tests are norm referenced. One exception is the criterion-referenced *Wiig Criterion-Referenced Inventory of Language* (CRIL) (Wiig, 1990), designed to be used

with individuals as old as 13 years. This instrument includes probes to assess performance in the areas of semantics, pragmatics, morphology, and syntax. The *Test of Adolescent Language* (second edition), *Woodcock Language Proficiency Battery, Fullerton Language Test for Adolescents,* and *Clinical Evaluation of Language Fundamentals–Revised* contain several subtests to assess skills in a variety of language areas, such as syntax and semantics. In contrast, the focus of the *Let's Talk Inventory for Adolescents* is to "probe speech act formulation ability in relation to communication function and intent and to audience (peer or authority/adult)" (Wiig & Semel, 1984, p. 526). That is, this instrument was designed to assess several pragmatic language skills of adolescents. The *Interpersonal Language Skills Assessment* and the *Test of Pragmatic Language,* as the names imply, also focus on pragmatic skills. *Evaluating Communicative Competence (Revised)* consists of 21 informal tasks designed to assess language processing, metalinguistic skills, and functional language use for a variety of purposes, including giving directions and storytelling. The five subtests of the *Test of Language Competence–Expanded Edition* are designed to assess semantic and syntactic skills, as well as pragmatic abilities. The last four instruments are tests of semantic ability only. The *Peabody Picture Vocabulary Test–Revised* examines receptive single-word vocabulary skills, whereas the *Expressive and Receptive One-Word Picture Vocabulary Tests: Upper Extensions* assess both expressive and receptive single-word vocabulary abilities. Neither of these tests encompasses the broader range of semantic skills included in *The Word Test–Adolescent* and the *Test of Word Knowledge.* These latter instruments include such tasks as defining words, explaining semantic absurdities, giving antonyms and synonyms, providing multiple meanings of words, using words and word expressions figuratively, and making categorical associations. Other tests that were not specifically designed to assess language may actually contain tasks that tap language skills and include norms for the adolescent years. Four such examples are the *Woodcock-Johnson Psycho-Educational Battery* (Woodcock & Johnson, 1977), the *Detroit Tests of Learning Aptitude* (Baker & Leland, 1967), the more recently revised *De-*

TABLE 11.7 Adolescent Language Tests

Test Name	Author(s)	Year
Clinical Evaluation of Language Fundamentals–Revised (CELF–R)	Semel, Wiig, and Secord	1987
Evaluating Communicative Competence–Revised	Simon	1986
Expressive and Receptive One-Word Picture Vocabulary Tests: Upper Extensions	Gardner and Brownell	1987
Fullerton Language Test for Adolescents (2nd ed.)	Thorum	1986
Interpersonal Language Skills Assessment	Blagden and McConnell	1984
Let's Talk Inventory for Adolescents (LTI-A)	Wiig	1982b
Peabody Picture Vocabulary Test–Revised (PPVT–R)	Dunn and Dunn	1981
Test of Adolescent Language (2nd ed.) (TOAL-2)	Hammill, Brown, Larsen, and Wiederholt	1987
Test of Language Competence–Expanded Edition (TLC)	Wiig and Secord	1989
Test of Pragmatic Language (TOPL)	Phelps-Terasaki and Phelps-Gunn	1992
Test of Word Knowledge (TOWK)	Wiig and Secord	1992
Wiig Criterion-Referenced Inventory of Language (CRIL)	Wiig	1990
Woodcock Language Proficiency Battery	Woodcock	1980
The Word Test–Adolescent	Zachman, Huisingh, Barrett, Orman, and Blagden	1989

troit Tests of Learning Aptitude–3 (Hammill, 1991), and the *Detroit Tests of Learning Aptitude–Adult* (Hammill & Bryant, 1991).

In comparison to the many language tests designed for use with younger children, there are very few tests for adolescents. Furthermore, the norms and construct validity of several of the tests have been questioned (Stephens & Montgomery, 1985). As a result of their review of several of these tests, Stephens and Montgomery listed six recommendations for using standardized tests with adolescents, recommendations that apply to testing of young children as well. Table 11.8 summarizes these recommendations. If we eliminate any of these tests because of questionable validity, our choices narrow even more. This is one reason

that nonstandardized testing and informal observation are used so frequently with adolescents. Other reasons are that many standardized tests examine only limited aspects of language behavior, and these tests alone do not yield sufficient information about patterns of language behaviors to allow us to develop specific intervention objectives. This topic is discussed in more detail in chapter 14. It is sufficient to say here that nonstandardized techniques are necessary when assessing the language skills of adolescents.

Nonstandardized Methods   Analysis of spontaneous language and assessment of language functioning within the language demands of an educational system are two broad, nonstandardized approaches to

TABLE 11.8   Recommendations for Using Standardized Tests with Adolescents

1. Standardized tests should constitute only part of the assessment process and test authors, themselves, make this recommendation.
2. More than one standardized test should be used . . . because variable performances across tests have been reported for some students.
3. If the testing times are widely spaced, such as 2 or 3 years apart, the results of in-depth standardized testing can contribute to demonstrating that an individual no longer needs special services; that is, his or her performance is not significantly different from that of peers.
4. If possible, clinicians should develop local norms.
5. Clinicians should be encouraged to cooperate with test constructors in the development of language tests.
6. It is the test user's responsibility to read, understand, and evaluate the manual accompanying a test and to stay current on the topic of standardized testing.

Source: Adapted from M. I. Stephens and A. A. Montgomery, A critique of recent relevant standardized tests, in *Topics in Language Disorders,* Vol. 5:3, pp. 21–45, with permission of Aspen Publishers, Inc., © 1985.

language assessment of adolescents. In contrast to using just one of these approaches, using both provides a more solid data base from which to identify an adolescent's competent and incompetent language skills and determine directions for intervention. Damico (1993) argues that assessment "activities used must be more *authentic,* more *functional,* and more *descriptive* than the assessment procedures previously employed with this population" (p. 29).

Analysis of Spontaneous Language.   It is impractical to attempt to analyze an adolescent's entire language behavior in any one day. Therefore, a limited but representative sample of spontaneous language is obtained for analysis. Specific factors related to obtaining language samples are discussed in chapter 14. There the focus is more on the younger child than on the adolescent with a suspected language disorder. However, the principles of obtaining a sample in varying communicative situations and of audio- or videorecording the sample apply in all instances. Here we discuss specific analysis techniques appropriate for adolescents.

The *Adolescent Conversational Analysis,* developed by Larson and McKinley (1987), is one of the few methods designed specifically for analyzing an adolescent's language sample. The authors suggest that it "is unique from [*sic*] other analyses in that it examines the adolescent's role both as a listener and a speaker, not simply as a speaker, during conversation" (pp. 107–108). Listener abilities that are analyzed are understanding the speaker's vocabulary and syntax, following the speaker's main ideas, listening in a nonjudgmental way, and signaling lack of understanding. Speaker abilities are divided into four aspects: language features, paralanguage features, communication functions, and verbal and nonverbal communication rules. Within each of these broad aspects, specific features of communicative functioning are noted and analyzed.

Elements of analysis for language features include the use of a variety of syntactic forms, occurrence of question forms, production of figurative language, evidence of nonspecific language, and occurrence of word retrieval problems, mazes, and false starts. Analysis of paralanguage behavior focuses on fluency, intelligibility, and suprasegmental features such as inflection, rate, and juncture. For the broad category of communication functions, specific functions used as analysis elements are giving information; getting information; describing ongoing events; persuading; expressing beliefs, feelings, and intentions; indicating readiness for additional communication; problem solving; and entertaining. The last of the four broad aspects, verbal and nonverbal communication rules, is divided further into verbal rules for topics and turns, verbal rules for politeness, and nonverbal rules. Seven verbal rules of topics and turns are analyzed (initiating conversations, choosing topics, maintaining topics, switching topics, taking turns, repairing conversations, and interrupting). Analysis of verbal rules of politeness focuses on appropriate quantity of talk, appearance of sincerity and honesty, making relevant contributions to the topic, expression of ideas clearly, and tactfulness. Lastly, four aspects of nonverbal rules are examined—gestures, facial expressions, eye contact, and proxemics (physical distance from partner).

Each of these communicative behaviors is judged as appropriate or inappropriate each time it occurs during a language sample. The tallies or frequency counts of both appropriate and inappropriate behaviors can be transferred to a profile form that summarizes an adolescent's strengths and weaknesses. This profile can lead to the development of specific intervention objectives and can form part of the basis of a valid and defensible intervention plan.

Simon's (1981b) model, shown in Figure 11.1, provides another guideline for analyzing an adolescent's language sample. As the sample is reviewed, instances of competent and incompetent use of each of the specific features of form, function, and style can be noted. To ensure that adequate opportunities occur in the sample for assessment of these communicative features, Simon (1981b, 1984) suggests that the examiner create a variety of communicative situations in which the adolescent can demonstrate skills in using Halliday's (1973, 1975) seven functions of language. Simon gives examples of role-playing situations, dialogue topics, and specific published materials that can be employed to elicit these different communicative functions.

An adolescent's language sample can also be analyzed in light of secondary-level communication competencies proposed by a number of state and local school systems. A relatively comprehensive list of competencies for high school graduates has been developed by Bassett, Whittington, and Staton-Spicer (1978). These competencies, shown in Table 11.9, are divided into four areas: communication codes, oral message evaluation, basic speech communication skills, and human relations. Within each area, several specific competencies are listed with examples of how each competency is employed in occupational, social, and political/civil situations. Communication competencies in both the role of speaker and listener are given, as are competencies for all parameters of language. As seen in the table, the area of communication codes includes such skills as listening effectively to spoken English (understanding directions given by a police officer), using words, pronunciation, and grammar appropriate for a situation (i.e., for a job interview), and employing appropriate nonverbal communication for a situation (using gestures to signal sympathy to a friend). Of the four competencies given for oral message evaluation, one involves being

able to distinguish facts from opinions, as in a political candidate's speech, and another requires recognizing when a listener has not understood a spoken message, as in knowing when a customer has not understood the directions for using a product. Among the basic speech communication skills listed are answering questions effectively, expressing and defending a personal point of view, and giving concise and precise directions. Three of the competencies in the human relations area are performing social rituals (such as making introductions), expressing feelings (such as stating dissatisfaction to a clerk), and describing another's point of view (such as stating the position of a supervisor who has given a recommendation about which one disagrees). Nineteen competencies are assessed in the four communication areas. This list of competencies provides a valuable guideline for analyzing an adolescent's communicative functioning in a variety of life situations. Deficits in specific areas can then be used to determine the direction of intervention.

Assessing the Educational System. As we indicated earlier in this chapter, language must work for an adolescent, and part of this process involves using it effectively in an academic setting. Success or failure in school significantly affects all aspects of life in adolescence, as well as in adult life. When an adolescent suspected of having a language disorder has particular difficulty with certain subject areas, Larson and McKinley (1987) believe that the student's educational environment, as well as his or her language skills, should be assessed. These authors suggest that such an assessment can help identify the source of the problem (either with the student or with the educational system), determine if the problem stems from the adolescent's lack of motivation or lack of skill, and indicate whether or not an intervention plan needs to include curriculum modification as well as more direct language intervention. In completing a curriculum analysis, the language of instruction, the language of the textbooks, the student's attitude toward specific subjects, and the student's ability to comprehend the language used in the curriculum are assessed.

To facilitate completing this assessment, Larson and McKinley (1987) developed the *Curriculum Analysis*

TABLE 11.9 Guidelines for Minimal Speaking and Listening Competencies for High School Graduates

Competencies	Application Examples		
	Occupational	Citizenship	Maintenance

I. *Communication codes.* This set of skills deals with minimal abilities in speaking and understanding spoken English and using nonverbal signs (e.g., gestures and facial expressions).

Competencies	Occupational	Citizenship	Maintenance
A. Listen effectively to spoken English	Understand directions given by job supervisor	Understand directions given on TV or radio on procedures necessary to vote	Understand weather bulletins broadcast on radio or TV
	Understand complaints and needs of customers	Understand directions to a jury from a judge.	Understand a doctor's directions for taking prescribed medication
	Understand suggestions and questions of fellow workers	Understand directions given by policemen	Understand a plumber's suggestions for preventive household maintenance
B. Use words, pronunciation, and grammar appropriate for situation	Use appropriate language during employment interviews	Use language understood by members of diverse groups at civic meetings	Describe an ailment so that a doctor can understand the symptoms
	Use words, pronunciation, and grammar which do not alienate co-workers	Use inoffensive words when expressing political views	Use language understood by a policeman when making a complaint
	Use words understood by co-workers	Use language understood by public officials	Use language understood by a banker when making a loan application
C. Use nonverbal signs appropriate for situation	Use appropriate gestures and eye contact during employment interviews	Use appropriate facial expressions and posture when expressing one's point of view at civic meetings	Use gestures which enhance a child's understanding of how to perform a household task
	Use appropriate facial expressions and tone of voice when conversing with a supervisor	Use appropriate nonverbal signs when campaigning for a political candidate	Use gestures which enhance a friend's understanding of how to play a game
	Use gestures which aid a co-worker in learning to perform a production task	Use appropriate nonverbal signs when engaging in informal discussions of political views with friends.	Use nonverbal signs to indicate sympathy to a friend

347

| | Application Examples | | |
Competencies	Occupational	Citizenship	Maintenance
D. Use voice effectively	Use sufficient volume when making a presentation to a large group in an on-the-job setting Use appropriate volume when conversing with a customer via telephone Speak with appropriate rate, volume, and clarity when conversing with your supervisor	Speak clearly and loudly enough to be heard in public debate or discussion Speak with appropriate rate, volume, and clarity when expressing views to an elected official Speak clearly and loudly enough to be heard and understood when giving testimony in court	Speak with appropriate rate, volume, and clarity in social conversations Speak with appropriate rate, volume, and clarity when reporting a fire or accident Speak with appropriate rate, volume, and clarity when soliciting funds for a charity

II. *Oral message evaluation.* This set of skills involves the use of standards of appraisal to make judgments about oral messages or their effects.

A. Identify main ideas in messages	Identify the task to be performed when given instructions orally Recognize performance standards for work assigned orally Recognize commitments, promises, threats, and commands	Select main ideas when listening to political speeches Identify key points in broadcast interviews with political candidates Identify critical issues in trial testimony	Obtain main ideas in messages concerning health-related news Identify main ideas in broadcast messages about tax return preparation Identify main ideas in a contract agreement
B. Distinguish facts from opinions	Obtain factual information about job opportunities Distinguish between facts and opinions in customer complaints Distinguish between facts and opinions in labor-management disputes	Distinguish between facts and opinions in political speeches Distinguish between evidence and opinion in testimony Distinguish between fact and opinion in newscasts	Distinguish facts from opinions in advertisements Distinguish facts from opinions with respect to effective illness treatment Distinguish facts from opinion regarding nutrition
C. Distinguish between informative and persuasive messages	Distinguish between informative and persuasive messages in a job interview Distinguish between informative and persuasive messages from a union organizer Distinguish between informative and persuasive messages of management	Identify when being subjected to propaganda Distinguish between informative and persuasive messages of politicians Distinguish between informative and persuasive messages of trial attorneys	Identify when being subjected to a sales presentation Distinguish between informative and persuasive messages about purchasing on credit Distinguish between informative and persuasive messages about non-prescription drugs

D. Recognize when another does not understand your message	Recognize lack of understanding in other employees Recognize when a job interviewer doesn't understand an explanation of work experience Recognize when a customer doesn't understand directions for product use	Recognize when another doesn't understand one's position on a public issue Recognize when a public official doesn't understand a request Recognize when a judge does not understand one's testimony	Recognize when another family member doesn't understand instructions Recognize when a doctor doesn't understand one's description of an illness Recognize when a salesperson doesn't understand a request

III. *Basic speech communication skills.* This set of skills deals with the process of selecting message elements and arranging them to produce spoken messages.

A. Express ideas clearly and concisely	Make a report to one's job supervisor Explain job requirements to a new employee State clearly relevant information about work experience when applying for a job	Describe a desired course of political action Describe an accident or crime to a policeman Explain citizens' rights to another	Explain an appliance malfunction to a repair person Explain an unfamiliar task to a child or other family member Explain one's values to a child or friend
B. Express and defend with evidence your point of view	Express and defend one's view in a union meeting Express and defend suggestions for changes in job conditions Express and defend reasons for job absence to one's supervisor	Express and defend one's view in a political discussion Express and defend one's innocence in court Express and defend one's position in a city council meeting	Express and defend one's refusal to accept unordered products or services Express and defend your faith or religion Express and defend your feelings in a family discussion
C. Organize (order) messages so that others can understand them	Use a chronological order to explain a complex business procedure to a co-worker Use a topical order when explaining production problems to a supervisor Use a problem-cause-solution order when making a suggestion to a supervisor	Use a topical order to explain political views Use a cause-effect order when giving an accident report Use a chronological order to explain a complaint to an elected official	Use a problem-cause-solution order to explain one's financial position when applying for a loan Explain to a child how to prevent accidents using a cause-effect order Use a chronological order to explain to a mechanic the development of an automobile malfunction

TABLE 11.9, *continued*

Competencies	Application Examples		
	Occupational	Citizenship	Maintenance
D. Ask questions to obtain information	Obtain information about correct job performance procedures	Obtain information from public officials about laws and regulations	Obtain information about interest rates for purchases bought on credit
	Obtain information about job benefits	Obtain information about another's evidence on a political issue	Obtain information about one's credit rating
	Obtain suggestions about how to improve your job performance	Obtain information about a political candidate's views	Obtain information about product safety
E. Answer questions effectively	Answer a potential employer's questions about your qualifications	Answer questions about one's position on public issues	Answer a doctor's questions about one's illness
	Answer customer questions	Answer questions of a census taker	Answer a tax auditor's questions
	Answer a supervisor's questions about one's job performance	Answer questions as a witness	Answer a child's questions so that the child understands
F. Give concise and accurate directions	Direct co-workers or subordinates in performing unfamiliar jobs	Give directions to another about the procedures necessary to vote	Teach a child how to play a game
	Instruct customers about product use	Give directions to another about the procedures necessary to file a tax return	Instruct repairpersons on how one wants some repair made
	Instruct an employee about improving job performance	Give directions to another about the procedures necessary to appear before the city council	Teach a child what to do in case of fire
G. Summarize messages	Summarize oral instructions given by a job supervisor	Summarize the position of a political candidate on a campaign issue	Summarize a public service message on auto safety
	Give a summary of customer suggestions to one's job supervisor	Summarize the arguments for and against a controversial issue	Summarize for family members a telephone conversation
	Summarize one's qualifications in a job interview	Summarize for another the laws/ regulations pertaining to some action	Summarize for family members the family financial position

350

IV. *Human relations*. This set of skills is used for building and maintaining personal relationships and for resolving conflict.

A. Describe another's viewpoint	Describe the viewpoint of a supervisor who disagrees with one's evaluation of job performance	Describe the viewpoint of a friend with whom one disagrees about public issues	Describe the viewpoint of a retail store manager to whom one returns merchandise
	Describe the viewpoint of a co-worker who disagrees with one's recommendations	Describe the viewpoint of a legislator who proposes a law one opposes	Describe the viewpoint of your spouse when one disagrees on a major decision
	Describe the viewpoint of union officials in a contract dispute	Describe the viewpoint of a jury member with whom one disagrees	Describe the viewpoint of a neighbor who complains about children's behavior
B. Describe differences in opinion	Describe differences in opinion with co-workers about work-related issues	Describe differences in opinion with a legislator about proposed legislation	Describe differences in opinion with spouse about child-rearing practices
	Describe differences in opinion with one's supervisor about the steps necessary to accomplish a goal	Describe differences in opinion with other jurors	Describe differences in opinion with a doctor regarding health care
	Describe differences in opinion with customers about product performance	Describe differences in opinion in a zoning hearing	Describe differences in opinion with spouse about the responsibility for household chores
C. Express feelings to others	Express personal reactions to changes in job conditions to one's supervisor	Express feelings of anger to your city councilperson	Express dissatisfaction to a store clerk
	Express satisfaction to a co-worker about his/her work	Express your positive reactions to an elected official's work	Express feelings of approval to a child for his/her school achievement
	Express feelings of dissatisfaction with co-workers regarding the quality of work interactions	Express feelings of disapproval regarding a legislator's position	Express feelings of sympathy to a friend whose parent has died
D. Perform social rituals	Introduce oneself at the beginning of a job interview	Introduce a motion at a public meeting	Make small talk in casual social settings
	Greet customers	Request an appointment with an elected official	Introduce strangers to one another
	Conclude a conversation with one's employer	Introduce a speaker at a political rally	Introduce oneself

Source: From "The Basics in Speaking and Listening for High School Graduates: What Should Be Assessed?" by R. Bassett, N. Whittington, and A Staton-Spicer, 1978, *Communication Education*, 27, pp. 298–302. Copyright 1978 by the Speech Communication Association. Reprinted by permission.

At the secondary education level, students are expected to acquire information independently, an expectation that language-disordered adolescents may not be able to meet without intervention.

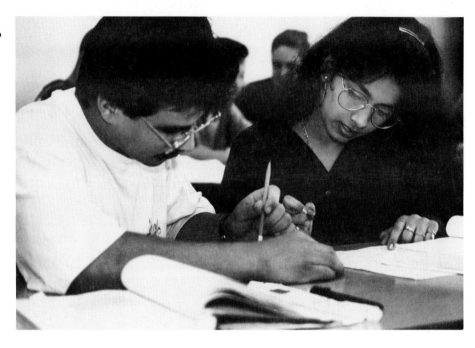

Form. This form is divided into three parts, all of which are completed for each course an adolescent finds especially difficult. The first section analyzes the textbook used in the course, and the second focuses on the course's organization and the student's comprehension of classroom lectures/instructions and examinations. The last section of the form asks the adolescent to answer "yes" or "no" to a list of questions designed to probe the adolescent's attitude toward the course. When the analysis is completed, it helps clarify what strategies can be employed to assist the adolescent in dealing with educational language levels.

Because many topics are repeated at different levels throughout elementary and secondary school, Prather (1984) suggests that educational materials, including texts, from earlier grades may be used to bridge a language gap in order for the student to acquire course content. Furthermore, the instructional materials used in the curriculum can indicate what vocabulary, verbal relationships, and grammar are expected at the various grade levels and in the various courses. Gruenewald and Pollak (1990) conceptualize the language

used in the educational process as consisting of an ongoing interactional triad among the teacher's language, the student's language, and the language concepts/content of the topic. This interactional triad is illustrated in Figure 11.2. The authors suggest that their triad can form the basis for analyzing the language required in a specific teaching-learning process and identifying where in the process a student might be encountering difficulties because of a mismatch between the "language of instruction" and the student's language abilities. *The Instructional Environment Scale* (Ysseldyke & Christenson, 1987) may also assist in examining the academic context in which a student is expected to function.

INTERVENTION

Unlike much of the intervention with language-disordered youngsters, who are often naive about the purposes and objectives of intervention, adolescents with language disorders must participate in planning their own intervention (Boyce & Larson, 1983; Ehren & Lenz, 1989; Klecan-Aker, 1985; Larson & McKinley,

Language content/concepts

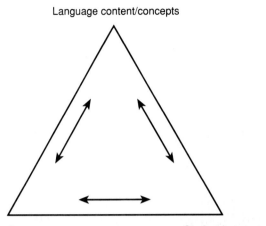

Teacher language   Student language

FIGURE 11.2   The Interaction of Language. (From *Language Interaction in Teaching and Learning* [2nd ed.] by L. Gruenewald and S. Pollak, 1990, Austin, TX: PRO-ED. Copyright 1990 by PRO-ED. Reprinted by permission.)

1985, 1987; McKinley & Larson, 1985; Prather, 1984; Schwartz & McKinley, 1984). As Larson and McKinley (1985) note, there can be "no 'hidden agenda' when providing services for adolescents" (p. 72). The purposes of any assessment, as well as the results of that assessment, must be shared with the adolescents (Larson & McKinley, 1985, 1987; McKinley & Larson, 1985), with explanations of why the assessed skills are important. In developing intervention plans, the adolescents themselves need to assist in establishing and prioritizing the objectives (Boyce & Larson, 1983; Klecan-Aker, 1985; McKinley & Larson, 1985, 1987; Prather, 1984). When adolescents recognize and accept that they have problems with communication and believe that intervention can help, they can often identify their own deficient communicative behaviors that they wish to improve and that are important to them. Reciprocally, involvement in setting their own objectives leads adolescents to accept responsibility for their problems and to realize that they have the major role in modifying their language skills. Such involvement can ultimately reduce or eliminate the motivational problems frequently observed when intervention is attempted with language-disordered ad-

olescents (Boyce & Larson, 1983; Klecan-Aker, 1985; Larson & McKinley, 1985, 1987; McKinley & Larson, 1985; Prather, 1984; Schwartz & McKinley, 1984).

Several principles guide the development of language intervention objectives for these adolescents. A number of authors (Buttrill, Niizawa, Biemer, Takahashi, & Hearn, 1989; Comkowycz et al., 1987; Ehren & Lenz, 1989; Larson & McKinley, 1985; Schwartz & McKinley, 1984; Wiig, 1989) advocate that objectives should emphasize showing the adolescents how to learn; that is, adolescents need to be taught strategies, rules, and techniques that will improve their communicative performances because these are the skills that can be generalized to daily language use. Part of intervention, then, includes discussions about and examples of other situations in which the learned strategies can be employed. The adolescents' conscious attempts to acquire strategies and to generate more examples of where else to apply the strategies enhance, in very practical ways, their metalinguistic and metacognitive skills—skills that are often deficient in language-disordered adolescents. Additionally, these activities stress the pragmatic aspects of language and make language functional for the adolescents. This approach contrasts with intervention objectives focusing on tutoring in academic content areas or remediating deficient skills.

Developing objectives that emphasize functional communication skills is another principle of language intervention for adolescents (Prather, 1984). These include the pragmatic language skills that promote positive human interactions, facilitate academic success, and allow people to operate on a day-to-day basis without recurring failures. It is also important to select objectives that will likely have immediate benefits for these adolescents in their interpersonal interactions. Mobbs, Reed, and McAllister (1993) asked normal adolescents to rank-order 14 communicative behaviors according to their relative importance in peer interactions. Table 11.10 shows the ranking in order from most to least important. This information may be useful in deciding which interpersonal communicative behaviors to emphasize in intervention to facilitate peer interactions. When intervention centers on practical and relevant language abilities, adolescents are

TABLE 11.10   Importance of Communicative Behaviors in Adolescents' Peer Interactions (in Order from Most to Least Important)

1. Taking the conversational partner's perspective.
2. Comprehending vocal tone indicating the speaker's mood.
3. Being tactful when giving an opinion about a topic.
4. Turn taking appropriately.
5. Using a pleasant vocal tone as opposed to an abrasive or hostile one.
6. Establishing and maintaining appropriate eye contact.
7. Comprehending nonverbal communication.
8. Using clarification and repair in conversation.
9. Selecting appropriate topics of conversation.
10. Communicating a point of view or a thought logically.
11. Relating a narrative cohesively and sequentially.
12. Comprehending humor.
13. Maintaining topics of conversation.
14. Using teenage or clique-specific slang or jargon.

Source: Adapted from Mobbs et al. (1993).

likely to recognize their importance and, therefore, to be motivated to acquire them. This is especially true if the purposes of the objectives are explained and if real-life examples of effective and ineffective communication are provided.

School systems' lists of secondary level communication competencies, referred to earlier in this chapter, can be utilized in selecting functional objectives. The competencies suggested by Bassett et al. (1978) can be particularly helpful and can even be used in developing ideas for intervention activities to achieve the objectives (see Table 11.9). To illustrate, these authors give the example of understanding a TV weather broadcast as one indication of their first competency (listening effectively to spoken language). In a small-group intervention setting, several functional objectives can be identified: (1) to understand meanings of words, such as "precipitation," "barometer," and "prevailing," as in "prevailing winds"; (2) to recognize cause–effect relationships based on the next day's forecast; (3) to identify specific differences between formal register, as used in a TV broadcast, and informal register inappropriate for such a communicative situation; (4) to select words, phrases, and sentences ap-

propriate for use in a formal communicative context such as giving a weather broadcast; and (5) to adopt a formal communicative style appropriately. We see that these objectives encompass semantic, syntactic, morphological, and pragmatic aspects of language at both the receptive and expressive levels. Yet, they center on a functional survival skill while promoting metalinguistic and metacognitive skills.

Activities for these objectives can include viewing a videotape of an actual weather broadcast and analyzing the vocabulary, syntax, morphology, and manner of presentation. As part of the analysis, the meanings of unknown words and nonverbal communicative behaviors can be explained, and the reasons for specific word choices, sentence structures, and other stylistic characteristics can be examined. The analysis can include examples and discussions of unacceptable communication alternatives. Implications of the forecast for dress and activities can also be discussed. Subsequently, the adolescents, as a group, can be asked to develop their own script for a TV weather broadcast. This script can be analyzed and revised, again with accompanying discussions about the rules, strategies, and techniques that need to be utilized. Finally, each student can take a turn giving the broadcast while the other students analyze the "performer's" communicative behaviors, either while the broadcast is being given or, more effectively, via a video replay. If we examine the competencies listed by Bassett et al. (1978), we see that the objectives and activities illustrated here address not only listening effectively to spoken language, but also using words and grammar appropriately for a specific context, employing appropriate nonverbal signs, using the voice effectively, identifying main ideas, distinguishing opinions and facts, expressing ideas concisely and clearly, and organizing and summarizing messages.

Schwartz and McKinley (1984) provide numerous suggestions for objectives, strategies, and activities that can be used in language intervention with adolescents, including skill development in the areas of listening, conversation, nonverbal communication, and asking questions. As one example of question-asking skills, Schwartz and McKinley suggest that students discriminate, on the basis of tone of voice, abrasively and nonabrasively asked questions, such as "Do we have to do all the problems on page 10?" said in an alienating way and again in a polite manner (p. 172). Once the adolescents are able to tell the difference between the questions and understand the effects the two ways of asking the same question have on listeners, these authors recommend that the students generate their own questions for information-seeking situations and practice saying them in nonabrasive ways. Schwartz and McKinley list realistic examples of information-seeking situations that adolescents are likely to encounter.

For many years, commercially published language intervention materials were available only for young children. Recently, materials designed for language-disordered adolescents, including computer software, have been published. They have eased the task of professionals serving adolescents with language disorders by providing easily accessed materials and activities that focus on pragmatic, semantic, and syntactic aspects of communication. These materials, however, do not determine intervention objectives or content. Rather, they provide tools that can be used to serve the purposes of the objectives and content.

When planning intervention objectives, the adolescent's developmental stage must be determined, and the strategies, activities, and objectives must correspond to his or her social-cognitive level (Larson & McKinley, 1987, 1988; McKinley & Larson, 1985). McKinley and Larson (1990) cite three developmental stages of adolescence referred to by Mitchell (1979) and suggest that the focus of intervention may differ, depending on the stage. Adolescents in Stage I (child adolescence or early adolescence), generally in the age range from about 11/12 to 13/14 years, may not have progressed to Piaget's formal thought level. As a result, they may require concrete learning situations (Larson & McKinley, 1987). For these adolescents, relationships with peers are beginning to take on greater importance (Cooper & Anderson-Inman, 1988). They also have several years of school ahead of them. Therefore, objectives that focus on language to improve social and academic performance may be appropriate (Larson & McKinley, 1993). In contrast, adolescents in Stage 3 (late adolescence or adult adolescence), typically between 16 and 18 years of age, may be able to learn from experiences employing formal operations and thought. Additionally, peer re-

lations are even more important than in early adolescence, and concern about vocational options and employment grows. For these adolescents, objectives that emphasize improving language in vocational, as well as social, situations may be more important (Larson & McKinley, 1993). Because adolescents in Stage 3 are approaching the end of secondary school, whether or not objectives that focus on language for academic performance are emphasized will likely relate to their plans to pursue further formal education and their academic records and abilities. For adolescents in the in between Stage 2 (middle adolescence), generally between 13 and 15 years, combinations of concrete and formal thought learning situations and experiences that bridge the concrete and formal operations levels may be required. In middle adolescence, peer relationships become important. Although several years of secondary school remain, vocational concerns may also emerge. For these reasons, intervention objectives that emphasize social, vocational, and academic language skills may be appropriate (Larson & McKinley, 1993). At all levels, however, intervention needs to utilize the adolescents' strengths and optimal learning modes to facilitate success (Prather, 1984; Schwartz & McKinley, 1984), which, in turn, enhances motivation.

One of the 1990 amendments to the Education of the Handicapped Act, now the Individuals with Disabilities Education Act (IDEA) (PL 101-476), emphasizes transition services for disabled students. This amendment requires educational systems to provide necessary support and services to promote coordinated, planned progression of disabled students (including language-disordered adolescents) from the school setting to postsecondary school pursuits such as employment or further education. A transition plan must be developed and implemented by the time a student is 16 years of age, but it can be developed earlier if necessary. Because language proficiency is critical to successful postsecondary pursuits, language intervention needs to be seen as an essential part of each student's transition program, and intervention objectives must reflect the vocational, academic, and social language skills necessary for a successful transition. This amendment provides an opportunity for professionals to increase and improve services for language-disordered students in the secondary schools. It may also help to break the cycle of neglect of language-disordered adolescents described earlier in this chapter.

According to Simon (1981a), intervention for language-disordered adolescents often involves considerable counseling about their communication problems. The time spent talking about their language disorders should not be viewed as a waste of valuable intervention time. Instead, counseling can help the students recognize the value of effective communication skills, assist them in setting priorities for intervention, promote metalinguistic awareness of communication, and help them cope more effectively with the problems stemming from their language disorders (Larson & McKinley, 1985).

Adolescents themselves have identified listener behaviors they believe to be nonsupportive (Baggett, 1969), behaviors that should be avoided when counseling students about their language problems. These include rushing adolescents as they try to talk about their concerns, avoiding the topic altogether, changing the topic as soon as it is introduced, avoiding eye contact, failing to respond as students talk, and arriving at conclusions before the adolescents finish their descriptions. In contrast, behaviors viewed as supportive include staying on the topic, taking the time to talk about students' concerns, listening to the students as they talk, asking questions, and providing ideas about ways to solve their problems (Baggett, 1969). These reported behaviors suggest valuable guidelines to employ when counseling adolescents about their language problems.

Traditional service delivery models are not effective for intervention with language-disordered adolescents (Buttrill et al., 1989; Comkowycz et al., 1987; Ehren & Lenz, 1989; Larson & McKinley, 1985, 1987; Larson, McKinley, & Boley, 1993; McKinley & Larson, 1985). Boyce and Larson (1983) give four reasons for the ineffectiveness of these traditional models:

1. When secondary students are removed from their classrooms for short periods of time twice a week, the usual daily schedules are disrupted.
2. Secondary students who need to walk in and out

of classrooms during class periods are viewed as different from their peers during a developmental period when conformity to the peer norm is important to them.
3. Intervention can be viewed as punitive because, in addition to the first two reasons, the adolescents "receive no credit for work that may be very difficult for them" (p. 23).
4. Establishing and maintaining relationships with service providers is difficult when these professionals are removed from the usual routine of the schools. Additionally, the traditional one-to-one intervention fails to promote communicative interactions and provide opportunities to practice new language skills in varied communicative contexts.

Alternative service delivery models for language-disordered adolescents have been proposed (Boyce & Larson, 1983; Comkowycz et al., 1987; Ehren & Lenz, 1989; Larson & McKinley, 1985, 1987; Larson et al., 1993; McKinley & Larson, 1985; Work, Cline, Ehren, Keiser, & Wujek, 1993). In these models, existing blocks of time in the school's daily schedule are frequently utilized for intervention. Students may be seen for an entire time period on a regularly scheduled basis, often five days a week, corresponding with other academic class schedules. As with other classes, the students are generally seen in groups, although these groups are much smaller than the usual academic class. Small-group sessions facilitate interaction and communication practice. Furthermore, students can work on comprehension, production, and metalinguistic skills simultaneously. To describe such an intervention format, supportive titles rather than punitive ones, are recommended, such as *Individualized Language Skills, Oral Communication Strategies,* and *Communication Skills* (Boyce & Larson, 1983; Larson & McKinley, 1985, 1987; McKinley & Larson, 1985). The Language Intervention Program for Secondary Students (LIPSS), implemented in Polk County Schools, Florida, selected the name *Exceptional Student Education-Language Arts,* because the class "is taught under the rubric of a state-designed curriculum framework" (Comkowycz et al., 1987, p. 204). A program in the Palo Alto Unified School District, California, chose the name *Language/Study Skills Class* (Buttrill et al., 1989).

Because the time frame in this service delivery model is similar to that of other classes adolescents take, the intervention period can actually be added as a course in the school's curriculum. In some instances, credit may even be given. The adolescents can be awarded grades, or their performances can be evaluated on a pass-fail basis. With this intervention format, students' efforts are recognized, intervention is not viewed as penalizing or stigmatizing, and functional communication strategies can be learned and practiced in interactive situations. This model resolves the problems of traditional service delivery formats. Furthermore, because the format fits into the daily academic schedule, intervention becomes an integrated, accepted part of the school routine.

Language-disordered adolescents' lack of motivation may be a barrier that needs to be dealt with if they are to accept services and if intervention is to be effective. The ideas presented here may lessen the problems associated with lack of motivation. In addition, specific performance contracts negotiated with the adolescents may enhance their motivation (Larson & McKinley, 1985, 1987; Prather, 1984; Schwartz & McKinley, 1984). Contracts need to establish clearly the behaviors to be demonstrated, the relevant time frame, and the methods of evaluation. The contract should focus initially on high success for behaviors that are important to the adolescent (Prather, 1984). However, Boyce and Larson (1983) believe that services should not be provided for an adolescent who "does not want responsibility [for the problem], denies the existence of a problem, and/or remains unmotivated to change" (p. 138). On the positive side, several authors point out that adolescents who recognize that they have communication problems, and who see and believe that intervention can help, rarely have motivational problems (Boyce & Larson, 1983; Prather, 1984).

SUMMARY

In this chapter we have seen that:

▶ Language continues to develop into adolescence as teenagers gain communicative competence.

▶ Many gaps remain in our knowledge of normal adolescent language development.

▶ These gaps make assessment of language-disordered adolescents an especially challenging process that must rely heavily on nonstandardized procedures.

▶ Fewer standardized language tests have been developed for adolescents than for youngsters, and the validity of several of these adolescent tests has been questioned.

▶ Intervention for language-disordered adolescents needs to:

▶ Focus on functional communication skills.

▶ Consider an adolescent's developmental stage.

▶ Teach communication strategies rather than academic content or improve skills.

▶ Deal with possible motivational problems.

▶ Modify traditional service delivery models to accommodate the needs of these adolescents.

If only one critical point emerges from this chapter, it is that language disorders negatively impact on adolescents' academic and personal successes in junior and senior high schools and limit their social, vocational, and educational opportunities as adults. To continue to neglect these language-disordered adolescents would be a sad professional commentary.

REFERENCES

Abkarian, G. G., Jones, A., & West, G. (1992). Young children's idiom comprehension: Trying to get the picture. *Journal of Speech and Hearing Research, 35,* 580–587.

Achenbach, T. (1970). Standardization of a research instrument for identifying associative responding children. *Developmental Psychology, 2,* 283–291.

Ackerman, B. (1982). On comprehending idioms: Do children get the picture? *Journal of Experimental Child Psychology, 33,* 439–454.

Albritton, T. (1984, November). *Secondary speech-language programs: Strategies for a new delivery system.* Paper presented at the Annual Convention of the American Speech-Language-Hearing Association, San Francisco.

Allen, R., & Brown, K. (1977). *Developing communication competence in children.* Skokie, IL: National Textbook.

Alley, G., & Deshler, D. (1979). *Teaching the learning disabled adolescents: Strategies and methods.* Denver: Love.

Aram, D., Ekelman, B., & Nation, J. (1984). Preschoolers with language disorders: 10 years later. *Journal of Speech and Hearing Research, 27,* 232–244.

Baggett, L. (1969, March). *Behavior that communicates understanding as evaluated by teenagers.* Paper presented at the American Personnel and Guidance Association Convention, Las Vegas.

Baker, H., & Leland, B. (1967). *Detroit tests of learning aptitude.* Indianapolis, IN: Bobbs-Merrill.

Bashir, A., Kuban, K., Kleinman, S., & Scavuzzo, A. (1983). Issues in language disorders: Considerations of cause, maintenance, and change. In J. Miller, D. Yoder, & R. Schiefelbusch (Eds.), *Contemporary issues in language intervention.* Rockville, MD: American Speech-Language-Hearing Association.

Bassett, R., Whittington, N., & Staton-Spicer, A. (1978). The basics in speaking and listening for high school graduates: What should be assessed? *Communication Education, 27,* 293–303.

Berman, A., & Siegal, A. (1975). *Delinquents are disabled: An innovative approach to the prevention and treatment of juvenile delinquency.* Paper presented at the Second International Scientific Conference on Learning Disabilities, Brussels.

Billow, R. (1975). A cognitive developmental study of metaphor comprehension. *Developmental Psychology, 11,* 415–423.

Blagden, C., & McConnell, N. (1984). *Interpersonal language skills assessment.* Moline, IL: LinguiSystems.

Blake, A. K. (1992). Speech-language pathologists in the schools. *Asha, 34,* 82.

Blalock, J. (1981). Persistent problems and concerns of young adults with learning disabilities. In W. Cruickshank & A. Silver (Eds.), *Bridges to tomorrow* (Vol. 2). Syracuse, NY: Syracuse University Press.

Bloom, L. (1988). What is language? In M. Lahey (Ed.), *Language disorders and language development.* Columbus, OH: Merrill/Macmillan.

Boyce, N., & Larson, V. Lord. (1981, November). *Language assessment of the adolescent.* Paper presented at the Annual Convention of the American Speech-Language-Hearing Association, Los Angeles.

Boyce, N., & Larson, V. Lord. (1983). *Adolescents' communication: Development and disorders.* Eau Claire, WI: Thinking Publications.

Bryan, T. (1977). Children's comprehension of nonverbal communication. *Journal of Learning Disabilities, 10,* 501–506.

Bryan, T., Donahue, M., & Pearl, R. (1981). Studies of learning disabled children's pragmatic competence. *Topics in Learning and Learning Disabilities, 1,* 29–39.

Buttrill, J., Niizawa, J., Biemer, C., Takahashi, C., & Hearn, S. (1989). Serving the language learning disabled adolescent: A strategies-based model. *Language, Speech, and Hearing Services in Schools, 20,* 185–203.

Camarata, S., Hughes, C., & Ruhl, K. (1988). Mild/moderate behaviorally disordered students: A population at-risk for language disorders. *Language, Speech, and Hearing Services in Schools, 19,* 191–200.

Chabon, S., Kent-Udolf, L., & Eglof, D. (1982). The temporal reliability of Brown's mean length of utterance (MLU-M) measure with post–Stage V children. *Journal of Speech and Hearing Research, 25,* 124–128.

Cole, P., & Wood, L. (1978). Differential diagnosis. In R. Martin (Ed.), *Pediatric audiology.* Englewood Cliffs, NJ: Prentice-Hall.

Comkowycz, S. M., Ehren, B. J., & Hayes, N. H. (1987). Meeting classroom needs of language disordered students in middle and junior high schools: A program model. *Journal of Childhood Communication Disorders, 11,* 199–208.

Cooper, D., & Anderson-Inman, L. (1988). Language and socialization. In M. Nippold (Ed.), *Later language development: Ages nine through nineteen.* Boston: Little, Brown.

Crystal, D., & Davy, D. (1975). *Advanced conversational English.* London: Longman.

Damico, J. (1985). Clinical discourse analysis: A functional approach to language assessment. In C. Simon (Ed.), *Communication skills and classroom success: Assessment of language-learning disabled students.* San Diego, CA: College-Hill Press.

Damico, J. (1993). Language assessment in adolescents: Addressing critical issues. *Language, Speech, and Hearing Services in Schools, 24,* 29–35.

Damico, J., & Oller, J. (1980). Pragmatic versus morphological/syntactic criteria for language referrals. *Language, Speech, and Hearing Services in Schools, 11,* 85–94.

Dent, C. H. (1984). The developmental importance of motion information in perceiving and describing metaphoric similarity. *Child Development, 55,* 1607–1613.

Despain, A. D., & Simon, C. (1987). Alternative to failure: A junior high school language development–based curriculum. *Journal of Childhood Communication Disorders, 11,* 139–179.

Donahue, M., & Bryan, T. (1984). Communicative skills and peer relations of learning disabled adolescents. *Topics in Language Disorders, 4,* 10–21.

Douglas, J. D., & Peel, B. (1979). The development of metaphor and proverb translation in children grades 1 through 7. *Journal of Educational Research, 73,* 116–119.

Duker, S. (1971). *Listening readings* (Vol. 2). Metuchen, NJ: Scarecrow Press.

Dunn, Lloyd, & Dunn, Leota. (1981). *Peabody picture vocabulary test–Revised.* Circle Pines, MN: American Guidance Service.

Ehren, B. J., & Lenz, B. K. (1989). Adolescents with language disorders: Special considerations in providing academically relevant language intervention. *Seminars in Speech and Language, 10,* 192–203.

Feuerstein, R. (1980). *Instrumental enrichment.* Chicago: Scott, Foresman.

Fowles, B., & Glanz, M. (1977). Competence and talent in verbal riddle comprehension. *Journal of Child Language, 4,* 433–452.

Gardner, H. (1974). Metaphors and modalities: How children project polar adjectives into diverse domains. *Child Development, 45,* 84–91.

Gardner, H., Kircher, M., Winner, E., & Perkins, D. (1975). Children's metaphoric productions and preferences. *Journal of Child Language, 2,* 125–141.

Gardner, M., & Brownell, R. (1987). *Expressive and receptive one-word picture vocabulary tests: Upper extensions.* Austin, TX: PRO-ED.

Gibbs, R. W. (1987). Linguistic factors in children's understanding of idioms. *Journal of Child Language, 14,* 569–586.

Grice, H. (1975). Logic and conversation. In P. Cole & J. Morgan (Eds.), *Syntax and semantics: Vol. 3. Speech Acts.* New York: Academic Press.

Gruenewald, L., & Pollak, S. (1990). *Language interaction in teaching and learning* (2nd ed.). Austin, TX: PRO-ED.

Hains, A., & Miller, D. (1980). Moral and cognitive development in delinquent and nondelinquent children and adolescents. *Journal of General Psychology, 137,* 21–35.

Hall, P., & Tomblin, J. B. (1978). A follow-up study of children with articulation and language disorders. *Journal of Speech and Hearing Disorders, 43,* 227–241.

Halliday, M. (1973). *Explorations in the functions of language.* London: Edward Arnold.

Halliday, M. (1975). *Learning how to mean: Explorations in the development of language.* London: Edward Arnold.

Hammill, D. (1991). *Detroit tests of learning aptitude* (3rd ed.). Austin, TX: PRO-ED.

Hammill, D., Brown, V., Larsen, S., & Wiederholt, J. L. (1987). *Test of adolescent language* (2nd ed.). Austin, TX: PRO-ED.

Hammill, D., & Bryant, B. (1991). *Detroit tests of learning aptitude–Adult.* Austin, TX: PRO-ED.

Hass, W., & Wepman, J. (1974). Dimensions of individual difference in the spoken syntax of school children. *Journal of Speech and Hearing Research, 17,* 455–469.

Havertape, J., & Kass, C. (1978). Examination of problem solving in learning disabled adolescents through verbalized self-instructions. *Learning Disabilities Quarterly, 1,* 94–100.

Honeck, R. P., Sowry, B. M., & Voegtle, K. (1978). Proverbial understanding in a pictorial context. *Child Development, 49,* 327–331.

Inhelder, B., & Piaget, J. (1958). *The growth of logical thinking from childhood to adolescence—An essay on the construction of formal operational structures.* New York: Basic Books.

Kessel, F. (1970). The role of syntax in children's comprehension from ages six to twelve. *Society for Research in Child Development Monographs, 35,* 1–95.

Klecan-Aker, J. (1985). Syntactic abilities in normal and language deficient middle school children. *Topics in Language Disorders, 5,* 46–54.

Klecan-Aker, J., & Hedrick, D. (1985). A study of the syntactic language skills of normal school-age children. *Language, Speech, and Hearing Services in Schools, 16,* 187–198.

Knapp, M. (1978). *Nonverbal communication in human interaction.* New York: Holt, Rinehart and Winston.

Larson, V. Lord, & McKinley, N. (1985). General intervention principles with language impaired adolescents. *Topics in Language Disorders, 5,* 70–77.

Larson, V. Lord, & McKinley, N. (1987). *Communication as-*

sessment and intervention strategies for adolescents. Eau Claire, WI: Thinking Publications.

Larson, V. Lord, & McKinley, N. (1988). Language disorders in the adolescent: Intervention. In D. Yoder & R. Kent (Eds.), *Decision making in speech-language pathology.* Burlington, Ontario: B. C. Decker.

Larson, V. Lord, & McKinley, N. (1990, November). *Adolescents with language disorders: An "action plan" for service delivery.* Poster session presented at the Annual Convention of the American Speech-Language-Hearing Association, Seattle.

Larson, V. Lord, & McKinley, N. (1993). Adolescent language: An introduction. *Language, Speech, and Hearing Services in Schools, 24,* 19–20.

Larson, V. Lord, McKinley, N., & Boley, D. (1993). Service delivery models for adolescents with language disorders. *Language, Speech, and Hearing Services in Schools, 24,* 36–42.

Lazar, R. T., Warr-Leeper, G. A., Nicholson, C. B., & Johnson, S. (1989). Elementary school teachers' use of multiple meaning expressions. *Language, Speech, and Hearing Services in Schools, 20,* 420–430.

Loban, W. (1976). *Language development: Kindergarten through grade twelve.* Urbana, IL: National Council of Teachers of English.

Lodge, D. N., & Leach, E. A. (1975). Children's acquisition of idioms in the English language. *Journal of Speech and Hearing Research, 18,* 521–529.

Lund, N. J., & Duchan, J. F. (1983). *Assessing children's language in naturalistic contexts.* Englewood Cliffs, NJ: Prentice-Hall.

Lund, N. J., & Duchan, J. F. (1988). *Assessing children's language in naturalistic contexts* (2nd ed.). Englewood Cliffs, NJ: Prentice-Hall.

McKinley, N., & Larson, V. Lord. (1983, November). *Adolescents' conversations with a friend and an unfamiliar adult.* Paper presented at the Annual Convention of the American Speech-Language-Hearing Association, Cincinnati.

McKinley, N., & Larson, V. Lord (1985). The neglected language disordered adolescent: A delivery model. *Language, Speech, and Hearing Services in Schools, 16,* 2–15.

McKinley, N., & Larson, V. Lord. (1990). Language and learning disorders in adolescents. *Seminars in Speech and Language, 11,* 182–191.

McKinley, N., & Larson, V. Lord (1991, November). *Seventh, eighth, and ninth graders' conversations in two experimental conditions.* Paper presented at the Annual

Convention of the American Speech-Language-Hearing Association, Atlanta.

Meltzer, L., Roditi, B., & Fenton, T. (1986). Cognitive and learning profiles of delinquent and learning disabled adolescents. *Adolescence, 21,* 581–591.

Miller, G. A., & Gildea, P. M. (1987). How children learn words. *Scientific American, 257,* 94–99.

Mitchell, J. (1979). *Adolescent psychology.* Toronto: Holt, Rinehart and Winston.

Mobbs, F., Reed, V. A., & McAllister, L. (1993, May). *Rankings of the relative importance of selected communication skills in adolescent peer interactions.* Paper presented at the Annual Conference of the Australian Association of Speech and Hearing, Darwin, Australia.

Morgan, D., & Guilford, A. (1984). *Adolescent language screening test.* Austin, TX: PRO-ED.

Neimark, E. (1980). Intellectual development in the exceptional adolescent as viewed within a Piagetian framework. *Exceptional Education Quarterly, 1,* 47–56.

Nichols, R., & Stevens, L. (1957). Listening to people. *Harvard Business Review, 35,* 85–92.

Nippold, M. (1985). Comprehension of figurative language in youth. *Topics in Language Development, 5,* 1–20.

Nippold, M. (1988a). Figurative language. In M. Nippold (Ed.), *Later language development: Ages nine through nineteen.* Boston: Little, Brown.

Nippold, M. (1988b). The literate lexicon. In M. Nippold (Ed.), *Later language development: Ages nine through nineteen.* Boston: Little, Brown.

Nippold, M. (1988c). Verbal reasoning. In M. Nippold (Ed.), *Later language development: Ages nine through nineteen.* Boston: Little, Brown.

Nippold, M. (1991). Evaluating and enhancing idiom comprehension in language-disordered students. *Language, Speech, and Hearing Services in Schools, 22,* 100–106.

Nippold, M. (1993). Developmental markers in adolescent language: Syntax, semantics, and pragmatics. *Language, Speech, and Hearing Services in Schools, 24,* 21–28.

Nippold, M., Cuyler, J., & Braunbeck-Price, R. (1988). Explanation of ambiguous advertisements: A developmental study with children and adolescents. *Journal of Speech and Hearing Research, 31,* 466–474.

Nippold, M., & Fey, S. (1983). Metaphoric understanding in preadolescents having a history of language acquisition difficulties. *Language, Speech, and Hearing Services in Schools, 14,* 171–180.

Nippold, M., Leonard, L., & Kail, R. (1984). Syntactic and conceptual factors in children's understanding of metaphors. *Journal of Speech and Hearing Research, 27,* 197–205.

Nippold, M., & Martin, S. (1989). Idiom interpretation in isolation versus context: A developmental study with adolescents. *Journal of Speech and Hearing Research, 32,* 59–66.

Nippold, M., Martin, S., & Erskine, B. (1988). Proverb comprehension in context: A developmental study with children and adolescents. *Journal of Speech and Hearing Research, 31,* 19–28.

Nippold, M., Schwarz, I., & Undlin, R. (1992). Use and understanding of adverbial conjuncts: A developmental study of adolescents and young adults. *Journal of Speech and Hearing Research, 35,* 108–118.

O'Connor, L., & Eldredge, P. (1981). *Communication disorders in adolescence: Program planning, diagnostics, and practical remediation techniques.* Springfield, IL: Charles C. Thomas.

O'Donnell, R., Griffin, W., & Norris, R. (1967). *Syntax of kindergarten and elementary school children: A transformational analysis.* Urbana, IL: National Council of Teachers of English.

Phelps-Terasaki, D., & Phelps-Gunn, T. (1992). *Test of pragmatic language.* Austin, TX: PRO-ED.

Pollio, M., & Pollio, H. (1979). A test of metaphoric comprehension: Preliminary data. *Journal of Child Language, 6,* 111–120.

Prather, E. (1984). Developmental language disorders: Adolescents. In A. Holland (Ed.), *Language disorders in children.* San Diego, CA: College-Hill Press.

Prather, E., Breecher, S., Stafford, M., & Wallace, E. (1980). *Screening test of adolescent language.* Seattle: University of Washington Press.

Prather, E., Brenner, A., & Hughes, K. (1981). A mini-screening language test for adolescents. *Language, Speech, and Hearing Services in Schools, 12,* 67–73.

Prinz, P. (1983). The development of idiomatic meaning in children. *Language and Speech, 26,* 263–272.

Prizant, B., Audet, L., Burke, G., Hummel, L., Maher, S., & Theadore, G. (1990). Communication disorders and emotional/behavioral disorders in children and adolescents. *Journal of Speech and Hearing Disorders, 55,* 179–192.

Reed, V. A. (1986). Language-disordered adolescents. In V. A. Reed, *An introduction to children with language disorders.* Columbus, OH: Merrill/Macmillan.

Reed, V. A. (1990, March). *Differences in the language skills of 8- and 14-year-old children.* Paper presented at the Annual Conference of the Australian Association of Speech and Hearing, Sydney.

Reed, V. A., & Miles, M. C. (1989). *Adolescent language disorders: A video inservice for educators.* Eau Claire, WI: Thinking Publications.

Reed, V. A., & Rasmussen, A. (1985, November). *Productive language skills of eight and fourteen year old children.* Paper presented at the Annual Convention of the American Speech-Language-Hearing Association, Washington, DC.

Rees, N., & Wollner, S. (1982, February). *A taxonomy of pragmatic abilities.* Madison, WI: Educational Teleconferencing Network.

Resnick, D. (1982). A developmental study of proverb comprehension. *Journal of Psycholinguistic Research, 11,* 521–538.

Reynolds, R., & Ortony, A. (1980). Some issues in the measurement of children's comprehension of metaphorical language. *Child Development, 51,* 1110–1119.

Roeber, E. (1980). *Development and validation of objective referenced test instrument for critical listening: Grades 4, 7 and 10.* Technical Report. Lansing: Michigan Department of Education.

Schwartz, L., & McKinley, N. (1984). *Daily communication: Strategies for the language disordered adolescent.* Eau Claire, WI: Thinking Publications.

Scott, C. M. (1984a). Adverbial connectivity in conversations of children 6 to 12. *Journal of Child Language, 11,* 423–452.

Scott, C. M. (1984b, November). *What happened in that: Structural characteristics of school children's narratives.* Paper presented at the Annual Convention of the American Speech-Language-Hearing Association, San Francisco.

Scott, C. M. (1988a). Producing complex sentences. *Topics in Language Disorders, 8,* 44–62.

Scott, C. M. (1988b). Spoken and written syntax. In M. Nippold (Ed.), *Later language development: Ages nine through nineteen.* Boston: Little, Brown.

Scott, C. M., & Rush, D. (1985). Teaching adverbial connectivity: Implications from current research. *Child Language Teaching and Therapy, 1,* 264–280.

Semel, E., & Wiig, E. (1980). *Clinical evaluation of language functions advanced level screening test.* San Antonio, TX: Psychological Corporation.

Semel, E., Wiig, E., & Secord, W. (1987). *Clinical evaluation of language fundamentals–Revised.* San Antonio, TX: Psychological Corporation.

Semel, E., Wiig, E., & Secord, W. (1989). *Clinical evaluation of language fundamentals–Revised: Screening test.* San Antonio, TX: Psychological Corporation.

Shultz, T., & Horibe, F. (1974). Development of the appreciation of verbal jokes. *Developmental Psychology, 10,* 13–20.

Shultz, T., & Pilon, R. (1973). Development of the ability to detect linguistic ambiguity. *Child Development, 44,* 728–733.

Simon, C. (1979). *Communicative competence: A functional-pragmatic approach to language therapy.* Tucson, AZ: Communication Skill Builders.

Simon, C. (1981a, November). *After is-verbing: Then what?* Paper presented at the Annual Convention of the American Speech-Language-Hearing Association, Los Angeles.

Simon, C. (1981b). *Communicative competence: A functional-pragmatic approach to language therapy.* Tucson, AZ: Communication Skill Builders.

Simon, C. (1984). Functional-pragmatic evaluation of communication skills in school-aged children. *Language, Speech, and Hearing Services in Schools, 15,* 83–97.

Simon, C. (1986). *Evaluating communicative competence–Revised.* Tucson, AZ: Communication Skill Builders.

Simon, C. (1987). *Classroom communication screening procedure for early adolescents.* Tempe, AZ: Communi-Cog Publications.

Spector, C. (1990). Linguistic humor comprehension of normal and language-impaired adolescents. *Journal of Speech and Hearing Disorders, 55,* 533–541.

Spekman, N. (1981). A study of the dyadic verbal communication abilities of learning disabled and normally achieving 4th and 5th grade boys. *Learning Disabilities Quarterly, 4,* 139–151.

Stephens, M. I., & Montgomery, A. (1985). A critique of recent relevant standardized tests. *Topics in Language Disorders, 5,* 21–45.

Tarnopol, L. (1970). Delinquency and minimal brain dysfunction. *Journal of Learning Disabilities, 3,* 200–207.

Thorum, A. (1986). *Fullerton language test for adolescents* (2nd ed.). Palo Alto, CA: Consulting Psychologists Press.

Tibbits, D. (1982). *Language disorders in adolescents.* Lincoln, NE: Cliff Notes.

Tomblin, J. B., Freese, P., & Records, N. (1992). Diagnosing specific language impairment in adults for the purpose of pedigree analysis. *Journal of Speech and Hearing Research, 35,* 832–843.

U.S. Department of Education (1991). *Thirteenth annual report to Congress on the implementation of the Individuals with Disabilities Education Act.* Washington, DC: U.S. Government Printing Office.

Valletutti, P., & Bender, M. (1982). *Teaching interpersonal and community living skills: A curriculum model for handicapped adolescents and adults.* Baltimore: University Park Press.

Vermont Department of Education. (1977). *Basic competencies: A manual of information and guidelines for teachers and administrators.* Montpelier, VT: State Department of Education.

Vermont Department of Education. (1979). *Basic competencies: Teacher's guide for basic competencies in reasoning.* Montpelier, VT: State Department of Education.

Wechsler, D. (1949). *Wechsler intelligence scale for children.* San Antonio, TX: Psychological Corporation.

Weiner, P. (1974). A language-delayed child at adolescence. *Journal of Speech and Hearing Disorders, 39,* 202–212.

Weiner, P. (1985). The value of follow-up studies. *Topics in Language Disorders, 5,* 78–92.

Werner, H., & Kaplan, B. (1963). *Symbol formation.* New York: Wiley.

Westby, C. (1984). Development of narrative language abilities. In G. Wallach & K. Butler (Eds.), *Language learning disabilities in school-age children.* Baltimore: Williams and Wilkins.

Westby, C. (1985). Learning to talk—talking to learn: Oral-literate language differences. In C. Simon (Ed.), *Communication skills and classroom success: Therapy methodologies for language-learning disabled students.* San Diego, CA: College-Hill Press.

Wiig, E. (1982a). *Identifying language disorders in adolescents.* Paper presented at the Gunderson Clinic, La Crosse, WI.

Wiig, E. (1982b). *Let's talk inventory for adolescents.* San Antonio, TX: Psychological Corporation.

Wiig, E. (1983, October-November). *Assessment and development of social communication skills in adolescents with language-learning disabilities.* Madison, WI: Educational Teleconferencing Network.

Wiig, E. (1989). *Steps to language competence: Developing metalinguistic strategies.* San Antonio, TX: Psychological Corporation.

Wiig, E. (1990). *Wiig criterion-referenced inventory of language.* San Antonio, TX: Psychological Corporation.

Wiig, E., & Fleischmann, N. (1980). Knowledge of pronominalization, reflexivization, and relativization by learning disabled college students. *Journal of Learning Disabilities, 13,* 571–576.

Wiig, E., Gilbert, M., & Christian, S. (1978). Developmental sequences in the perception and interpretation of lexical and syntactic ambiguities. *Perceptual and Motor Skills, 44,* 959–969.

Wiig, E., & Harris, S. (1974). Perception and interpretation of nonverbally expressed emotions by adolescents with learning disabilities. *Perceptual and Motor Skills, 38,* 239–245.

Wiig, E., & Secord, W. (1989). *Test of language competence–Expanded edition*. San Antonio, TX: Psychological Corporation.

Wiig, E., & Secord, W. (1992). *Test of word knowledge*. San Antonio, TX: Psychological Corporation.

Wiig, E., & Semel, E. (1973). Comprehension of linguistic concepts requiring logical operations. *Journal of Speech and Hearing Research, 16,* 627–636.

Wiig, E., & Semel, E. (1974). Logicogrammatical sentence comprehension by adolescents with learning disabilities. *Perceptual and Motor Skills, 38,* 1331–1334.

Wiig, E., & Semel, E. (1975). Productive language abilities in learning disabled adolescents. *Journal of Learning Disabilities, 8,* 578–586.

Wiig, E., & Semel, E. (1984). *Language assessment and intervention for the learning disabled* (2nd ed.). Columbus, OH: Merrill/Macmillan.

Winner, E. (1979). New names for old things: The emergence of metaphoric language. *Journal of Child Language, 6,* 469–491.

Winner, E., Engel, M., & Gardner, H. (1980). Misunderstanding metaphor: What's the problem? *Journal of Experimental Child Psychology, 30,* 22–32.

Winner, E., Rosenstiel, A., & Gardner, H. (1976). The development of metaphoric understanding. *Developmental Psychology, 12,* 289–297.

Wood, M. (1982). *Language disorders in school-age children.* Englewood Cliffs, NJ: Prentice-Hall.

Woodcock, R. (1980). *Woodcock language proficiency battery.* Hingham, MA: Teaching Resources.

Woodcock, R., & Johnson, M. (1977). *Woodcock-Johnson psycho-educational battery.* Hingham, MA: Teaching Resources.

Work, R., Cline, J., Ehren, B. J., Keiser, D., & Wujek, C. (1993). Adolescent language programs. *Language, Speech, and Hearing Services in Schools, 24,* 43-53.

Ysseldyke, J., & Christenson, S. (1987). *The instructional environment scale.* Austin, TX: PRO-ED.

Zachman, L., Huisingh, R., Barrett, M., Orman, J., & Blagden, C. (1989). *The word test–Adolescent.* Moline, IL: LinguiSystems.

· Chapter 12 ·

Children with Acquired
Language Disorders

Steven H. Long

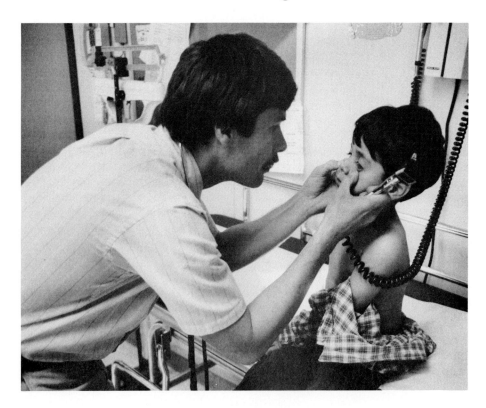

OBJECTIVES

Upon completion of this chapter, the reader should be able to:

▶ Understand the definitions of acquired aphasia in children and discuss its etiologies.

▶ Discuss the basic concepts of language recovery in children as a function of physiological restitution and normal language development.

▶ Describe the general characteristics of the language of children with acquired aphasia.

▶ Discuss principles of language assessment and intervention for children with acquired aphasia.

Most children learn to talk, read, and write only once and then use those abilities for the rest of their lives. For a special group of children, however, the experience of language acquisition is at least partially repeated. These children sustain some type of brain injury that pushes them down the ladder of language development and forces them to climb it again. Fortunately, nature is able to heal or compensate for much of the damage that occurs. But recovery is not complete, and the changes children undergo create enormous stress on them and their families. Professionals must be available to help interpret and explain these changes, as well as to provide intervention that complements the natural recuperation process.

AN OVERVIEW OF ACQUIRED CHILDHOOD APHASIA

Definition

Historically, the term *aphasia* has been used to describe two different conditions in children. From chapter 5 we know that the terms *developmental* or *congenital* aphasia have sometimes been used to describe children who show language impairment without sensory dysfunction, mental retardation, or other neurological damage. These, however, are older labels. In more recent clinical and research literature, these terms have commonly been replaced by *developmental language disorder* or *specific language impairment*. In contrast, the terms *acquired* aphasia or *childhood* aphasia refer to children who have a language disorder stemming from a disease or accident that alters neurological functioning. Children with acquired aphasia begin to develop language normally

but then lose all or part of their communicative abilities as a result of the neurological damage they sustain.

Types of Brain Injury

Brain injuries occur in localized and diffuse forms. *Localized* or *focal* lesions are confined to specific areas of the brain and result from penetrating injuries (such as gunshot wounds), vascular lesions (strokes or hemorrhages), or tumors. *Diffuse* lesions are spread out over many brain regions and usually result from traumatic head injuries or poisoning. In all types of brain injury, nerve cells are killed in one of three ways:

1. Directly, as a result of mechanical shearing or lack of oxygen carried by blood.
2. Indirectly, as a result of the degeneration of their connections with other nerve cells.
3. Inadvertently, as a result of electrical overstimulation associated with the interruption of blood flow.

Nerve cell death caused by overstimulation has been discovered relatively recently and appears amenable to early drug treatment (Almli & Finger, 1992). Thus, in the future, it may be possible to reduce the amount of permanent damage caused by certain kinds of brain injuries.

Traumatic Brain Injury Every year about 1 million American children and adolescents suffer brain injuries as a result of motor vehicle accidents, falls, sports accidents, and abuse. About 165,000 require hospitalization and 16,000 to 20,000 incur damage that is moderate to severe (Savage, 1991). Different terms are used to describe the neurological damage that results from accidents involving the head. **Closed head injury** indicates that a child has suffered diffuse rather than focal brain injury as a result of a blow to the head. The other frequently used term, **traumatic brain injury,** can be defined as

> an insult to the brain, not of a degenerative or congenital nature but caused by an external physical force, that may produce a diminished or altered state of consciousness, which results in impairment of cognitive abilities or physical functioning. It can also result in the disturbance of behavioral or emotional functioning. These impairments may be either temporary or permanent and cause partial or total functional disability or psychosocial maladjustment. (National Head Injury Foundation, cited by Savage, 1991, p. 3)

Traumatic brain injury should not be confused with *minimal brain dysfunction,* an older term for children with behavioral evidence of neurological dysfunction but no history of injury (see chapter 7). Professionals often use the terms *head injury* and *traumatic brain injury* interchangeably. The latter is more specific and leaves no doubt that a child's problems are the result of injury to the brain, not the head (Savage, 1991).

Traumatic brain injury results from several causes, which are more likely among particular age groups. Infants and toddlers are generally hurt through falls or abuse. Older preschoolers suffer falls, while young school-age children suffer injuries through sports and accidents involving them as pedestrians, bike or skateboard riders, or passengers. Adolescents sustain the most accidents, primarily as the result of motor vehicle accidents. Beginning in the preschool years, boys become two to four times more likely than girls to suffer a traumatic brain injury (Savage, 1991).

Children and adolescents with traumatic brain injury are more numerous than is generally realized. Estimates are that approximately 4% of all children in kindergarten through 12th grade have experienced some type of head trauma. Among children enrolled in special education programs, this figure jumps to somewhere between 8 and 20% (Savage, 1991).

Automobile accidents causing head injury in children are more likely to occur at low speeds. The rotational acceleration to which their brains are subjected is, therefore, likely to be less than that of adolescents and adults involved in high-speed crashes. Damage may be confined to the cortex of the brain, whereas in adolescents and adults it can extend into the white matter. In addition, children are less likely to develop contusions and hematomas (Ewing-Cobbs, Fletcher, Landry, & Levin, 1985). On the other hand, infants with head injury often have a poorer outcome. They are *more* susceptible to hematomas, may have white matter damage because their brains have little myelination, and, in cases where the trauma is caused by abuse, may be delayed in receiving medical attention (Ylvisaker, 1989).

Classification of brain injury is based on scores from the Glasgow Coma Scale (GCS), shown in Table 12.1, which measures eye opening, motor responses, and verbal responses. The scale and corresponding severity ratings are as follows:

13–15   mild brain injury

9–12   moderate brain injury

3–8   severe brain injury

Although initial GCS scores generally predict which children will die or have a poor outcome from an ac-

TABLE 12.1 The Glasgow Coma Scale	Best Eye Opening		Best Motor Response		Best Verbal Response	
	4	Spontaneous	6	Obeys commands	5	Oriented
	3	To speech	5	Localizes to pain	4	Confused
	2	To pain	4	Flexion—withdrawal to pain	3	Inappropriate words
	1	None	3	Abnormal flexion to pain	2	Incomprehensible
			2	Extension to pain	1	None
			1	None		

Source: Adapted from Teasdale and Jennett (1974).

cident, the ratings do not necessarily correlate with the level of difficulty that surviving children will experience in motor performance, education, and socialization (Haley, Cioffi, Lewin, & Baryza, 1990; Savage, 1991). The GCS was originally developed for use with adults. Evaluation of motor and verbal responses is, therefore, difficult with young children and infants because of the lack of developmental scoring (Haley et al., 1990).

Strokes and Tumors   The most common causes of aphasia in adults are relatively uncommon in children. For example, in 1989, the death rate for cerebrovascular disease in the United States was 4 per 100,000 for children under 15 years of age. The comparable figure for adults age 65 and older was 2,296. Similarly, the death rate for cancerous tumors of all kinds was 9 per 100,000 for children, while for adults it was 3,853 (National Center for Health Statistics, 1992). Obviously, in comparison to the incidence of traumatic injuries, vascular lesions are rarely seen. Yet, when they do occur and produce unilateral damage to the left hemisphere, they result in aphasic symptoms that are comparable to those seen in adults (Satz & Bullard-Bates, 1981).

More than one third of childhood strokes occur during the first 2 years of life. The usual causes of stroke in children are cardiac disease, vascular occlusion, sickle cell disease, vascular malformation, and hemorrhage. Blockage of a cerebral artery may result from trauma, infection, or cellular changes, or it may occur for no discernible reason. It frequently causes a sudden hemiplegia in a child and may be accompanied by seizures. In sickle cell anemia, deformed red blood cells cause vascular obstruction, leading to a crisis in which coma and seizures occur. Cerebral hemorrhage is often produced by the rupture of malformed blood vessels. Children with this condition are at risk for recurrence throughout their lives (Millikan, McDowell, & Easton, 1987).

Landau-Kleffner Syndrome   The least frequent cause of acquired aphasia in children is *Landau-Kleffner syndrome,* in which a convulsive disorder, indicated by abnormal electroencephalogram (EEG) tracings, occurs at about the same time as a breakdown in language. The condition has been profiled as follows (Bishop, 1985; Cooper & Ferry, 1978; Gordon, 1990; Miller, Campbell, Chapman, & Weismer, 1984):

▷ It has a low incidence. As of 1984, only 94 cases had been reported in the literature. By 1985, the number had increased to 119.
▷ Age of onset ranges from 1½ to 13 years.
▷ Language regression may be gradual or sudden.
▷ All children show abnormal EEG results, and over two thirds experience some type of seizure before, simultaneous with, or after the language regression.
▷ Affected children show such a severe disturbance in auditory comprehension that they appear deaf, but there is typically no loss of hearing sensitivity for pure tones.
▷ Males are affected twice as often as females.
▷ Changes in aphasia, seizures, and EEG findings do not correlate well. Some children stop having seizures and show normal EEG tracings but continue to exhibit aphasia. Others show the opposite pattern.

Associated Problems

Children with acquired aphasia are certain to have other problems as a result of their brain injuries. The number and extent of these difficulties vary widely from one injured child to the next. However, studies suggest some general characteristics of children in three etiological categories: those with traumatic brain injury, those with Landau-Kleffner syndrome, and those with vascular lesions. Findings for these three groups are shown in Table 12.2. The impairments associated with acquired aphasia can have a significant impact on the procedures used for evaluating and treating the language disorder. For example, perceptual and motor difficulties may make it necessary to adapt test materials and procedures. Behavioral disturbances may interfere with attempts to include a child in group instruction or recreation.

LANGUAGE DEVELOPMENT AND LANGUAGE RECOVERY

The same kinds of brain injuries can affect both children and adults. Yet, it is commonly believed that the effects of these injuries on language are different for

TABLE 12.2 Associated Physical, Cognitive, Perceptual Motor, Behavioral, and Social Problems in Children with Acquired Aphasia

Etiology	Traumatic Brain Injury	Landau-Kleffner Syndrome	Vascular Lesion
Gross and fine motor	▷ Severe TBI: spasticity, ataxia, delayed motor milestones ▷ Mild TBI: fine motor and visuomotor deficits, reduction in age-appropriate play and physical activity	▷ Gross and fine motor skills are usually good, sometimes superior	▷ Hemiparesis on side opposite brain injury
Cognitive	▷ Problems with long- and short-term memory, conceptual skills, problem solving ▷ Reduced speed of information processing ▷ Reduced attending skills	▷ Normal performance intelligence in most cases	▷ Lower scores on standardized intelligence tests, with performance scores higher than verbal scores
Perceptual motor	▷ Visual neglect, visual field cuts ▷ Motor apraxia, reduced motor speed, poor motor sequencing	▷ Normal hearing sensitivity to pure tones but may not respond to speech stimuli ▷ Long-term effects: difficulty understanding speech in competing noise situations; difficulty with tasks that challenge visual perception and visual memory	▷ Visual neglect, motor apraxia ▷ Visual discrimination problems in cases of crossed aphasia (right hemisphere lesion)
Behavioral	▷ Impulsivity, poor judgment, disinhibition, dependency, anger outbursts, denial, depression, emotional lability, apathy, lethargy, poor motivation	▷ Inattention, withdrawal, aggressiveness, temper outbursts, nightmares, refusal to respond, hyperactivity	▷ Inattention, distractibility
Social	▷ Does not learn from peers, does not generalize from social situations ▷ Behaves like a much younger child, withdraws ▷ Becomes distracted in noisy surroundings and becomes lost even in familiar surroundings	▷ May have periods of social withdrawal	▷ May have periods of social withdrawal (elective mutism reported in one case)

Sources: Burd, Gascon, Swenson, & Hankey, 1990; Cooper & Ferry, 1978; DePompei & Blosser, 1987; Haley et al., 1990; Martins, Ferro, & Trindade, 1987; Mantovani & Landau, 1980; McNaughton, 1991; Miller, Campbell, Chapman, & Weismer, 1984; Satz & Bullard-Bates, 1981; Shoumaker, Bennett, Bray, & Curless, 1974; Worster-Drought, 1971; Ylvisaker, 1989.

the two age groups. The prevailing view has been that children with acquired aphasia differ in at least three respects:

1. They have a lower incidence of aphasia.
2. They present different language symptoms.
3. They recover faster and more fully than adults.

These assertions, though generally true, have been reinterpreted slightly in recent years. A key issue has been the validity of the *progressive laterality hypothesis,* which maintains that cerebral dominance is not present at birth but develops slowly over the course of childhood (Lenneberg, 1967). If it is true that language has not yet fully lateralized in preadolescents, then it is understandable that damage to the dominant hemisphere (usually the left one) would not produce aphasia or would produce only mild symptoms. Moreover, the absence of cerebral dominance suggests that higher-level functions, including language, are less localized in a child's brain. This means that uninjured parts of the brain might be able to assume the functions previously handled by injured regions. This notion relates to the concept of neurological *plasticity* and is raised later in this chapter. However, anatomical and electrophysiological studies indicate that **lateralization** is present very early in life, leading to the suggestion that brain asymmetry exists from the moment of birth (Kinsbourne & Hiscock, 1977; Molfese, Freeman, & Palermo, 1975; Wada, Clarke, & Hamm, 1975). The lower incidence of aphasia in children is explained by the fact that children are less susceptible to brain tumors and cerebrovascular accidents (strokes). When children do sustain unilateral damage to the left hemisphere of the brain, their risk of aphasia is approximately the same as that of adults. Also, like adults, they are far more likely to acquire aphasia from a left-sided than a right-sided brain injury (Satz & Bullard-Bates, 1981).

The language symptoms of children with aphasia are thought to be different from those of adults. Satz and Bullard-Bates (1981) reviewed the major clinical studies from the previous century and concluded that the only consistent finding is that the majority of children exhibit a nonfluent aphasia pattern. They tend to be mute immediately following a brain injury. As speech returns, it is sparse and effortful and does not usually contain **paraphasia** (fluent misnamings or sound substitutions) or **jargon** (unintelligible sequences of syllables). In all other respects, children appear to show the same language disturbances found among adults with aphasia. They have disorders of auditory comprehension, writing, reading, and naming. Unlike adults, variation in symptoms has not yet been related to factors such as the site and extent of brain damage, the etiology (head trauma, stroke, tumor, etc.), or the age of the child.

Although the symptoms of children with aphasia are similar to those of adults, the prognosis for the two groups is considerably different. When all cases of acquired aphasia are taken together, about 75% of children show dramatic spontaneous recovery of language that is unrelated to their recovery of motor function (Satz & Bullard-Bates, 1981). The rate of recovery is considerably lower for children with aphasia secondary to convulsive disorder, about 33% (Cooper & Ferry, 1978). Recovery is rarely complete. One fourth or more of children with brain injuries show residual aphasia more than a year **postonset**, and even when they appear to be clinically recovered from the aphasia, they continue to show deficits on tests of intelligence and academic achievement (Satz & Bullard-Bates, 1981). The strong recovery of some children with aphasia raises two questions:

1. Why do other children not recover as well?
2. Why do children recover so much better than adults?

Recovery in adults with aphasia has been related to several factors, such as age, type of aphasia, etiology, and severity of injury (Sarno, 1981). These factors also have been presumed to affect recovery in children. In particular, it has been claimed that children with vascular lesions do not recover language as well as children who suffer traumatic injuries (Dennis, 1980). However, other investigators believe that the research conducted to date has not clearly differentiated the influence of one factor versus another (Satz & Bullard-Bates, 1981).

For adults who suffer strokes, younger age is regarded as a positive prognostic factor (Sarno, 1981). The same might, therefore, be true for children with vascular lesions, though research has not yet confirmed it. Among children who suffer traumatic brain injuries, age interacts with factors such as anatomical development, type of injury, and state of language development. Toddlers and young children appear to recover best because (1) their brains withstand injury better than those of infants, (2) they have established certain spoken language skills and sometimes written language skills prior to injury, and (3) they still have enough plasticity for functional reorganization of the brain to occur. Children who acquire aphasia secondary to convulsive disorder (Landau-Kleffner syndrome) generally recover better when onset occurs at older ages. This has been attributed to the syndrome's disruption of further language development (Bishop, 1985).

Explanations of better recovery in children remain speculative. It has been suggested that as the brain matures, specific areas become "committed" to particular functions. The biological process by which this occurs is still unclear, though it appears to involve a complex interaction of new cell growth, death of unneeded cells, and the spreading and retraction of axons. If an injury occurs before all areas are committed, language functions seem to be able to transfer to the uncommitted brain tissue (Almli & Finger, 1992; Hécaen, 1976; Janowsky & Finlay, 1986). Some studies indicate that after age 5, children's patterns of recovery from aphasia become increasingly like those of adults (Wetherby, 1985). Thus, children's brains appear to have greater plasticity but slowly lose the capacity for functional reorganization over the course of childhood.

LANGUAGE CHARACTERISTICS OF CHILDREN WITH ACQUIRED APHASIA

Because children with acquired aphasia often recover much of their premorbid communicative ability, we cannot give a single description of their language characteristics. Aphasiologists characterize the first 3 months to 1 year following brain injury as a period of spontaneous recovery during which the nervous system is able to recover a number of functions without any type of intervention (Sarno, 1981). Language impairment is most pronounced during this **acute** period. After the phase of spontaneous recovery,

children with acquired aphasia will likely be left with residual language difficulties that affect interpersonal communication to some degree but, in most cases, have their greatest impact on academic performance. In the following sections, we will delineate the common language characteristics during the acute recovery period and afterward. Distinctions will be drawn between the behaviors of children with traumatic brain injury, vascular lesions, and Landau-Kleffner syndrome.

Acute Recovery Period

Comprehension   A wide range of comprehension impairments is found among children with acute aphasia. In general, the severity of the comprehension disorder corresponds to the severity of the injury. For example, a child with a severe traumatic brain injury will usually show more difficulty at first than a child with a mild traumatic brain injury. Similarly, a massive stroke or hemorrhage will produce more devastating effects than a small one. A study of 57 children and adolescents with mild to moderate-severe closed head injury found that more than 18% had poor auditory comprehension of syntactically complex sentences but only 2% had trouble understanding single words (Ewing-Cobbs et al., 1985).

Children with vascular lesions also show individual variability in their comprehension problems. Dennis (1980) described a 9-year-old girl who, immediately following a left-sided stroke, was impaired in her auditory comprehension of words and simple commands. Her reading comprehension of the same content was better but suffered interference if she read aloud. In a larger investigation, two of eight children with left-sided nontraumatic brain injuries exhibited problems of auditory comprehension (Hécaen, 1976).

The most serious comprehension impairments are found in children with Landau-Kleffner syndrome. The impairment ranges from limited ability to understand commands to complete obliviousness to speech (Landau & Kleffner, 1957; Mantovani & Landau, 1980; Miller et al., 1984; Pearce & Darwish, 1984; Shoumaker et al., 1974; Worster-Drought, 1971). These children may not even respond appropriately to nonspeech auditory stimuli, which has led some investigators to label the condition as an auditory **agnosia**, an inability to make sense of sound (Stein & Curry, 1968).

Word Retrieval   Difficulties with word retrieval are frequently observed in children with acquired aphasia. They may appear as an inability to name pictures and objects or as excessive hesitation and nonspecific word use in spontaneous speech. One study found that a relatively small percentage (9%) of children and adolescents with mild to moderate-severe head injuries were hampered in confrontation naming; a larger number (more than 18%) had trouble retrieving words in a specific category (Ewing-Cobbs et al., 1985). In their spontaneous speech, children and adolescents with traumatic brain injury produce significantly fewer words and fewer different words than control subjects when first evaluated after their injury. Significant improvement in vocabulary usage occurs for most children during the first year following injury, but some continue at a lower level (Campbell & Dollaghan, 1990). In general, some word-finding difficulty can be expected in closed head injury cases, regardless of the severity of the injury or the age of the child (Dennis, 1992).

Few studies have documented lexical difficulties in children with left-sided vascular lesions, though such problems are evident in many forms of aphasia in adults (Albert, Goodglass, Helm, Rubens, & Alexander, 1981). The 9-year-old girl previously described had a number of word-finding impairments 2 weeks after a stroke. She produced semantic paraphasias ("bottle" for "cup"), phonemic paraphasias (/sheks/ for "scotch tape"), and random misnamings. Perseverative responses were common. Her ability to write names was better than her ability to speak them (Dennis, 1980). Problems in naming have been reported in other children with nontraumatic brain injuries. Paraphasia may be somewhat less common than it is in adults with aphasia (Hécaen, 1976).

Children with Landau-Kleffner syndrome show word substitutions and word-retrieval problems in spontaneous speech (Landau & Kleffner, 1957; Shoumaker et al., 1974). These problems are similar to those of children with language-learning disabilities. The most common signs of word-finding difficulty are filled pauses ("uh", "um"), word and phrase revisions, substitution of semantically or phonologically related words for the intended words, and overuse of indefinite reference terms ("this," "that," "thing," "stuff") (Miller et al., 1984).

Syntax   Children with aphasia tend to be nonfluent. Many of them do not speak at all for a time immediately following injury. This **mutism** lasts for varying lengths of time but eventually gives way to speech characterized by a reduced syntax (Satz & Bullard-Bates, 1981). When evaluated soon after sustaining traumatic brain injury, children and adolescents show significant differences on a number of global measures of spontaneous speech: a smaller number of utterances produced, a shorter MLU, a smaller percentage of complex utterances, and a larger percentage of utterances with mazes (Campbell & Dollaghan, 1990). Performance is also impaired on various structured communication tasks such as object description, sentence repetition, and formulation of sentences containing target words. Writing tends to be even more impaired than speaking. In a group of children with closed head injury, sentence copying was poor in about one out of five children and dictation was deficient in nearly one of three (Ewing-Cobbs et al., 1985).

Case studies of children who suffer strokes suggest a similar pattern of syntactic deficits. A child who suffered a massive left-sided stroke was impaired, two weeks postonset, in describing the use of common objects, repeating sentences, and formulating sentences with target words. Much of the difficulty was still present at 3 months postonset (Dennis, 1980). Another child, a 5-year-old who exhibited a crossed aphasia (resulting from a right hemisphere lesion), was initially mute. Over the next 3 months, syntax progressed to single words, then two- and three-word combinations with lengthy delays between words, then short phrases, and finally, short sentences (Burd et al., 1990).

Children with Landau-Kleffner syndrome may become mute or show speech limited to grunts, gestures, and isolated vowels and consonants (Miller et al., 1984). Shoumaker et al. (1974) described three children whose speech fluctuated over the course of the disorder but, at its worst, was limited to a few words. McNaughton (1991) reported on a 6-year-old boy who inconsistently produced about 30 word approximations that could be understood only by familiar listening partners. He also developed a repertoire of 15 idiosyncratic gestures such as drawing the letter *M* in the air to signify "McDonalds" or drawing a grid in the air to request a game of tic-tac-toe. A Dutch girl has been described who experienced seizures and aphasia from 5 to 8 years. Measurements of MLU and number of words spoken fluctuated as she experienced language breakdown, recovery, another breakdown, and another recovery (van de Sandt-Koenderman, Smit, van Dongen, & van Hest, 1984).

Speech Production   Problems of speech intelligibility are found in many children with acquired aphasia. Damage to motor planning regions of the brain or to cranial nerve pathways may produce sound substitutions and omissions or slurred speech, the symptoms of apraxia of speech or dysarthria. Differential diagnosis of these or other articulatory impairments is difficult during the period of acute recovery (Jaffe, Mastrilli, Molitor, & Valko, 1985). Problems may also emerge in speech prosody, the normal use of pitch, loudness, rate, and rhythm.

Immediately after traumatic brain injury, one evaluation of children and adolescents showed reduction in the percentages of consonants produced correctly in spontaneous speech. Most of the children recovered their articulation skills during the first year. Improvement in articulation was generally the earliest and strongest of all gains in expressive language (Campbell & Dollaghan, 1990). Articulation problems have also been observed in children with left-sided nontraumatic brain injuries (Dennis, 1980; Hécaen, 1976). Even greater speech disturbances are reported for children with Landau-Kleffner syndrome. A variety of misarticulations may occur, and prosody may resemble that of deaf children, that is, a high fundamental frequency used with little variation in intonation (Cooper & Ferry, 1978; Miller et al., 1984; McNaughton, 1991; van de Sandt-Koenderman et al., 1984; Worster-Drought, 1971)

Later Recovery and Residual Language Impairment

Though it is plain that children with aphasia recover more fully than adults, recent findings also indicate that children experience some persistent language impairment. This appears to be true regardless of the etiology of the aphasia. In one study, children and adolescents were evaluated for a year following traumatic brain injury. They showed marked improvement over that time but still had residual deficits in spontaneous conversation (Campbell & Dollaghan, 1990). Another study examined the performance of children 1 to 7 years after closed head injury. Persistent problems were found in several areas of school performance and academic achievement (Ylvisaker, 1989).

Children's recovery from vascular lesions shows a similar pattern. There appears to be a strong initial recovery of language functions. The 9-year-old girl in Dennis' (1980) report was evaluated at 2 weeks and 3 months following her stroke. She improved dramatically in articulation and lexical comprehension but made lesser gains in expressive language and comprehension of more complex material. Despite their early progress, most children remain impaired to some degree well after the original injury. For example, an evaluation of 11 children and adolescents with nontraumatic brain injuries more than a year postonset found that they were able to communicate verbally and engage in conversation but still exhibited residual language and academic difficulties (Cooper & Flowers, 1987). The spontaneous spoken language of these children is less elaborated syntactically and contains more errors in the complex sentences that are produced (Aram, Ekelman, & Whitaker, 1986). Naming is slower than in normal subjects, but the pattern of errors produced is generally similar to that of normal children and does not resemble the **dysnomia** (difficulty in retrieving names or words) of adults with aphasia (Aram, Ekelman, & Whitaker, 1987). Unfortunately, time alone does not solve these problems. Follow-up of young adults who experienced strokes as children has shown a wide range of language impairments, with resulting effects not only on their academic performance but on their social lives as well (Watamori, Sasanuma, & Ueda, 1990).

Children with Landau-Kleffner syndrome also show long-term language disability. Review of the literature shows that language difficulties either recurred or persisted beyond 6 months in 94% of the reported cases (Miller et al., 1984). It is clear, then, that all children with acquired aphasia can be expected to exhibit some language difficulty well after the time of their brain damage and probably into adulthood.

Academic Achievement

Given the amount of recovery that children with acquired aphasia often achieve, there is a tendency to view many of them as fully recovered. It is apparent, however, that the effects of brain damage are widespread and can be a subtle influence on a child's performance, particularly at school. Even intelligence testing may not be sensitive to certain deficits incurred by children with head injury and consequently may not be predictive of academic success. In one study, seven children were given intelligence and achievement tests a year after their accidents. Although they all had IQs above 100, only one child was maintaining a normal pace of improvement in achievement scores (Ylvisaker, 1989).

Classroom performance can be affected in many different ways. Table 12.3 shows the results of one follow-up study of children with acquired aphasia. As can be seen, deficits were detected on several formal language tests, as well as on measures of academic achievement. However, such deficits do not automatically result in school failure. Shoumaker et al. (1974) described a teenage boy who developed Landau-Kleffner syndrome when he was 8 years old. He continued to attend regular school despite the disorder, and his grades ranged from poor to fair. Furthermore, only three of the nine patients described in another study experienced academic difficulties later in life (Mantovani & Landau, 1980).

Writing skills appear to be especially susceptible to impairment as a result of brain injury. Hécaen (1976) reported on the language symptoms of eight children and adolescents who suffered left-sided nontraumatic brain injuries. Two of them showed reading difficulties, and six had problems with writing. Written language skills seem to be more affected in younger children with closed head injury than in adolescents. This may be due either to the effect of the injury on

TABLE 12.3 Residual Language and Academic Problems of Children with Acquired Aphasia

Language Ability Tested	Number of Children Scoring More Than Two Standard Deviations Below the Mean
Comprehension of single words	9/15
Comprehension of spoken sentences	7/15
Comprehension of contextual spoken language	4/15
Oral production of sentences of varying grammatical complexity	9/15
Recall of vocabulary within a semantic category (word fluency)	4/15
Single word picture labeling	8/15

Achievement Test	Number of Children Scoring More Than One Standard Deviation Below the Mean
Reading recognition	3/15
Reading comprehension	5/15
Spelling	8/15
Arithmetic	12/14

Source: Adapted from Cooper and Flowers (1987).

acquiring new skills or to the greater writing experience of adolescents, which makes their writing more
resistant to disruption (Ewing-Cobbs et al., 1985).

Much of the research documenting academic difficulties among children with acquired aphasia has relied on standardized language or achievement tests to
measure their abilities. But these tests do not reflect
the full extent of the problems these children experience in the classroom. A survey of the teachers of severely head-injured students indicated an even wider
range of academic difficulties, especially with more
complex tasks requiring processing and integration of
information (Ylvisaker, 1989). The results of this survey are summarized in Table 12.4. Clearly, the problems these children can face in school are extensive
and cut across all academic areas.

The academic problems created by brain damage
are not limited to deficits in specific skills. It is not
uncommon to find a disturbance of metacognitive
and metalinguistic functions. Ylvisaker and Szekeres
(1989) have identified seven problems:

1. Limited *self-awareness* of communication problems, which leads to reluctance or unwillingness
to work on them.
2. Poor *planning* of language responses, resulting
in disorganized, haphazard narratives.

3. Difficulty in *initiating* conversations.
4. Problems in *inhibiting* inappropriate remarks.
5. Failure to *self-monitor* situations and conversations, resulting in inappropriate behavior or
poor comprehension.
6. *Self-evaluations* that are too general ("it's okay"
or "it's all wrong") and that, therefore, do not
lead to constructive responses.
7. *Lack of flexibility* in considering various solutions to problems.

Thus far, metacognitive/metalinguistic problems have
been described in detail only for children with closed
head injuries. However, children with vascular lesions
and Landau-Kleffner syndrome have also been de-
picted as having difficulties with narrative organization, awareness of their impairments, and timely
initiation of speech (Dennis, 1980; McNaughton,
1991). Future studies may reveal the full extent of metacognitive deficits in these populations.

DIFFERENCES BETWEEN DEVELOPMENTAL AND ACQUIRED LANGUAGE DISORDERS IN CHILDREN

Throughout this chapter, we have noted that children
with acquired aphasia are a unique population be-

TABLE 12.4 Academic Diffi-culties Reported by Teachers of Children with Severe Head Injuries

Reading	▷ 25% of the children had difficulty with reading vocabulary. ▷ 50% had difficulty with rate of reading. ▷ 70% had difficulty with higher levels of comprehension. ▷ 90% had trouble comprehending written passages of substantial length.
Auditory comprehension	▷ 70% showed deterioration in auditory comprehension when the amount of language was increased. ▷ 25% performed more poorly on a standardized comprehension test when stimuli were presented at a rapid rate.
Expressive language	▷ 14% had difficulty expressing simple ideas. ▷ 75% had difficulty expressing complex ideas in both spoken and written forms. ▷ Recall of vocabulary within a semantic category (word fluency) was below normal limits.
Writing	▷ 75% scored below the 15th percentile on a timed writing test.
Memory	▷ 77% showed deficits in long-term recall of verbal material.
Attention	▷ 60% were distracted by auditory and visual stimuli in the classroom.

Source: Adapted from Ylvisaker (1989).

cause they have developed and then lost a competence with language. The evidence of rapid recovery of skills makes it apparent that children do not relearn language following a brain injury (Geschwind, 1974). They appear instead to reaccess some of the abilities that existed premorbidly, to compensate for some of the abilities that are lost, and to resume acquiring new skills.

Compared to children with developmental language disorders, children with acquired aphasia differ in attitude, in profile of abilities, and in pattern of improvement. DePompei and Blosser (1987) have noted the following characteristics in children with closed head injury:

▷ They have previous successful experiences in social and academic settings.
▷ Before their injury, they had a self-concept of being normal.
▷ They have many discrepancies in ability levels.
▷ They show inconsistent patterns of performance.
▷ During recovery they are likely to show great variability and fluctuation.
▷ They have greater problems in generalizing, structuring, and integrating new information.

Intervention for children with acquired aphasia cannot rely on the same strategies that are used for developmental language disorders. The differences in the experiences of these children and in our expectations for their rate of progress should lead us to organize intervention programs that cater to their special needs while recognizing their commonality with other children.

IMPLICATIONS FOR ASSESSMENT AND INTERVENTION

Assessment

The prevalence of acquired aphasia in children is significantly lower than either the prevalence of developmental language disorders or the prevalence of aphasia in adults. As a result, few tests have been developed specifically to evaluate childhood aphasia. It is possible to administer norm-referenced tests that are used to identify developmental language disor-

ders. These will at least establish how children with acquired aphasia compare to their typically developing peers. However, these tests cannot be used to answer questions about rate or pattern of recovery, as can tests constructed for adults with aphasia. It is tempting to administer a battery of tests to compare a child's performance across different modalities (e.g., speaking, listening, writing). However, in most instances the tests have been standardized on different populations, and any conclusions about patterns of impairment must, therefore, be severely limited (Swisher, 1985). Two tests are adaptations of instruments originally devised for use with adults. The adaptation of the *Neurosensory Center Comprehensive Examination for Aphasia* (Gaddes & Crockett, 1975) provides norms for children from 6 to 13 years of age. The *Porch Index of Communicative Ability in Children* (Porch, 1979) has norms for children from 3 to 12 years. These tests cannot be interpreted in the same fashion as their adult counterparts, and questions remain about whether the aphasia models they are based upon can be validly applied to children (Spreen & Risser, 1981). Nevertheless, they may prove useful in assessment, if only as a criterion-referenced measure of a child's behavior during the period of spontaneous recovery.

The assessment process for children with aphasia needs to be multidisciplinary. Among the professionals who may be involved are a classroom teacher, nurse, occupational therapist, parent, pediatrician, physical therapist, psychologist, recreational therapist, and speech-language pathologist. To synthesize information from a variety of sources (tests, interviews, observations) and facilitate team decision making, a common rating scale may be used to track a child's progress (Bagnato et al., 1988).

Social and Legislative Influences

Children with traumatic brain injury are now included in the category of "other health impaired" in the federal laws on education for disabled children and, thus, are eligible for services from public school systems. However, the cost of such services is prohibitive for many smaller schools. Consequently, many children with mild and moderate traumatic brain injury are not served. Furthermore, children with nontraumatic

Because federal laws do not define education, professionals may disagree on what constitutes educational services for children with traumatic brain injury.

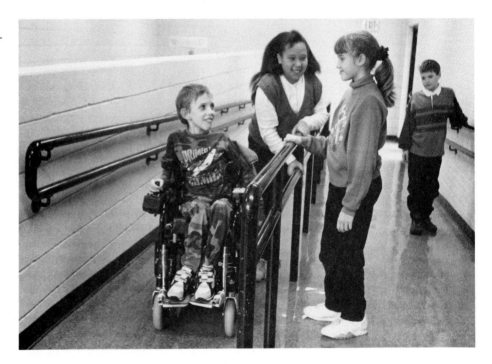

brain injuries resulting from stroke, infection, poisoning, and other causes are not included in the definition of traumatic brain injury and, therefore, may not receive services (Savage, 1991).

Interestingly, these federal laws do not define education, with the result that education and rehabilitation professionals may disagree on what are appropriate services for a child. A plan for therapy that is deemed necessary by rehabilitation personnel may be rejected or severely reduced by public schools on the grounds that it is not strictly necessary for educational purposes (Savage, 1991). Economy may be a factor in the acceptance, rejection, or modification of these plans.

Nonspeech Options

A full discussion of alternative/augmentative communication strategies and devices is beyond the scope of this chapter, but some mention must be made of their relevance to children with acquired aphasia. During the early stages of recovery, all expressive modalities may be impaired or speech may be unintelligible, thereby requiring the use of an alternative/augmenta-

tive device. The immediate need is to establish reliable signals for "yes" and "no." Depending on the child's level of cognitive, linguistic, and motoric functioning, it may be practical to use writing, head nodding or shaking, pointing to printed words, or eye blinking (Jaffe et al., 1985).

The use of alternative/augmentative communication devices with children who have acquired aphasia will differ in certain ways from their use with children who have developmental problems (Jaffe et al., 1985):

▷ The rapid rate of recovery of children with acquired aphasia means that the systems will become outdated more quickly; they must be constantly reevaluated.

▷ Children will be very sensitive at first to overstimulation; the amount of material included in a communication board or other device must be quite small at first, then gradually enlarged.

▷ Children may reject devices with synthetic speech because these do not sound like their own voices, which they heard before they were injured.

▷ Children with severe frontal lobe damage and generalized cognitive deficits will have difficulty initiating communication in any form, including alternative/augmentative devices.

Despite these factors, alternative/augmentative communication may be highly desirable and effective for certain children with aphasia. Children with Landau-Kleffner syndrome are especially promising candidates. Some of these children may incur a "double dissociation": between auditory input and meaning and between meaning and expression. In these cases, a visually based alternative/augmentative communication device might tap their underlying linguistic abilities and result in markedly better language acquisition (Miller et al., 1984). Several dramatic successes have been reported in the literature. Pearce and Darwish (1984) described a 6-year-old child with Landau-Kleffner syndrome who learned to use a nonverbal communication system with Blisssymbolics, introduced in chapter 1. In 6 months he learned about 200 symbols, after which sign language was introduced to meet his expanding communicative needs. By 8 years of age he was able to combine 4 or 5 signs in an utterance; in contrast, he could produce only 10 to 15 differentiated monosyllabic words in a structured setting. Cooper and Ferry (1978) described a 13-year-old child who had developed aphasia along with convulsive disorder at 4 years of age. He was able to speak only a few single words, and these were minimally intelligible. However, he readily signed, gestured, and used fingerspelling. Another child they evaluated was previously diagnosed as mentally retarded but responded dramatically to a TC approach (described in chapter 9) and was able to demonstrate above-average performance intelligence. A third child suffered seizures from 2½ to 7 years and did not produce useful language until 10 years of age. At that time he received instruction in manual communication and, within 6 months, acquired a vocabulary of over 200 signs.

Cooper and Ferry (1978) caution, however, that not all children with Landau-Kleffner syndrome have facility with gesture; thus, "manual communication cannot be considered a panacea for this population" (p. 183). As another example of the use of alternative/augmentative communication systems, one child who achieved only partial success was described by McNaughton (1991). After a year of intervention a 6-year-old boy was able and willing to use a communication board with a graphic display in a limited way. However, he used the board only if he was unable to communicate his message through a combination of speech approximations, idiosyncratic gestures, and pointing. Best results were, therefore, obtained by combining the child's idiosyncratic communication strategies with the alternative/augmentative device.

Behavior Disorders

Behavior disorders associated with brain injury can be either active or passive. Children and adolescents with an active disorder are likely to be described as aggressive, impulsive, disinhibited, or antisocial. Those with a passive disorder may be called slow or said to lack drive and motivation (Eames, 1988). The behavioral outcome in each type of child is the result of an interaction among the effects of the brain injury, the behavioral predispositions of the individual (e.g., a tendency toward aggressiveness or depression), and the adjustment made to the new situation created by the accident (e.g., new living quarters, parent–child relationships, school, peer group). All of these factors must be considered in understanding a child's behavior and developing an intervention plan to deal with it. In addition, certain types of behavior problems may be driven by neurological damage and, therefore, may require drug treatment along with behavioral intervention (Eames, 1988).

Children who suffer head injuries are often described as impulsive and aggressive, factors that predispose them to injury (Klonoff, 1971). However, many of the children who have mild behavioral and cognitive disturbances following head injury may have demonstrated these problems before their accidents (Mahoney, D'Souza, & Haller, 1983), suggesting again the influence of preinjury predispositions.

Intelligibility

Children with acquired aphasia who also present a speech production problem may require intervention so that efforts to promote language recovery are not hindered by poor intelligibility. Improvements in intelligibility allow these children to display linguistic abilities without frustration, thereby improving and encouraging conversational interaction (Fey, 1986). Gains in intelligibility will also benefit any other intervention strategies that require judgments about the correctness of children's attempts to master target forms.

Problems of aphasia, dysarthria, and apraxia of speech can coexist in children with traumatic brain injury. During the early stages of recovery, treatment is limited to facial and oral stimulation and feeding therapy. If a child is alert but unintelligible, alternative/augmentative communication devices may prove useful. Later, usually 1 year or more postonset, severe **hypernasality** may be treated by fitting a palatal lift **prosthesis** or performing palatal surgery. Articulatory impairments are usually amenable to phonetic placement approaches or drill designed to increase gradually the length and complexity of phonetic units that a child can produce (Jaffe et al., 1985).

Development versus Remedial Logic

Depending on the age at which a child acquires aphasia, professionals may apply different models of recovery. Preschool children are likely to be learning fundamental syntactic and phonological skills at the time of their injury. Consequently, a developmental model likely remains appropriate, and may be used to select goals and teaching strategies for these children (Ylvisaker & Holland, 1984). With older children and adolescents, a model based on observed patterns of physiological recovery may be more useful. Table 12.5 presents a three-stage model of recovery, listing some of the symptoms and intervention strategies relevant to each stage.

Facilitating versus Compensatory Intervention

Children with acquired aphasia are still in the process of learning language when their brain injury occurs. Consequently, the goal for intervention must be not only to restore what was lost but also to facilitate the new learning that was interrupted. Haley et al. (1990) describe this in terms of four objectives:

1. Restoration of function.
2. Compensation for function.
3. Adaptation of the environment to facilitate function.
4. Normal acquisition of developmental skills.

In the late stages of recovery, the role of the professional is to assist children in compensating for skills that are lost or to help in adapting the environment. Many techniques and strategies can be applied in this process, some of which are listed in Table 12.6.

Returning to School

Special education services designed primarily for children with mental retardation, learning disabilities, or emotional disturbances may not be appropriate for children with acquired aphasia. On the other hand, full-time mainstreaming into a regular education classroom may be overwhelming for a child who has been in a hospital environment for several months (DePompei & Blosser, 1987). Because the federal education laws allow children with traumatic brain injury to be designated as "other health impaired," school personnel are required to develop customized programs that meet children's individual needs (Ylvisaker, Hartwick, & Stevens, 1991). The rapid rate of recovery of many children with brain injuries means that their Individualized Educational Programs must be reviewed and modified more frequently than those of other children (Savage, 1991; Ylvisaker et al., 1991).

To function effectively in school, children must be able to cope with demands for attention, concentration, and socialization. Cohen, Joyce, Rhoades, & Welks (1985) suggest that as a prerequisite to returning to school a child must be able to do the following:

▷ Attend to a task for 10 to 15 minutes.
▷ Tolerate 20 to 30 minutes of general classroom stimulation, such as movement, noises, and visual distractions.
▷ Function within a group of two or more students.
▷ Engage in meaningful communication through speech, gesture, or the use of an alternative/augmentative communication device.
▷ Follow simple directions.
▷ Show potential for learning.

TABLE 12.5   Stages of Recovery in Closed Head Injury

Stage	Symptoms	Intervention Strategies
Early	▷ Responds to stimulation but can be easily over-stimulated. ▷ Disoriented to person, place, time, and own condition. ▷ Inconsistent memory function, especially for recent events. ▷ Inconsistent comprehension of speech. ▷ Uses simple gestures to communicate. ▷ Speech may be unintelligible, echolalic, perseverative, halting.	Control amount and type of stimulation child receives ▷ Counsel family members. ▷ Determine and provide stimuli to which child is most appropriately responsive. ▷ Reassess frequently. ▷ Modify environment to suit needs of child; provide familiar pictures, objects, music, etc. ▷ Verbally orient child to time and place.
Middle	▷ Alert and more oriented but still confused about schedules and own condition. ▷ Limited attention span and concentration. ▷ Information processing and language comprehension limited to small amounts and to simple concepts and words. ▷ Speaks but may require prompting. ▷ Loses train of thought while talking and has difficulty with word retrieval.	Begin practice of cognitive and communicative functions ▷ Structure child's day and provide ongoing orientation by means of schedule and logbook. ▷ Schedule intervention in group and individual sessions. ▷ Work on attending behavior, memory function, and information processing by gradually increasing length and complexity of tasks. ▷ Ensure high success rate, vary activities, and use video to maintain child's motivation. ▷ Focus on improving comprehension of longer and more complex stimuli.
Late	▷ Well oriented as long as a routine is followed. ▷ Difficulty in shifting from one task to another. ▷ Capable of learning new skills and information, though slowly and with effort. ▷ Difficulty with comprehension of nonliteral language (metaphors, jokes). ▷ Disorganization evident at all levels of language; has difficulty focusing on main points or staying on topic. ▷ Few syntactic errors; mild word-finding problems.	Begin to teach compensatory strategies and use of alternative communication devices ▷ Practice deductive reasoning and problem solving (e.g., "Twenty questions"). ▷ Vary activities and discussions to encourage cognitive flexibility (e.g., change rules of a game slightly). ▷ Practice self-monitoring and require child to request clarification of information that is not understood. ▷ Compensate for poor memory with associative strategies and memo books. ▷ Practice analyzing information for major points.

Source: Adapted from Ylvisaker and Holland (1984).

Successful return to school also requires the involvement and cooperation of professionals at both the hospital and school, as well as family members and individuals in the community. Ylvisaker et al. (1991) have drawn attention to many areas that require planning and follow-up:

1. The parents must be prepared for their role as advocates for their child's education. They must obtain information about medical and social aspects of brain injury, entitlement to special education under federal laws, and cost sharing between schools and insurance companies.

TABLE 12.6 Compensatory Teaching Strategies

Socialization and emotional support	▷ Plan small-group activities with unimpaired children to facilitate interaction skills.
	▷ Schedule time for rest and emotional release. Encourage child to discuss problems as they come up.
Instruction	▷ Give instructions both verbally and in writing. Repeat or paraphrase them as necessary. If understanding is critical, ask the student to repeat information or respond to a few questions about the instructions.
	▷ Encourage student to self-monitor comprehension and to request repetition or rephrasing of instructions.
	▷ Develop a verbal system (e.g., calling student's name) or a nonverbal system (e.g., posting a symbol or picture) for cuing the student to attend, respond, or change some aspect of behavior.
	▷ Allow additional time for processing of instructions, responding to questions, and completing assignments.
	▷ Provide child with a buddy to assist in following classroom directions, completing assignments, and traveling within the school.
Assistive devices	▷ Allow and encourage the use of calculators, tape recorders, and computers.
	▷ Have the student maintain a schedule and logbook tracking all classes, appointments, assignments and due dates, and room locations. Include pictures of persons who are not readily identified.
	▷ Provide maps for finding locations within the school.
Modification of materials	▷ As far as possible, structure the physical environment to reduce distractions and allow freedom of movement.
	▷ Use enlarged print in reading materials, and supplement texts with pictures and other resources (e.g., vocabulary lists, outlines of key points) to facilitate comprehension.
	▷ Cover parts of the page during reading and look at exposed areas systematically; use a finger or index card to help in scanning.
	▷ Modify assignments and tests according to the student's abilities by reducing the amount of reading or the number of problems.

Sources: Adapted from DePompei and Blosser (1987), Haarbauer-Krupa, Henry, Szekeres, and Ylvisaker (1985), and Ylvisaker et al. (1991).

2. Children with brain injuries must maintain peer relationships that are as close to normal as possible. Friends and classmates should be informed about the child's condition, and about how it affects and does not affect participation in various games and activities. Children who are willing can be involved in explaining their injuries to their peers.

3. Children should be prepared for the demands of school before they return. Environmental conditions such as noisy classrooms and crowded hallways can be simulated in the hospital, and children can be encouraged to visit their schools before they return full time. Special instructional materials (e.g., large-print books, modified worksheets) and procedures should be tested

and evaluated before they are used on a regular basis.

4. Teachers and other school staff should be educated about the child's condition, needs, and abilities. One individual should be appointed as case manager to coordinate the services provided by the school.

5. The need for vocational rehabilitation should be considered from an early age. Efforts should be made to provide work experiences for children with brain injuries so that they develop normal expectations for and attitudes about employment.

6. Children who are discharged from the hospital during the summer months will require special planning to see them through the period until school begins.

7. Physical, health, or cognitive problems may prevent some children from attending school. In this case they are entitled to homebound services from the school system, which require special coordination efforts.

Plainly, the transition back to school is a challenge to friends, parents, school personnel, and, most of all, the child. Professionals should be ready to help organize and assist in this crucial process.

SUMMARY

In this chapter, we have seen that:

▶ Acquired aphasia is a condition in which a child begins to develop language and then loses all or part of that ability due to a brain injury.

▶ The major causes of acquired aphasia in children are closed head injury, vascular lesions, and convulsive disorder (Landau-Kleffner syndrome).

▶ Besides causing aphasia, brain injuries can produce impairments of gross and fine motor skills, cognition, perception, and social behavior.

▶ Children, like adults, have a dominant hemisphere for language function. Therefore, they are more likely to acquire aphasia from a left-sided than a right-sided brain injury. Unlike adults, most children spontaneously recover a substantial portion of their premorbid communicative ability.

▶ The stronger recovery of children is thought to be due to the plasticity of the nervous system in early life. Regions of the brain that are not fully committed are able to take on functions previously served by damaged nerve tissue.

▶ During the acute recovery period, children with acquired aphasia may show a dramatic loss of language abilities. In the most severe cases, they may be mute and completely unresponsive to speech stimuli.

▶ Most children recover much of their ability to comprehend and produce language during the first year following their injury. Thereafter, they are often plagued with residual communicative difficulties that can seriously affect their academic performance.

▶ Assessment and intervention for children with acquired aphasia is a multidisciplinary endeavor. It must be planned with consideration of each child's intelligibility, behavior problems, preferred modality, and changing needs over the course of recovery.

▶ The aims of intervention are to assist in the restoration of some language functions and the acquisition of skills whose development was interrupted, and to help children compensate for other functions that remain impaired. Compensation may be achieved by using alternative/augmentative communication devices or by modifying learning materials and instructions.

▶ The transition back to school is a complex undertaking that requires considerable cooperation, organization, and sensitivity to the host of physical, educational, and social problems a child will encounter.

Children with acquired aphasia pose special challenges to professionals working with language disorders. Over the course of recovery, these children gradually exchange medical problems for social and educational ones. In most instances, professionals working in hospital settings hand over the intervention to school personnel. There are opportunities for

confusion as these changes in service occur. This problem is best avoided by increasing everyone's awareness and understanding of these children's capabilities, disabilities, and needs.

REFERENCES

Albert, M. L., Goodglass, H., Helm, N. A., Rubens, A. B., & Alexander, M. P. (1981). *Clinical aspects of dysphasia.* New York: Springer-Verlag.

Almli, C. R., & Finger, S. (1992). Brain injury and recovery of function: Theories and mechanisms of functional reorganization. *Journal of Head Trauma Rehabilitation, 7,* 70–77.

Aram, D. M., Ekelman, B. L., & Whitaker, H. (1986). Spoken syntax in children with acquired left and right hemisphere lesions. *Brain and Language, 27,* 75–100.

Aram, D. M., Ekelman, B. L., & Whitaker, H. (1987). Lexical retrieval in left and right lesioned children. *Brain and Language, 31,* 75–100.

Bagnato, S. J., Mayes, S. D., Nichter, C., Domoto, V., Hamann, L., Keener, S., Landis, C., Savina, J., & Telenko, A. (1988). An interdisciplinary neurodevelopmental assessment model for brain-injured infants and preschool children. *Journal of Head Trauma Rehabilitation, 3,* 75–86.

Bishop, D. V. M. (1985). Age of onset and outcome in "acquired aphasia with convulsive disorders" (Landau-Kleffner syndrome). *Developmental Medicine and Child Neurology, 27,* 705–712.

Burd, L., Gascon, G., Swenson, R., & Hankey, R. (1990). Crossed aphasia in early childhood. *Developmental Medicine and Child Neurology, 32,* 539–546.

Campbell, T. F., & Dollaghan, C. A. (1990). Expressive language recovery in severely brain-injured children and adolescents. *Journal of Speech and Hearing Disorders, 55,* 567–581.

Cohen, S. B., Joyce, C. M., Rhoades, K. W., & Welks, D. M. (1985). Educational programming for head injured students. In M. Ylvisaker (Ed.), *Head injury rehabilitation: Children and adolescents.* Austin, TX: PRO-ED.

Cooper, J. A., & Ferry, P. C. (1978). Acquired auditory verbal agnosia and seizures in childhood. *Journal of Speech and Hearing Disorders, 43,* 176–184.

Cooper, J. A., & Flowers, C. R. (1987). Children with a history of acquired aphasia: Residual language and academic im-

pairments. *Journal of Speech and Hearing Disorders, 52,* 251–262.

Dennis, M. (1980). Strokes in childhood I: Communicative intent, expression, and comprehension after left hemisphere arteriopathy in a right-handed nine-year-old. In R. W. Rieber (Ed.), *Language development and aphasia in children.* New York: Academic Press.

Dennis, M. (1992). Word finding in children and adolescents with a history of brain injury. *Topics in Language Disorders, 13,* 66–82.

DePompei, R., & Blosser, J. (1987). Strategies for helping head-injured children successfully return to school. *Language, Speech, and Hearing Services in Schools, 18,* 292–300.

Eames, P. (1988). Behavior disorders after severe head injury: Their nature and causes and strategies for management. *Journal of Head Trauma Rehabilitation, 3,* 1–6.

Ewing-Cobbs, L., Fletcher, J. M., Landry, S. H., & Levin, H. S. (1985). Language disorders after pediatric head injury. In J. K. Darby (Ed.), *Speech and language evaluation in neurology: Childhood disorders.* Orlando, FL: Grune & Stratton.

Fey, M. E. (1986). *Language intervention with young children.* Boston: College-Hill Press.

Gaddes, W. H., & Crockett, D. J. (1975). The Spreen-Benton aphasia tests, normative data as a measure of normal language development. *Brain and Language, 2,* 257–280.

Geschwind, N. (1974). Disorders of higher cortical function in children. In N. Geschwind (Ed.), *Selected papers on language and the brain.* Dordrecht, Holland: D. Reidel.

Gordon, N. (1990). Acquired aphasia in childhood: The Landau-Kleffner syndrome. *Developmental Medicine and Child Neurology, 32,* 270–274.

Haarbauer-Krupa, J., Henry, K., Szekeres, S. F., & Ylvisaker, M. (1985). Cognitive rehabilitation therapy: Late stages of recovery. In M. Ylvisaker (Ed.), *Head injury rehabilitation: Children and adolescents.* Austin, TX: PRO-ED.

Haley, S. M., Cioffi, M. I., Lewin, J. E., & Baryza, M. J. (1990).

Motor dysfunction in children and adolescents after traumatic brain injury. *Journal of Head Trauma Rehabilitation, 5,* 77–90.

Hécaen, H. (1976). Acquired aphasia in children and the ontogenesis of hemispheric functional specialization. *Brain and Language, 3,* 114–134.

Jaffe, M. B., Mastrilli, J. P., Molitor, C. B., & Valko, A. S. (1985). Intervention for motor disorders. In M. Ylvisaker (Ed.), *Head injury rehabilitation: Children and adolescents.* Austin, TX: PRO-ED.

Janowsky, J. S., & Finlay, B. L. (1986). The outcome of perinatal brain damage: The role of normal neuron loss and axon retraction. *Developmental Medicine and Child Neurology, 28,* 375–389.

Kinsbourne, M., & Hiscock, M. (1977). Does cerebral dominance develop? In S. J. Segalowitz & F. A. Gruber (Eds.), *Language development and neurological theory.* New York: Academic Press.

Klonoff, H. (1971). Head injuries in children: Predisposing factors, accident conditions, and sequelae. *American Journal of Public Health, 61,* 2405–2417.

Landau, W. M., & Kleffner, F. R. (1957). Syndrome of acquired aphasia with convulsive disorder in children. *Neurology, 10,* 915–921.

Lenneberg, E. (1967). *Biological foundations of language.* New York: Wiley.

Mahoney, W. J., D'Souza, B. J., & Haller, J. A. (1983). Long-term outcome of children with severe head trauma and prolonged coma. *Pediatrics, 71,* 756–761.

Mantovani, J. F., & Landau, W. M. (1980). Acquired aphasia with convulsive disorder: Course and prognosis. *Neurology, 30,* 524–529.

Martins, I. P., Ferro, J. M., & Trindade, A. (1987). Acquired crossed aphasia in a child. *Developmental Medicine and Child Neurology, 29,* 96–100.

McNaughton, D. (1991). Augmentative and alternative communication intervention for a child with acquired aphasia with convulsive disorder: A case study. *Journal of Speech Language Pathology and Audiology, 15,* 35–41.

Miller, J. F., Campbell, T. F., Chapman, R. S., & Weismer, S. E. (1984). Language behavior in acquired childhood aphasia. In A. L. Holland (Ed.), *Language disorders in children: Recent advances.* San Diego: College-Hill Press.

Milliken, C. H., McDowell, F., & Easton, J. D. (1987). *Stroke.* Philadelphia: Lea & Febiger.

Molfese, D. L., Freeman, R. B., & Palermo, D. S. (1975). The ontogeny of brain lateralization for speech and non-speech stimuli. *Brain and Language, 2,* 356–368.

National Center for Health Statistics. (1992). *Health, United States, 1991.* Hyattsville, MD: Public Health Service.

Pearce, P. S., & Darwish, H. (1984). Correlation between EEG and auditory perceptual measures in auditory agnosia. *Brain and Language, 22,* 41–48.

Porch, B. E. (1979). *Porch index of communicative ability in children.* Palo Alto, CA: Consulting Psychologists Press.

Sarno, M. T. (1981). Recovery and rehabilitation in aphasia. In M. T. Sarno (Ed.), *Acquired aphasia.* New York: Academic Press.

Satz, P., & Bullard-Bates, C. (1981). Acquired aphasia in children. In M. T. Sarno (Ed.), *Acquired aphasia.* New York: Academic Press.

Savage, R. C. (1991). Identification, classification, and placement issues for students with traumatic brain injuries. *Journal of Head Trauma Rehabilitation, 6,* 1–9.

Shoumaker, R. D., Bennett, D. R., Bray, P. F., & Curless, R. G. (1974). Clinical and EEG manifestations of an unusual aphasia syndrome in children. *Neurology, 24,* 10–16.

Spreen, O., & Risser, A. (1981). Assessment of aphasia. In M. T. Sarno (Ed.), *Acquired aphasia.* New York: Academic Press.

Stein, L. K., & Curry, E. K. W. (1968). Childhood auditory agnosia. *Journal of Speech and Hearing Disorders, 28,* 361–370.

Swisher, L. (1985). Language disorders in children. In J. K. Darby (Ed.), *Speech and language evaluation in neurology: Childhood disorders.* Orlando, FL: Grune & Stratton.

Teasdale, G., & Jennett, B. (1974). Assessment of coma and impaired consciousness: A practical scale. *Lancet, 2,* 81–84.

van de Sandt-Koenderman, W. M. E., Smit, I. A. C., van Dongen, H. R., & van Hest, J. B. C. (1984). A case of acquired aphasia and convulsive disorder: Some linguistic aspects of recovery and breakdown. *Brain and Language, 21,* 174–183.

Wada, J. A., Clarke, R., & Hamm, A. (1975). Cerebral hemispheric asymmetry in humans. *Archives of Neurology, 32,* 239–246.

Watamori, T. S., Sasanuma, S., & Ueda, S. (1990). Recovery and plasticity in child-onset aphasics: Ultimate outcome at adulthood. *Aphasiology, 4,* 9–30.

Wetherby, A. M. (1985). Speech and language disorders in children—an overview. In J. K. Darby (Ed.), *Speech and language evaluation in neurology: Childhood disorders.* Orlando, FL: Grune & Stratton.

Worster-Drought, C. (1971). An unusual form of acquired aphasia in children. *Developmental Medicine and Child Neurology, 13,* 563–571.

Ylvisaker, M. (1989). Cognitive and psychosocial outcome following head injury in children. In J. T. Hoff, T. E. Anderson, & T. M. Cole (Eds.), *Mild to moderate head injury.* London: Blackwell Scientific.

Ylvisaker, M., Hartwick, P., & Stevens, M. (1991). School reentry following head injury: Managing the transition from hospital to school. *Journal of Head Trauma Rehabilitation, 6,* 10–22.

Ylvisaker, M., & Holland, A. L. (1984). Head injury. In W. H. Perkins (Ed.), *Language handicaps in children.* New York: Thieme-Stratton.

Ylvisaker, M., & Szekeres, S. F. (1989). Metacognitive and executive impairments in head-injured children and adults. *Topics in Language Disorders, 9,* 34–49.

· Chapter 13 ·

Language and Other Special Populations of Children

Steven H. Long

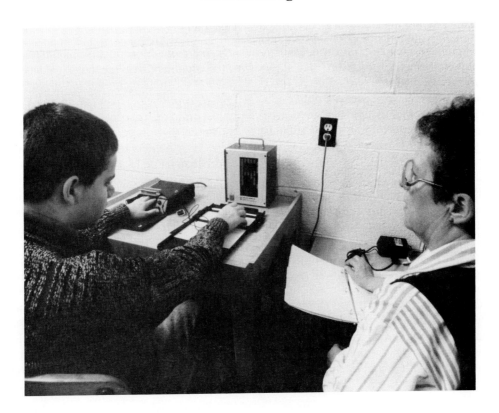

Upon completion of this chapter, the reader should be able to:

▶ Discuss definitions of giftedness and factors that affect estimates of its prevalence among children.

▶ Describe general characteristics of the spoken and written language of gifted children.

▶ Discuss issues in assessment and intervention with gifted children who also have physical, sensory, or learning disabilities.

▶ Discuss the definitions, causes, and prevalence of visual impairment in children.

▶ Describe characteristics of the spoken language of blind children.

▶ Discuss general principles of intervention with blind children and their parents.

▶ Understand the etiology and types of cerebral palsy and other neuromotor disorders.

▶ Understand the general speech and language characteristics of children with cerebral palsy.

▶ Discuss the general aims of intervention for children with cerebral palsy.

▶ Discuss possible causes of delayed language development in children with cleft palate.

LANGUAGE AND GIFTED CHILDREN

It may surprise some readers to find a discussion of gifted children in a text about disorders of language. There are at least three reasons, however, why it is relevant to describe this population. First, gifted children, like children with language impairments, are exceptional. The psychometric procedures for identifying both groups of children are quite similar, and *gifted education* is commonly viewed either as a branch of *special education* or as a parallel division of education. Second, children with exceptional abilities are sometimes disruptive in the classroom because they are not sufficiently challenged by the style and pace of the curriculum (McCluskey & Walker, 1986). Hence, they may be referred for evaluation by a school psychologist, speech-language pathologist, or other professional. Third, and most important, the population of gifted children overlaps with three other groups: bilingual-bicultural children, children with physical or sensory handicaps, and children with learning disabilities. One of the issues noted by experts in gifted education as most important to that field is how best to identify and serve gifted children who are economically disadvantaged or who have some handicap that limits the expression of their abilities (Cramer, 1991). To some extent, therefore, professionals who serve children with language disorders have an important role to play in assessment and educational planning for children who are gifted.

An Overview of Giftedness

Definition In popular thinking, there seems to be little argument that some individuals are more able than others. Our language has a number of words—*gifted, genius,* and *talented* among them—to distinguish those with exceptional abilities. Among scholars, however, there is considerable dispute over the concept of *giftedness* and whether it reflects anything more than natural variation, the effects of practice, and the advantages of being raised in a privileged environment (Howe, 1990). One thing is clear: There is no single definition of *giftedness*. The difficulty in defining this term is much like the problem of defining *disordered* or *impaired*. Children may be viewed as disordered if they display characteristics that will hinder them from achieving socially valued goals such as getting along with peers, gaining an education, or finding a job (Fey, 1986). Similarly, children may be considered gifted if they show superior abilities in domains that society values: speech and language, writing, music, athletics, art, and others. In 1972, the U.S. Office of Education created the following definition of gifted and talented children that emphasized the idea of social value:

> Gifted and talented children are those identified by professionally qualified persons who by virtue of outstanding abilities are capable of high performance. These are children who require differentiated educational programs and services beyond those normally provided by the regular school program in order to realize their contribution to self and society. (Marland, 1972, p. 2)

This definition is deliberately broad and calls attention to the special educational needs of these children. Another definition of giftedness, based on opinions contributed by a panel of experts in the field, is shown in Table 13.1. This definition is more detailed and reflects the evolution of thinking among educators from the 1970s to the 1990s. Three major refinements have been made:

1. Giftedness is defined as a potential ability as well as a demonstrated ability. This subtle change is needed to justify efforts at early identification of gifted children whose skills are not yet well developed.

TABLE 13.1   A Consensus Definition of Giftedness by Experts in Gifted Education

1. Giftedness is the potential for exceptional development of specific abilities as well as the demonstration of performance at the upper end of a talent continuum; it is not limited by age, gender, race, socioeconomic status, or ethnicity.
2. A Gifted Child is one who is developmentally advanced in one or more areas; he or she has potential or demonstrated ability in general intellectual ability, specific academic aptitude, leadership, creative productive thinking, or the visual and performing arts; because of this potential or demonstrated ability, the child requires differentiated education services in order to function at the level appropriate to his or her potential.
3. A Gifted Adult is one who shows unusual skill, ability, or talent in one or more areas of intellect, leadership, or in the visual or performing arts; he or she makes independent and creative contributions to a field.

Source: Cramer (1991, p. 88).

2. The definition contains a warning against biased judgments. This is consistent with the opposition to stereotyping and discrimination at all levels of education.
3. Separate characteristics are described for a gifted child and a gifted adult. The distinction is primarily one of potential versus performance. It is also suggested that a feature of giftedness in mature individuals is independent and creative work.

In principle, children may display giftedness in several different ways. They may score very highly on general tests of intelligence, suggesting that they are developmentally advanced in a number of areas. Or they may achieve high scores on tests of aptitude in only one or two domains, such as visuospatial abilities or mathematics. Another possibility is that they will not distinguish themselves on any formal test but will manifest their special abilities through their behavior in natural surroundings. Table 13.2 lists some of the behavioral characteristics of gifted children that can be observed informally. As with their performance on standardized tests, gifted children may display exceptional behaviors in all or just a few of the categories shown. Of particular relevance to this chapter is the number of references in the table to language and language-related skills.

Prevalence   Neither of the definitions of giftedness just reviewed have any official or legal standing. They are merely attempts to delineate the concept in a way that is logical and consistent with observed characteristics. In many educational systems, however, giftedness is a category of placement. The responsibility for setting eligibility criteria is left to the states or, in some cases, to local school districts. Although not all gifted children perform well on tests, most states rely on standardized instruments for identification and placement in special educational programs. For example, one state has the following criteria: (1) a score of 130 or more on the *Wechsler Intelligence Scale for Children–Revised* (WISC–R) Full Scale or Verbal and (2) a rank of not less than the 95th percentile on national norms on two or more of the mathematics, language

TABLE 13.2 Behavioral Characteristics of Gifted Children

Category	Behavior
Communication	▷ Has unusually advanced vocabulary for age or grade level; uses terms in a meaningful way; has verbal behavior characterized by richness of expression, elaboration, and fluency. ▷ Demonstrates a flair for dramatic or oral presentations.
Learning	▷ Has quick mastery and recall of facts. ▷ Has rapid insight into cause–effect relationships; tries to discover the how and why of things; asks many thought-provoking questions (as distinct from information or factual questions). ▷ Learns from experience and seldom repeats mistakes. ▷ Transfers learning easily from one situation to another.
Motivation	▷ Becomes absorbed and involved in certain topics or problems; is persistent in seeking task completion; displays long attention span. ▷ Strives toward perfection; is self-critical; is not easily satisfied with work. ▷ Often is self-assertive (sometimes even aggressive); stubborn in beliefs.
Creativity/sensitivity	▷ Displays a great deal of curiosity about many things; constantly asks questions about anything and everything. ▷ Displays much intellectual playfulness; fantasizes; imagines ("I wonder what would happen if . . . "). ▷ Is unusually aware of impulses and more open to the irrational (freer expression of feminine interest for boys, greater than usual independence for girls); shows emotional sensitivity.
Leadership	▷ Carries responsibility well; can be counted on to fulfill promises and usually does it well. ▷ Is self-confident with peers as well as adults; seems comfortable when asked to show work to the class. ▷ Adapts readily to new situations; is flexible in thought and action and does not seem disturbed when the normal routine is changed.

Sources: Adapted from Alexander and Muia (1982) and Renzulli and Hartman (1971).

arts, science, and social science sections of the *Iowa Test of Basic Skills* (ITBS) (Fehrenbach, 1991).

Because of variation in definitions and eligibility criteria, prevalence estimates for giftedness can range from 2% to almost 90% (Fenstermacher, 1982; Lilly, 1979; Mitchell & Erickson, 1978; Sanderlin & Lundy, 1979). Very high estimates are nearly always based on definitions that focus on children's potential for achievement, not their actual achievement. Some ed-

ucators, especially in the United States, are reluctant to recognize a category of "gifted children" because it smacks of elitism and therefore runs contrary to the democratic, egalitarian principles of America (Mills & Durden, 1992). Individuals who share this view prefer to highlight the latent abilities all children have if provided stimulation and educational opportunity. This opinion is supported by psychological research indicating that most children's abilities can be accelerated beyond what is currently considered average by means of well-designed programs of instruction and encouragement (Howe, 1990). In the following discussion, we will be using *gifted* in its more narrow sense of children who appear to excel without special instruction.

Language Characteristics of Gifted Children

One of the most striking features of gifted children is their **precocious** language development. If provided with a normal home environment, many of these children talk early and learn to read before they start school (Freeman, 1986). Parents often note advanced language skills as one of the first indicators of giftedness in their children. As shown in Table 13.3, one survey found that the characteristic mentioned most frequently by parents was expressive language; 4 of the top 12 traits were skills or interests involving oral and written language.

Other than its faster rate, there is no evidence that the language learning of gifted children differs from that of typically developing children. Thus, it is likely

TABLE 13.3   Skill Categories Mentioned Most Often by Parents of Gifted Preschool Children

Rank Item	Skill
1	Language: expressive-productive
2	Memory
3	Abstract thinking
4	Ahead of peers
5	Curiosity
6	Language: receptive-comprehensive
7	Motor
8	Nomination (comments by others)
9.5	Awareness of the environment
9.5	Special knowledge (e.g., dinosaurs, foreign languages)
11	Early interest in books and reading
12	Word and symbol recognition

Source: Adapted from Louis and Lewis (1992).

that a developmental model can be used to predict their language skills. Gifted preschool children may produce and understand language at a level that would be expected of elementary school children, and gifted children between 5 and 10 years of age may show language skills that resemble those of middle and high school children.

It should be remembered, however, that advanced language ability is not a requirement of giftedness. A child may be gifted in musical, artistic, athletic, mathematical, or social skills and display ordinary verbal abilities. One of the main features of handicapped gifted children is the discrepancy between their superior abilities in one domain and their mediocre or even deficient skills in another (Waldron, Saphire, & Rosenblum, 1987). Therefore, we cannot speak of the "language of gifted children" as though they were a homogeneous group. The following discussion refers only to those children who display precocious verbal skills as a component of their giftedness.

Oral Language   Gifted children are often said to be precocious talkers. One frequently cited milestone is the age at which first words are spoken. For example, one study of 37 gifted children reported that half of them said their first words before they were 1 year old and five of them began to talk as early as 6 months of age (Price, 1976). There are two problems, however, in interpreting the first-word phenomenon: (1) the source of information is usually the parents, who may be biased in their recall by their present belief that the child is gifted, and (2) there are no established criteria for what constitutes a first word, in contrast to a phonetically consistent form, a **protoword**, or any of the other vocalizations routinely produced by infants after about 7 months of age (Fletcher, 1979). What may be a more reliable indicator of advanced verbal development is the rate at which a child progresses from single words to word combinations or the rate at which vocabulary is acquired during the single-word period. Recall that typically developing children make the transition from single words to syntax over a period of about 6 to 12 months. During this time their rate of vocabulary growth is slow compared to what it will be after syntax is well established (Garman, 1979).

Gifted children may exceed both of these expectations by moving rapidly beyond single words to syntax and/or by acquiring a large vocabulary—well in excess of 50 words—before they begin to combine words.

Once a child is producing syntax, the most conspicuous sign of verbal giftedness is the amount and sophistication of vocabulary. In all children, lexical development can be judged from a series of quantitative and qualitative changes that occur:

▷ The number of different words used increases.
▷ Word usage becomes more specific and adult-like.
▷ Vocabulary knowledge extends into an increasing number of semantic fields.
▷ There is greater knowledge of structural relationships among words, indicated by the production of synonyms, antonyms, definitions, and subordinate and superordinate terms.

Gifted children are likely to be advanced in all of these respects. Both their comprehension and production vocabularies will be larger than average. For example, in one study of fourth- to seventh-grade students, gifted children were identified by teachers' reports, reading comprehension scores, and scores on the *Peabody Picture Vocabulary Test,* a measure of receptive vocabulary. Their average vocabulary score was 130, two standard deviations above the test mean (Winne, Woodlands, & Wong, 1982). With the growth of vocabulary comes an increase in the precision with which words are used. Typical children between 1½ and 3 years of age produce a number of semantic mismatches—overextensions, underextensions, and outright misnamings (e.g., "bowl" used to talk about a toy telephone) (Crystal, 1981). Gifted children are conspicuous by the fact that they produce fewer of these mismatches. They are also less likely to rely on personal and indefinite pronouns to establish reference, being able instead to use the appropriate lexical item (Guilford, Scheuerle, & Shonburn, 1981).

Many factors influence the vocabulary that children learn, but a general developmental trend is for them to learn words across a wider range of semantic fields (Crystal, 1981, 1982). For example, we expect that much of a child's early vocabulary will pertain to fields such as man (e.g., "mommy," "brother," "boy," "police-man"), body ("tummy," "arm," "sick"), clothing ("put on," "coat," "shoe"), food ("banana," "eat," "cook"), and moving ("come," "go," "take"). Not until children are older do we find them using many words in fields such as religion ("church," "rabbi," "altar"), business ("insurance," "advertise," "secretary"), world ("continent," "soil," "equator"), or money ("check," "invest," "expensive"). Gifted children, though, are often exceptions to this rule and will amaze adults by their command of such advanced vocabulary. A sophisticated vocabulary, though, is not always an indicator of giftedness. It is possible for a child's knowledge of words in particular categories to be accelerated through specialized instruction and practice (Howe, 1990). Parents may be impressed by an ability to name state capitals, colors, or insects, but such rote knowledge is commonly found in children who do not meet psychometric criteria for giftedness (Louis & Lewis, 1992).

As vocabulary is learned, children also begin to sort out the relationships among words. Thus, they become able not only to retrieve individual words (e.g., "big") but also to retrieve words that are similar in meaning ("huge," "giant"), that are opposite in meaning ("little," "tiny"), or concepts that have some hierarchical relationship (size, dimension). This progression in vocabulary knowledge is often related to conceptual growth, particularly to the development of abstract thinking. Knowledge of antonyms, synonyms, and related vocabulary indicates that children have identified an abstract linkage among words. This paves the way for them to acquire higher-order vocabulary, such as "vehicle," "furniture," or "beverage." Conceptual development is also reflected in the ability to define words. Very young children may define "clock" by pointing to the object. Later in development, they may describe its function ("It wakes you up") or attributes ("It's round, and it's got hands"). Eventually, they are able to give both a class name and a specific attribute or property ("an instrument for telling time") (Litowitz, 1977). Gifted children are frequently advanced in their knowledge of abstract vocabulary and of word relationships. This is shown in their spontaneous use of higher-order words, their ability to paraphrase, and their ability to define words, a task included in the verbal portion of many intelligence tests (Freeman, 1979; Namy, 1967; Weiser, 1965, cited by Swafford, 1986).

Precocious vocabulary development is a striking feature of the language of gifted children. In contrast, advanced syntactic abilities may not be as dazzling but are further indications of oral language proficiency. Several measures have been used to examine the syntactic skills of gifted children. By asking children to explain the meaning of nonsense words embedded in sentences (e.g., "We saw a *trog* car"), researchers have found that gifted children are more sensitive to syntactic constraints on meaning (Williams & Tillman, 1968). Gifted children were better able to infer what the sense of a word must be based on its position within a sentence. They also perform superiorly on imitation tasks in which sentence stimuli are constructed to represent a wide range of sentence types (commands, questions, statements) and syntactic forms (passive sentences, complex sentences, expanded phrases, etc.) (Guilford et al., 1981). Studies of spontaneous speech have also shown evidence of precocious syntax. Four-year-old gifted children displayed an MLU that is above the average for their age, while gifted children in the fifth grade used longer sentences and a higher proportion of complex sentences than their typically developing peers (Guilford et al., 1981; Jensen, 1973). Also impressive is the fact that 92% of the utterances spoken by gifted 4-year-olds were free of syntactic errors compared to 74% of the utterances of their typically developing peers (Guilford et al., 1981; Lee, 1974). Among typically developing children, it is still common at that age to find errors involving forms such as pronouns, determiners, irregular inflections, auxiliary verbs, adverbs, and subject-verb agreement (Crystal, Fletcher, & Garman, 1989). Gifted children appear to be accelerated in their mastery of these potentially troublesome syntactic structures.

Differences in language use are often mentioned as a characteristic of gifted children. As noted in Table 13.2, these children are noted for their persistent and insightful question asking and for their skill in producing narratives and other oral presentations. In a formal analysis of language functions, Jensen (1973) found that gifted fifth-grade students were more likely to converse about general, scientific, or practical concerns, while their typically developing peers tended to

talk about personal experiences, perceptions, and preferences. There is little research directly comparing the pragmatic language skills of gifted and typically developing children. Following the general principle that gifted children show normal but accelerated development, we might anticipate that they would be superior in their skills of referential communication, conversational repair, and topic management. Future study may provide us with more insight into these matters.

Reading and Writing The literature on giftedness is divided on the significance of early reading ability. Many authors assert that early reading is characteristic of gifted children (Freeman, 1979, 1986; Price, 1976). But in a survey of parents of preschoolers believed to be gifted, only 16% mentioned an early interest in books and reading. Even when early reading was reported, it was not predictive of whether the child was actually gifted (Louis & Lewis, 1992). This is consistent with research suggesting that early reading is not strongly related to intellectual ability and is probably attributable to child-rearing practices (Jackson, 1988; Jackson, Donaldson, & Cleland, 1988).

There is better agreement that once they begin to read, many gifted children show an exceptional enthusiasm for books and quickly become extremely able readers. In a study of 8th-, 10th-, and 12th-grade students, it was discovered that gifted students made more frequent use of effective strategies such as rereading, inferring, predicting, and relating to content area. Average readers, on the other hand, were more often concerned about word pronunciation and made more inaccurate summaries of what they were reading (Fehrenbach, 1991). The more effective strategies used by gifted children enable them to read with greater comprehension than their peers. This provides them with a tremendous advantage in all academic areas, especially as they advance in school and reading becomes a principal method of acquiring new information (Bashir, 1989).

In comparison to their oral expression and reading skills, the writing ability of many gifted children is less impressive, although the content of what they write is frequently above average (Namy, 1967). Nevertheless, the form of their writing often resembles that of their typically developing peers. They may write in simple sentences and use a limited vocabulary (Mindell & Stracher, 1980). The discrepancy between writing and other language skills is usually explained in terms of motivation. Good writing requires a command of form—punctuation, spelling, organization—that is unnecessary for other language behaviors. Writing is also a motor skill that must be learned and integrated with the pace at which thinking occurs. Many gifted children appear to be put off by the work that is demanded for writing and by the way it slows self-expression (Freeman, 1979; McCluskey & Walker, 1986). Consequently, they may not practice their writing sufficiently to develop a level of skill equal to their other language abilities.

Language in Disadvantaged or Disabled Gifted Children

One of the top priorities recently identified by a panel of experts in gifted education was the issue of special populations of gifted children (Cramer, 1991). Three of the subgroups specifically identified were as follows:

1. Children from economically disadvantaged backgrounds, the majority of whom are members of racial/ethnic minorities.
2. Children with intellectual, motor, or sensory handicaps.
3. Children who are underachieving because of learning disabilities superimposed on a high level of intelligence.

There has been little study of these subgroups, and they have proven difficult to identify and serve.

Disadvantaged children who are also gifted are frequently not recognized. Perhaps because they anticipate and actively look for signs of giftedness in their children, white middle-class parents are far more likely to seek specialized evaluation and educational services for their preschoolers. In one study, 118 parents contacted a gifted child clinic seeking to have their children tested. Nearly equal numbers of boys and girls were referred. All the families were white middle-class, and the majority of parents were college educated (Louis & Lewis, 1992). The parents of disadvantaged children may not perceive giftedness, or they may lack the means or motivation to pursue special services.

When they begin school, disadvantaged children should have an equal opportunity to be recognized as gifted. Research has shown, however, that teachers' judgments of individual students are swayed by gender, race, and social class background (Brophy & Good, 1974; Minner, 1990). Identification is also made difficult by differences in the verbal behavior of disadvantaged students, even those who are gifted. Whereas gifted children from affluent families tend to use language in imaginative play and to comment on past or future events, gifted disadvantaged children are likely to express needs, monitor their own actions, and identify present actions and objects (Tough, 1977). Therefore, they may not adhere to the profile of a gifted child, which emphasizes verbal creativity and elaboration, as we have seen. Cultural differences and test biases, as discussed in chapter 10, may also inhibit Hispanic-American, African-American, and Asian-American children from exhibiting their competencies fully.

Studies in the psychobiology of intelligence suggest that as a general principle, specific abilities can function independently of one another (Freeman, 1986). Hence, it is possible for an individual to have a profile of abilities in which all are superior; or to have a few superior and the rest average; or even to have some superior, some average, and others inferior. An extreme and well-publicized example of discrepant ability levels is found in the **idiot savant**, an individual whose measured general intelligence is in the range of mental retardation but who evidences a specific talent, such as sculpture, music, or feats of recall. In contrast to the individual's many deficiencies, the single high ability is astonishing. Another example of discrepancy is a child with a severe disabling condition, such as cerebral palsy or autism, who nonetheless possesses superior intellectual or other abilities. We are becoming increasingly aware of such individuals as we learn to assist their communication with alternative/augmentative devices and techniques such as facilitated communication, as discussed in chapter 8. Another central problem in identifying gifted children who are disabled has been to find a nonbiased means of assessment.

A different category of children with discrepant abilities are those described as *underachievers*. These children function at levels that are roughly age appropriate, but they are hindered by learning disabilities or adverse social or emotional conditions that prevent them from realizing their full potential (Alexander & Muia, 1982; Fox, Brody, & Tobin, 1983). Formally, these children are identified by the inconsistency between their scores on IQ or achievement tests and their actual classroom performance (National Joint Committee on Learning Disabilities, 1989). Informally, these children often call attention to themselves because of personality and behavioral disturbances. Researchers have found that gifted children who do not achieve often lack self-confidence, have lower self-concepts, may have difficulty forming social relationships, and exhibit aggression (Schiff, Kaufman, & Kaufman, 1981; Waldron et al., 1987). Those gifted underachievers who have learning disabilities are often verbally superior, in contrast to most children with learning disabilities, who are linguistically deficient and perform better on nonverbal tasks. Perhaps as a result, gifted underachieving children are frequently not referred to be assessed for learning disabilities until they reach the third grade or beyond (Schiff et al., 1981).

Implications for Intervention

Professionals who serve children with language disorders have a different role to play with various subgroups of gifted children. With advantaged children who are verbally gifted, professionals in most educational settings defer to a teacher who has been charged with developing a gifted education program. That program will vary from one school to another but likely will consist of some combination of *acceleration* approaches, which attempt to provide a curriculum that matches gifted children's abilities, and *grouping* approaches, which separate gifted children from other students during certain instructional periods so that they can work at a faster pace (VanTassel-Baska, 1992). Teaching methods tend to focus less on

content, which gifted children find easy to master, and more on synthesis and creative processing of information (Freeman, 1986).

With disadvantaged gifted students, professionals have more responsibility in evaluating their abilities and interpreting issues of language difference to other educators. Gifted children with bilingual-bicultural backgrounds require attention to matters of nonbiased assessment and nonstandard dialect, as discussed in chapter 10. They also may need help in understanding and adjusting to their own giftedness. As we observed earlier, these children are much less likely to be identified by their families. Thus, most disadvantaged gifted children have never been told that they are gifted and have received little reinforcement for their exceptional abilities. Because of their cultural background as well as peer pressure, they may find it difficult to display their verbal abilities. This is a delicate issue that calls for sensitivity to a child's age, peer group, family, and ethnic group. For some children, it may be prudent to let them develop their language skills quietly through reading and writing rather than force them into special programs that create problems in psychosocial development.

Gifted children who have physical, sensory, or learning disabilities are frequently referred for intervention because of what they cannot do. Common sense dictates that professionals should try to take advantage of these children's giftedness in compensating for their deficiencies. For example, gifted children can often be taught *workaround* strategies, that is, alternative ways of accomplishing tasks they find difficult. Technology can assist these students in several ways. For children with physical or sensory handicaps, alternative/augmentative devices may be the key to all teaching efforts. For those with learning disabilities, computers, calculators, and other specialized electronic devices offer assistance with vexing tasks such as spelling, calculating, and handwriting. The psychological profile of these students indicates that they are hindered by their own frustration and lack of confidence. They may benefit from cognitive training, discussed in chapter 7, that reduces impulsive responding and promotes alternative methods of rehearsal and problem solving.

LANGUAGE AND CHILDREN WITH VISUAL IMPAIRMENT

Judged by their progress through major language milestones, few children with visual impairment as their sole disability will meet the criteria for a language disorder. Due to their sensory deficit, however, these children acquire language differently from sighted children, which often leads to a request for professional evaluation and consultation. In addition, until complete developmental and sensory evaluations can be performed, there will be a concern that a child with visual impairment may also have hearing impairment or intellectual deficits. In that event, the prognosis for normal development of language is considerably poorer. Most congenitally deaf-blind children do not develop normal communicative competence (Freeman & Blockberger, 1987). All children with mental retardation will have difficulty with language; visual impairment merely adds to that burden and raises a serious obstacle to intervention efforts.

An Overview of Visual Impairment

Definition and Cause A number of terms are used by professionals in medicine, education, and rehabilitation to describe loss of vision. *Blindness* has no fixed definition. It is possible to measure vision in different ways (Dekker & Koole, 1992). The standard optometric test is a measure of visual acuity for objects at a distance. However, many individuals with visual impairment cannot see at a distance but do possess some near vision. Furthermore, vision does not operate independently of other sensory and cognitive systems. It is possible to have some functional vision if the nervous system is able to augment a very weak visual signal with information gained from other sensory channels and from previous experiences.

The American Foundation for the Blind recommends that the term *blind* be used to refer to individuals with no usable sight. Persons with usable vision, no matter how little, should be described as *visually impaired, partially sighted,* or *low vision* (Sardegna & Otis, 1991). Within the category of blindness, distinctions are made between individuals who do and do not have light perception and between those who can and cannot detect movement, as when a hand is waved

in front of the face. Blindness may be congenital, with onset at birth or shortly after, or **adventitious,** occurring later in life. Children who become blind after 5 years of age retain visual memories and are able to visualize as an adjunct to thinking (Sardegna & Otis, 1991). Among children with visual impairment and no other deficits, language development is seriously affected only in children with congenital blindness who have no pattern recognition (Freeman & Blockberger, 1987). In the remainder of this section, we will limit the discussion to children who are congenitally blind. Children with lesser degrees of visual impairment can be expected to show greater parallels with the language development of sighted children. Children with visual impairment along with mental retardation or a physical handicap will have wide-ranging language impairments.

Congenital blindness results from diseases or conditions that are either inherited or occur in utero. Damage may affect either nonneural (lens, cornea, iris) or neural (retina, optic nerve) portions of the visual system. Certain conditions, such as retinitis pigmentosa, are degenerative, so that vision will become worse as a child grows older. Recent improvements in obstetric and **neonatal** care now allow many extremely premature infants to survive. These infants, however, are at risk of auditory and visual impairments (Allen & Capute, 1986). U.S. surveys taken in 1986 and 1989 indicated that about 2,200 legally blind babies were born and survived beyond 1 month of age. This figure compares to a total of more than 3.7 million infants living beyond 1 month in each of those years (Kirchner, Berman, & Dimitrova, 1992).

Language Characteristics of Blind Children

Few developmental differences are observed between typically developing and blind children during the first 4 months of life. At that point, sighted children begin to attend to their hands, which in turn encourages manual exploration of the environment. In contrast, children who are blind rely on others to present objects for them to manipulate. They tend to mouth objects for a slightly longer time than sighted children, probably as compensation for the loss of visual information about what they are holding (Sardegna & Otis,

1991). Blind children are generally delayed in walking and symbolic play (Fraiberg, 1977). If they are encouraged to become physically active, however, they show few differences from sighted children in gross motor skills. They have good spatial orientation and can participate in many normal games and sports. Without this encouragement and opportunity, they may develop stereotypical movements such as rocking, head swaying, and poking or rubbing of the eyes (Sardegna & Otis, 1991).

To understand how language develops in blind children, it is crucial to consider the role that vision plays in typical language development. During their first year, sighted children develop preverbal communication routines that are mediated largely through sight. Recall that:

▷ Early exchanges between parents and infants are regulated through eye contact and head turning (Brazelton, Koslowski, & Main, 1974).

▷ Shared attention is achieved by the parent and infant each watching the other's eye movements (Bruner, 1975).

▷ Systematic use of gesture is an important early form of intentional communication and overlaps with children's first use of meaningful words (Bates, Camaioni, & Volterra, 1975; Fogel, 1980).

Blind children also develop routines with their parents but do so through a more laborious auditory-tactile process. For example, while it is possible to observe when a child is attending auditorily, the cues—cocking the head or becoming still—are subtle and easily missed (Urwin, 1984). Therefore, the mother tends to talk more and use touch and body contact to maintain a link with the child. Mother and child play games involving repetition and anticipation, comparable to peekaboo, but using touching, tickling, stroking, and other forms of contact instead of visual cues. The infant's vocalizations are actively encouraged to the point where idiosyncratic routines may develop. These vocal routines, though they also occur in sighted children, are especially important to the development of blind children because they serve as both an emotional link to the caretaker and a key sensory experience (Urwin, 1984). Pointing and reaching

for sources of sound are delayed in these children. Not surprisingly, therefore, the onset of meaningful speech occurs slightly later than in sighted children.

Children who are blind become more developmentally heterogeneous as they grow older. Many factors have an impact on their language development, including the degree of visual loss, the presence of other impairments, and the response of caretakers to their impairments. Nevertheless, certain behaviors occur with sufficient frequency in these children to be considered generally characteristic.

Syntax The syntactic development of blind children differs little from that of sighted children. They are slightly delayed in beginning to use word combinations but, by age 3, their MLUs are comparable to those of their typically developing peers (Landau & Gleitman, 1985). Utterance length may be less representative of syntactic competence than it is in typically developing children because of blind children's tendency to echo phrases they hear before they have productive control of the syntax of those phrases.

Semantics As vocabulary is learned, the contexts and functions of words tend to be restricted. Words first learned in the context of routine activities, such as eating or bathing, may not be used outside those contexts until a child is much older. Typically developing children commonly overextend the meanings of early words, for example, using "juice" to refer to all potable liquids. Most of these overextensions are based on visual similarities among objects. As might be expected, blind children rarely overextend the meanings of words they acquire (Andersen, Dunlea, & Kekelis, 1984).

A number of early-developing concepts are closely linked to visual experiences. Thus, children who are blind may be slow to understand or use words such as "dirty," "clean," "open," "shut," "in," "out," "up," and "down." This delay appears to be due exclusively to the lack of sensory experience. Concepts and words that can be learned through other sense information, such as "sticky," "sweet," "hot," "cold," and "big," are readily learned (Sardegna & Otis, 1991).

Blind children may display a type of egocentrism in the learning of words that are not substantial. Action words may be used only to refer to actions they are performing and not to actions involving other people or objects (Andersen et al., 1984). For example, the words "up" and "down" may be used only to request or describe the child's own movement and not as general locative terms (Urwin, 1984). Relational vocabulary, such as "more" or "no," may be used only in expressing personal needs and not in commenting on changes of state in the environment (Andersen et al., 1984).

In typically developing children, vision facilitates awareness of themselves as separate from others and from their environment (Sardegna & Otis, 1991). Delays in a blind child's internal representation of self may be responsible for the pronominal reversals and confusions they often display (Fraiberg & Adelson, 1977). For example, one child requested a drink by saying, "I want some juice. She wants some juice" (Kitzinger, 1984, p. 142). Alternatively, pronoun confusion may be viewed as a problem with understanding deictic language, where meaning changes according to the speaker's perspective. Other deictic words, such as "here," "there," "this," and "that," also present difficulties to blind children (Andersen et al., 1984).

Echolalia   A characteristic of blind children's communication that draws frequent comment is their use of imitation. As in children with autism, this behavior is described as *echolalia* when it appears to occur in an automatic and unthinking way, that is, when the listener believes the speech was repeated without communicative intent (Howlin, 1982; Prizant & Rydell, 1984). A high proportion of blind children's utterances may be echoic. In one study of a 3-year-old girl, the percentage of echoed utterances in spontaneous speech was 20.7% with her mother and 35.7% with an adult she knew slightly (Kitzinger, 1984).

Echoed utterances may appear more unusual than they really are. Lacking sight, blind children must find substitutes for many communicative behaviors that are typically accomplished with nonverbal visual signals. For example, repetition frequently serves the function of acknowledgment, which sighted children perform nonverbally by looking, nodding the head, changing facial expression, and so on. Sighted children are known to produce **monologues** that serve the purposes of verbal rehearsal, dramatic play, and direction of their own actions (Piaget, 1926; Weir, 1970). Yet this speech is typically accompanied by movement, especially with the hands, that gives the words a context. Kitzinger (1984) gives an example of and a commentary about a blind girl's monologue in which she produces different voices but gives no other clues about the purpose of her language:

> Some of Betty's [the blind child's] echoed comments gave the impression that she had incorporated wholesale, without modification, aspects of others' speech:
>> Betty is sitting on her potty and the following "conversation" takes place.
>> **Betty:** (with echoed intonation) Pull down your pants. You're too big for the potty.
>> **Betty:** (in her own voice) I'm too big for the potty.
>> **MK** [the adult]: Who says that?
>> **Betty:** (calling out) Ann! Ann!
>> **MK:** Does Ann say you are too big for the potty?
>> **Betty:** (with echoed intonation) Ann's toilet is never . . . (unintelligible) . . . on the potty.
> Betty seems to be relaying some former experience prompted by the context. It was said without any apparent intention of communicating something to me but had the quality of play of a sighted child, perhaps with a doll as a prop. Had she used such a prop a shared context would have been provided and the purpose of these utterances would have been clearer. (p. 142)

Pragmatics   Blindness has some inevitable consequences for the way in which children use language. For example, language is used less often to name or request objects that are remote and cannot be touched. Certain features of language may develop earlier or to a greater extent because they serve a compensatory role. Rising intonation may be used from an early age to keep a conversation going. Sighted children typically use eye contact for the same purpose. Blind children may show greater knowledge and use of people's names, for this gives them the ability to initiate social interactions even when they cannot locate the conversational partner (Urwin, 1984).

Unusual nonverbal mannerisms may develop in blind children because they cannot observe certain behaviors during conversation. For obvious reasons, they have more difficulty in adjusting their vocal loudness to suit the distance of the listener. Therefore, they tend to speak at a constant, loud level (Freeman & Blockberger, 1987). Blind children tend to nod their heads less often but to smile more often. They may have eyebrow movements that appear inappropriate because these are not used to indicate interest or give emphasis to what is being spoken (Parke, Shallcross, & Anderson, 1980).

Implications for Intervention

Unlike many other groups of children with language disorders, there is some question whether language intervention is necessary for blind children. Most professionals agree, however, that intervention is needed to monitor and interpret the child's language acquisition because it can be expected to follow a different developmental path. Freeman and Blockberger (1987) suggest that intervention with blind children and their families should have three objectives:

1. Helping the child gain information through sources other than vision.
2. Helping the parents to interact with the child in ways that are stimulating and enjoyable.
3. Modifying those behaviors of the child that bring negative attention and reduce communicative effectiveness.

During the first year of life, the child will be quite dependent on the parents for stimulation. Obviously, sound and touch must be used to fill in the gaps left by the child's lack of vision. With sighted infants it is possible to have interactions that are mostly nonverbal. While it should not be necessary to talk all the time, mothers of blind children do talk more and have more frequent physical contact with them (Urwin, 1984).

The interests and concerns of the parents must be considered. Some parents may worry mainly about the child's physical independence and therefore emphasize early motor experiences. Other parents may focus on trying to normalize the child's learning by providing an enriched environment for manual exploration and auditory and tactile stimulation (Urwin, 1984). Both sets of goals are important and can be used to facilitate the acquisition of language.

Superficially, some blind children may resemble children with autism because of their stereotyped movements, echolalia, and pronoun confusions. We have seen, however, that each of these behaviors is an understandable consequence of the lack of vision. In general, they will become less frequent as the children grow and become more independent. Professionals can be useful by providing an interpretation of the behaviors and by preventing negative reactions when they occur. For example, when blind children echo for no clear purpose, the natural reaction is to redirect the conversation. By doing this, however, we are not reinforcing the child's attempt to communicate through available means. It is important to try to discern the child's intent and then respond appropriately to it (Kitzinger, 1984).

Blind children are a small population, and it is, therefore, difficult to develop good instincts for working with them and their families. Despite their training, many professionals may tend to overcompensate for the visual impairment rather than relying on a style of interaction that is generally effective with children. On the other hand, some necessary modifications are easily forgotten because visual ability is so easily assumed. Table 13.4 lists some suggestions that may facilitate interactions with blind children.

On the whole, progress in language acquisition cannot always be judged accurately by comparing blind children to the developmental milestones of typically developing children. Some early communicative behaviors are delayed because they must be mediated through touch or hearing, which are less efficient sources of information. As a general guideline, professionals should always ask themselves whether a child's behavior is reasonable and even understandable in view of the sensory deficit.

LANGUAGE AND CHILDREN WITH NEUROMOTOR IMPAIRMENT

Unlike many of the other populations of children discussed in this text, children with neuromotor impairment do not present unique symptoms of language disorder. This does not mean that they are free of communication difficulties. Their language problems, though, are not the direct result of the neuromotor

TABLE 13.4   Suggestions for Interacting with
Blind Children

▷ Talk in a normal voice.

▷ Provide verbal signals to substitute for nonverbal cues. For example, narrate what you are doing when you introduce or change materials.

▷ Make sure that drawers, cabinet doors, and other obstacles are either fully open or shut.

▷ Feel comfortable using "sighted" words such as "see," "look," or "pretty." Blind children will interpret these appropriately in relation to their abilities.

▷ Tell the child when you are going to move to another part of the room.

▷ Don't be surprised if the child reacts negatively to being suddenly held or picked up. This is not a rejection of affection but a response to being interrupted unexpectedly.

▷ State your name when you approach the child unless you are well known. Don't expect that the child will recognize your voice.

▷ Don't use toy miniatures unless the child has previous experience with them. Remember that most representational toys rely on visual analogy with the real objects.

Sources: Adapted from Sardegna and Otis (1991) and van Kleek and Richardson (1988).

disorders that interfere with posture and movement. Instead, these children are impaired communicators because of conditions that frequently coexist with neuromuscular disorders: mental retardation, hearing impairment, visual impairment, and seizure disorders. They may also suffer from general delays because motoric disabilities interfere with their abilities to explore the environment and to speak, gesture, and engage in social interaction.

Children with Cerebral Palsy

The most common neuromotor disorder in children is **cerebral palsy**. This condition has no single cause and includes many different types and distributions of muscular impairment. The common elements in cerebral palsy are as follows:

▷ It is caused by an injury to the brain.

▷ It appears very early in life, either at birth or during the preschool years.

▷ The damage to the brain does not become worse over time, though an individual's capability for functional movement may deteriorate (Boone, 1972; Scherzer & Tscharnuter, 1990).

Etiology and Types of Cerebral Palsy   The causes of cerebral palsy are classified by when they occur: during pregnancy (prenatal), during birth (perinatal), or during the first few years of life (postnatal). Prenatal events, such as infection, physical injury, or substance abuse, may cause injury to the fetus or disrupt the normal development of the nervous system. During delivery, the major risks are lack of oxygen (anoxia), infection, and cerebral hemorrhage (Scherzer & Tscharnuter, 1990). Postnatal causes include cerebrovascular accidents, brain infection, and trauma. We see that there is overlap between the etiological categories of postnatal cerebral palsy and acquired childhood aphasia. The latter is discussed in chapter 12.

Estimates of the incidence of cerebral palsy vary between 1 and 6 children per 1,000 (Copeland & Kimmel, 1989; McDonald & Chance, 1964). Recent studies indicate two opposite trends in the frequency of the disorder. The number of perinatal cases appears to be declining, probably as the result of improvements in obstetric care and fetal monitoring equipment used during delivery. On the other hand, improvements in neonatal medicine have increased the survival of low-birth-weight (premature) babies, who have an elevated risk of cerebral palsy (Skidmore, Rivers, & Hack, 1990).

Different types of cerebral palsy are distinguished by the nature of the movement disorder and the portion of the body it affects. Tables 13.5 and 13.6 show the two systems of classification. It is also common for professionals to rate the severity of symptoms as mild, moderate, or severe. Roughly a third of all cases are considered to fall into each severity category (Scherzer & Tscharnuter, 1990). The number of severe cases may be increasing, however, due to the rise in the number of low-birth-weight babies. Prematurely born children with cerebral palsy tend to show more severe involvement (Franco & Andrews, 1977).

Associated Problems   Rarely are the problems of children with cerebral palsy limited to their neuro-

TABLE 13.5   Classification of Cerebral Palsy by Neuromuscular Characteristics

Type	Frequency	Characteristics
Spastic	50%	▷ Increased muscle tone ▷ Exaggerated stretch reflex ▷ Slow, effortful, jerky voluntary movement
Athetoid	10%	▷ Involuntary movements when volitional actions are attempted ▷ Fluctuating muscle tone: normal at rest, increased with voluntary movement ▷ Involuntary movement increases with stress or distraction
Ataxic	5–10%	▷ Disturbed equilibrium leading to problems of balance ▷ Normal reflexes and muscle tone
Rigid	1%	▷ Simultaneous contraction of all muscle groups, producing constant muscle tone ▷ Slow, effortful voluntary movement; involuntary movement may be better
Mixed	30%	▷ Combination of more than one type; most commonly spasticity and athetosis ▷ One type usually predominates

Sources: Adapted from Boone (1972), Copeland and Kimmel (1989), and Scherzer and Tscharnuter (1990).

motor difficulties. Table 13.7 summarizes information on some of the most commonly associated problems. In children with multiple handicaps, it is exceedingly difficult to judge the contribution of each impairment to the total disorder. For example, we might expect children with cerebral palsy to be slightly delayed in their cognitive development because of the limitations imposed on their physical exploration of the environment. If these children are also visually impaired, their ability to learn through observation will be compromised, leading to much greater restrictions on cognitive growth. And if these children are further affected by seizures, the pace of learning can slow markedly, or even regress, if the seizures are severe enough to produce brain damage.

Language Characteristics of Children with Cerebral Palsy   There is no pattern of communication deficits that is always identified with cerebral palsy. Every child with this condition has a profile of lan-

TABLE 13.6   Classification of Cerebral Palsy by Limb Distribution

Type	Frequency	Description
Monoplegia	Rare	One limb involved
Hemiplegia		Arm and leg involved on only one side
Paraplegia	Very rare	Only legs involved
Quadriplegia		Trunk and all limbs involved
Diplegia		All limbs involved but lesser involvement of arms

Sources: Adapted from Boone (1972), Copeland and Kimmel (1989), and Scherzer and Tscharnuter (1990).

TABLE 13.7 Associated Problems in Children with Cerebral Palsy

Mental retardation	Between 50% and 75% are estimated to be intellectually impaired (Cruickshank, 1976). Testing is difficult or impossible with some children because of their inability to produce reliable verbal or other motor responses.
Orthopedic problems	Nearly all children have some orthopedic problem stemming from an imbalance in muscle forces. Physical therapy is prescribed to facilitate the development of motor reflexes and reduce the imbalances. Bracing is used to stabilize limbs, permitting greater mobility, and to counteract muscular pressure that leads to bone deformities. If these therapies are ineffective, surgery may be recommended to restore muscle balance or stabilize certain joints (Boone, 1972).
Feeding problems	Feeding problems result from abnormal development of oral reflexes and damage to the cranial nerves that supply the muscles of the face and mouth. Dental problems may also develop. Children will have difficulty with all phases of eating: sucking, chewing, and swallowing. Problems can be reduced through customized feeding programs that include precise positioning, relaxation and desensitization exercises, and special procedures for introducing food into the mouth (Inge, 1992).
Hearing loss	Estimates of hearing loss vary from 5% to 40% of children with cerebral palsy (Boone, 1972; Nober, 1976). Both conductive and sensorineural losses are found.
Seizures	Seizures occur commonly, especially in children of the spastic type (Boone, 1972). Anticonvulsant medications are often prescribed to control seizure activity. Some medications can adversely affect attention.
Visual impairment	Visual problems can result in an expressionless appearance and are associated with poor head control. Perception of color is better than perception of shape. Spatial perception is frequently poor, causing difficulty in reaching for objects (Jan, Groenveld, Sykanda, & Hoyt, 1987).

guage skills that is derived from the severity of the neuromotor disorder, the number of associated problems, and the manner in which all of these impairments interact. Several other chapters in this text contain discussions of language characteristics that are potentially relevant to children with cerebral palsy. Children with mental retardation are described in chapter 6; children with learning disabilities in chapter 7; children with hearing impairment in chapter 9; children with acquired aphasia in chapter 12; and children with visual impairment in this chapter. If a child

with cerebral palsy comes from a bilingual-bicultural family, then chapter 10 is also pertinent.

A key to predicting the language deficits and potential of children with cerebral palsy is to assess their ability to compensate. Table 13.8 shows a simple outline of five resources for language learning and suggests how a child can compensate for the loss of each. For example, children with neuromotor disorders are denied normal opportunities for physical exploration of the environment. In typically developing children, this exploration increases their knowledge of the

TABLE 13.8 Compensation for Loss of Language Learning Resources

Resource	Compensation
Physical exploration	Hearing, sight, intelligence
Hearing	Sight, physical exploration, intelligence
Sight	Hearing, physical exploration, intelligence
Intelligence	Social interaction
Social interaction	Intelligence

world and leads to preverbal communicative interactions. Children with cerebral palsy need to compensate through vicarious experience, which is most effective if they possess normal hearing, sight, and intelligence.

Children with both cerebral palsy and mental retardation must work harder to compensate. As a rule, children with mental retardation require additional language stimulation, which can be brought about through greater social interaction. However, social interaction will be made more difficult by the children's **motor impairment**. If adjustments are made—by pro-

viding extra time and structuring the interaction so that only simple motor responses are required—then a child with both of these conditions may still acquire considerable language.

Compensation becomes extremely difficult if, along with cerebral palsy and mental retardation, a child also has a sensory deficit. Whether hearing or sight is impaired, two of the normal means of compensation—physical exploration and intelligence—are not fully available. Therefore, the child is reduced to a very small window of experience and can be expected to show severe problems in the acquisition of language.

A child with cerebral palsy may have a language disorder as well as problems with speech.

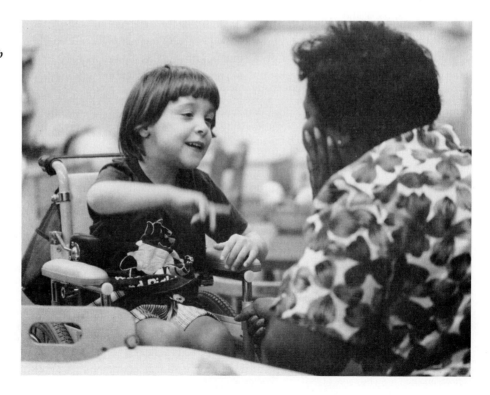

Even when a child with cerebral palsy is capable of learning language, there remain serious problems in how that language can be encoded. Depending on the nature and extent of the child's neuromotor impairment, the ability to speak or use the hands to communicate (through gesture, writing, or signing) may be seriously compromised. The primary speech impairment in cerebral palsy is **dysarthria**, produced by neuromuscular damage affecting the systems for respiration, phonation, and articulation. The likelihood of dysarthria increases with the amount of upper limb involvement. Thus, it is uncommon in children with **hemiplegia** or **paraplegia** and is most frequent and severe in children with **quadriplegia** (Thompson, 1988). The major symptoms of dysarthria found in children with different types of cerebral palsy are shown in Table 13.9. There may also be articulatory symptoms, such as difficulty with speech initiation or inconsistent error patterns, that are better attributed to an apraxia of speech (a neurological disorder that affects the ability to plan speech movements). Regardless of the diagnosis, the effect on language acquisition will be to reduce the child's ability for self-expression. Communication may still be possible, but never at the speed or level of sophistication of the child's typically developing peers.

The role of speech practice in advancing the development of language is unclear. The rewards for language use are undoubtedly fewer for children with cerebral palsy, which may reduce their motivation to learn. We do not know whether the ability to speak is also an important element in certain mechanisms of language learning, for example, imitation and verbal rehearsal. One study of adolescents with cerebral palsy found that they scored low on tests of receptive vocabulary and same-different phoneme discrimination. The investigators suggested that the children were less able to store phonological information because of their speech production difficulties. This memory weakness may cause a specific impairment in the learning of vocabulary (Bishop, Byers Brown, & Robson, 1990). Though some children with cerebral palsy are able to develop high levels of language competence despite their limited speaking ability, they appear to be exceptions to the general rule.

Implications for Intervention Children with cerebral palsy have multiple disabilities that require

TABLE 13.9   Symptoms of Developmental Dysarthria in Children with Cerebral Palsy

Subsystem	Nonspeech Problems	Speech Problems
Respiration	▷ Reversed breathing (simultaneous muscle movements for inhalation and exhalation) ▷ Rapid, shallow breathing ▷ Involuntary movement of respiratory muscles	▷ Short phrasing (small number of words spoken per breath) ▷ Frequent inspiration ▷ Decreased rate of speech
Phonation	▷ Incomplete approximation of vocal folds ▷ Involuntary spasms of vocal folds ▷ Increased or decreased tension of vocal folds, depending on type of cerebral palsy	▷ Breathy voice ▷ Decreased loudness but with sudden bursts ▷ Reduced variation in pitch but with sudden pitch breaks
Resonance	▷ Inadequate velopharyngeal closure	▷ Hypernasality
Articulation	▷ Weakness in articulatory muscles ▷ Reduced range of motion ▷ Variation in muscle tone ▷ Abnormal jaw and tongue reflexes	▷ Middle vowels are most accurate, front and back vowels more difficult ▷ Consonant manner errors predominate, especially with fricatives and affricates ▷ Final consonant sounds are more difficult ▷ More severe problems in individuals with athetosis than in those with spasticity

Source: Adapted from Edwards (1984) and Thompson (1988).

intervention from a number of cooperating professionals. The goals of language intervention can vary considerably, depending on the type, distribution, and severity of each child's neuromotor impairment and the number of associated problems. For instance, a child with mild spastic hemiplegia and moderate hearing loss might require only amplification and short-term articulation therapy. But a child with severe athetoid quadriplegia and mental retardation would most likely be a candidate for a simple alternative/augmentative communication device. In all cases, language intervention has three purposes:

1. To compensate for impaired motor and sensory functions.
2. To facilitate the development of motor speech skills and cognitive-linguistic abilities.
3. To modify the environment so that the child is able to communicate more independently.

Because cerebral palsy is usually detected at birth or soon afterward, early intervention is possible and desirable, especially for efforts at compensation and facilitation. Environmental adaptations that move a child in the direction of independence naturally become more important in later years.

A central component of all intervention for children with cerebral palsy is the development of a program for proper handling and positioning. Abnormal variations in muscle tone usually result in undesirable movements and postures that inhibit skill development. By handling and positioning these children properly, muscle tone is more normalized and the body is better stabilized to allow standing and limb movement (Inge, 1992). Occupational and physical therapists will usually be in charge of developing the program, but everyone interacting with a child will be expected to assist in its implementation.

Compensation for sensory impairments must begin with auditory and visual assessment. Depending on the extent of any losses that are discovered, three avenues of intervention are available: (1) amplification of input by means of hearing aids and glasses; (2) training to improve specific subskills such as visual tracking, scanning, use of peripheral vision, sound localization, and sound discrimination; and (3) use of alternative input sources, such as vibrotactile units that convert sound into vibrations felt on the skin (Marchant, 1992).

Motor speech skills are best facilitated in the context of feeding. Special exercises and feeding techniques have been developed to reduce the interference of oral **reflexes** during biting, chewing, and swallowing (Morris & Klein, 1987). These procedures are implemented during infancy, before a child is expected to talk, in order to provide a better foundation for oral motor skills. Once the child's motor and sensory abilities have been attended to, language and cognitive development are promoted through a home program of stimulation and social interaction. The task of the professional is often to help interpret the child's communicative behaviors, which may be ambiguous at first glance, and to offer steadfast encouragement to the parents, who must continue to provide stimulation even when there may be little response in return.

The chief adaptation that can be made to help the communication of children with cerebral palsy is to introduce an alternative/augmentative device. At one time, nonspeech communication systems were considered a last resort, to be attempted only after all attempts at training speech had been exhausted. That attitude has changed dramatically in recent years due to improvements in technology and changes in public attitudes toward the disabled. The argument that the general public will be put off by alternative/augmentative communication devices or unable to understand them has lost most of its force. As useful as these devices can be, it should be remembered that, by themselves, they can only facilitate language form and not its content or use. Studies of the conversational acts employed by alternative/augmentative system users have shown that many types of acts are absent. The general tendency is for these individuals to produce mainly responses to information requests (Lewis & Ripich, 1984; Udwin & Yule, 1991).

Children with cerebral palsy require intervention in almost all aspects of their lives. Because the intervention is so pervasive, it imposes a particular burden on the family of the child. Professionals should be especially sensitive to parents' need to be the child's primary caretakers. Morris (1987) has distinguished between vertical and horizontal approaches with regard to relating to parents. In the *vertical approach,* the professional acts as an authority who dictates to the parents. In the *horizontal approach,* the parents and professional work together on equal terms to identify and solve the child's problems. Parents are acknowledged as the best source of information about their child's daily abilities and problems. They are asked questions such as "What are your goals?" and "What would you like to see changed?" The horizontal approach has greater ecological validity in that it provides the professional with better access to information about the child's everyday routine. This should improve the outcome of language intervention, as well as letting the family participate more fully in decisions about the child.

Also not to be forgotten are the nonaffected siblings of a child with cerebral palsy. Given the demands made on the time and resources of the parents by the disabled child, siblings can easily develop feelings of resentment and jealousy. One solution may be to involve siblings as change agents. This approach has been used successfully to improve both the physical status and the daily living skills of children with cerebral palsy (Craft, Lakin, Oppliger, Clancy, & Vanderlinden, 1990). Similar successes may be possible with communication goals.

Communication of Other Children with Neuromotor Impairment

Although cerebral palsy is the most common form of neuromotor impairment, it is not the only one. Other neurological diseases and injuries can impair a child's ability to communicate. A brief summary of some of those conditions is presented here.

Muscular Dystrophy   In contrast to cerebral palsy, **muscular dystrophy** is a progressive disorder that produces weakness and wasting of muscles (Cutler, 1992). The earliest signs of the condition are problems of balance and motor coordination. Over time the arms, legs, and face are affected, so that eventually children are unable to walk or talk. There are several types of muscular dystrophy, most of which are genetically determined metabolic disorders that result in poor oxygenation and nutrition of muscle tissue (Warfel &

Schlagenhauff, 1980). Duchenne muscular dystrophy, the most common type, has its onset in early childhood. Boys are affected almost exclusively and most children are wheelchair bound by age 10 (Jung et al., 1989). Children frequently die within 10 to 15 years after the first symptoms are observed, usually as the result of respiratory or acute infections (Mullins, 1979).

Most studies of children with Duchenne muscular dystrophy indicate that they generally have lowered intellectual functioning. Verbal abilities appear consistently lower than performance abilities in young children, but there is more balance among some older children. This suggests that language deficits, especially in reading and spelling, persist in a proportion of these children (Dorman, Hurley, & D'Avignon, 1988). Speech production abilities are related to the progress of the disorder. As muscular degeneration occurs, it affects the respiratory, phonatory, and articulatory systems, producing a gradually worsening dysarthria. Intervention is usually targeted at each child's specific language difficulties and at achieving the best possible compensation for the motor speech disorder. Alternative/augmentative communication systems may be used when intelligible speech becomes impossible.

Spina Bifida   Spina bifida refers to a range of defects caused by a cleft in the spinal column. It is the most common central nervous system malformation. The spinal cord, the protective sheath around it, or the vertebrae of the spine can be affected. The defects usually occur in the lower portions of the spinal column. Milder forms of spina bifida do not affect the spinal cord itself and can, if necessary, be corrected by surgery. The most severe form of the disorder, spina bifida myelomeningocele, is caused by a large opening in the vertebral column through which the spinal cord and nerve roots protrude. Surgery, performed to repair the open defects, typically results in the loss of sensation and voluntary movement below the level of the vertebral anomaly. About 75% of children with spina bifida myelomeningocele also have hydrocephalus and are, therefore, at risk for mental retardation (Bergsma, 1979; Mullins, 1979; Sadler, 1990).

Speech and language disturbances in children with spina bifida result primarily from any associated mental retardation (Byrne, Abbeduto, & Brooks, 1990; Tew, 1991). As in children with cerebral palsy, the motor impairment severely reduces the opportunities for physical exploration and may therefore contribute to cognitive delays.

Spinal Cord Injury The most common cause of spinal cord injury is trauma from motor vehicle and sports accidents. Typically the injury results in fracture and dislocation of the cervical vertebra. The spinal cord is compressed, and the blood supply may be reduced by damage to the anterior spinal artery. Sudden quadriplegia can occur if the head is severely flexed or extended. Recovery can be improved by steroid treatment if it is administered shortly after the accident (Cutler, 1992).

There are typically no direct effects on speech and language from a spinal cord injury. If a child sustains head trauma in the same accident, then acquired aphasia may result, as discussed in chapter 12.

LANGUAGE AND CHILDREN WITH CLEFT PALATE

There is no question that children with cleft palate have unique problems in mastering phonetic skills. The patterns of articulation and resonance that are characteristic of these children are strongly related to the severity of the cleft and the adequacy of the result achieved by corrective surgery. This relationship is captured in the commonly used phrase *cleft palate speech,* which indicates that the quality of speech is determined in most respects by the nature of the structural deficit. The question raised here is whether there is such a thing as *cleft palate language,* that is, a differentiated pattern of language disability that is exclusive to children with orofacial anomalies.

An Overview of Cleft Palate

Cleft lip, cleft palate, and related disorders are congenital malformations of the midface and oral cavity. A variety of forms occur, ranging from a small notch of the lip to a total cleavage affecting the lip, bony palate,

soft palate, and other facial structures. Genetic factors are the most important influence on the development of clefts, but certain drugs and environmental pollutants have also been implicated (McWilliams, Morris, & Shelton, 1984). In some instances, clefting occurs as part of a larger syndrome, which can include mental retardation and other disabilities as concomitant problems (Jung et al., 1989).

Incidence figures vary, depending on the range of clefting that is included. McWilliams et al. (1984) offer the "safe, conservative estimate" that 1 child out of every 750 is born with cleft lip, cleft palate, or both. For reasons not yet known, the frequency of clefting is lowest for African-Americans and grows progressively higher for white Americans, Asian-Americans, and certain groups of Native Americans (Chung & Myrianthopoulos, 1968; Oka, 1979; Ross & Johnson, 1972). The occurrence of combined cleft lip and palate is nearly twice as great for males, but females have a higher incidence of isolated cleft palate (Oka, 1979).

One of the major complications of palatal clefting is the elevated risk it brings for middle ear disease and conductive hearing loss. This problem exists for most children both before and after surgical repair of the palatal opening. It is caused by a combination of obstruction, structural anomaly, and muscle weakness, all of which affect the functioning of the eustachian tube (McWilliams et al., 1984). Vigilance in diagnosing and treating middle ear disease in children with clefts appears to bring the frequency of conductive hearing loss in line with that of typically developing children (Broen, Doyle, Moller, & Prouty, 1991).

Language Characteristics of Children with Cleft Palate

The effect of cleft palate on language development is best conceived as a set of interacting risk factors. Individually, the impact of these factors is probably quite limited. Collectively, however, they appear capable of disrupting the normal processes of language acquisition. The variables often identified as significant will now be considered.

Mental Retardation The risk of mental retardation is high only among children who have clefts as part of a syndrome that includes other anomalies. Among children whose only anomaly is a cleft, there is a slight tendency for those with isolated cleft palate to score lower on intelligence tests (McWilliams et al., 1984). The differences in performance are very small, however.

Hearing Loss   Because of their risk of developing middle ear disease, children with cleft palate are virtually certain to experience fluctuating conductive hearing loss. In one study, children followed for 9 to 24 months were found to have depressed hearing on 16% of the days (Broen et al., 1991). The frequency of hearing loss is probably even higher for children who are not monitored so closely.

Surgery and Recuperation   Surgery for cleft lip is usually performed at about 3 months of age. The repair of the palate is commonly postponed until later, but in most cases it is completed before 2 years of age (McWilliams et al., 1984). Thus, children with cleft lip and palate must undergo two surgeries in their first 2 years of life. Postsurgically, they must be somewhat limited in their activities to protect the wound and prevent infection. The effects of these experiences on language development are not well known and seem likely to vary among children. Nevertheless, they do appear to alter, at least temporarily, the normal patterns of parent–child interaction and motor exploration. One study found that children with cleft palate only scored lower on developmental scales of activity and imaginative play between 6 and 24 months (Starr, Chinsky, Canter, & Meier, 1977). These developmental delays may slow progress in certain aspects of language acquisition.

Disruption in Speech Production   Palatal surgery is typically performed at about the time a child is starting to talk. Studies of the prelinguistic vocalizations of babies with cleft palate show that they pro-duce fewer oral sounds and more nasals and **glottals** (Devers & Broen, 1991; Grunwell & Russell, 1987; O'Gara & Logemann, 1988). Following the surgery, which facilitates oral sound production, there probably must be a reorganization of the motor schemes for producing speech (Broen et al., 1991). This may cause a delay in the acquisition and use of meaningful vocabulary.

Unintelligible Speech   Nearly all children with cleft palate will have reduced speech intelligibility, especially until the cleft has been surgically corrected and they have had time to adjust to the changes in the speech mechanism. This poor intelligibility will hinder parents and other conversational partners from responding appropriately to children's speech attempts. The number of successful communicative interactions will be diminished, and language learning may be curbed.

Studies on the language development of children with cleft palate have been conducted for over 50 years. The main findings of this research are that these children do display mild delays in language acquisition. In early childhood, both language comprehension and production are affected. After the preschool years, the problems tend to become expressive (McWilliams et al., 1984). Vocabulary learning may be one of the more consistent areas of deficit. Compared to their typically developing peers, children with cleft palate who are just beginning to talk tend to use words that begin with different sounds. For some children this may reflect an avoidance of sounds they find difficult to produce (Estrem & Broen, 1989). Cumulative records of the vocabulary used during the second year of life have shown that children with clefts consistently lag behind in lexical acquisition (Broen et al., 1991). As they grow older, the gap in language abilities gradually closes. The problems that remain often appear related to interpersonal factors, such as concerns about appearance and peer acceptance.

SUMMARY

In this chapter we have seen that:

▶ *Giftedness* has no sanctioned definition. Experts generally describe it as either the potential or actual demonstration of exceptional abilities.

▶ Not all gifted children have exceptional verbal abilities. Those who do follow typical developmental paths but at an accelerated rate.

▶ Three special populations of gifted children are those from disadvantaged backgrounds, those with physical or sensory disabilities, and those with concomitant learning disabilities.

▶ Intervention with disabled gifted children is designed to help them compensate for their impairments. The superior intelligence of these children may facilitate the use of technology and cognitive teaching strategies.

▶ The major variables in visual impairment are degree of loss and age of onset. Children with no useful sight from birth are described as congenitally blind and show a different pattern of language development.

▶ The early language development of blind children is affected by the unavailability of vision to guide early mother–infant interactions.

▶ The major differences in blind children's language are semantic and pragmatic. Words are used more restrictively and may be acquired later if the underlying concept is visual. Language functions related to sight are also delayed. Unusual or inappropriate nonverbal behaviors may develop.

▶ Echolalia is not uncommon in blind children and is used to compensate for nonverbal, visually mediated behaviors that are not available to blind children.

▶ Intervention with blind children should help to compensate for sensory loss, facilitate parent–child interaction, and reduce the frequency of inappropriate behaviors.

▶ Cerebral palsy is a set of nonprogressive neuromotor disorders caused by brain damage during fetal development or infancy.

▶ There is no standard profile of language disability in children with cerebral palsy. Deficits result from the combined effect of neuromotor impairment, seizures, sensory loss, and mental retardation.

▶ Language intervention in cases of nonprogressive neuromotor impairment aims to compensate for those motor and sensory functions that will remain impaired, to stimulate cognitive-linguistic abilities, and to modify the environment so that the child can function more independently within it.

▶ Neuromotor disorders other than cerebral palsy have different effects on speech and language abilities. Progressive disorders cause steady deterioration of function. Some disorders have little or no effect on communication.

▶ Children with cleft palate who do not have other physical anomalies exhibit mild delays in language acquisition that are in most cases outgrown.

▶ Hearing loss, time spent in surgery and recuperation, structural changes in the speech mechanism, and unintelligible speech are the most conspicuous factors affecting the language development of children with clefts.

In this chapter we have examined four groups of children who present very different language characteristics. Their needs for language intervention may extend from comprehensive services to no services at all. Professionals must be prepared to encounter a range of associated problems and ability levels. They should be careful not to assume that certain competencies are present. Nor should they restrict their expectations of what these children can accomplish.

REFERENCES

Alexander, P. A., & Muia, J. A. (1982). *Gifted education: A comprehensive roadmap.* Rockville, MD: Aspen.

Allen, M. C., & Capute, A. J. (1986). Assessment of early auditory and visual abilities of extremely premature infants. *Developmental Medicine and Child Neurology, 28,* 458–466.

Andersen, E. S., Dunlea, A., & Kekelis, L. S. (1984). Blind children's language: Resolving some differences. *Journal of Child Language, 11,* 645–664.

Bashir, A. S. (1989). Language intervention and the curriculum. *Seminars in Speech and Language, 10,* 181–191.

Bates, E., Camaioni, L., & Volterra, V. (1975). The acquisition of performatives prior to speech. *Merrill-Palmer Quarterly, 21,* 205–216.

Bergsma, D. (1979). *Birth defects compendium* (2nd ed.). New York: Alan R. Liss.

Bishop, D. V. M., Byers Brown, B., & Robson, J. (1990). The relationship between phoneme discrimination, speech production, and language comprehension in cerebral-palsied individuals. *Journal of Speech and Hearing Research, 33,* 210–219.

Boone, D. R. (1972). *Cerebral palsy.* Indianapolis, IN: Bobbs-Merrill.

Brazelton, T., Koslowski, B., & Main, M. (1974). The origins of reciprocity: The early mother–infant interaction. In M. Lewis & L. Rosenblum (Eds.), *The effect of the infant on its caregiver.* New York: Wiley.

Broen, P. A., Doyle, S., Moller, K., & Prouty, J. (1991, November). *Early language development in children with cleft palate.* Paper presented at the Annual Convention of the American Speech-Language-Hearing Association, Atlanta.

Brophy, J., & Good, T. (1974). *Teacher–student relationships.* New York: Holt, Rinehart and Winston.

Bruner, J. (1975). The ontogenesis of speech acts. *Journal of Child Language, 2,* 1–19.

Byrne, K., Abbeduto, L., & Brooks, P. (1990). The language of children with spina bifida and hydrocephalus: Meeting task demands and mastering syntax. *Journal of Speech and Hearing Disorders, 55,* 118–123.

Chung, C., & Myrianthopoulos, N. (1968). Racial and prenatal factors in major congenital malformations. *American Journal of Human Genetics, 20,* 44–66.

Copeland, M. E., & Kimmel, J. R. (1989). *Evaluation and management of infants and young children with developmental disabilities.* Baltimore: Paul H. Brookes.

Craft, M. J., Lakin, J. A., Oppliger, R. A., Clancy, G. M., & Vanderlinden, D. W. (1990). Siblings as change agents for promoting the functional status of children with cerebral

palsy. *Developmental Medicine and Child Neurology, 32,* 1049–1057.

Cramer, R. H. (1991). The education of gifted children in the United States: A Delphi study. *Gifted Child Quarterly, 35,* 84–91.

Cruickshank, W. (1976). The problem and its scope. In W. Cruickshank (Ed.), *Cerebral palsy: A developmental disability.* Syracuse, NY: Syracuse University Press.

Crystal, D. (1981). *Clinical linguistics.* New York: Springer-Verlag.

Crystal, D. (1982). *Profiling linguistic disability.* London: Edward Arnold.

Crystal, D., Fletcher, P., & Garman, M. (1989). *Grammatical analysis of language disability* (2nd ed.). London: Cole & Whurr.

Cutler, R. W. P. (1992). Neurology. In E. Rubentein & D. D. Federman (Eds.), *Scientific American medicine.* New York: Scientific American.

Dekker, R., & Koole, F. D. (1992). Visually impaired children's visual characteristics and intelligence. *Developmental Medicine and Child Neurology, 34,* 123–133.

Devers, M. C., & Broen, P. A. (1991, November). *Prelinguistic vocalizations of infants with and without cleft palate.* Paper presented at the Annual Convention of the American Speech-Language-Hearing Association, Atlanta.

Dorman, C., Hurley, A. D., & D'Avignon, J. (1988). Language and learning disorders of older boys with Duchenne muscular dystrophy. *Developmental Medicine and Child Neurology, 30,* 316–327.

Edwards, M. (1984). *Disorders of articulation: Aspects of dysarthria and verbal dyspraxia.* New York: Springer-Verlag.

Estrem, T., & Broen, P. A. (1989). Early speech production of children with cleft palate. *Journal of Speech and Hearing Research, 32,* 12–23.

Fehrenbach, C. R. (1991). Gifted/average readers: Do they use the same reading strategies. *Gifted Child Quarterly, 35,* 125–127.

Fenstermacher, G. D. (1982). To be or not to be gifted: That is the question. *Elementary School Journal, 82,* 299–303.

Fey, M. (1986). *Language intervention with young children.* San Diego, CA: College-Hill Press.

Fletcher, P. (1979). The transition into language: Introduction. In P. Fletcher & M. Garman (Eds.), *Language acquisition.* New York: Cambridge University Press.

Fogel, A. (1980). Gestural communication during the first six months. In A. P. Reilly (Ed.), *The communication game.* Piscataway, NJ: Johnson & Johnson.

Fox, L. H., Brody, L., & Tobin, D. (1983). *Learning-disabled/*

gifted children: Identification and programming. Austin, TX: PRO-ED.

Fraiberg, S. (1977). *Insights from the blind*. London: Souvenir Press.

Fraiberg, S., & Adelson, E. (1977). Self representation in language and play. In S. Fraiberg (Ed.), *Insights from the blind*. London: Souvenir Press.

Franco, S., & Andrews, B. (1977). Reduction of cerebral palsy by neonatal intensive care. *Pediatric Clinics of North America, 24*, 639–645.

Freeman, J. (1979). *Gifted children: Their identification and development in a social context*. Baltimore: University Park Press.

Freeman, J. (1986). Up-date on gifted children. *Developmental Medicine and Child Neurology, 28*, 77–80.

Freeman, R., & Blockberger, S. (1987). Language development and sensory disorder: Visual and hearing impairments. In W. Yule and M. Rutter (Eds.), *Language development and disorders*. Philadelphia: J. B. Lippincott.

Garman, M. (1979). Early grammatical development. In P. Fletcher & M. Garman (Eds.), *Language acquisition*. New York: Cambridge University Press.

Grunwell, P., & Russell, J. (1987). Vocalisations before and after cleft palate surgery: A pilot study. *British Journal of Disorders of Communication, 22*, 1–17.

Guilford, A., Scheuerle, J., & Shonburn, S. (1981). Aspects of language development in the gifted. *Gifted Child Quarterly, 25*, 159–163.

Howe, M. J. A. (1990). *The origins of exceptional abilities*. Cambridge, MA: Basil Blackwell.

Howlin, P. (1982). Echolalic and spontaneous phrase speech in autistic children. *Journal of Child Psychology and Psychiatry, 23*, 281–293.

Inge, K. J. (1992). Cerebral palsy. In P. J. McLaughlin & P. Wehman (Eds.), *Developmental disabilities: A handbook for best practices*. Boston: Andover Medical.

Jackson, N. E. (1988). Precocious reading ability: What does it mean? *Gifted Child Quarterly, 32*, 200–204.

Jackson, N. E., Donaldson, G. W., & Cleland, L. N. (1988). The structure of precocious reading ability. *Journal of Educational Psychology, 80*, 234–243.

Jan, J. E., Groenveld, M., Sykanda, A. M., & Hoyt, C. S. (1987). Behavioural characteristics of children with permanent cortical visual impairment. *Developmental Medicine and Child Neurology, 29*, 571–576.

Jensen, J. (1973). Do gifted children speak an intellectual dialect? *Exceptional Children, 39*, 337–338.

Jung, J. H., Gagne, J., Godden, A. L., Leeper, H. A., Moon, J. B., & Seewald, R. C. (1989). *Genetic syndromes in communication disorders*. Austin, TX: PRO-ED.

Kirchner, C., Berman, J., & Dimitrova, G. (1992, June). *The youngest of all: Trends in the rate and number of newborn infants with blindness or visual impairment*. Paper presented to the Association for Education and Rehabilitation of the Blind and Visually Impaired, Los Angeles.

Kitzinger, M. (1984). The role of repeated and echoed utterances in communication with a blind child. *British Journal of Disorders of Communication, 19*, 135–146.

Landau, B., & Gleitman, L. (1985). *Language and experience: Evidence from the blind child*. Cambridge, MA: Harvard University Press.

Lee, L. (1974). *Developmental sentence analysis*. Evanston, IL: Northwestern University Press.

Lewis, B. A., & Ripich, D. (1984). Pragmatic language of cerebral-palsied adult speakers and augmentative communication device users in a group interaction. *Developmental Medicine and Child Neurology, 26*, 239.

Lilly, M. (Ed.). (1979). *Children with exceptional needs: A survey of special education*. New York: Holt, Rinehart and Winston.

Litowitz, B. (1977). Learning to make definitions. *Journal of Child Language, 4*, 289–304.

Louis, B., & Lewis, M. (1992). Parental beliefs about giftedness in young children and their relation to actual ability level. *Gifted Child Quarterly, 36*, 27–31.

Marchant, J. M. (1992). Deaf-blind handicapping conditions. In P. J. McLaughlin & P. Wehman (Eds.), *Developmental disabilities: A handbook for best practices*. Boston: Andover Medical.

Marland, S. (1972). *Education of the gifted and talented: Report to the Congress of the United States by the U.S. Commissioner of Education*. Washington, DC: U.S. Office of Education.

McCluskey, K. W., & Walker, K. D. (1986). *The doubtful gift*. Kingston, Ontario: Ronald P. Frye.

McDonald, E. T., & Chance, B. (1964). *Cerebral palsy*. Englewood Cliffs, NJ: Prentice-Hall.

McWilliams, B. J., Morris, H. L., & Shelton, R. L. (1984). *Cleft palate speech*. Philadelphia: B. C. Decker.

Mills, C. J., & Durden, W. G. (1992). Cooperative learning and ability grouping: An issue of choice. *Gifted Child Quarterly, 36*, 11–16.

Mindell, P., & Stracher, D. (1980). Assessing reading and writing of the gifted: The warp and woof of the language program. *Gifted Child Quarterly, 24*, 72–80.

Minner, S. (1990). Teacher evaluations of case descriptions of LD gifted children. *Gifted Child Quarterly, 34*, 37–45.

Mitchell, P., & Erickson, D. (1978). The education of gifted and talented children: A status report. *Exceptional Children, 45,* 12–16.

Morris, S. E. (1987). Therapy for the child with cerebral palsy: Interacting frameworks. *Seminars in Speech and Language, 8,* 71–86.

Morris, S. E., & Klein, K. D. (1987). *Pre-feeding skills: A comprehensive resource for therapists.* Tucson, AZ: Therapy Skill Builders.

Mullins, J. (1979). *A teacher's guide to management of physically handicapped students.* Springfield, IL: Charles C. Thomas.

Namy, E. (1967). Intellectual and academic characteristics of fourth grade gifted and pseudogifted students. *Exceptional Children, 34,* 15–18.

National Joint Committee on Learning Disabilities. (1989). Issues in learning disabilities: Assessment and diagnosis. *Asha, 31,* 111–112.

Nober, E. H. (1976). Auditory processing. In W. Cruickshank (Ed.), *Cerebral palsy: A developmental disability.* Syracuse, NY: Syracuse University Press.

O'Gara, M. M., & Logemann, J. A. (1988). Phonetic analyses of the speech development of babies with cleft palate. *Cleft Palate Journal, 25,* 122–134.

Oka, S. (1979). Epidemiology and genetics of clefting: With implications for etiology. In H. Cooper, R. Harding, W. Korgman, M. Mazaheri, & R. Millard (Eds.), *Cleft plate and cleft lip: A team approach to clinical management and rehabilitation of the patient.* Philadelphia: W. B. Saunders.

Parke, K., Shallcross, R., & Anderson, R. (1980). Differences in coverbal behavior between blind and sighted persons during dyadic communication. *Journal of Visual Impairment and Blindness, 74,* 142–146.

Piaget, J. (1926). *Language and thought of the child.* New York: Harcourt, Brace and World.

Price, E. (1976). How 37 gifted children learned to read. *Reading Teacher, 30,* 44–48.

Prizant, B. M., & Rydell, P. J. (1984). Analysis of functions of delayed echolalia in autistic children. *Journal of Speech and Hearing Research, 27,* 183–192.

Renzulli, J., & Hartman, R. (1971). Scale for rating behavioral characteristics of superior students. *Exceptional Children, 38,* 243–248.

Ross, B., & Johnson, J. (1972). *Cleft lip and palate.* Baltimore: Williams and Wilkins.

Sadler, T. W. (1990). *Langman's medical embryology* (6th ed.). Baltimore: Williams and Wilkins.

Sanderlin, O., & Lundy, R. (1979). *Gifted children.* New York: A. S. Barnes.

Sardegna, J., & Otis, T. P. (1991). *The Encyclopedia of blindness and vision impairment.* New York: Facts on File.

Scherzer, A. L., & Tscharnuter, I. (1990). *Early diagnosis and therapy in cerebral palsy* (2nd ed.). New York: Marcel Dekker.

Schiff, M., Kaufman, A., & Kaufman, N. (1981). Scatter analysis of WISC-R profiles for learning disabled children with superior intelligence. *Journal of Learning Disabilities, 14,* 400–404.

Skidmore, M. D., Rivers, A., & Hack, M. (1990). Increased risk of cerebral palsy among very low-birthweight infants with chronic lung disease. *Developmental Medicine and Child Neurology, 32,* 325–332.

Starr, P., Chinsky, R., Canter, H., & Meier, J. (1977). Mental, motor, and social behavior of infants with cleft lip and/or cleft palate. *Cleft Palate Journal, 14,* 140–147.

Swafford, K. M. (1986). Language and gifted children. In V. A. Reed, *An introduction to children with language disorders.* Columbus, OH: Merrill/Macmillan.

Tew, B. (1991). The effects of spina bifida upon learning and behavior. In C. M. Bannister & B. Tew (Eds.), *Current concepts in spina bifida and hydrocephalus.* London: MacKeith Press.

Thompson, C. K. (1988). Articulation disorders in the child with neurogenic pathology. In N. J. Lass, L. V. McReynolds, J. L. Northern, & D. E. Yoder (Eds.), *Handbook of speech-language pathology and audiology.* Philadelphia: B. C. Decker.

Tough, J. (1977). *The development of meaning.* New York: Halsted Press.

Udwin, O., & Yule, W. (1991). Augmentative communication systems taught to cerebral-palsied children—a longitudinal study. II. Pragmatic features of sign and symbol use. *British Journal of Disorders of Communication, 26,* 137–148.

Urwin, C. (1984). Language for absent things: Learning from visually handicapped children. *Topics in Language Disorders, 4,* 24–37.

van Kleeck, A., & Richardson, A. (1988). Language delay in the child. In N. J. Lass, L. V. McReynolds, J. L. Northern, & D. E. Yoder (Eds.), *Handbook of speech-language pathology and audiology.* Philadelphia: B. C. Decker.

VanTassel-Baska, J. (1992). Educational decision making on acceleration and grouping. *Gifted Child Quarterly, 36,* 68–72.

Waldron, K. A., Saphire, D. G., & Rosenblum, S. A. (1987). Learning disabilities and giftedness: Identification based on self-concept, behavior, and academic patterns. *Journal of Learning Disabilities, 29,* 422–427.

Warfel, J., & Schlagenhauff, R. (1980). *Understanding neurologic disease.* Baltimore: Urban & Schwarzenberg.

Weir, R. H. (1970). *Language in the crib.* The Hague: Mouton.

Williams, C., & Tillman, M. (1968, February). *Word associations for selected form classes of children varying in age and intelligence.* Paper presented at the Annual Meeting of the American Educational Research Association, Chicago.

Winne, P. H., Woodlands, M. J., & Wong, B. Y. L. (1982). Comparability of self-concept among learning disabled, normal, and gifted students. *Journal of Learning Disabilities, 15,* 470–475.

· Part Three ·

Language Assessment and Intervention

· Chapter 14 ·

Assessment and Diagnosis

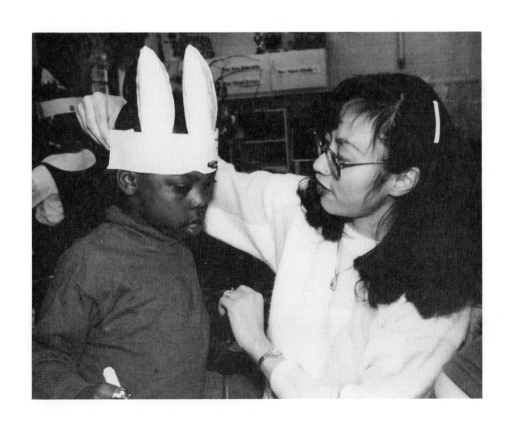

Upon completion of this chapter, the reader should be able to:

▶ Define the various terms associated with assessment and diagnosis.

▶ Describe the objectives of the assessment and diagnostic process and the general issues related to achieving the objectives.

▶ Understand the differences between screening and assessment and diagnosis, and the issues relevant to false-positive and false-negative results of screening procedures.

▶ Perceive assessment and diagnosis as ongoing processes and understand the documentation of intervention efficacy as part of the ongoing assessment process.

▶ Describe the procedures and tools that can be used in assessment and diagnosis and the ways in which these procedures and tools facilitate the process.

▶ Discuss the strengths and weaknesses of norm-referenced standardized testing.

▶ Discuss aspects of language sampling and analysis.

▶ Describe various procedures for assessing pragmatic skills.

▶ Describe the importance of valid, reliable intelligence testing as part of the total assessment and diagnosis of language-disordered children and understand issues related to accurate intelligence testing of this population.

The assessment and diagnostic process is the first step in helping children with language disorders. Information obtained from this process is used to identify children for whom language intervention is appropriate and to provide directions for that intervention. In this chapter, the various terms used to describe the process and the objectives to be achieved are discussed. The procedures and tools employed in assessment and diagnosis are reviewed, with special attention to language sampling and assessment of pragmatic skills. A section on intelligence testing and on the problems involved when a child has a language impairment is also included.

TERMINOLOGY

In chapter 4, we examined the issues related to classification and categorization. Our discussion of terminology here embodies many of those issues. The terms used to describe the process of examining a child with a suspected language disorder depend on the purposes of the examination.

Miller (1983) identifies two approaches to assessment with different purposes. One, the *descriptive* approach, emphasizes the description, or consequences, of a child's language behaviors. The aims of this approach are (1) to identify problematic areas in the child's language performance and (2) to specify both the patterns of language performance that the child possesses and those that are missing from the child's repertoire. The outcomes of this approach are guidelines for developing appropriate intervention strategies and, as Miller suggests, possible identification of other underlying or associated problems. That is, language behaviors may be indicators of primary or secondary etiological factors for which intervention beyond that for the language problem is necessary.

Several terms are used to characterize this descriptive approach (Nation & Aram, 1977). The word *examination* suggests an activity involving an inventory of a child's behaviors, whereas *appraisal* implies interpretation of findings as well as an inventory of strengths and weaknesses. Both *evaluation* and *assessment* convey interpretive and descriptive activities, but *assessment* seems to be the more inclusive term, implying "a description of the nature, severity, and prognosis of the problem as well as a plan of remediation" (Nation & Aram, 1977, p. 11). *Assessment* is one of the terms used in the title of this chapter, not because it is currently popular, but because it conveys the meaning that most closely characterizes the descriptive approach.

The second approach discussed by Miller (1983) is the *causative* approach. This approach is allied with the medical model, and its aim is to identify the etiology of a child's language disorder. This approach implies that knowing the etiology of the problem can lead to specific intervention plans. Although the descriptive approach may lead to the identification of an underlying cause, the focus of the two approaches differs. With the causative approach, there is an emphasis on the diagnosis of the language disorder and its etiology. We have seen that, in reality, it may not always be possible to diagnose the etiology. In other instances, the etiology may indicate a larger condition of which a language disorder is only part, as in the case of **microcephaly** and concomitant brain damage that results in mental retardation and an associated language problem. Such a diagnosis of the cause falls within the realm of medicine and the physician. Knowing the etiology may or may not alter significantly the intervention program, nor may it necessarily make the intervention more effective, as many language characteristics of one primary etiology overlap those of another etiology.

There are, however, instances when diagnosing the cause of a problem, or at least identifying cause-related factors, can influence the intervention strategies and the professionals involved in implementing a coordinated intervention program. One obvious example is a language disorder stemming from a hearing loss. In other situations, recognizing a child's language behaviors as being characteristic of a specific diagnostic category, such as those behaviors observed in children with autism, can lead to appropriate diagnostic team efforts and ultimately to effective medical, therapeutic, and/or educational intervention. From this viewpoint, diagnosis and the activities that go into the search for possible underlying causes are seen as important parts of the process, albeit not to the exclusion of describing a child's language behavior. Hence, the term *diagnosis* is included in the title of this chapter.

OBJECTIVES OF THE ASSESSMENT AND DIAGNOSTIC PROCESS

The assessment and diagnostic process has been compared to the scientific method of inquiry, in which questions to be answered or hypotheses to be tested are formulated, specific procedures to answer the questions or test the hypotheses are selected, data are collected according to the procedures, data are analyzed, and the results are used to recommend a plan of intervention (Meitus & Weinberg, 1983; Nation & Aram, 1977; Wiig & Semel, 1984). At the root of and critical to the process are the questions to be asked. These questions direct what we want to find out and guide how we proceed. Ultimately, they can determine what we find. If the right questions or enough questions are not asked, the correct answers will not be discovered. In this sense, the questions become the objectives for the assessment and diagnostic process.

We previously alluded to some of the objectives of the process. Lund and Duchan (1988) have succinctly listed the common objectives of an assessment and diagnostic process for children with suspected language disorders in the form of five questions. In Table 14.1 these are restated as objectives. A discussion of each of these objectives follows.

Determining If a Child Has a Language Problem

Some children seen for assessment and diagnosis have been referred by other professionals (e.g., physicians, psychologists, regular or special education teachers) or by their parents. Other children have been identified as part of a screening program. A *screening* typically involves a brief examination of several parameters of communication. Screening procedures are generally superficial and are designed to serve large numbers of children in a short time. Therefore, the results of a screening cannot satisfy the objective of determining whether or not a child has a language

---

TABLE 14.1   Objectives of the Assessment and Diagnostic Process

1. To determine whether or not a child has a language problem.
2. To identify the cause of the problem.
3. To identify the deficit areas.
4. To describe the regularities in the child's language behaviors.
5. To decide what is recommended for the child.

Source: Adapted from Lund and Duchan (1988).

problem. Rather, the purpose of a screening is to detect children whose language performances during this brief examination differ sufficiently from normal expectations to warrant concern and additional investigation. The results of a screening may raise concerns, but they cannot confirm or reject those concerns. Having concerns raised, however, leads to referral for full assessment and diagnosis.

Because of the federal education laws emphasizing early identification of children with disabilities, screening programs are becoming increasingly common. One problem with screenings is the degree to which professionals can have confidence that a screening program is detecting the right children. That is, children with normal language skills are not identified as candidates for full assessment, yet children with possible language problems are. When children with normal language skills are identified by a screening process as potentially language disordered, these results are termed *false positives*. In chapter 5 we indicated that when children who do have language disorders are not identified, these results are termed *false negatives*. No one screening process is infallible, although combinations of different procedures may reduce the margin of error. The issue, therefore, becomes the direction in which to err. A process that leads to too many false positives has the potential to swamp the service delivery system. As Tomblin and his colleagues (Tomblin, Hardy, & Hein, 1991) point out, a screening process that results in a 60% false-positive error rate will generate, from a mass screening that identified 1,800 children as suspect and requiring full assessment and diagnostic procedures, 1,350 children who turn out to have normal language skills and 900 who are found to have impaired language skills. As we will see later, a full assessment and diagnostic process takes a fair amount of a professional's time. Therefore, completing full assessments on children who do not need them consumes valuable professional resources. False negatives, on the other hand, risk missing children who need language intervention. If 1,000 children are screened but the screening process has a false-negative error rate of 10%, 100 children who have language impairments will be thought to have adequate language skills and will likely not receive intervention. Given the now well-established relationship between language impairments and academic and social problems, this is a significant failure on the part of the system and has negative consequences for the children.

Another problem with screening processes is that subtle language problems that can interfere with academic performance may be missed. Most screening procedures consist of relatively gross and superficial measures of language performance. Otherwise, they become too lengthy for professionals who must see large numbers of children in a short time. A recurring theme in this text has been the need to stress or challenge a child's language performance if these subtle problems are to be identified (Lahey, 1990). When screening procedures fail to challenge children's language performances, professionals run the risk of increasing the false-negative rate. On the other hand, even normal children's language performances will deteriorate under conditions that stress their language systems too much. In such cases, professionals run the risk of increasing the false-positive rate. The answer is, of course, to determine the balance between too little and too much challenge to the child's system. Unfortunately, we do not know exactly what that balance should be or how to achieve it, although, as we have indicated previously in this text, narrative production may provide some of the answers to this dilemma for older preschool children and for school-age children and adolescents. It does not, however, provide all of the answers.

As is obvious from this discussion, not all children referred for assessment and diagnosis have language impairments. In some cases, they are seen because of false-positive screening results. In other cases, a child may be referred by another professional as part of that individual's eliminative diagnostic process. That is, the referral source's operational plan may be that if a child does not have a language disorder, then the child does not have some other condition. Certain etiologies may then be eliminated from further consideration. Referrals may also come from people who are concerned about a child's communicative behavior but who are unaware of the language expectations for children at different ages. Some children seen for assessment and diagnosis may be *late bloomers,* that is, who are showing early but temporary delays in language development and who will outgrow their delays without residual problems.

In determining whether or not a child has a language problem, it is necessary to find out whether that child is demonstrating language behaviors that deviate from those typical of children of that age and to ascertain whether any differences, if they exist, are significant ones that will likely not be resolved if left alone. Procedures often involve exploring a child's performances on a variety of language tasks and in a variety of situations and comparing the performances to some standards or norms. Parental/caregiver reports of children's language performances are other important tools used to determine the presence or absence of a language disorder. Issues related to identification of children with language impairments, standards used for comparison, and prediction are involved in achieving this first objective. These issues were presented in chapters 4 and 5, and readers may wish to review these discussions.

Identifying the Cause of the Problem

The second objective—to identify the cause of the problem—refers to our previous discussion of etiologies and the diagnostic approach, and we will not repeat it here. Case history information, gathered from an interview with the child's primary caregivers, a case history questionnaire, reports from other professionals, and/or information obtained by achieving the other objectives of the assessment and diagnostic process are the usual methods of achieving this objective, if it is possible to do at all. In some instances, attention to possible causes or cause-related factors can alert professionals to the need to make referrals to other professionals for additional examination.

In some instances, it may be possible to identify maintaining factors instead of a cause or cause-related factors. Although maintaining factors do not cause a child's language problem, they can hinder a child's progress in language growth even with intervention. One example might be recurring ear infections. Another might relate to child–parent/caregiver interac-

tions, as discussed in chapter 5, that serve to slow even further a child's language learning. Even though the assessment and diagnostic process may not result in the identification of causal or cause-related factors, it may highlight maintaining factors that can be addressed in intervention.

Identifying Deficit Areas

The third objective is to determine the parameters of language that may be deficient in a child and the mode(s)—comprehension and/or production—in which the deficits occur. Some children may have difficulties producing age-appropriate sentences, although they may have no problems understanding syntactic constructions or comprehending and using the semantic and pragmatic systems. Other children may have problems with all aspects of language. Standardized and nonstandardized testing and observation in all parameters of language are the procedures typically employed to achieve this third objective. Knowledge of a child's specific deficit areas can help determine the broad focus or foci of an appropriate intervention plan.

Describing the Regularities in the Child's Language

Although achieving the third objective may identify broad areas of language deficits, more specific, descriptive information about a child's language skills is necessary to develop an effective and comprehensive intervention plan (Fey, 1986; Lahey, 1988; Lund & Duchan, 1988; Owens, 1991). The fourth objective is to describe patterns of language skills within each of the parameters of language. These are the regularities that comprise the child's language system in terms of the patterns both present and absent. Rarely can the results of standardized tests lead to a description of a child's language patterns. Analyses of a child's language behaviors when communicative situations and stimuli are systematically varied typically result in more useful information than that which comes from standardized testing. To achieve this fourth objective, nonstandardized methods followed by in-depth analyses of the results may be the most revealing procedures to employ.

Another aspect of this objective is discovering a child's potential to improve performance, the extent to which a child can improve performance, and the circumstances under which improved performance can be obtained (Coggins, 1991; Olswang & Bain, 1991). Different contexts with differing cues and support may elicit better language performance. After the regularities in a child's language performance have been identified through assessment, the professional can systematically manipulate contextual support and/or cues for a child and observe what conditions, if any, result in more advanced responses or even more attempts at responses. Support can be manipulated "by changing the consequences following a child's response, by changing the antecedent events preceding a child's response, or by modifying the task" (Olswang & Bain, 1991, p. 260). Of these methods, changing the antecedent events may be most frequently used. This method often results in changed performance and may provide the most information about what situations produce change (Olswang & Bain, 1991). Common ways in which antecedent events can be manipulated are shown in Table 14.2. The information gained from these procedures is used to indicate which children may benefit the most from interven-

tion and change their behaviors most easily and what methods might best be used to facilitate change.

Deciding What to Recommend

The last objective involves more than just deciding whether or not a child needs intervention. It involves deciding whether or not a child can benefit from intervention (Olswang & Bain, 1991). If intervention is warranted, it involves deciding on the form of intervention (i.e., direct intervention delivered by a professional; indirect intervention delivered through another agent, such as parents or teachers, and guided and monitored by the professional; or a combination). It also involves deciding on the appropriate setting for intervention (e.g., in a separate room such as a resource room or clinic room, in a special class, in the classroom or preschool, in the home, or a combination of settings) and, if in a separate resource/clinic room, whether the child should be seen individually, in a group, or a combination of both. When intervention is necessary, specific sequential language goals that evolve directly from a child's deficit areas, the regularities in the child's language system, and the types of context/cues that result in improved performance and that take into account the possible causal and/or maintaining factor(s) must be identified. These goals

TABLE 14.2 Examples of Manipulating Antecedent Events	Types of Manipulation	Explanations/Examples
	Modality change	Present stimuli in a visual rather than an auditory form.
	Progressive addition of modalities	Present stimuli in one modality (e.g., auditory), add a second modality for bimodal stimuli (e.g., auditory plus visual), add a third modality for multimodal stimuli (e.g., auditory plus visual plus tactile).
	Multiple presentations of stimuli before child responds	Present stimuli one or more times (e.g., say the word or sentence several times) before asking the child to respond; can be combined with previous approach.
	Provide models/hints for target response	Present an example of the expected response for the child to imitate; present the first part (or last part) of the expected response; tell the child to think about producing the target response before asking the child to produce it; tell the child a critical feature of the correct response.

Source: Adapted from Olswang and Bain (1991, p. 260).

form the framework of an intervention plan designed for an individual child. Recommendations must specify a series of goals to be incorporated into a comprehensive plan if the intervention is to be successful. Recommendations may also include referrals to other professionals who can assist the child or the child's caregivers. When intervention is not recommended, the plans for follow-up need to be determined. Children's progress without intervention is then monitored at regular intervals to ensure that they are progressing adequately (McDermott, 1985; Olswang & Bain, 1991). The recommendations from the assessment and diagnostic process specify the follow-up times and the criteria against which progress will be evaluated. It is not enough simply to recommend or not recommend intervention.

Assessment and diagnosis are continuing processes. The recommendations made as a result of an initial diagnostic and assessment process should not be considered etched in stone. It may be inappropriate to adhere unbendingly to such recommendations once intervention commences. We learn more about a child as we work with that child over time than we can determine in the few hours spent on initial assessment and diagnosis. The child also changes. We need to be prepared to change our minds or our hypotheses as new information about a child comes to light. Because diagnosis and assessment are ongoing processes, we need to be constantly "searching for new patterns and ready to change hypotheses and approaches when the child's performance so indicates. It makes every interaction with a child a part of the ongoing assessment of language and communication" (Lund & Duchan, 1988, p. 13). When intervention has not been initially recommended or when one form of intervention has been specified, we also need to be prepared to change course if the child does not improve.

The ongoing nature of assessment includes documenting the efficacy of intervention. If there are no significant changes in the child's language as a result of intervention, we need to do something different. Bain and Dollaghan (1991) write that a significant change "is a change in client performance that (a) can be shown to result from treatment rather than from maturation or other uncontrolled factors, (b) can be shown to be real,

rather than random, and (c) can be shown to be important, rather than trivial" (pp. 264–265).

During intervention, a child's performance is probed at regular intervals in systematic ways on tasks that were not directly targeted in intervention, that is, on exemplars of the desired behavior that were not presented during intervention (Bain & Dollaghan, 1991; Fey, 1986). The child's performance on some behaviors that have not been intervention goals is also measured regularly. If performance improves on intervention objectives but not on behaviors that have not been targeted, the changes on the target objectives can be viewed as resulting from intervention and not from other factors. Determining whether a change is real or random is more difficult. It involves using valid and reliable procedures to measure performance, yet the same norm-referenced, standardized tests cannot be administered repeatedly over short periods of time because the child's performance is likely to improve just from practice with the test, not because the ability or skill being measured has improved (McCauley & Swisher, 1984b). The tests, therefore, no longer accurately measure the behavior in question. Professionals are left with using procedures that they develop themselves and whose validity and reliability cannot always be ensured (Bain & Dollaghan, 1991). Factors to consider in determining if a change is important include (1) the magnitude of the change in relation to the amount of intervention time needed to achieve it and the child's unique characteristics; (2) the impact of the change on the child's life; and (3) the opinions/ratings of unbiased adults who have observed the child's performance on the language behavior in question before and after intervention on the targeted objective (Bain & Dollaghan, 1991).

From the foregoing discussion, we can see that assessment is not truly distinct from intervention. Assessment and intervention are *dynamic, interactive* processes in all of our efforts to assist children with language disorders.

TOOLS AND PROCEDURES

A variety of tools and procedures are employed in the diagnosis and assessment of children with suspected language disorders. In combination, the results obtained are used to accomplish the objectives of the process. One procedure or tool is insufficient for a thorough diagnosis and assessment. Instead, it is from analyzing and synthesizing the information obtained from a number of tools and procedures that the goals for an effective and comprehensive intervention program can be determined.

Case History Information

The purpose of a case history is to gather "information about antecedent and continuing conditions related to the communication difficulty and whatever predisposing, precipitating, and maintaining factors may be present" (Peterson & Marquardt, 1981, p. 22). Such information can assist in specifying the nature of the language disorder, what may be included in an intervention plan, and the possible causes or cause-related factors of the problem. It may help in deciding whether to intervene directly, intervene indirectly, or wait and monitor a child's development. For example, case history information may reveal family histories of language and/or learning problems or other factors that place a child at risk for continuing language problems. Having this information would no doubt influence what is recommended for the child. Another child may be found to have a history of recurring middle ear infections, or otitis media, in which case the intervention plan would ensure that the child received regular audiological assessments to monitor the hearing status. For still another child, case history information may indicate delays in achieving early milestones in all areas of development. Combined with other information obtained during the diagnostic and assessment process or from a multidisciplinary assessment, the child may be identified as mentally retarded and qualified for early intervention services or other special education services. Language intervention often involves teaching a child's parents/caregivers more effective ways of encouraging their child's language acquisition. Case history information can provide clues to the effectiveness of caregiver–child interactions and to possible guidelines for working with the caregivers as part of a child's total intervention program.

Three procedures are commonly used to obtain case history information: (1) reports from other professionals, (2) case history questionnaires, and (3) interviews. Information from other professionals' reports may assist in putting the child's language problem in perspective and help in sorting through a variety of interacting factors that may be related to the language problem.

Parents or other adults who know the child, such as teachers or social workers, are often asked to complete a case history questionnaire, usually before the child is seen for assessment and diagnosis. Although there is no standard format for case history questionnaires, information about a child's environment and family, medical and educational history, early developmental history, and any past communication assessments and intervention is typically requested. For school children, information about their academic performance and classroom behavior is important. As we saw in chapter 5, parental/caregiver reports of a child's language behaviors can aid in the early identification of language impairment, and there are several tools to obtain this information. In addition, questionnaires often provide space for the informants to give their general impressions about the problem. Standard identifying information (such as name, age, birthdate, referral source, address, telephone number, and date) is also requested. When older children or adolescents are to be seen for assessment and diagnosis, they may be asked to supply some of this information, as well as obtaining the information from the adults in their lives (Larson & McKinley, 1987; Wiig & Semel, 1984). This procedure may lead to an understanding of how the child or adolescent views the problem and how it is affecting his or her life. It can also help identify possible conflicting views of the problem held by the adults and the child. Furthermore, the child's or adolescent's written responses can be analyzed for possible signs of reading or writing difficulties. All this information can significantly affect the overall recommendations for the child and the specific ways in which an intervention plan is implemented.

A common practice is to obtain the written responses on a case history questionnaire and then to interview the informants. Because written information is already available, the interview is not an iteration of the questionnaire. Instead, this information is used to provide guidelines to areas that need to be explored in more depth during the interview. If the diagnosis and assessment involves older children or adolescents, they, too, should be interviewed (Larson & McKinley, 1987; Wiig & Semel, 1984). Not only is this a way of gathering case history information in more depth, the child's or adolescent's communicative behaviors during the interview may provide valuable insights into the possible areas of language deficit.

What to Assess

Before assessment information is obtained from interaction with or observation of a child, the behaviors, skills, and interactions to be assessed must be determined. Most assessment and diagnostic procedures include evaluating a child's abilities with the syntactic, semantic, morphological, phonological, and pragmatic components of the language system in terms of both comprehension and production skills. During the assessment, the situations in which these skills are demonstrated are systematically varied to provide a broad base of information regarding the child's deficits and specific patterns of language competencies. The effects of one component of language on others, as the first component is assessed under several conditions, are also examined.

Observation of a child in a variety of settings is an essential feature of the assessment and diagnostic process. Because the language-learning environment can significantly affect a child's language skills, that environment is often assessed. We indicated that case history information may provide clues to the effectiveness or ineffectiveness of the child's environment for language learning. However, further information about the environment may be important. Observations of child–caregiver interactions and visits to the child's home may be included in the assessment and diagnosis. Dialectal and sociological influences on a child's communicative behaviors need to be identified. Observations of a child in the classroom and during peer interactions are valuable in making valid decisions about a child's communicative performance. Observation helps ensure that decisions about inter-

vention and about what intervention emphasizes are socially valid for children.

Although the exact relationship between cognition and language is not known, cognitive abilities do play a part in language performance. Therefore, assessment of a child's cognitive level and behaviors, as they may relate to language, is often included.

Information about a child's abilities in areas other than language can help clarify the nature of the language problem, lead to an appropriate diagnosis, and delineate a number of the recommendations to include in an intervention plan. For these reasons, a child's behavior and developmental gross and fine motor, perceptual, adaptive, and general social skills may be assessed. Recall from chapter 5 that several of these areas may be able to help predict which toddlers with expressive language delay are likely to catch up without intervention and which are not. According to Peterson and Marquardt (1981), information about a child's "motor and perceptual functioning as well as language skills provide information on neurological integrity and maturation" (p. 158).

A child's hearing level and oral structures and movements are also generally assessed. In other chapters, we have discussed the importance of adequate auditory functioning for language acquisition. Examination of a child's oral structures and functions provides knowledge about the child's ability to produce the sounds that make up the phonological system of language.

Methods of Assessment

Several methods of obtaining information about the language behaviors of children are typically employed in an assessment and diagnosis. Norm-referenced standardized tests, language sampling, and criterion-referenced procedures are common methods. In a comprehensive assessment and diagnostic process, one method is not used to the exclusion of others (Emerich & Haynes, 1986).

Norm-Referenced Standardized Testing   A *standardized test* is one in which there is a "specified procedure for obtaining and analyzing information, in an effort to ensure objectivity, reliability, and validity"

(Carrow-Woolfolk & Lynch, 1982, p. 236). For most standardized language tests, the stimuli for obtaining responses from a child are developed by the author(s) of the test and included with the test itself. The procedures for using the stimuli, recording responses, and judging the adequacy of responses are specified in the instructions. Most standardized tests are also *norm-referenced,* that is, they provide a means for comparing the child's score to some standard of performance. A representative group of children without language disorders has typically been given the test, and their performances are those to which a specific child's score is compared. To allow for comparison, the child's raw score (usually the number of correct responses or errors) is generally converted to one or more other types of scores that reflect some sort of ranking or norm (e.g., age equivalencies, percentile ranks, or standard scores). The idea behind raw score conversion is to give some indication of the child's performance compared to those of peers so that the child's performance can be judged as falling within or outside the limits of this normal range. In chapter 4 we discussed the concerns regarding the use of age-equivalency scores as the standard to which we compare a child's performance (e.g., Lahey, 1988, 1990; Lawrence, 1992; McCauley & Demetras, 1990).

There has been a proliferation of norm-referenced standardized tests in recent years. Numerous tests to measure children's comprehension of various aspects of the morphological, semantic, and syntactic systems are on the market. Tests designed to examine children's use of these systems are also available, as are tests to measure children's skills with the phonological system. There are fewer norm-referenced standardized tests in the area of pragmatics, partly because the importance of this aspect of communication has been recognized more recently than that of the other areas and partly because of the inherent difficulties in developing valid and reliable tests for this area. As Owens (1991) writes, "The nature of pragmatics makes formal testing difficult" (p. 56).

There are several reasons for test proliferation. The assessment and diagnostic process for a child suspected of having a language disorder is a demanding and time-consuming task. Consequently, there is an ongoing search to find easier and quicker methods of achieving its objectives. The use of tests is often viewed as a way of easing the task. The emphasis on accountability and documentation has also provided an impetus for test development in the belief that numbers and norms are evidence of fulfilling these responsibilities. However, good assessment and diagnosis requires the ability to make judgments, based on extensive knowledge, about a child's performance. Those who lack the knowledge, or who lack confidence in their knowledge and abilities to make these judgments, may turn to tests as the sole answers to their dilemmas, thus creating a demand for standardized tests.

Although there are problems in overdependence on the use of standardized tests, these tools do serve several purposes. If they are selected carefully and employed correctly, and if the results are interpreted properly, language tests can help determine whether or not a child has a language problem and, in some instances, provide information about language areas that might be deficient. As we recall, these are two objectives of the assessment and diagnostic process. However, tests must be selected that are appropriate in terms of the characteristics of the norming population to which the child's performance will be compared. If a test has been normed on middle-class children of certain ages, the norms cannot be used to judge the performances of children from other socioeconomic groups or of other ages. Furthermore, tests must demonstrate validity and reliability if they are to be useful at all. These aspects of test selection cannot be taken lightly. Although we will not discuss these psychometric concepts here, serious concerns have been raised about the validity and reliability of a number of commonly used standardized tests of language skills (e.g., McCauley & Swisher, 1984a; Muma, 1983, 1984; Reed & Holmes, 1981; Ribner, Becker, Marks, Kahn, & Wolfson, 1983; Stephens & Montgomery, 1985). Finally, if tests are employed to help identify areas of deficit, then those that examine skills in the specific areas in question must be chosen.

Standardized tests are tools. They do not direct or determine the assessment process. We select and use them because we want to accomplish an objective and we believe they will assist us. We do not use them because they are available. We use a hammer because we want to accomplish a carpentry objective, and we believe the hammer is the tool we need. We use a measuring cup because we want to accomplish a cooking objective, and we believe the cup is the tool we need. However, it could be that a saw would be a better tool for our carpentry objective or a food processor would be better for our cooking objective. In the same way, a tool other than a standardized test or a different standardized test could be better for accomplishing the specified objectives. Sometimes we may have to use more than one tool (e.g., a hammer and a saw to complete the carpentry objective or a measuring cup and a food processor to complete our cooking objective). This means, of course, that we must clearly know what our objectives are before selecting the tools to accomplish them.

Standardized tests alone rarely yield enough information to describe a child's patterns or regularities of language behavior or to decide on the specifics of an intervention plan (Lieberman & Michael, 1986; Reed, 1992). For the most part, standardized tests do not contain a sufficient number of items examining a single feature in a wide variety of contexts to describe the content of performance or determine whether or not that feature should be a target for intervention. What standardized tests may indicate are which skills appear to be suspect and which ones need to be examined in more detail.

Some of the common errors in and misconceptions about test use that have been highlighted here are listed in Table 14.3. As Lieberman and Michael (1986) have stated, "Let the clinician beware" (p. 71).

Because standardized tests rarely provide sufficient information to develop intervention objectives, a more detailed description of the child's language is needed. To accomplish the objectives of describing a child's language patterns and determining specific intervention recommendations, we use other tools, such as language sampling and/or criterion-referenced procedures.

Language Sampling   Our discussion in chapter 11 of assessment for adolescents suspected of having language disorders included an overview of language sampling as it applies to these older students. Here we focus on general principles of language sampling and

TABLE 14.3   Common Errors and Misconceptions in Using Standardized Tests

1. Assuming that test scores demonstrate professional accountability.
2. Using tests to cover for insufficient knowledge or confidence.
3. Misinterpreting various types of test scores.
4. Using tests with children not represented in the norming sample.
5. Administering tests with inadequately demonstrated validity and reliability.
6. Using tests that do not measure the desired skills or abilities.
7. Employing tests without being clear about the objectives to be accomplished.
8. Using tests to identify specific intervention objectives for children.

its use with younger children. Although language sampling is frequently employed, there is no universally agreed-on method for eliciting and analyzing a language sample. The sample used for analysis must, however, be an accurate representation of what the child does and can do with language.

Eliciting the Sample.   Unstructured, free play is frequently used to elicit samples of language from children. Children with language disorders may be reticent, especially with someone unfamiliar to them. If they do talk, it is possible that what they say will not be indicative of their usual communication. In an unstructured, free-play context, a comfortable communicative environment is created in which a child is encouraged, but not pressured, to talk. A child may be more apt to communicate when the focus is on activities rather than on talking, when the activities are unstructured and of the child's own choosing, and when the adult's language relates to the child's utterances and the activities and contains few yes/no question forms and imperatives such as "Tell me . . . ," at least in the initial stages of the interaction (Hubbell, 1977; Lahey, 1988; Lee, 1974; Longhurst & Grubb, 1974; Miller, 1978).

Pictures and requests for a child to tell a story are sometimes used to elicit a language sample. There are drawbacks to these activities, however, as a child may give brief, labeling responses (Lahey, 1988) or use repetitious linguistic structures. The result may well be a sample that lacks the quantity and quality representative of the child's usual language functioning. Activities must be interesting and appropriate for a child's age and cognitive level (Lee, 1974; Lund & Duchan, 1988; Miller, 1981). Toys that represent people and environments familiar to a child (toy house, cars, eating utensils, a doll family) and toys with moving or broken parts may be better stimuli for eliciting language than pictures or stories alone. The decision on whether to present several toys together or one at a time depends on the child. Some children become overwhelmed, distracted, and, therefore, silent if too many toys are available, whereas other children need several toys to play with, especially if some of the toys are not interesting to them. If one strategy is not working, change to the other, but remember that it is always easier to add toys than to take some away.

Miller (1981) cautions that materials and activities must not serve "as a substitute for interaction with the child" (p. 11). The examiner and child should play and talk together in a relaxed, natural, child-directed free-play situation. The examiner can comment on what he or she is doing and what the child is doing, respond in a spontaneous way to the child's attempts at communication and activities, ask occasional open-ended questions about the child's activities and intentions, and even be silent periodically while engaging in play with the child (Lund & Duchan, 1988; McLean & Snyder-McLean, 1978). Although the examiner's language should be natural for the situation, Lee (1974) suggests that the examiner attempt to elicit increasingly complex language from the child by introducing these forms into his or her own language and creating situations in which the child's usual and logical responses would include these forms.

Another caution about what materials to use when eliciting a language sample comes from the literature on the effects of shared knowledge between listener and speaker on the level of language children use. Liles (1985) found that children used more sentences and more of certain types of cohesive devices in their narratives when the listener did not know the content of the narratives, that is, when the speaker and listener had no shared knowledge. Masterson and Kamhi (1991) found that children's sentences tended to be more complex when they had limited contextual support, such as in playing with pictures and props. The presence of pictures and toys during a language sample elicitation period may actually decrease the level of a child's language because both the examiner and the child can see the objects and participate in the events, thereby creating a condition of shared knowledge. Shared knowledge between listener and speaker reduces informational demands on a speaker.

There is a recent suggestion in the literature that more structured contexts for eliciting language may be effective, particularly for certain types of language behaviors, and in some instances may result in higher level language use by a child. For example, two studies on toddlers' uses of communicative intentions in unstructured and structured situations found that the structured contexts elicited more requests for objects or actions than the unstructured contexts (Coggins, Olswang, & Guthrie, 1987; Wetherby & Rodriguez, 1992). With regard to communicative intentions involving comments on objects or actions, when multiple communicative situations were included in a structured context, Wetherby and Rodriguez (1991) found that children produced the same number of comments about objects or actions in both the structured and unstructured contexts. It may be that when several situations for producing communicative intents are included in structured contexts, structured contexts for sampling communicative intentions may be more effective and time efficient than unstructured contexts. As another example, Evans and Craig (1992) found that an interview context in which school-age children were asked open-ended questions about their family, school, and free-time activities elicited more and longer utterances, and more that were syntactically and semantically complex, than a free-play context. These authors concluded that the interview context was a valid and reliable method of eliciting a language sample from school-age children and was more efficient than a free-play context because it took less time.

At some point during a sampling procedure, it is necessary to challenge the child's language system (Lahey, 1990). Although we may initially want to create a relaxed environment with the idea of encouraging the child to "open up," such an environment may not place sufficient language demands on the child to tap his or her maximum potential or stress the language system. The examiner will, therefore, need to modify expectations for the child in order to encourage the child to use higher levels of language in more communicatively demanding contexts.

Because of the nature of language in interactions, the examiner's language and the activities will place constraints on what language will be elicited from a child. As a result, some vocabulary, morphological forms, syntactic structures, and pragmatic behaviors that are within a child's language repertoire may not be elicited. This is always one of the dangers in language sampling. Systematically varying the activities and the language directed to the child is one way to offset possible contamination of the sample. Another way is to sample the child's language in a variety of contexts and with a variety of people. It may be possible for a highly skilled examiner alone to elicit an adequate sample for analysis. However, since language normally changes as conversational partners and contexts change, valuable information about a child's ability to modify language forms and content appropriately may be lost if a sample is obtained only as the child interacts with the examiner in the testing situation. Several authors suggest that two different contexts for eliciting a sample are the minimum, with general agreement that the more varied the contexts, the better (Cole, Mills, & Dale, 1989; Lahey, 1988; Owens, 1991). A child may also feel more comfortable and, therefore, may be more talkative when interacting with familiar people in familiar environments. For these reasons, a number of authors recommend involving parents, siblings, or other children during the elicitation of a language sample and collecting samples as a child interacts with them in different situations (Cole, 1982; Lahey, 1988; Larson & McKinley, 1987; Lund & Duchan, 1988; McLean & Snyder-McLean, 1978; Muma, 1978; Owens, 1991; Roth & Spekman, 1984a, 1984b, among others).

An examiner cannot always be sure that a sufficient number of occurrences of specific communicative behaviors will occur during a child-directed free-play sample to allow for analysis. Consequently, it may be necessary to impose certain linguistic forms and activities on the child to elicit these language behaviors. Lund and Duchan (1988) provide several examples of elicitation techniques. One technique is referred to as *patterning*. In using this strategy, the examiner begins a series of comments that have a similar structure. Once the pattern is set, the examiner stops, with the intent that the child will continue the pattern. As an example, the examiner might look in a grab bag and remove toys one at a time, each time saying, "I have a _____." After several examples, the bag can be offered to the child with a verbal or nonverbal prompt to continue. Another technique is *role playing,* in which the examiner and the child act out certain events (Staab, 1983). Puppets may be used if the child is reticent or unable to assume one of the roles. Not only may situations and roles be devised to elicit certain language forms, such as the infinitive structure "I'm going to huff, and to puff, and to blow your house down" in the *Three Little Pigs,* but they may be developed to evaluate a child's ability to modify language forms for different listeners. Games can also be used to elicit specific language behaviors, such as the question "Do you have a _____?" in "Go Fish" or, as Lund and Duchan suggest, prepositions in an adaptation of "Hide and Seek" where the child finds objects by guessing their locations.

Video narration has recently been described as another means of eliciting language samples (Dollaghan, Campbell, & Tomlin, 1990). In video narration, a child talks about events in a video, either as the video is shown or afterward. As we have seen, conversations and other language sampling techniques are subject to variability because of differences in contexts, and sampling methods may not be sufficient to elicit certain language behaviors. Advantages of video narration include (1) content stability, which tends to standardize the content of language and reduces interference from extraneous and uncontrolled factors; (2) potentially high interest value; (3) production of all utterances by the child, rather than splitting the speaking time between the child and the examiner; and (4) high processing demands that stress the child's language system. An obvious disadvantage of video narration is that it is a monologue, offering no information about dyadic communication skills, such as turn taking or conversational repair. Dollaghan et al. (1990) also report that some young children may become so engrossed in the video that they forget the task of narration. However, video narration may provide a valuable adjunct to other sample elicitation techniques and may overcome some of the problems associated with these procedures (Dollaghan et al., 1990).

Sample Length.   There is no one correct answer to the questions of how long a sample should be for an adequate analysis or whether length should be measured in time or by number of utterances. The length of the sample depends on the child's language level, age, willingness to talk, and fatigue level; the time that can be devoted to the task; and the analysis techniques to be used. Recommendations regarding the number of utterances range from 50 to 100 (Hannah, 1977; Lahey, 1988; Lee, 1974; Owens, 1991; Tyack & Gottsleben, 1974). Generally, 30 minutes is suggested as the minimum amount of time to spend obtaining a language sample (Crystal, Fletcher, & Garman, 1976; Lahey, 1988; Miller, 1981). Miller (1981) writes that with "a transcript that includes everything the child and the adult said for 30 minutes we have the ability to perform several kinds of analyses, the choice of which will depend upon our specific goals for assessment" (p. 13).

Recording the Sample.   Rarely is it possible for an examiner who is busy interacting with a child to record in writing what the child says and does as the events are happening. Yet, a verbatim transcription that includes contextual information is essential for analysis. The usual method is to audiotape the interactions to preserve the events for later transcription and analysis. While audiorecording, it is essential that the examiner make handwritten notes on the contexts in which a child's utterances occur. These notes contain information about the objects in the environment; the child's nonverbal behaviors; the events that happen before, during, and after the child's statements; and the time of each interaction. This information is used later to interpret the child's utterances in terms of communicative behaviors such as the functions, intentions, and semantic relations expressed. As videotaping equipment becomes more accessible, its use can

reduce the need to hand-record contextual information and increase the accuracy with which pragmatically relevant information can be retained for later analyses. Simultaneous audio- and videorecording is recommended whenever possible (Owens, 1991).

Transcription and Analysis.   Once a sample is recorded, it needs to be transcribed for analysis. The format into which a language sample is transcribed depends on the analysis method to be used. One method is to break the sample into separate utterances for analysis and then to determine the child's MLU, using Brown's (1973) procedures for calculating the average number of morphemes occurring in the child's utterances. These rules for determining MLU are found in Appendix E. This method allows assignment of a child's linguistic level to a stage of language development characterized by length and acquisition of specific grammatical features, as discussed in chapter 3. To complete such an analysis, a transcription of consecutive utterances is needed. In addition to MLU, the occurrence of grammatical morphemes in obligatory contexts is noted.

Carrow-Woolfolk and Lynch (1982) suggest that a child's MLU can be used to decide what additional methods of analysis may be employed. These authors recommend that for a child whose MLU is below 1.00, the child's lexicon should be specified and the semantic intentions and pragmatic functions present in the child's language repertoire should be analyzed. For a child whose MLU falls between 1.00 and 2.5, they suggest that the lexicon should again be specified and that the child's semantic intentions, semantic relations, grammatical morphemes, and pragmatic functions should be analyzed. A transcription that includes context notes, the adult's or other conversational partners' comments, the child's utterances, and even comments regarding nonverbal behaviors is needed. A number of authors have developed procedures that can be useful in completing these in-depth transcriptions and subsequent analyses (e.g., Lahey, 1988; Miller, 1981; Ochs, 1979). Crystal's (1982) *PRISM-L* and *PRISM-G* and Lahey's (1988) content/form analysis provide techniques for examining aspects of semantics. Another approach for analyzing lexical usage is the *Type-Token Ratio* (TTR), that is, the ratio of the number of different words in a sample to the total number of words. Lee's (1974) *Developmental Sentence Types* analysis procedure for presentence utterances can also provide valuable information about children's development of early language.

When a child's MLU is above 2.5 morphemes, Carrow-Woolfolk and Lynch (1982) suggest that, in addition to the semantic relations and functions/intentions of the child's communicative behaviors, the morphosyntactic forms present in the language patterns should be analyzed. To complete these linguistic analyses, consecutive utterances, as well as context and pragmatic notations, must be transcribed. Lee's (1974) *Developmental Sentence Scoring* (DSS) procedure, Tyack and Gottsleben's (1974) *Language Sampling, Analysis, and Training Procedure* (LSAT), Hannah's (1977) *Applied Linguistic Analysis, II,* Crystal et al.'s (1976) *Language Assessment, Remediation, and Screening Procedure* (LARSP), and Miller's (1981) *Assigning Structural Stage* (ASS) are some of the methods available to analyze a child's morphosyntactic patterns.

We have indicated previously in this text that MLU as a measure of language development may be less reliable for children older than 3 to 3½ years of age (Klee, 1985; Klee & Fitzgerald, 1985; Scarborough, Wyckoff, & Davidson, 1986; Wells, 1985). It is also particularly susceptible to variation dependent on the context used to sample the language (Evans & Craig, 1992; Klee, Schaffer, May, Membrino, & Mougey, 1989). Therefore, other analysis methods may be more accurate measures of language for children over age 3 to 3½ years.

In examining language performance in school-age children, we may see analyses based on terminal units (T-units), or in some cases communication units (C-units). Hunt (1965) devised the T-unit as a way of segmenting samples of school-age children's written work into units for analysis. One T-unit consists of an independent or main clause with all of its modifiers, including any dependent, or subordinate, clauses attached to it. In contrast, the C-unit was used by Loban (1976) to analyze spoken language. The definition of a C-unit is the same as that of a T-unit, except that in transcription of a sample, single words and phrases (i.e., not clauses, which have a subject and a finite

verb) can be included in the sample to be analyzed if they are appropriate responses to an examiner's statements or question. The T-unit excludes these forms from analysis, largely because this unit was devised for written language that generally does not include such structures. A difficulty with analyzing samples based on C-units is that any utterance that contains a coordinating conjunction (e.g., "and," "but") used to conjoin two or more independent clauses is broken into separate units for analysis. For example, "But the boy didn't like the pie and he ordered a different one the next time" would be two analysis units, "But the boy didn't like the pie" and "And he ordered a different one the next time." Therefore, technically no analysis unit can consist of a compound sentence, a problem that could affect analysis, interpretation of results, and decisions about intervention.

Whichever analysis procedure an examiner chooses to use, the regularities in the child's communicative behaviors must be abstracted in order to identify the specific target skills that need to be included in a language intervention plan. Different procedures provide different types of information, and it may be necessary to use several analysis procedures (Klee, 1985; Klee & Paul, 1981).

Computer-Assisted Analysis.   Increasingly, the computer is being used as a tool in assessment and intervention. Several computer programs have been developed to assist in analyzing language samples. Among these are *Systematic Analysis of Language Transcripts* (SALT) (Miller & Chapman, 1983), *Lingquest 1* (Mordecai & Palin, 1982), and *Computerized Profiling* (Long & Fey, 1993). For the most part, these programs focus on analysis of the morphosyntactic aspects of language, although some provision may be made for limited analyses of semantic characteristics. For example, the SALT program can complete a TTR and provide an alphabetized list of word roots. Computerized Profiling can perform analyses based on both the LARSP and DSS procedures. Of these programs, Lingquest I performs the least comprehensive analysis. In using computerized programs, the utterances for analysis are entered into the computer according to the format specified by the program. In most instances, some analysis of each utterance is required as it is entered. For example, the computer needs to know where one utterance ends and another begins. It may also need to know that "is" in the sentence "She is running" is an auxiliary verb and not a copula, and that "she" is a subjective pronoun. Unless these structures are coded initially, the computer cannot accurately perform further analyses. Accuracy in entering the initial data is essential, and computerized programs do not eliminate the need for some analysis by the professional. What they do do is perform subsequent analyses quickly and, in some instances, allow for several different kinds of analysis once the initially analyzed utterances are entered. They also complete the analyses in systematic ways so that performances can be compared for the same child at different times or for different children.

Assessing Pragmatic Skills   As part of an assessment and diagnostic process, it is important to evaluate not only a child's semantic, syntactic, and morphological regularities, but pragmatic skills as well. However, only a few published instruments are available for this task. Several nonstandardized procedures for assessing children's pragmatic skills have been suggested (Johnson, Johnston, & Weinrich, 1984; Lahey, 1988; Simon, 1984), but overall, methods for analyzing the pragmatic aspects of language are less well developed than those for analyzing morphosyntactic performance.

Roth and Spekman (1984a) suggest that one reason for the limited number of systematic pragmatic assessment procedures is the lack of an organizational framework to guide the assessment process. To fill this gap, these authors propose an organizational framework (1984a) and procedures (1984b) for the assessment of pragmatic abilities. Central to their framework is context since it is "a variable that affects the type and form of communicative intentions conveyed, the information that must be presupposed, and the manner in which conversations are organized" (p. 3). In any context, three broad aspects of pragmatic skills are then examined: communicative intentions, presuppositions, and social organization of discourse.

Communicative Intentions.   Assessment of communicative intentions is especially important for both young, preverbal children and verbal toddlers, as we saw in chapter 5. Assessment of these intentions in preschoolers and school-age children is no less important. Communicative intentions can be assessed in terms of the range of intentions comprehended and used by a child and the forms in which the intentions are conveyed (Roth & Spekman, 1984a). Sets of intentions and functions identified by Dore (1975) and Halliday (1975) can be used as guidelines in examining how many different intentions and functions are present in a child's communicative patterns. Because intentions can be expressed by nonverbal and/or linguistic means, the manner in which a child codes the range of functions and intentions also needs to be determined. Roth and Spekman additionally recommend that the degree of explicitness a child employs to express these functions and intentions, such as direct imperatives, permission directives, or hints, be examined. It may be possible to assess many elements of communicative intentions via analysis of a language sample. However, contrived situations, such as giving a child broken pencils or only one part of a toy to use, or putting desired objects in a closed, clear plastic container, may be used to create opportunities to examine a child's range of communicative intentions and the degree of sophistication in expressing them (Roth & Spekman, 1984b). Wetherby and Rodriguez (1992) have identified 12 situations they call *communicative temptations* that can be used to assess the communicative intentions of young children. These are listed in Table 14.4 and may provide ideas for the types of strategies that can be employed with toddlers to elicit communicative intents. Wetherby and Rodriguez suggest that the more effective communicative temptations may be the activities with balloons, bubbles, jar, wind-up toy, books, and blocks in the box.

Presuppositions.   Presupposition abilities can be assessed in terms of the informativeness of a child's messages and the modifications a child makes in the messages in response to social context variables (Roth & Spekman, 1984a). Aspects of informativeness to assess include the topics a child chooses to talk about, whether or not what is stated is new information or something already known, and the linguistic forms (e.g., cohesive devices, deictic references, and direct/

TABLE 14.4 Communicative Temptations to Elicit Communicative Intentions in Young Children

Communicative Temptation	Explanation
Desired food	Examiner eats a desired food item (e.g., a cookie) as the child watches but does not offer any to the child.
Wind-up toy	Examiner activates a wind-up toy, lets it wind down, and hands it to the child.
Blocks in a box	Child is given four blocks, one at a time, to drop in a box and is then immediately given a small animal figure to drop in the box.
Books	Examiner gives the child a book and encourages him/her to look at the book and turn the pages; the examiner then repeats this process with a second book.
Bubbles	Examiner opens a jar of bubbles, blows bubbles, closes the jar, and gives the closed jar to the child.
Social games	Examiner initiates a familiar and unfamiliar game (e.g., patty-cake, peek-a-boo) with the child and continues until the child expresses pleasure; examiner then discontinues the game and waits.
Balloon	Examiner blows up a balloon, deflates it slowly, either hands the deflated balloon to the child or holds it to own mouth, and waits.
Disliked food/ toy	Examiner offers the child a disliked food item or toy and waits.
Jar	In front of the child, examiner places a desired food item or toy in a clear jar/container that the child cannot open, closes the container, puts it in front of the child, and waits.
Jello	The child's hands are placed in a cold, wet, sticky substance (e.g., jello, paste, pudding).
Ball	Examiner rolls the ball to the child and, after the child returns the ball three times, the examiner rolls a different object to the child.
Bye-bye	Examiner waves and says "bye-bye" to objects as they are removed in the first four situations but does not do so when the items are removed in the remaining situations.

Source: Adapted from Wetherby and Rodriguez (1992, p. 132).

indirect article reference forms) the child employs. Social context variables that influence communication refer to social rules governing behaviors in different situations, listener characteristics, and the available modes for communication, that is, visual and auditory channels, as in face-to-face interactions, or auditory-only channels, as in telephone conversations (Roth & Spekman, 1984a). A child's abilities to alter communicative content and form as each of these variables is systematically manipulated can also be included as part of the assessment process. One procedure that can be employed is a modification of the barrier game in which a child attempts to get a listener to choose an abstract object, construct a drawing, or arrange objects in a predetermined order only on the basis of the child's verbal instructions (Roth & Spekman, 1984b; Simon, 1984). Changing communicative partners with respect to age, degree of familiarity, or social status and varying the amount and quality of listener feedback given to a child during a referential communication task are other suggested assessment procedures. To assess a child's use of cohesive devices, such as deictic references and definite/indefinite article references, storytelling activities with special attention to narrative analysis (Johnston, 1982; Roth & Spekman, 1984b) and having the child answer carefully formulated questions about a story, such as the techniques developed by Warden (1976) and Maratsos (1974), can be used (Roth & Spekman, 1984b).

Narrative analysis is increasingly a part of the assessment and diagnostic process. Owens (1991) suggests that Applebee's (1978) narrative levels, as presented in chapter 3, can provide an appropriate framework for analyzing narratives of preschool children, while story grammar analysis, such as that of Stein and Glenn (1979) presented in chapter 1, can be used with school-age children. In using story grammar for narrative analysis, special attention to the structural patterns and the associated structural properties of narratives is warranted. Glenn and Stein (1980) have identified seven structural patterns of narratives that differ in the complexity of their structural properties. These patterns are listed in order of complexity in Table 14.5 and can be used to evaluate the degree of complexity evidenced in a child's narrative skills. In examining this table, it may be helpful to also review Table 1.4 in chapter 1. Recall that narrative production may be a method of challenging a child's language system in areas other than the structure of the narratives themselves.

Social Organization of Discourse.   According to Roth and Spekman (1984a), the third broad aspect of pragmatic abilities to assess is a child's "ability to function in, and contribute to, the ongoing stream of discourse or conversation" (p. 7). Specific behaviors to evaluate are the amount of a child's social speech (speech addressed to a listener) versus nonsocial speech (speech that does not obligate a listener to respond, such as monologues) and the child's abilities to maintain a topic of conversation, to initiate and terminate conversations, and to repair communication breakdowns. A child's turn-taking skills are also assessed. Dyadic communication portions of a language sample may provide the necessary information to assess many of these skills. In chapter 5 we saw one on-line method of assessment that can be used with young children in group situations to examine their social, interactive

TABLE 14.5   Structural Patterns and Properties of Narratives

Structural Patterns	Structural Properties
Descriptive sequence	A chain of setting statements with no temporal or causal links.
Action sequence	A setting statement with action statements functioning as attempts; action statements are chronologically but not causally chained.
Reaction sequence	A setting statement, an initiating event, and several action (attempt) statements in order of direct cause–effect relation, i.e., first action directly causes next action, but with no goal direction.
Abbreviated episode	A setting statement and either an initiating statement followed by a consequence or an event statement followed by a consequence. Goal direction is either explicit or implicit.
Complete episode	A setting statement and two of three components (initiating event, internal response, attempt) followed by a consequence. Goal direction is present.
Complex episode	Multiple episodes or expansion of complete episodes. Reaction statements and internal plans may be included.
Interactive episode	More than one character and separate episodes, with each influencing the others.

Source: Adapted from Glenn and Stein (1980).

communication with peers (Rice, Sell, & Hadley, 1990). Recall that Fey's (1986) interactionist approach (chapter 4) emphasizes how children use language in social-conversational situations. Fey developed a coding system, based on those of Dore (1979) and Chapman (1981), to describe and classify each conversational act a child produces during an interactive interchange, with some acts reflecting assertiveness and others reflecting responsiveness. Examples of this coding system are requests for information (RQIN), requests for attention (RQAT), statements (ASST), disagreements (ASDA), responses to requests for information (RSIN), responses to requests for clarification (RSCL), and responses to requests for attention (RSAT). The frequency of occurrence of these different acts during the interchange is used to classify a child into one of four profiles of social-conversational participation (e.g., active conversationalist, passive conversationalist, inactive communicator, verbal non-communicator) (see chapter 4). Basic goals are determined from a specific child's profile (Fey, 1986). When samples of naturalistic dyadic communication have failed to elicit discourse elements of interest, role playing and contrived communicative situations may be needed to create opportunities to assess a child's skills. For example, an examiner may purposefully give vague instructions to a child or use a nonverbal cue indicating a lack of understanding, such as a puzzled expression, to evaluate a child's reactions (Roth & Spekman, 1984b).

Data obtained with these procedures can provide valuable information about a child's possible areas of deficit and the regularities in the child's communicative repertoire. This information is critical in deciding what to recommend and in developing a specific intervention plan.

Criterion-Referenced Testing   Criterion-referenced testing is one form of nonstandardized testing. However, the term *nonstandardized* does not describe a process for which the procedures are random, disorganized, and unstructured. Instead, *nonstandardized testing* refers to activities for which the examiner's behaviors, the stimulus materials, the ways that the stimuli are manipulated, and the methods of recording responses are determined by the examiner

rather than by some external source, such as an administration protocol that accompanies a standardized test (Carrow-Woolfolk & Lynch, 1982). In non-standardized testing, it is the examiner who structures and organizes the assessment procedures on the basis of the child's individual needs. In Siegel's (1975) opinion, "the best 'instrument' available is a clinician who has some knowledge of recent research and theory in language, some experience in describing and dealing with important communication behaviors, and some reservoir of confidence in his or her own abilities to observe behavior, develop hypotheses, and change ideas and approaches when necessary" (p. 213).

In *criterion-referenced testing,* the examiner determines the methods and procedures before testing but, importantly, also determines the standard of performance required. "The purpose of criterion-referenced measures is to provide information about the performance of individuals or groups of individuals relative to certain tasks or goals" (Lahey, 1988, p. 141). This form of testing assists in learning how well a specific language skill is established in a child's communicative behavior. Criterion-referenced testing is valuable both in initial assessment to help determine intervention objectives and in intervention to measure a child's progress toward acquisition of targeted language skills and to evaluate intervention efficacy.

Leonard, Prutting, Perozzi, and Berkley (1978) propose three rationales for employing criterion-referenced, clinician-constructed tasks to supplement standardized language testing. The first rationale is to examine in more detail those features of language that appeared troublesome for a child on a standardized instrument. We have indicated that few standardized tests assess a sufficient number of items for a specific linguistic feature to determine whether or not that feature is truly present in or absent from the child's language patterns. For example, the *Test for Auditory Comprehension of Language* (TACL) (Carrow, 1973) assesses a child's ability to interpret only three regular noun plurals. Of these, two items assess the /z/ allomorph and one item assesses the /s/ allomorph. To assess a child's skills with this feature in more depth, more regular noun plural items could be selected so that root word endings are varied and more opportunities to respond to items examining all three regular allomorphs, including /əz/, are provided. Items might include "drums," "dogs," "cakes," "lips," "horses," and "dishes." In designing the task, a child could be asked to select one picture from three (two of which are related decoys) that represents the noun plural in question. Such a task would be consistent with the task used in the TACL.

A second rationale focuses on examining some aspects of language that standardized tests omit. As we have seen, pragmatic skills are relatively untapped by standardized tests. Therefore, clinician-constructed measures such as those suggested in the previous section may allow examination of these aspects of language functioning.

The last rationale provided by Leonard et al. (1978) is to "determine the scope of a child's difficulty with a particular feature of language" (p. 374). Specifically, the tasks or stimuli used to assess a feature may create problems for the child rather than the child having difficulty with the feature itself. In order to discern the reasons for a child's problem, a task or stimulus different from the ones used on a standardized test to assess the feature can be devised. This is not unlike modifying antecedent events, which we discussed earlier in this chapter with regard to intervention efficacy. For example, the pictures provided with a standardized test may be unclear or confusing. It is possible that changing the pictures may elicit correct responses. As another example, a child may not be able to deal with sentence completion tasks, such as "Here is a dog. Here are two _____," which are used in several standardized tests. Yet, the same child may be able to use many of the same morphological forms in other types of tasks.

PHONOLOGICAL ASSESSMENT

The primary focus of this chapter, as of this book, has been on the semantic, pragmatic, syntactic, and morphological aspects of language. However, as children's uses of speech sounds are viewed more and more as an aspect of language, some mention of phonological assessment, albeit brief, is appropriate.

The traditional approach to assessing a child's sound-production skills involves an articulation test typically designed to have the child say each sound as it occurs at the beginning, middle, and end of single words. Each of the child's sound productions is judged as correct or incorrect, and if incorrect, the type of error made (e.g., omission of the sound, substitution of one sound for another, distortion of the sound) is noted. Unfortunately, this procedure has not provided sufficient information to describe patterns or regularities in performance when, among other problems, many more sound errors occur in spontaneous speech than on single-word articulation tests or when children's misarticulations appear inconsistent from one production to the next. More recently, a different approach to assessing children's sound-production skills—the phonological process approach—has gained attention.

The purpose of the phonological process approach is to identify those error patterns or consistencies that a child uses in producing the sounds as they occur in the lexicon, syntactic structure, and morphological units of the language. Several authors have used different sets of phonological processes (e.g., Hodson, 1986; Ingram, 1976; Shriberg & Kwiatkowski, 1980; Weiner, 1978). There is, at present, no one agreed-on set of phonological processes that includes those in children's normal phonological development or disordered development. Recall from chapter 3 that some phonological processes that have been identified are weak syllable deletion, in which an unstressed syllable in a word is omitted ("tato" for "potato"); assimilation, in which one sound causes a change in another sound, as when the "t" in "cat" causes the "k" sound to be produced as a "t" as well ("tat" for "cat"); stopping, in which stop sounds are substituted for continuant sounds ("tee" for "see"); backing, in which back sounds are substituted for front sounds ("gay" for "day"); and consonant cluster reduction, in which one or more elements of a consonant cluster are omitted ("top" for "stop"). Just as there is no standard set of phonological processes, there is no standard method of assessing for these processes. However, despite the set of processes and the assessment procedure employed, the emphasis is on analysis to discover the rules or strategies that comprise an individual child's phonological system. Once discovered, these regularities lead to intervention to modify the child's processes in a direction that more closely resembles the adult phonological rule system.

Intelligence testing for children with impaired or different language is a challenging task for psychologists.

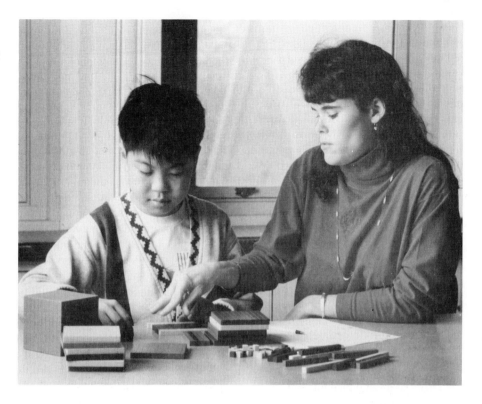

INTELLIGENCE TESTING

Results of intelligence tests administered by qualified psychologists can contribute important information to that obtained during a comprehensive assessment and diagnostic process for a child with a suspected language disorder. In previous chapters we described the language characteristics of special populations of children. Although their unique communicative behaviors and considerations were highlighted, assessment of language abilities alone rarely leads to differential diagnoses. Within any one special population there is individual variation in the language characteristics the children demonstrate, and as we have seen, there can be some overlap in the language characteristics associated with one of these conditions and those of other conditions. However, when results obtained from valid intelligence testing are combined with those obtained from language assessment, the possibilities of arriving at differential diagnoses through professional team efforts increase considerably.

Recall that in identification of language-disordered children, one standard to which children's language performances are sometimes compared is mental age (MA). In fact, some diagnoses are predicated on a child's intelligence level, such as specific language impairment (Camarata & Swisher, 1990), learning disability, and mental retardation. In chapter 7 we saw that one of the criteria used in identifying learning-disabled children is at least normal intellectual functioning despite some language comprehension and/or expression problems. These children also typically demonstrate areas of strengths and weaknesses in their language or language-related skills, some of which may even fall within or above the normal range. In contrast, mentally retarded children demonstrate overall delays in developmental skills in comparison to their chronological age (CA). These delays are observed in their intellectual functioning, as well as in all aspects of communicative behaviors, although in many instances language may be the most depressed skill area (Bateman & Wetherel, 1965). Although many autistic children may obtain overall intelligence test scores that place them in the retarded range, they may perform better than retarded children and better than might be predicted on the basis of their overall IQ scores on certain cognitive tasks, such as concrete discriminations (Maltz, 1981), and worse than retarded children on other tasks, such as symbolic play activities (DeMyer, 1976). When the results of analyses of these specific tasks are paired with the language patterns that emerge from a language assessment and diagnostic process, children whose problems stem primarily from autism can likely be discriminated from those children whose language patterns in conjunction with their intellectual skills primarily reflect mental retardation or learning disabilities.

Although differential diagnosis itself does not result in the development of child-specific, individually designed intervention plans, it does have implications for educational and therapeutic intervention. The intervention for a severely involved cerebral-palsied child with normal intelligence needs to be quite different from that of a cerebral-palsied child who is also mentally retarded. Similarly, a hearing-impaired child with normal intelligence must not be misdiagnosed as mentally retarded and provided with the types of services appropriate for children with limited cognitive functioning. Bilingual-bicultural children whose language patterns represent language differences do not require language intervention programs designed for children with language disorders, nor should their language differences cause them to be diagnosed as mentally retarded if they are not. If, however, a bilingual-bicultural child demonstrates a language disorder or some additional special condition, such as a learning disability, intervention and programs to meet the specific needs of that child must be determined.

Intelligence testing for children with impaired or different language is a challenging task for psychologists. It is unfortunate that in the past, children with normal or above-average intelligence but with language differences or disorders—such as hearing-impaired, bilingual-bicultural, and cerebral-palsied children—were misdiagnosed as mentally retarded and placed in classrooms for low-functioning children. A major reason for these misdiagnoses stems from the nature of the commonly used intelligence tests. Historically, the *Stanford-Binet Intelligence Scale* (Terman & Merrill, 1973), which yielded a single IQ score, has been recognized as heavily based on language and language-related abilities. When this test is given to a child with a language disorder or difference, the resulting IQ score reflects the child's language skills rather than the child's intellectual potential. Although the fourth edition of this test (Thorndike, Hagen, & Sattler, 1985) has attempted to address concerns about gender and ethnic biases (Aiken, 1988), it continues to have a relatively heavy language component. In contrast, the *Wechsler Intelligence Scale for Children-Revised* (WISC-R) (Wechsler, 1974) and the *Wechsler Preschool and Primary Scale of Intelligence* (WPPSI) yield separate IQ scores for the performance and verbal portions, as well as a full-scale combined IQ score. As with the Stanford-Binet, the verbal scale tends to reflect a child's language abilities or disabilities. The performance scale is generally a more accurate indication of a language-disordered child's intellectual level, although cautions are appropriate even in interpreting the performance IQ as valid. When instructions are given orally, a child with language comprehension problems can be at a severe disadvantage in completing the performance tasks accurately because the instructions may not be understood. For example, in one study, the WISC-R performance IQ scores of hearing-impaired children increased about 20 points when the examiner's oral instructions were supplemented with manual communication (Sullivan, 1978).

An extremely unfortunate situation for language-different and language-disordered children was the description and subsequent use of an early edition of the *Peabody Picture Vocabulary Test* (PPVT) (Dunn, 1965) as a measure of intellectual functioning. Rather than assessing intellectual level, the PPVT and its new edition, the *Peabody Picture Vocabulary Test-Revised* (PPVT-R) (Dunn & Dunn, 1981), actually assess receptive single-word vocabulary. Fortunately, the authors of the PPVT-R no longer refer to the test as a measure of intelligence, although some texts on psychological assessment continue to list it as such (Aiken, 1988). As a receptive vocabulary test, the PPVT-R has recently been criticized as racially and/or economically biased for use with low-income African-American preschool and school-age children who speak BEV (Washington & Craig, 1992). In this study, the children as a group scored at approximately the 10th percentile rank and more than one standard deviation below the mean for the test. If these concerns are raised about the PPVT-R when it is used as a measure of receptive vocabulary, we could hypothesize about the detrimental impacts if the test is used as a measure of intelligence with these children.

The *Kaufman Assessment Battery for Children* (K-ABC) (Kaufman & Kaufman, 1983) is becoming an increasingly popular intelligence test. It assesses the ability, in children as young as 2½ years, to problem-solve using simultaneous or sequential mental processes. Achievement tests for reading and arithmetic are also included. "Based on extensive research on neuropsychology and cognitive psychology, the K-ABC is said to be especially appropriate for determining the mental abilities of preschool, minority, and exceptional children" (Aiken, 1988, p. 172).

There are several alternative intelligence tests that minimize the language loading seen in some of the tests, such as the Stanford-Binet, WISC-R, WPPSI, and *Peabody Picture Vocabulary Test.* Two such tests are the third edition of the *Columbia Mental Maturity Scale* (Burgemeister, Blum, & Lorge, 1972) and the *Arthur Adaptation of the Leiter International Performance Scale* (Arthur, 1955). Maltz (1981) particularly recommends use of the last test with autistic children because it is reportedly sensitive to their cognitive characteristics. The *Hayes-Binet* adaptation of the *Stanford-Binet Intelligence Scale* may be an acceptable alternative for visually impaired children, although concerns about the language ability of these children remain. The *Coloured Progressive Matrices* (Raven, 1963), a test based mostly on visual perception, is also sometimes used with communicatively impaired or language-different children. Along with the *Coloured Progressive Matrices,* the Cattells' IPAT *Culture-fair Intelligence Test* (Cattell & Cattell, 1973) is generally viewed as culture free and minimizes test bias for bilingual-bicultural children with different language styles. One of the few measures that has been normed specifically for hearing-impaired children is the *Hiskey-Nebraska Test of Learning Aptitude* (Hiskey, 1966). An examiner can choose to give either verbal or pantomimed instructions. However, if verbal instructions are used with a hearing-impaired child, the norms for normally hearing children must be used.

Although standardized tools for assessment of intelligence are supposed to be given in specific ways, with little room for deviation from stated protocols, their uses with language-disordered or language-different children may require special precautions in giving the tests or modifications of instructions, materials, or administration procedures if relatively accurate estimates of intelligence are to be obtained. For example, for a cerebral-palsied child with severe oral and motor involvements, testing materials may need to be cut apart and placed so that the child merely has to look at the stimuli to respond. Or the examiner may need to change the procedures to allow for multiple-choice responses instead of oral or motor target responses. A number of intelligence tests have timed subtests that are inappropriate for children with motor handicaps, and many of the tests that minimize language loading emphasize the visual modality, which renders them unsuitable for children with visual impairments. In some cases, children with sensory impairments may be given only one scale of the WISC-R or the WPPSI, for example, the verbal scale to children with visual impairments or the performance scale to children with hearing impairments. For a hearing-impaired child who is visually oriented, appropriate visual cues may facilitate optimal performance, but distracting visual information may adversely affect the child's performance. In administering test items that use a picture response format, an examiner should avoid looking at any specific picture after giving a test stimulus or placing his or her hand in such a way as to direct inadvertently the hearing-impaired child's responses (Davis & Hardick, 1981). Because a hearing-impaired child will often change a response if asked to repeat it, even though the original response may have been correct, an examiner should avoid asking such a child to indicate a response a second time (Davis & Hardick, 1981).

These are only a few examples of the modifications and precautions necessary when testing these special children. However, an insightful psychologist who understands the impacts language problems can have on intelligence test results, who carefully selects the most appropriate tests, and who is willing to adapt to the special needs of these children can often obtain valid estimates of their intellectual functioning, even for difficult-to-test autistic children (DeMyer, 1976).

SUMMARY

In this chapter we have seen that:

► Assessment and diagnosis needs to accomplish five objectives, and several procedures and tools are employed to achieve them.

► Screenings are brief examinations of children's communicative performances, the results of which can raise concerns about children's language but cannot determine if children have language problems; screening procedures need to reduce false-negative and false-positive results as much as possible.

► Causal and cause-related factors may or may not be able to be identified from an assessment and diagnostic process; it is, however, important to consider them and to look for maintaining factors.

► The regularities in a child's language must be identified to develop intervention objectives; language sampling, criterion-referenced testing, and clinician-constructed tasks are generally the most valid procedures; assessing a child's regularities in phonological production is part of the process.

► Assessment and diagnosis is an ongoing process; evaluation of intervention efficacy is part of this process.

► Norm-referenced, standardized tests are tools and cannot be used alone to achieve the objectives of assessment and diagnosis; professionals must be careful not to misuse or misinterpret standardized tests.

► Factors to consider in language sampling include the methods used to elicit the sample, the settings and communicative partners involved, the length of the sample, the ways to record the sample, and the transcription and analysis procedures used; methods of transcription and analysis vary, depending on the purpose of the analysis and the general communicative level of the child.

► Assessing pragmatic and narrative skills is an essential part of the assessment and diagnostic process and generally requires the use of nonstandardized approaches.

► Intelligence testing is an important aspect of a child's total assessment; obtaining valid results when children have language problems is a challenging task for psychologists, requiring careful test selection and possibly involving modification of usual procedures.

The diagnostic and assessment process for a child with a suspected language problem involves gathering information about the child from a variety of sources and procedures. All of these lead to accomplishing the five objectives of the diagnostic and assessment process.

REFERENCES

Aiken, L. (1988). *Psychological testing and assessment* (6th ed.). Boston: Allyn and Bacon.

Applebee, A. (1978). *The child's concept of story.* Chicago: University of Chicago Press.

Arthur, G. (1955). *Arthur adaptation of the Leiter international performance scale.* Chicago: Stoelting.

Bain, B., & Dollaghan, C. (1991). The notion of clinically significant change. *Language, Speech, and Hearing Services in Schools, 22,* 264–270.

Bateman, B., & Wetherel, J. (1965). Psycholinguistic aspects of mental retardation. *Mental Retardation, 3,* 8–13.

Brown, R. (1973). *A first language: The early stages.* Cambridge, MA: Harvard University Press.

Burgemeister, B., Blum, L., & Lorge, I. (1972). *Columbia mental maturity scale* (3rd ed.). San Antonio, TX: Psychological Corporation.

Camarata, S., & Swisher, L. (1990). A note on intelligence assessment within studies of specific language impairment. *Journal of Speech and Hearing Research, 33,* 205–207.

Carrow, E. (1973). *Test for auditory comprehension of language.* Hingham, MA: Teaching Resources.

Carrow-Woolfolk, E., & Lynch, J. (1982). *An integrative approach to language disorders in children.* New York: Grune & Stratton.

Cattell, R., & Cattell, A. (1973). *IPAT culture-fair intelligence test*. Champaign, IL: Institute for Personality and Ability Testing.

Chapman, R. (1981). Exploring children's communicative intents. In J. Miller, *Assessing language production in children*. Baltimore: University Park Press.

Coggins, T. (1991). Bringing context back into assessment. *Topics in Language Disorders, 11,* 43–54.

Coggins, T., Olswang, L., & Guthrie, J. (1987). Assessing communicative intents in young children: Low structured observation or elicitation tasks? *Journal of Speech and Hearing Disorders, 52,* 44–49.

Cole, K., Mills, P., & Dale, P. (1989). Examination of test-retest and split-half reliability for measures derived from language samples of young handicapped children. *Language, Speech, and Hearing Services in Schools, 20,* 259–268.

Cole, P. (1982). *Language disorders in preschool children*. Englewood Cliffs, NJ: Prentice-Hall.

Crystal, D. (1982). *Profiling linguistic ability*. London: Edward Arnold.

Crystal, D., Fletcher, P., & Garman, M. (1976). *The grammatical analysis of language disability: A procedure for assessment and remediation*. London: Edward Arnold.

Davis, J., & Hardick, E. (1981). *Rehabilitative audiology for children and adults*. New York: Wiley.

DeMyer, M. (1976). Motor, perceptual-motor and intellectual disabilities of autistic children. In L. Wing (Ed.), *Early childhood autism*. London: Pergamon Press.

Dollaghan, C., Campbell, T., & Tomlin, R. (1990). Video narration as a language sampling context. *Journal of Speech and Hearing Disorders, 55,* 582–590.

Dore, J. (1975). Holophrase, speech acts, and language universals. *Journal of Child Language, 2,* 21–40.

Dore, J. (1979). Conversational acts and the acquisition of language. In E. Ochs & B. Schieffelin (Eds.), *Developmental pragmatics*. New York: Academic Press.

Dunn, Lloyd. (1965). *Peabody picture vocabulary test*. Circle Pines, MN: American Guidance Service.

Dunn, Lloyd, & Dunn, Leota. (1981). *Peabody picture vocabulary test–Revised*. Circle Pines, MN: American Guidance Service.

Emerich, L., & Haynes, W. (1986). *Diagnosis and evaluation in speech pathology* (3rd ed.). Englewood Cliffs, NJ: Prentice-Hall.

Evans, J., & Craig, H. (1992). Language sample collection and analysis: Interview compared to freeplay assessment contexts. *Journal of Speech and Hearing Research, 35,* 343–353.

Fey, M. (1986). *Language intervention with young children*. San Diego, CA: College-Hill Press.

Glenn, C., & Stein, N. (1980). *Syntactic structures and real world themes in stories generated by children*. Urbana: University of Illinois Center for the Study of Reading.

Halliday, M. (1975). *Learning how to mean: Explorations in the development of language*. London: Edward Arnold.

Hannah, E. (1977). *Applied linguistic analysis, II*. Pacific Palisades, CA: SenCom Associates.

Hiskey, M. (1966). *Hiskey-Nebraska test of learning aptitude*. Lincoln: University of Nebraska Press.

Hodson, B. (1986). *The assessment of phonological processes–Revised*. Austin, TX: PRO-ED.

Hubbell, R. (1977). On facilitating spontaneous talking in young children. *Journal of Speech and Hearing Disorders, 42,* 216–231.

Hunt, K. (1965). *Grammatical structures written at three grade levels*. Urbana, IL: National Council of Teachers of English.

Ingram, D. (1976). *Phonological disability in children*. London: Edward Arnold.

Johnson, A., Johnston, E., & Weinrich, B. (1984). Assessing pragmatic skills in children's language. *Language, Speech, and Hearing Services in Schools, 15,* 2–9.

Johnston, J. (1982). Narratives: A new look at communication problems in older language-disordered children. *Language, Speech, and Hearing Services in Schools, 13,* 144–155.

Kaufman, A., & Kaufman, N. (1983). *Kaufman assessment battery for children (K-ABC)*. Circle Pines, MN: American Guidance Service.

Klee, T. (1985). Clinical language sampling: Analysing the analyses. *Child Language Teaching and Therapy, 1,* 182–198.

Klee, T., & Fitzgerald, M. (1985). The relation between grammatical development and mean length of utterance in morphemes. *Journal of Child Language, 12,* 251–269.

Klee, T., & Paul, R. (1981). A comparison of six structural analysis procedures: A case study. In J. Miller, *Assessing language production in children*. Baltimore: University Park Press.

Klee, T., Schaffer, M., May, S., Membrino, I., & Mougey, K. (1989). A comparison of the age–MLU relation in normal and specifically language-impaired preschool children. *Journal of Speech and Hearing Disorders, 54,* 226–233.

Lahey, M. (1988). *Language disorders and language development*. New York: Merrill/Macmillan.

Lahey, M. (1990). Who shall be called language disordered? Some reflections and one perspective. *Journal of Speech and Hearing Disorders, 55,* 612–620.

Larson, V. Lord, & McKinley, N. (1987). *Communication as-*

sessment and intervention strategies for adolescents. Eau Claire, WI: Thinking Publications.

Lawrence, C. (1992). Assessing the use of age-equivalent scores in clinical management. *Language, Speech, and Hearing Services in Schools, 23,* 6–8.

Lee, L. (1974). *Developmental sentence analysis.* Evanston, IL: Northwestern University Press.

Leonard, L., Prutting, C., Perozzi, J., & Berkley, R. (1978). Nonstandard approaches to the assessment of language behaviors. *Asha, 20,* 371–379.

Lieberman, R., & Michael, A. (1986). Content relevance and content coverage in tests of grammatical ability. *Journal of Speech and Language Disorders, 51,* 71–81.

Liles, B. (1985). Cohesion in the narratives of normal and language-disordered children. *Journal of Speech and Hearing Disorders, 28,* 123–133.

Loban, W. (1976). *Language development: Kindergarten through grade twelve.* Urbana, IL: National Council of Teachers of English.

Long, S., & Fey, M. (1993). *Computerized profiling (Macintosh Version 1.0, MS-DOS Version 7.1).* San Antonio, TX: Psychological Corporation.

Longhurst, T., & Grubb, S. (1974). A comparison of language samples collected in four situations. *Language, Speech, and Hearing Services in Schools, 5,* 71–78.

Lund, N., & Duchan, J. (1988). *Assessing children's language in naturalistic contexts* (2nd ed.). Englewood Cliffs, NJ: Prentice-Hall.

Maltz, A. (1981). Comparison of cognitive deficits among autistic and retarded children on the Arthur Adaptation of the Leiter International Performance Scales. *Journal of Autism and Developmental Disorders, 11,* 413–426.

Maratsos, M. (1974). Preschool children's use of definite and indefinite articles. *Child Development, 45,* 446–455.

Masterson, J., & Kamhi, A. (1991). The effects of sampling conditions on sentence production in normal, reading-disabled, and language-learning-disabled children. *Journal of Speech and Hearing Research, 34,* 549–558.

McCauley, R., & Demetras, M. (1990). The identification of language impairment in the selection of specifically language-impaired subjects. *Journal of Speech and Hearing Disorders, 55,* 468–475.

McCauley, R., & Swisher, L. (1984a). Psychometric review of language and articulation tests for preschool children. *Journal of Speech and Hearing Disorders, 49,* 34–42.

McCauley, R., & Swisher, L. (1984b). Use and misuse of norm-referenced tests in clinical assessment: A hypothetical case. *Journal of Speech and Hearing Disorders, 49,* 338–348.

McDermott, L. (1985). Service alternatives: In *Caseload issues in schools: How to make better decisions* (pp. 18–24). Rockville, MD: American Speech-Language-Hearing Association.

McLean, J., & Snyder-McLean, L. (1978). *A transactional approach to early language training.* Columbus, OH: Merrill.

Meitus, I., & Weinberg, B. (1983). *Diagnosis in speech-language pathology.* Baltimore: University Park Press.

Miller, J. (1978). Assessing children's language behavior: A developmental process approach. In R. Schiefelbusch (Ed.), *Bases of language intervention.* Baltimore: University Park Press.

Miller, J. (1981). *Assessing language production in children.* Baltimore: University Park Press.

Miller, J. (1983). Identifying children with language disorders and describing their language performance. In J. Miller, D. Yoder, & R. Schiefelbusch (Eds.), *Contemporary issues in language intervention.* Rockville, MD: American Speech-Language-Hearing Association.

Miller, J., & Chapman, R. (1983). *SALT: Systematic analysis of language transcripts.* Madison: Language Analysis Laboratory, Waisman Center, University of Wisconsin.

Mordecai, D., & Palin, M. (1982). *Lingquest 1 & 2.* Napa, CA: Lingquest Software.

Muma, J. (1978). *Language handbook: Concepts, assessment, intervention.* Englewood Cliffs, NJ: Prentice-Hall.

Muma, J. (1983, November). *Language assessment: How valid is the process?* Paper presented at the Annual Convention of the American Speech-Language-Hearing Association, Cincinnati, OH.

Muma, J. (1984). Semel and Wiig's CELF: Construct validity? *Journal of Speech and Hearing Disorders, 49,* 101–104.

Nation, J., & Aram, D. (1977). *Diagnosis of speech and language disorders.* St. Louis, MO: C. V. Mosby.

Ochs, E. (1979). Transcription as theory. In E. Ochs & B. Schieffelin (Eds.), *Developmental pragmatics.* New York: Academic Press.

Olswang, L., & Bain, B. (1991). When to recommend intervention. *Language, Speech, and Hearing Services in Schools, 22,* 255–263.

Owens, R. (1991). *Language disorders: A functional approach to assessment and intervention.* New York: Merrill/Macmillan.

Peterson, H., & Marquardt, T. (1981). *Appraisal and diagnosis of speech and language disorders.* Englewood Cliffs, NJ: Prentice-Hall.

Raven, J. (1963). *Coloured progressive matrices.* San Antonio, TX: Psychological Corporation.

Reed, V. A. (1992). Associations between phonology and other language components in children's communicative performance: Clinical implications. *Australian Journal of Human Communication Disorders, 20,* 75–87.

Reed, V. A., & Holmes, A. (1981). Australian children's performances on the Test for Auditory Comprehension of Language. *Australian Journal of Human Communication Disorders, 9,* 24–35.

Ribner, S., Becker, L., Marks, S., Kahn, P., & Wolfson, F. (1983). A validation study of the elementary and advanced screening tests of the Clinical Evaluation of Language Functions (CELF). *Language, Speech, and Hearing Services in Schools, 14,* 215–222.

Rice, M., Sell, M., & Hadley, P. (1990). The social interactive coding system (SICS): An on-line, clinically relevant descriptive tool. *Language, Speech, and Hearing Services in Schools, 21,* 2–14.

Roth, F., & Spekman, N. (1984a). Assessing the pragmatic abilities of children: Part 1. Organizational framework and assessment parameters. *Journal of Speech and Hearing Disorders, 49,* 2–11.

Roth, F., & Spekman, N. (1984b). Assessing the pragmatic abilities of children: Part 2. Guidelines, considerations, and specific evaluation procedures. *Journal of Speech and Hearing Disorders, 49,* 12–17.

Scarborough, H., Wyckoff, J., & Davidson, R. (1986). A reconsideration of the relation between age and mean utterance length. *Journal of Speech and Hearing Research, 29,* 394–399.

Shriberg, L., & Kwiatkowski, J. (1980). *Natural process analysis.* New York: Wiley.

Siegel, G. (1975). The use of language tests. *Language, Speech, and Hearing Services in Schools, 6,* 211–217.

Simon, C. (1984). Functional-pragmatic evaluation of communication skills in school-aged children. *Language, Speech, and Hearing Services in Schools, 15,* 83–97.

Staab, C. (1983). Language functions elicited by meaningful activities: A new dimension in language programs. *Language, Speech, and Hearing Services in Schools, 14,* 164–170.

Stein, N., & Glenn, C. (1979). An analysis of story comprehension in elementary school children. In R. Freedle (Ed.), *New directions in discourse processing* (Vol. 2, pp. 53–120). Norwood, NJ: Ablex.

Stephens, M., & Montgomery, A. (1985). A critique of recent relevant standardized tests. *Topics in Language Disorders, 5,* 21–45.

Sullivan, P. (1978). *A comparison of administration modifications on the WISC-R perfomance scale with different categories of deaf children.* Unpublished doctoral dissertation, University of Iowa, Iowa City.

Terman, L., & Merrill, M. (1973). *Stanford-Binet intelligence scale.* Boston: Houghton Mifflin.

Thorndike, R., Hagen, E., & Sattler, J. (1985). *Stanford-Binet intelligence scale* (4th ed.). Chicago: Riverside.

Tomblin, J. B., Hardy, J., & Hein, H. (1991). Predicting poor-communication status in preschool children using risk factors present at birth. *Journal of Speech and Hearing Research, 34,* 1096–1105.

Tyack, D., & Gottsleben, R. (1974). *Language sampling, analysis, and training.* Palo Alto, CA: Consulting Psychologists Press.

Warden, D. (1976). The influence of context on children's use of identifying expressions and references. *British Journal of Psychology, 67,* 101–112.

Washington, J., & Craig, H. (1992). Performance of low-income, African American preschool and kindergarten children on the PPVT-R. *Language, Speech, and Hearing Services in Schools, 23,* 329–333.

Wechsler, D. (1974). *Wechsler intelligence scale for children–Revised.* San Antonio, TX: Psychological Corporation.

Weiner, F. (1978). *Phonological process analysis.* Baltimore: University Park Press.

Wells, G. (1985). *Language development in the pre-school years.* New York: Cambridge University Press.

Wetherby, A., & Rodriguez, G. (1992). Measurement of communicative intentions in normally developing children during structured and unstructured contexts. *Journal of Speech and Hearing Research, 35,* 130–138.

Wiig, E., & Semel, E. (1984). *Language assessment and intervention for the learning disabled* (2nd ed.). New York: Merrill/Macmillan.

· Chapter 15 ·

Language Intervention

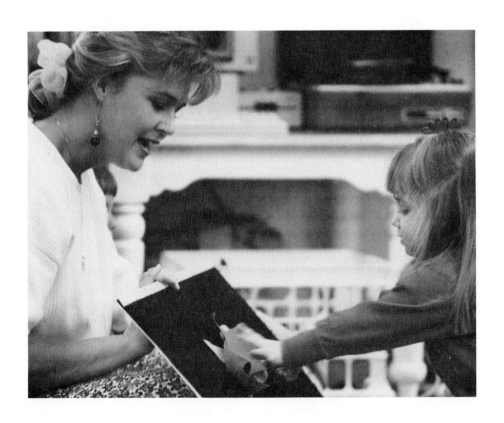

Upon completion of this chapter, the reader should be able to:

▶ Identify considerations in planning and implementing language intervention and discuss how these influence intervention decisions.

▶ Describe various approaches to intervention, and discuss the ways in which they overlap and affect other decisions about interventions.

▶ Describe methods of highlighting intervention targets in order to increase the salience of the rules and regularities to be discovered.

▶ Describe facilitating and elicitation techniques that can be employed in language intervention.

In previous chapters, we discussed a number of intervention considerations. Many of these considerations are appropriate for other children and situations and should be viewed as having applications beyond the specific instances cited. However, no two language-disordered children are exactly alike in the language abilities and disabilities they manifest. Therefore, each child's language intervention plan is developed individually. The plan is based initially on the results of the diagnosis and assessment process and later on the ongoing assessment that is part of any intervention program. There is no one recipe for language intervention. Instead, there are multiple factors and approaches that must be considered in planning.

CONSIDERATIONS IN INTERVENTION

Normal versus Not So Normal Processes

Many of the approaches in language intervention are based on language behaviors and developmental patterns observed in normal children (Olswang & Bain, 1991). Owens (1991) states, "Language intervention strategies should closely approximate the natural process of language acquisition" (p. 177). This approach implies an assumption that what is good and works for normal children is good and works for children with language problems. The problem is, of course, that language-disordered children are not learning language normally, and it is possible that what works for normal language-learning children may not work for language-disordered children.

Connell (1987) compared the effectiveness of two commonly used intervention techniques (modeling and imitation) in teaching a language form to both normal and language-disordered children. The normal language-learning children gained most from the modeling technique. In contrast, the language-disordered children benefited more from the imitation technique. In a later investigation, Connell and Stone (1992) reported that the normal language-learning children in their study learned a morphological rule easily from either modeling or imitation, whereas the language-disordered children showed little learning as a result of the modeling technique but significantly greater acquisition of the morpheme as a result of the imitation technique. Apparently, the modeling technique that worked for the normal children did not work for the children with language problems.

One approach to intervention places an emphasis on naturalistic child-directed environments "closely resembling normal mother–child interaction" (Yoder, Kaiser, & Alpert, 1991, p. 155). Such an approach is based largely on the knowledge that normal children learn language by actively exploring their environments and interacting communicatively with others. Yet, not all language-impaired children may benefit optimally from this strategy. We have seen previously in this text that some children with language problems may demonstrate communicative behaviors that lead observers to label them as unresponsive and/or passive in communicative situations (Fey, 1986; Hadley & Rice, 1991; Paul, 1991; Paul, Looney, & Dahm, 1991; Skarakis-Doyle, MacLellan, & Mullin, 1990). These children may not be able to take full advantage of such a "naturalistic" environmental strategy.

It is likely that at least some language-disordered children need approaches that differ from normal language-learning in order to benefit most from intervention. This means that we may need to modify the normal process somewhat in order to effect language change as efficaciously as possible. Doing more of what is normal by applying the normal process model fully to intervention for language-disordered children may not be totally appropriate (Olswang & Bain, 1991).

Rules and Regularities

One of the more widely accepted principles of language intervention is that it should allow a child to discover the rules or regularities of the linguistic units, concepts, and contexts that occur in the environment (Lahey, 1988; Lahey & Bloom, 1977; Leonard, 1973; Owens, 1991). An objective of intervention is, therefore, to create and/or capitalize on situations and experiences so that the child can discover the regularities. An attempt is made to reduce the complexities seen in usual language learning situations so that the child's task in identifying the regularities is simplified. Multiple repetitions of systematically controlled but varied events may help facilitate the desired discoveries. For example, if the goal is to help a child discover the meaning of "more" to express recurrence, one activity might involve a musical jack-in-the-box controlled by an adult. After an initial presentation of the toy's action, hopefully to the child's delight, the adult allows the child to play with it momentarily, then closes the lid, gives it back to the child for a moment, and finally says to the child, "More. More." After a slight pause, the adult repeats the sequence. After the whole process is repeated several times, the adult begins to pause for longer periods of time between saying "More" and opening the box, with the aim that the child will request "more." Should that happen, the adult immediately opens the box.

Although the child may begin to use "more" in this situation, we cannot be sure exactly what the child has discovered about its meaning. It may be that the child has linked the little doll, the action of popping up, or the action of winding the handle with the word. Consequently, other events that highlight the regularities of "more" need to be introduced into intervention. The jack-in-the-box activity might be followed by a treat, such as juice, during which the child is given sip-sized amounts of juice in a glass. After the child drinks the juice, the adult asks "more?" and more is poured. The intention is that the child will start to use the expression appropriately after the adult begins to pause between asking if the child wants more and supplying it. Additional events clearly illustrating the desired discoveries are also necessary. A pragmatic emphasis is inherent in such an intervention approach. In this example, the inclusion of communicative intents in the form of Halliday's (1975) regulatory function or Dore's (1975) requesting action intention is obvious. The child discovers that the behaviors of others can be regulated and desires can be met through the appropriate use of language.

Different types of intervention objectives (e.g., semantic, morphological or syntactic, pragmatic) may require different approaches in helping children discover the rules and regularities. Connell (1989), for instance, reported that an intervention approach that employed *induction* (discovering a general rule from observing individual cases) facilitated semantic objectives. In contrast, an intervention approach that employed *deduction* (applying a general or known rule to a new or unknown situation) facilitated morphosyntactic objectives.

Although this principle of assisting children to discover the regularities applies to language intervention for preschoolers, school-age children, and adolescents alike, it is especially applicable for younger children who have not acquired metalinguistic skills in order to talk about and analyze language. For older children and adolescents with some metalinguistic abilities, explanations of the regularities to be discovered may help them focus on the rules. Incorporating some use of writing or written practice may even assist older children in identifying the regularities and reinforcing the interaction between oral and written language (Johnson, 1985). However, these explanations and analyses are no substitutes for actual practice in contextually appropriate situations.

Usefulness of the Intervention Content

This discussion brings us to another consideration in language intervention. Language-disordered children must learn to communicate, not just learn the forms and content of language. Cole (1982) writes that children should draw the following conclusions about language:

Through language, they can influence what other people do.

They can use language to get what they want and to reject what they do not want.

They can use language to call attention to what they find interesting or important.

Through language, they can represent their needs, desires, and ideas.

Their use of language facilitates establishment and maintenance of interpersonal relationships.

Language assists them in gaining new information, in sharing prior experiences, and in making projections about the future.

They can use language to resolve conflicts, defend their viewpoints, and protect their own interests.

Through interpreting what others say, they can benefit from another person's experiences and gain insights into someone else's ideas and feelings. (p. 101)

Intervention, therefore, needs to stress useful language. In suggesting criteria to be used to select which words should first be taught to language-disordered children, Lahey and Bloom (1977) make a strong case for emphasizing words that have broad applications for children in many different communicative situations. The more frequently children can use a word, the more useful the word is for them. For example, the word "no" has far broader uses than the word "yes." With "no," a child can comment on the disappearance of objects and events, express nonexistence, reject unwanted events and objects, and deny. With "no," a child can learn to exercise some control or to regulate the environment. The word, therefore, has important pragmatic and semantic value for the child. In contrast, the applicability of "yes" is more limited. As Lahey and Bloom point out, affirmation is the usual state of affairs, and "yes" is necessary only as a response to another's question about a desire or the truth. "Yes" is only a child-responding word, whereas "no" is both a child-responding and a child-initiating word. Holland (1975) supports this notion of usefulness when she writes that the words to be included

in intervention should be "maximally exploitable" (p. 519).

This principle of usefulness is one of the major reasons for the present emphasis on the pragmatic aspects of language. In planning content and forms to stress in intervention, the ways in which children can employ them in their daily environments are always considered. Teaching children how to communicate may, in fact, be the primary focus of intervention in some instances. Recall that some language-impaired youngsters seem uninterested in communication and communicative interactions. Helping these children to discover that language is useful for a variety of functions and intentions, and then teaching them how to employ language to accomplish these purposes, can be important intervention objectives.

When it is appropriate to emphasize syntax and morphology, the usefulness of the forms for the child is important in selecting what grammatical features to teach. This includes the unique and definitive meanings the forms can encode for a child, the efficiency with which certain forms can communicate (e.g., one utterance encoding two ideas, as in a sentence with a relative clause, such as "I like the boy who plays nicely" rather than two utterances to express the ideas, such as "I like the boy." "He plays nicely."), and the variety of ways the forms can provide for encoding functions and intentions (e.g., direct versus indirect requests).

Developmental and Nondevelopmental Intervention

Language intervention plans are often strongly grounded in normal language development. We have encountered this notion elsewhere in this text. Normal language developmental patterns can guide the sequences of objectives planned for language-disordered children (e.g., Cole, 1982; Fey, 1986; Holland, 1975; Lahey, 1988; Lahey & Bloom, 1977; McLean & Snyder-McLean, 1978; Miller & Yoder, 1972, 1974; Owens, 1991). A rationale behind a developmental approach is that a particular language skill has antecedents that provide the bases for the acquisition of the higher-level skill. New language skills are built on previously acquired skills, and earlier-acquired abilities influence the learning of later-developing ones. Information from normal language development assists us, therefore, in deciding what skills need to be learned before other skills can be acquired.

In many cases, a developmental approach to language intervention is warranted. There is limited evidence that developmental approaches are more successful and potentially promote generalization more than nondevelopmental approaches (Bryen & Joyce, 1985; Dyer, Santarcangelo, & Luce, 1987). Besides providing a rationale for selecting initial goals of intervention, a developmental approach is a way of guiding ongoing intervention.

Examples of using a developmental approach in choosing intervention goals for syntax or morphology include (1) focusing on relative clauses to modify objects of sentences before relative clauses to modify subjects of sentences, for which an embedding process is required; (2) emphasizing the present progressive verb inflection (ing) before past tense verbs or third-person present tense regular verb inflections ("runs"); and (3) introducing the allomorph /z/ to pluralize nouns before the allomorphs /s/ and /əz/. In using Clark's (1973) proposed developmental concepts derived from her Semantic Feature Hypothesis to guide intervention goals in the semantic area, the positive term of antonym word pairs or the term in these pairs that represents the greater change from a child's status quo might be introduced first. For example, "big" and "new" might be taught before "little" and "old." Similarly, words with fewer semantic features and broader applicability ("big") would be chosen as intervention targets before words having more features and more specific applications ("tall"). Because normal children generally use semantic relations expressing nomination, recurrence, and nonexistence before those indicating attributes of objects, the former types of semantic relations might be emphasized in intervention before entity + attributive ("car big") and attributive + entity ("big car") relations. For intervention focusing on pragmatic aspects of language, utterances that encode only one function per utterance would be stressed prior to those that encode two or more functions per utterance. Intervention for conversational turn-taking skills might begin with the language precursors of reciprocal interactions at the nonverbal level, if the child lacks these

skills, before introducing verbal turn-taking activities. In helping children learn to maintain a topic in conversation, intervention might first focus on having the children use one, possibly two, contingent responses and later include objectives for several contingent responses. Furthermore, contingent responses involving repetitions of part of an adult's previous utterance (focus/imitation devices) might be encouraged before contingent responses involving the addition of new information (substitution/expansion devices).

Normal developmental data need to be viewed, however, as providing guidelines rather than prescriptions for language intervention (Fey, 1986; Lahey, 1988; Owens, 1991). Furthermore, although a developmental approach is likely the more frequently used strategy for planning intervention, there may be occasions where deviations from usual developmental sequences are appropriate. As we saw in chapter 8, intervention with autistic children may not always follow developmental sequences. Fey (1986) suggests that characteristics of a specific child, such as intellectual level or level of comprehension for a particular language skill, may also indicate the occasional use of nondevelopmental strategies. Another example relates to normal children's tendency to use irregular past tense verbs before regular past tense verbs (Brown, 1973). However, this sequence is rarely used in intervention. The former ability probably reflects lexical learning rather than discovery of morphological rules represented by acquisition of the latter skills. Therefore, if past tense verbs are to be an intervention focus, regular past tense verbs should be taught with the objective of having a child discover the morphological rules before irregular past tense verbs were emphasized. In other instances, a child or the child's parents/caregivers or teachers may have immediate communication needs that require a nondevelopmental approach. However, most professionals recommend a return to a developmental approach as soon as possible and suggest that normal developmental sequences be used within a larger objective that itself may not be in developmental sequence.

Comprehension or Production

In chapter 1, we saw that the relationship between language comprehension and production is not well understood. We do know, however, that comprehension skills do not always precede, nor are they always superior to, production skills. However, some professionals recommend that comprehension objectives be introduced before production objectives. They propose that a child needs to understand the meaning behind a word or an utterance before being expected to use it and that comprehension activities additionally heighten a child's attention to the rules and regularities to be discovered. Having children rotely produce specific forms without understanding their meanings or purposes certainly does not lay the groundwork for generalization to everyday use.

In contrast to the comprehension approach, others suggest that intervention focus on production, with comprehension included as a concomitant goal. A rationale behind this approach is that comprehension develops concurrently with production if language intervention is done with an emphasis on meaning, as well as linguistic forms, as systematic input is provided by the adult. That is, language intervention that focuses on using appropriate forms to represent content in various contexts and for different purposes (Lahey, 1988) likely improves production skills as well as comprehension skills.

At present, there is no agreement on which intervention approach is more effective. However, two studies looking at language-impaired children's learning of different aspects of language suggest that these children may need opportunities to produce intervention targets in order to incorporate these targets in their expressive language. Dollaghan's (1987) study focused on lexical acquisition. She investigated normal and language-impaired children's ability to fast-map the meanings of words. She found that normal and language-impaired children were equally able to infer word meaning from limited, structured exposures. However, the language-impaired children could not produce the words following limited exposure, whereas the majority of the normal language-learning children could. Connell and Stone (1992) focused on morphological acquisition. In their study, normal and language-impaired children were taught several morphemes. Both groups learned to comprehend their meanings. However, the language-impaired children were able to use the morphemes only if they had previously been asked to produce utterances containing the morphemes. From these two studies, it would seem that training involving comprehension resulted in comprehension of the targets; training involving comprehension alone did not result in production; and production practice resulted in use of the targets.

A production approach may be more appropriate for some intervention objectives, whereas a comprehension approach may be more effective for others. It is important not to assume that one approach is always superior to the other. This is true as an orientation toward language intervention for children generally and likely applies to individual children in their own intervention programs. At one point in a child's intervention, it may be appropriate to emphasize comprehension before production for a specific language goal. At a different point in intervention, for another language goal, it may be more appropriate to stress production. The approach selected depends on the child, the language goal, and the child's changing needs during intervention.

Focus of Intervention

Whether initial intervention focuses on pragmatic, semantic, and/or morphosyntactic skills depends on an individual child's needs identified in the diagnostic and assessment process. Very young prelinguistic children may first need to develop intentional and nonverbal communicative interactions and cognitive skills associated with language learning, such as participation in joint action routines, symbolic play with accompanying symbolic gestures, or gestural requests for objects. For other children, developing social interactive discourse skills may be most immediate. Discovering morphological or syntactic rules and regularities may be appropriate for other language-disordered children, whereas developing semantic skills may be most important for still others. Children may often need intervention in more than one area and/or may need to strengthen their associations among the areas. Intervention for specific language patterns is individualized for each child.

Although it may be appropriate to focus intervention on one aspect of language, this does not preclude attention to the other aspects of language. In fact, in a review of studies investigating various approaches to teaching language-disordered children linguistic skills, Leonard (1981) concluded:

> Training approaches that focus only on particular linguistic forms are likely to result in the child's use of these forms, and little more. Approaches that provide exposure to, and practice with linguistic features in addition to those serving as the major focal points of training are likely to result in somewhat broader linguistic gains. (p. 110)

Intervention plans need to attend to all aspects of language simultaneously, even though one aspect may receive greater emphasis. As indicated previously, language skills emphasized in intervention also need to be useful. In focusing on syntax, it makes little sense to have a child produce syntactic sequences containing words whose meanings are unknown to the child or to use sentences in which the semantic relations among the words are typically nonsensical (e.g., "The tree is walking."). Intervention with a syntactic focus also needs to help a child realize the ways linguistic forms can be used for communication. As an example, yes/no question transformations can be used to gain information ("Can it bark?"), request objects or permission ("Can I have it?"), or direct another's actions ("Can you get a chair?"). Even though another child's intervention may contain a pragmatic focus, form and content must match the aspects of use being emphasized. If an objective of intervention is to help a child express instrumental functions (Halliday, 1975), logical forms might include a reaching or pointing gesture paired with an object's name, the phrase "want _____," or the sentence "I want _____." The specific form selected for the child would, of course, depend on the child's level of syntactic proficiency. Similarly, intervention with a semantic focus must include relationships among meanings of words, as expressed in morphological and syntactic forms, and use of the word meanings in appropriate contexts. When all aspects of language are kept in mind in planning and executing intervention, a primary focus on one aspect may well facilitate a child's learning of the other secondary aspects concurrently. This is likely true, however, only if intervention is not limited to drill work. Instead, intervention needs to encourage a child's use of a specific target in human interactions.

The focus of intervention may interact with the strategies used to promote language learning (Olswang & Bain, 1991). Earlier, we noted Connell's (1989) work suggesting that inductive strategies might be more effective for semantic objectives, whereas deductive strategies might work better for morphosyntactic objectives. In planning intervention, therefore, it is necessary to decide what strategy is likely to be most facilitative for the focus of intervention (Olswang & Bain, 1991).

Although intervention may begin with a greater focus on one aspect of language than others, the focus may shift several times. As a child progresses, an initial emphasis on pragmatic skills may shift to semantic or morphosyntactic skills. Ongoing intervention is a fluid process, the focus of which changes to meet the child's changing needs. As the focus changes, so do the strategies.

Controlling Complexity

When intervention focuses on one aspect of language, it is important to control the complexity of the other aspects that are simultaneously included. It is unreasonable to expect a language-disordered child to use a new word in a multiword utterance containing a new syntactic form to express a new function all at the same time. Even children who are acquiring language normally do not do this. They tend to use simpler, earlier-acquired syntactic structures to encode new ideas or content and to express earlier-acquired content in new syntactic forms (Bloom, Miller, & Hood, 1975; Slobin, 1973). Similarly, we can expect children to use newly acquired intentions and functions in old, well-established linguistic forms to express well-known content.

In using this information for intervention, a new morphological or syntactic structure would initially be presented in a situation where the child could use well-established words in highly stabilized, perhaps even routinized, contexts. For semantics, intervention would first involve new words or new semantic relations used in familiar morphosyntactic forms and contexts. For improvement of pragmatic skills, the child would initially be encouraged to apply the new skills to old linguistic forms in familiar interactions. Even controlling the phonological content of words being taught with a focus on semantics may influence how easily the words are acquired (Leonard, 1984). Recall that Leonard and his colleagues (Leonard, Schwartz, Morris, & Chapman, 1981; Schwartz & Leonard, 1982) found that young children acquired new words more quickly when the words contained sounds already in their repertoires than when the words contained sounds the children had not yet used. As a child starts to demonstrate acquisition of the new target language behavior, less established aspects of the other language components can be gradually introduced.

Reinforcement

Reinforcement is a powerful factor in language intervention. As Mowrer (1982) points out: "There can be no doubt that the most widely known procedure for increasing and sustaining a behavior is the application of positive reinforcement following a behavior. It is also one of the most effective means of changing behavior" (p. 207). There are two types of *positive reinforcers,* which are defined solely by their effects in increasing the frequency of behaviors. The two types are *primary reinforcers,* such as food, which are biologically determined, and *secondary reinforcers,* which become reinforcing through their associations with primary reinforcers. Although primary reinforcers are occasionally employed in language intervention when a child is unresponsive to secondary reinforcers, secondary reinforcers are typically used. Common types of secondary reinforcers are tokens, verbal praise, and natural consequences of appropriate language use. Natural consequences include gaining and sustaining an adult's attention, having desires and needs met, and engaging in pleasurable human interactions.

In recent years, there has been an increased realization of the reinforcing effects that natural consequences of language use have in language intervention. Meline (1980) points out that the "power of language lies within the functions it serves" (p. 95). When successful communication occurs and a child's purposes and intents are fulfilled because of the language the child used, those language behaviors are naturally reinforced. The child learns that appropriate language use is a powerful tool in controlling the environment.

The current emphasis on natural language reinforcers evolved, in part, from a recognition of the limitations that tokens and verbal praise as reinforcers have in language intervention, particularly in the generalization of language behaviors to everyday use. In fact, Hubbell (1977) concluded from his review of the literature that responses to another's talking that are typically viewed as positive reinforcers, such as indicating approval verbally or touching the speaker in an affectionate manner, actually decrease the probability that further talking will occur. Hubbell surmised that these behavioral responses constrained further talking because they interrupted the verbal interaction that was taking place. Furthermore, Spradlin and Siegel (1982) have suggested that the reinforcers often used in language intervention bear "little resemblance to those that are provided in the outside environment" (p. 5). These authors express a specific concern about the effects these artificial forms of reinforcement have on generalization of language skills. They write that if "generalization is to occur, the child should be offered the kinds of reinforcers during training that will be available in the nontraining environment" (p. 5).

Arguments can be made, however, for sometimes employing primary reinforcers or tokens and/or verbal praise in language intervention. Some severely impaired children appear to have so few social needs and desires that finding naturalistic secondary forms of reinforcment can be difficult, if not impossible (McCormick & Goldman, 1984). There are also aspects of language, such as the use of specific grammatical features, that do not have ready naturalistic reinforcers. Among these grammatical features are many of the auxiliary verbs and the copula "to be." Artificial and contrived reinforcers can help to increase the salience of certain language features, aiding a child in discovering more readily the rules that govern their uses.

If these forms of reinforcement are employed in language intervention, there should be a consistent move toward eventually replacing them with natural reinforcers. This can be accomplished either by gradually eliminating the artificial reinforcers and introducing the naturalistic ones or by pairing the artificial and naturalistic reinforcers so that the latter take on the characteristics of the former. When this occurs, the artificial reinforcers are no longer necessary. Using artificial reinforcers also requires that considerable attention be given to the generalization of language skills. In contrast, naturalistic reinforcers by themselves tend to facilitate generalization.

Generalization

Generalization of language skills learned in intervention to effective use in everyday situations is the major objective of language intervention plans. Unfortunately, lack of generalization is too often a problem. In fact, it is sufficiently problematic that Owens (1991) suggests that generalization be planned before implementing intervention. All too often, children use language skills learned in intervention only in those situations and not in other contexts. Not surprisingly, the types of reinforcement employed, as just discussed, may be one reason generalization fails to occur. To reiterate, natural reinforcers, or at least a combination of natural and artificial reinforcers, may be more conducive to generalization than artificial reinforcers alone. Spradlin and Siegel (1982) cite other reasons that generalization may not occur. Materials used to stimulate language, such as objects and pictures, may be employed repeatedly. Or a child may be asked to use the specific language skills only with the same adult, often in the same relatively sterile room. In other cases, the focus of intervention may ignore certain aspects of language, or the language skills emphasized may not be functional and useful for a child. That is, they lack ecological validity for the child.

Although generalization is often a problematic area of language intervention, some evidence suggests that children will spontaneously generalize the use of specific language skills emphasized in intervention to other skills that closely resemble them (e.g., Gray & Fygetakis, 1968; Hegde, 1980; Hegde, Noll, & Pecora, 1979; Leonard, 1974; Wilcox & Leonard, 1978). This form of generalization is referred to as *response class generalization*. For example, a child may receive intervention targeting the copula "is" and generalize its use to the auxiliary "is" in similar types of sentences,

even though the latter skill was not an intervention target. However, there may be limitations on response class generalization. One of these limitations may involve typical developmental sequences seen in normal children (Wilcox & Leonard, 1978). If the nontargeted skills are normally developed much later than the targeted skill, response class generalization may not be observed. Additionally, the nontargeted skills may need to share many of the topographical features, such as phonological and grammatic similarities, of the targeted skill in order for generalization to occur (Leonard, 1981). For this reason, a child may generalize use of the copula "is" to the auxiliary "is" but not to the copula "was."

Another positive factor in generalization involves the contexts to which targeted language skills may spontaneously generalize. When contexts differ only slightly from the situation used in intervention to teach a language skill, some generalization to those different contexts without specific intervention has been observed (Gray & Fygetakis, 1968; Hegde et al., 1979; Hester & Hendrickson, 1977). On the negative side, however, when contexts differ in several respects from the one in which a skill was originally targeted, little generalization may take place (e.g., Mulac & Tomlinson, 1977; Zwitman & Sonderman, 1979). In reviewing the literature in this area, Leonard (1981) concludes:

> There is little evidence that the child's use of the trained form will extend to speaking situations that bear little resemblance to the training/testing situation. Additional training using a variety of settings, verbal and visual stimuli, and interactants seems to be necessary to achieve this level of usage. (p. 114)

Although limited spontaneous response class generalization and generalization to slightly different contexts may be observed for some language skills, it appears that language intervention needs to attend specifically to the process of generalization. We have seen that effective control of reinforcers is an important factor in promoting generalization. Spradlin and Siegel (1982) concur with Leonard (1981) on other factors that are important to generalization:

1. Employ different stimuli to elicit the targeted language behavior.

2. Employ a variety of contexts in which the targeted language behavior is to be used.

3. Employ different people with whom the targeted behavior is to be used. These people include other children, parents, classroom teachers, and other adults.

To employ parents and other adults effectively in an intervention plan, these people will probably need training in facilitating generalization. As we have seen previously in this text, parents/caregivers are essential partners in intervention. Olswang, Kriegsmann, and Mastergeorge (1982) describe a successful intervention plan in which a child's teacher was trained to assist in increasing a language-disordered child's use of requesting behaviors. Spradlin and Siegel (1982) suggest that in natural environments parents can be shown how to (1) create situations so that learning language accomplishes things more effectively and efficiently than nonlanguage use; (2) postpone reinforcements and give appropriate verbal models when a child indicates a communicative attempt nonverbally; (3) respond appropriately to a child's attempts at communication; and (4) arrange opportunities in the environment for a child to use specific language responses.

Connell (1982) adds another component. He suggests that generalization can also be facilitated by *contrast training*. In this procedure, sentences that require a targeted language skill are contrasted with "minimally different sentences" that do not require that skill. The concept behind this approach is to provide "the learner with grammatical and contextual information concerning the obligation of linguistic forms" (p. 235). The intent is for the child to generalize appropriately to sentences that obligate a specific language skill but not overgeneralize to sentences in which the skill should not be used. Although Connell limits his discussion of contrast training to syntax, this approach may be applicable to semantic, morphological, and/or pragmatic aspects of language.

Child Characteristics

The individual characteristics of each child influence not only the focus of intervention, but also many of the other decisions that are made about intervention (Carrow-Woolfolk, 1988). For a child with attention difficulties, a nondistracting intervention environment may be considered appropriate. For a child with communicative interactive difficulties without attention problems, a group setting, classroom, or preschool setting may be chosen. The combinations are numerous. Unfortunately, we have only limited empirically derived information to provide guidelines for matching specific child characteristics with intervention approaches and/or strategies.

Some of the factors that have been considered are age and nonverbal intelligence level, as well as level of language functioning; the latter includes amount of verbal behavior generally and types of language needs or the focus of intervention. We need to be aware, however, that these factors may not be discrete. Age, cognition, and language level/focus of intervention may interact. For example, older children can be expected to have greater language functioning and, therefore, intervention needs that focus on morphosyntactic structures. Similarly, more cognitively advanced children can be expected to have greater language functioning. Conclusions from several articles in the literature (Cole & Dale, 1986; Connell, 1987; Friedman & Friedman, 1980) have suggested that higher-functioning language-impaired children (age and/or cognitive skill and/or language level) benefit more from naturalistic, conversational approaches and that lower-functioning language-impaired children benefit more from didactic, structured approaches. More recently, the results of a study by Yoder et al. (1991) seem to challenge some of these findings. These authors found that lower-functioning language-impaired children made greater progress with a naturalistic approach, whereas higher-functioning children progressed more with a didactic, structured approach. In attempting to integrate their findings with the earlier ones, Yoder and his colleagues suggested that subject differences and the resulting language intervention goals may have contributed to the discrepant findings. To reiterate, higher-functioning children are more likely to have intervention objectives that focus on morphosyntactic structures. Therefore, the type of language goal may interact with the effectiveness of different approaches. Yoder et al. write, "Future studies should control the type of language goal while investigating which treatment methods are most efficient for which children" (p. 166). At present, we do not know exactly how level of functioning, type of intervention objective, and intervention approach interact. We do know, however, that we need to consider such interactions in making intervention decisions.

Another characteristic to be considered is the child's interests, which affect the activities employed. Activities need to reflect the child's interests and cognitive level. When a child is presented with different toys and situations, it may be possible for the adult to follow the child's lead in deciding what is interesting and stimulating for the child at the moment and create the logical opportunities to use a targeted language skill in that context. Holland (1975) provides an example of how language intervention can capitalize on a child's momentary interests:

> I observed a therapy session in which a gifted clinician was teaching "more." She had prepared for the session by amassing quantities of similar small items to use in conjunction with her own utterance "more _____" and had plans eventually to demand the word from the child. However, the child, hyperactive and of limited verbal skills, became fascinated by a box of Kleenex in the room. The clinician began pulling tissues from the box, accompanying each pull with her utterance "more Kleenex." Eventually, when clinician and child had scattered tissues around the room the clinician introduced the utterance "more throw," accompanied by the two of them creating a snowfall of tissues. In this manner the child learned "more." (pp. 517–518)

Unfortunately, some language-disordered children demonstrate so little interest in their environments that an approach focusing on child-oriented activities is useless. For these children, the adult may need to create interesting situations artificially through structured reinforcement schedules, parallel and intersecting play activities, and/or careful control of stimuli presentations. In other instances, specific targeted language behaviors, such as some morphosyntactic structures, may necessitate more adult-oriented activities. The point is that both child-oriented and adult-oriented activities can be appropriate, depending on the individual child's status and the language behavior to be emphasized. Successful language intervention depends, in part, on the ability to determine which approach is appropriate under the circumstances and a willingness to employ each as the situations demand.

Metalinguistics

We have seen that toddlers and preschoolers possess only rudimentary metalinguistic skills, at best, and that the beginning of relatively sophisticated metalinguistic skills emerges in the early school years. Therefore, for young children it is inappropriate to base intervention strategies on metalinguistic skills. That is, we do not teach a word's meaning, a discourse rule, or a morphosyntactic structure by explaining the meaning or the rule to a toddler or preschooler. Rather, we teach by example. This does not mean, however, that we must avoid referring to a regularity. In fact, such references may actually help a young child focus on the regularity and promote development of metalinguistic skills. Such reference is not unusual in parent–preschooler interactions, although it may not correspond to parent–toddler interactions. Parents of normal preschoolers occasionally comment to their children that certain words have specific meanings, that some things can be said to some people and not to others, and that some ways of saying a sentence are right and others are wrong. What the developmental information about toddlers' and preschoolers' metalinguistic skills does imply is that intervention strategies that depend on metalinguistic skills are not appropriate. In contrast, intervention for school-age children and adolescents may not only use metalinguistics as a strategy but may also include the improvement of metalinguistic abilities as an objective.

APPROACHES TO INTERVENTION

In this section we discuss various approaches to intervention. Although we divide this section into four subsections, it will become apparent that the topics are not autonomous. Rather, aspects of each discussion interact with aspects of the others.

Direct and Indirect Intervention

Previously in this text, reference has been made to direct and indirect intervention. The basic difference between the two approaches is who acts as the primary agent of language change for a child (Olswang & Bain, 1991). In *direct intervention,* the professional is the primary change agent. The professional plans the objectives of intervention and the strategies to be employed and interacts directly with the child. Others, such as parents/caregivers and teachers, are typically involved in the planning and may even assist the professional in implementation, but the professional retains the role of major change agent (Olswang & Bain, 1991; Wilcox, 1989). In *indirect intervention,* the professional also plans the objectives, again typically with parents/caregivers and/or teachers, and decides on specific strategies for implementation. However, individuals other than the language professional, such as parents/caregivers and/or teachers, carry out the plans. The professional works with these individuals to show them how to carry out the plans and monitors the implementation and the child's progress. The professional generally does not work directly with the child. In chapter 5 we discussed the necessity to train parents/caregivers for indirect intervention with toddlers and preschoolers. The same is true when teachers or day-care providers are the primary agents of change. In some cases, a combination of direct and indirect intervention may be warranted, or intervention may change from one approach to another as the objectives and the child's language behavior change.

There is little empirical information to help us in deciding which approach is most effective under what conditions. Olswang and Bain (1991) point out that identifying the purpose of intervention at a specific point in time may assist in deciding which approach may be more effective. They suggest that direct intervention may be more appropriate when the aim is to establish a new language behavior and that indirect intervention may be more appropriate when the aim is to stabilize, generalize, or extend a language behavior that the child already demonstrates or that has been established as a result of direct intervention. In situations where both direct and indirect intervention are occurring, certain objectives to establish specific behaviors may require direct intervention and other objectives to extend or generalize different language behaviors may involve indirect intervention.

Group and Individual Intervention

In chapter 11, we suggested that for language-disordered adolescents, group intervention may be more effective than individual, or one-to-one, intervention. This belief is somewhat counter to the more traditional view. For many years it was thought that a one-to-one setting was the most effective format. With this format, extraneous environmental distractions could be controlled, allowing a child to focus on the desired stimuli. Language learning, it was believed, would be promoted quickly.

The rationale behind a one-to-one structure for language intervention may, in part, be valid. Reducing distractions can increase the salience of the provided stimuli to promote learning of the targeted language rules and regularities. However, language is an interactive, interpersonal behavior. As such, many of the reasons cited for employing group intervention with language-disordered adolescents also apply to young children. Young children learn language by interacting with their environments and the people in them. A one-to-one intervention format often limits the number of events and contexts in which language teaching can occur and restricts the number of people with whom the language can be used. In contrast, small-group intervention formats for young children can provide situations for language learning not present in individual intervention settings. In light of our previous discussions of reinforcement and generalization, we can see how a group format might furnish opportunities for naturalistic reinforcers to occur and promote generalization. Each child in a small group is exposed to a variety of stimuli, experiences, contexts, and people that are not available in one-to-one situations. A number of adults, including parents, could participate, providing the children opportunities to use language with different adults as well as other children. This format could also be used to help train parents and teachers in strategies to be employed in indirect intervention.

The decision as to whether a child will benefit more from a group setting or an individual format depends on the specific child. Some children, particularly those who are hyperactive, distractible, or inattentive or those who show little interest in interacting with people, may initially require one-to-one intervention. For other children, a small-group setting may be more appropriate. Furthermore, the type of setting from which a specific child will benefit may change as the child's behaviors and language skills change. Children who initially require individual intervention can progress to a group setting. Children initially seen in a group setting may later need intervention for specific skills best learned in a one-to-one format. Again, there is no fixed rule as to which format must be used throughout a child's intervention program. Instead, flexibility in providing a child with the appropriate setting at a particular point is the key.

The decision regarding the structure of a child's intervention does not always involve a choice between a group or an individual format (Hubbell, 1977). In many instances, a combination of the two can be effective. Targeted language skills can be presented in an undistracting, one-to-one situation and then used in the variety of contexts and with the variety of people present in a group setting.

Three Language-Teaching Methods

"Contemporary language teaching methods may be characterized along a continuum from highly structured didactic teaching to naturalistic child-oriented interventions" (Yoder et al., 1991, p. 155). As Fey (1986) points out, many highly structured, didactic language-teaching methods may fail to incorporate language-learning situations, activities, and consequences that occur in the actual environment. Although these methods may be beneficial in establishing certain types of language behaviors, they may have difficulty in promoting generalization and in making language useful. The naturalistic methods, on the other hand, may fail to provide sufficiently salient or frequent exemplars for a child to discover and/or practice the desired language behaviors. Another problem is that intervention objectives may be so broad or general that determining the efficacy of intervention is troublesome. Children who have difficulty attending to their environments may find naturalistic methods overwhelming, and those who are uninterested in their environments may continue

to be uninterested when this teaching method is employed.

Because of the problems associated with both highly structured and naturalistic methods, many professionals have tried to adopt methods somewhere in between. Fey (1986) terms these hybrid intervention methods. These methods attempt to bring to intervention environments and/or activities that are as natural as possible but still provide sufficient opportunities for the adults to control and manipulate the teaching situations in order to ensure adequate exemplars, opportunities for response, practice, and generalization.

Olswang and Bain (1991) have presented three commonly adopted language teaching methods: milieu teaching, joint action routines, and inductive teaching. As the authors explain, these methods share some similar features and incorporate procedures found in other methods as well. However, they vary in terms of the degree of structure involved.

Milieu Teaching   Of the three methods, milieu teaching is least structured. Natural consequences of communication as reinforcements, activities determined by the child's interests and attention, conversational contexts for teaching, and intervention in the child's usual environment (home, preschool, classroom) are characteristics of the milieu teaching approach. Opportunities for targeted language behaviors are dispersed throughout a session. Olswang and Bain (1991) identify three procedures used in milieu teaching, although these procedures can also be employed in other teaching approaches. The procedures are incidental teaching, mand-model teaching, and delay.

Incidental Teaching.   In incidental teaching, the child determines the activity or topic, and the adult works the language teaching into it. The activity or topic lasts only as long as the child is interested in and reinforced by it. During this period, the adult may use a variety of techniques, discussed later in this chapter, to elicit specific language behaviors. Incidental teaching was introduced in chapter 6.

Mand-Model.   This procedure was also introduced in chapter 6. Unlike incidental teaching, it is a more adult-oriented procedure. The adult chooses a time to direct the child's attention to an object or activity and asks for (mands) a response from the child or provides a prompt for a response. If the child gives an appropriate response verbally, the adult reinforces the response and then gives the child the desired object or allows the activity to proceed. If the child's response is incomplete or incorrect, models of the target response or other elicitation techniques are used.

Delay.   When a child wants an object out of reach or desires certain events to occur, the adult looks questioningly at the child but waits, usually for about 15 seconds (Olswang & Bain, 1991), before responding. Obviously, the adult is waiting for an appropriate response from the child before complying. If the child does not respond, the adult may provide a model of the target response or use other elicitation techniques and wait again. Generally, the sequence is repeated only twice before complying with the child's desires. Too many repetitions without a successful outcome may do nothing more than increase a child's frustration. However, if too many unsuccessful outcomes occur, immediate reevaluation of the teaching approaches and strategies being employed is warranted.

Delay is an important intervention procedure even when used with other language teaching methods. Language-disordered children may not be able to respond as quickly as normal language-learning children. They may need more time to understand what is expected, to process the stimuli, and/or to retrieve and generate a response.

One of the major difficulties with milieu teaching is the dispersed nature of the opportunities for learning.

Joint Action Routines   This teaching method is sometimes known as *script therapy*. The idea is to create interactive, systematic repetitions of events in which each partner has predictable language and behavioral patterns to complete. The routines can reflect usual events in a child's environment or they can be created. These routines are socially based and incorporate the need to communicate. They focus on specific themes or topics, such as craft activities in which the adult and child interact and the child has to ask for needed materials. Joint action routines are purported

to reduce demands on a child so that the child can focus on the language tasks required. As the child becomes familiar with specific routines, the expectations for language use gradually change to more advanced skills. A problem with this method of language teaching is the manner in which the routines are or are not modified to increase the level of language expected from a child and the strategies employed to elicit the higher-level language behaviors. Generalizing the routines to novel situations can also be problematic.

Inductive Teaching   Inductive teaching is the most structured and adult-oriented method discussed here. The ideas related to inductive teaching are not unlike those presented in our discussion of rules and regularities earlier in this chapter. The adult manipulates meaningful communicative interactions so that the child begins to identify patterns (or regularities) and hypothesize a rule to govern the language associated with the patterns. Olswang and Bain (1991) identify three elements of inductive teaching:

1. The communicative interactions are arranged to allow the child to discover that a pattern exists. Connell's (1982) concept of contrast training applies here. The important features that contrast meaningful situations linguistically are highlighted.
2. The child discovers that the meaningful context or communicative interaction is associated with the pattern and, in fact, explains the pattern. The child learns that the patterns involved affect meaning.
3. The child hypothesizes "the rule that captures the nature of the correspondence between the observed pairs of stimuli. The assumption of this procedure is that the induction process is an innate one so that by this step, if the preceding ones have been arranged correctly, hypothesizing the rule will occur automatically" (Olswang & Bain, 1991, pp. 81–82).

We have seen, however, that although it is necessary to figure out the rules and regularities in order to learn language, merely knowing the rules and regularities may not be enough to produce them.

In practice, it is not unusual to see professionals using elements of all three methods. Each has its merits and drawbacks. The merits need to be matched to the child and the intervention objectives. These different methods or elements of these methods may suit different children and different language objectives. What we do not know yet is how to match these variables unfailingly. We do know that we need to try.

Service Delivery Models

Previously in this text, particularly in chapter 7, we have introduced ideas related to different models of delivering language intervention services to children. Several models have been described in the literature, and a number of terms have been used. In 1983, the Committee on Language, Speech, and Hearing Services in the Schools, a committee of the American Speech-Language-Hearing Association, described four service delivery models for the school setting: indirect services (commonly referred to as the *consultation model,* direct services (self-contained classroom), direct services (resource room), and direct services (itinerant). We can note some similiarities with our previous discussion of direct and indirect intervention approaches. As federal education laws have increasingly influenced service delivery in education, with emphases on integration and mainstreaming of children with special needs into the regular education environment as much as possible, the four types of models just listed have been modified. There has been an increasing trend to provide language intervention

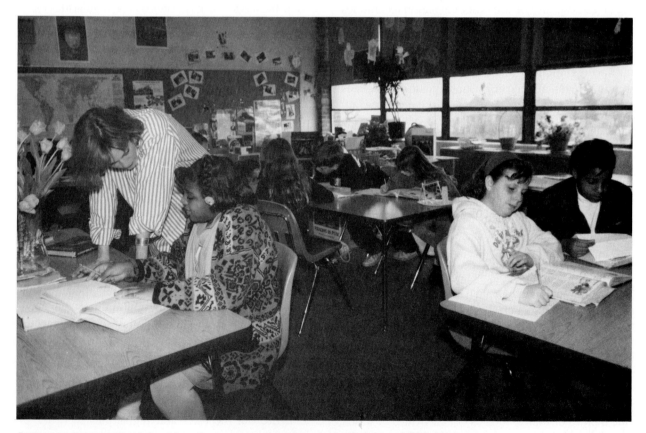

Language intervention takes place in a variety of settings, including in a child's classroom.

in children's classrooms or other usual environments. These services are sometimes delivered by an adult other than the professional; in this case, they are considered indirect interventions and fall into the category of consultation services because of the consultative role that the language professional plays. In some situations, children may work with the language professional in their classrooms during other activities, such as free reading, art, or group discussions. These services would be considered direct intervention but not necessarily consultative or collaborative. In still other cases, the language professional delivers the services in the classrooms, generally in collaboration with the regular educator or other professionals, aides, or parents/caregivers. Forms of delivery in these instances may include team teaching or turn teaching with the teachers. In the latter situation, each of the professionals may teach part of the curriculum, depending on their areas of expertise. Although this is considered to be a collaborative model, direct intervention is being provided by the language professional. As whole language approaches, as discussed in chapter 1, are being integrated more fully into educational curricula, we see language professionals increasingly using team or turn teaching. Strengths that have been attributed to collaborative, and even consultative, service delivery models are the ecological validity of the language intervention and the promotion of generalization. In descriptions of how collaborative approaches to services had been implemented in school systems in four different parts of the United States (Borsch & Oaks, 1992; Brandel, 1992; Montgomery, 1992; Roller, Rodriquez, Warner, & Lindahl, 1992), one obvious feature was the variations that occurred in the programs. As Ferguson (1992) noted, "Program designs are as individual as those who participate in their development; there is no single correct program" (p. 361).

Another obvious feature was that the educational systems had not completely abandoned the use of what has come to be known as the *traditional pull-out* model even though collaborative approaches had been implemented. *Pull-out* means that a child leaves the typical educational routine to receive services from a specialist. At the extreme, pull-out might be complete. The child would receive all education in a self-contained classroom and might again be pulled out for other special services, such as language intervention. Typically, however, the child participates in the usual educational routine most of the time, leaves it temporarily for special services, and then returns. In chapter 11, we discussed why this model was not appropriate in secondary school for adolescents with language disorders. This model has also been criticized for various other reasons, discussed in chapter 7. Two of the biggest criticisms relevant to language intervention have been the limited contextual support for language learning and the difficulties in generalizing language skills to the naturalistic environment. Others have interpreted pull-out to mean that the child is seen individually by the professional. However, pull-out does not equate to individual intervention and does not preclude group intervention, which can take place within a pull-out model. Therefore, the issues related to pull-out are not essentially issues related to individual versus group intervention approaches, as discussed earlier. It is likely that some language-disordered children at certain times during their language intervention benefit from language teaching that takes place in a less distracting environment in which the targeted rules and regularities can be made more salient and language teaching techniques can be used more consistently.

Most professionals now agree that pull-out is insufficient as the sole model for language intervention. It can, however, be used successfully in combination with both consultative and collaborative models. Service delivery does not have to be seen as all or nothing with regard to models. Rather, it is viewed as requiring several models, with each contributing differently to different children with differing language needs at different times.

In the introduction to this section on approaches to language intervention, we indicated that the topics to be discussed were not totally autonomous. We can see that decisions regarding group or individual intervention and those regarding direct or indirect intervention would interact with service delivery models and language teaching methods. For example, certain language teaching methods could be used more effectively in group than individual intervention and in collaborative service delivery models when the language professional works directly with the child. In planning language intervention for an individual child, these variables are all considered and influence the decisions made, decisions that are constantly reevaluated and modified if necessary.

HIGHLIGHTING INTERVENTION TARGETS

For whatever reasons, language-disordered children have not learned language incidentally in the same ways as normal children. When a specific language feature is chosen as a target for intervention, it may be necessary to highlight the regularities of the feature in order for a language-disordered child to discover the general rule from exposure to particular instances. Lahey (1988) refers to this highlighting procedure as enhancing the salience of the language patterns from which the child is to discover the rules. Several techniques can be employed to increase the salience of language features. Earlier we indicated that limited use of techniques involving metalinguistic skills may be helpful. Other techniques discussed here are multiple exposures to the language feature targeted, suprasegmental and rate variations, reduction in the complexity of an adult's utterances containing the language feature, and input modality variations.

Multiple Exposures

Normal children learn language without observing explicitly designed, multiple repetitions of events that illustrate content and context that are simultaneously paired with an adult's carefully chosen utterances containing systematic examples of specific linguistic forms. However, for a language-disordered child, controlling these examples and increasing the frequency of the child's exposure to the targeted language feature are ways to enhance the feature's salience. The technique of multiple exposures can be used for any aspect of language targeted for intervention in order to assist the child to discover the appropriate rules. In targeting the early-developing regulatory function, for example, a game similar to "Simon Says" can be employed. The adult can first direct the activities of the child via utterances such as "You hop," "You jump," or "Hop," "Jump." After multiple examples, the child be-

comes the director and orders the adult, who obeys readily. A subsequent activity can employ dolls, one for the child and one for the adult. During play, the adult repeatedly tells the doll to perform acts, such as "Go to bed," and follows each command with the consequent action, such as putting the doll in a cradle. After multiple sequences, the adult can cue the child by asking, "What do you want your doll to do? Tell him" or "Tell my doll what to do." Gentle sabotage can be an effective intervention technique. When things do not go according to plan, the most efficient and effective way of correcting the situation is language. A caution is, however, warranted. Although gentle sabotage may work, sabotage that creates frustration in the child will not work and is unfair to the child. Gently sabotaging a child's play with cars and trucks by moving another vehicle to block the movement of the child's toy can help the child realize that his or her verbalizations can regulate the adult's behavior. The adult can say "Move" or "Don't" and then move the vehicle. Desirable toys can be placed in sight but out of reach of the child. The adult can even talk about the seen but unreachable toys. If the child points to one of them, a gestural regulatory behavior, the adult can reach for a toy, pause (seen as delay in the milieu teaching approach), cue the child with "Get toy?" and pause again to wait momentarily for the child's order. In a 30-minute period with activities such as these, it is possible to generate 50 to 100 examples of the regulatory function paired with linguistically appropriate structures and corresponding content.

The examples given at the beginning of this chapter to illustrate discovery of the meaning of "more" can also be used to demonstrate the technique of multiple exposures in semantically focused intervention. In a morphological or syntactic focus, such as one aimed at discovering the regularities for the copula "is" to form interrogatives, multiple exposures to the target can be accomplished during guessing games ("Is it a dog?" or "Is it red?"). For example, the adult and child can take turns hiding objects in a box. After each object is hidden, the adult can engage in a sequence, such as asking, "Is it blue?"; looking in the box; saying, "No"; asking, "Is it red?"; looking again; saying "No"; asking, "Is it green?"; looking again; saying "Yes"; and finally, removing the green object. (This activity assumes, of course, that the child knows colors.)

Suprasegmental and Rate Variations

Lahey (1988) also suggests that varying suprasegmental or prosodic features—such as stress and intonation—and modifying rate of input to a child may increase the salience of the target. In targeting interrogative reversals, as in the previous example, the adult could stress the "is" to highlight its location in the syntactic sequence ("*Is* it blue?"; "*Is* it red?"; "*Is* it green?"). In the example with "more," the word "more" could be stressed in utterances like "*More* juice," "*More* jump," and "*More* toys." Some morphological markers, such as possessive, plural, and third-person singular present tense verb inflections, can be prolonged as well as stressed.

Although mothers have been found to modify the prosodic features of their language addressed to normal language-learning children (Berko Gleason & Weintraub, 1978; Broen, 1972; Brown, 1973), the effectiveness of this technique in intervention for language-disordered children has not been consistently substantiated. Each child responds differently; for some it may help, and for others it may hinder learning the targets. It should, therefore, be used with care. If used at all, it probably should be employed only on a temporary basis, with a return to language input with normal prosodic characteristics as quickly as possible.

Modifying the rate of language input to a child is another possible way of enhancing salience. As with prosodic modifications, mothers tend to use slower rates when talking to children than when talking to adults (Broen, 1972). In fact, mothers talk even more slowly to younger children than to older children (Broen, 1972). Recall that some of the research on children with specific language impairments suggests that these children may have problems processing rapidly changing sequences of auditory stimuli (e.g., Lubert, 1981; Tallal & Piercy, 1973, 1974, 1975). It may be that presenting the rate of language models more slowly increases the likelihood that a language-disordered child will discover the desired rule. Pausing between utterances may also give children time to understand a previous utterance before being confronted with a new one. In addition, pausing may provide the child with time to generate a response. However, Rice, Buhr, and Oetting (1992) found that inserting a pause before words for which language-impaired children were to fast-map the meanings did not help the children to learn the meanings. Again, without empirical confirmation, these techniques should be used only if a child appears to respond positively to them.

Reducing the Complexity of Language

Earlier in this chapter we indicated that when intervention focuses on one aspect of language, it is important to control the complexity of the other aspects that are simultaneously included. It is also important to control the overall complexity of the language that is used as input to a child. Not only do mothers talking to their normally developing children reduce their rates of speech and vary the prosodic features of the language, they also reduce the overall complexity of their language by using short, simple utterances. A similar technique may be effective in highlighting the systematic patterns from which a child is to learn the governing rules. Instead of using long, complex utterances that can hide the elements to be discerned, pairing short, simple utterances with appropriate content and context appears to be a logical approach. To illustrate, we can refer again to the "more" example. The utterances "more" and "more juice" were used instead of "Do you want more juice?", "Tell me you want more juice," or "I want some more juice. Would you like some more juice, too?" Notice, also, the utterances used in the examples for targeting the regulatory function of language and the interrogative reversal of the copula "is."

In addition to controlling the length and morphosyntactic complexity of language models, an adult must use words that are well within a child's semantic repertoire. If the child does not understand the meaning of an adult's model, it is doubtful that the child will discern anything from the utterance. Excessive, complex utterances can potentially do as much to slow a child's progress as failure to provide a sufficient number of exposures to the intervention targets.

Input Modality Variations

Some children may benefit from intervention that employs input modalities in addition to the auditory modality. This technique relates to the idea of modifying antecedent events, which was discussed in the previous chapter. Gestures paired with specific linguistic forms can often increase the salience of the target. The meanings of words, such as "here," "there," and "give," can be enhanced when the words are supported with an adult's gestures. Gestures can highlight a number of pragmatic intents and functions, such as reaching for desired objects as "I want the _____" or "Want _____" is said. Gestures can also reinforce turn-taking skills. In intervention designed to pair "all gone," "no," "no _____," or "gone" with the object relations of disappearance and nonexistence, an adult can raise his or her hands in the classic "I don't know/ Where is it" gesture, adopt a puzzled facial expression, and move his or her head in a searching manner as the appropriate linguistic forms are modeled. Negative head shakes can also highlight negative markers in targets such as "The dog is *not* big."

In previous chapters, the possible use of manual communication paired with oral language with children who are not hearing impaired was discussed. Using a manual sign in conjunction with an auditory model may help a language-disordered child initially attend to the intervention target. However, its use should be discontinued as soon as possible when working with children whose sole problems appear to be in the area of language.

Graphically displayed symbols have also been used occasionally to enhance the salience of a specific target. The symbols are typically presented in conjunction with auditory input and then gradually eliminated as a child begins to demonstrate awareness of the target. The *Fokes Sentence Builder* (Fokes, 1976, 1977) is an example of this method. Such an approach is probably most appropriate for older language-disordered children and for morphosyntactic intervention goals.

FACILITATING TECHNIQUES TO ELICIT AND TEACH LANGUAGE TARGETS

The previous sections have focused on a number of factors that must be considered in planning language intervention. Here we discuss the adult's behaviors that can be used to elicit and teach target language skills. Techniques range from direct to indirect. Some of the techniques have evolved from observations of mothers' verbal behaviors that seem to promote language learning in their normally developing children. The efficacy of some of the techniques has been examined empirically for teaching a few language behaviors; other techniques have not been studied. For the most part, however, the decisions about which techniques may be effective are left to the adult who is working with a specific child. Certain approaches would seem more appropriate than others for some children at specific points in an intervention sequence. Sufficient flexibility is needed so that when one technique or combination of techniques is not working, other techniques can be selected. Typically, several techniques are used simultaneously.

The techniques included here are not listed in preferential order or, for the most part, in hierarchical order. Furthermore, the list is not complete. The techniques discussed here are those that have been cited in the literature most frequently. Examples of each technique are included. However, because the examples are designed to illustrate a specific technique, they may appear more stilted and exaggerated than they would be when used in true language intervention situations.

Self-Talk

In **self-talk**, an adult talks aloud about objects in the immediate environment and about actions that are occurring at the moment. It is important that the topics be in context at the moment to parallel the situations in which children typically begin to talk. The language the adult uses needs to correspond closely to the child's language level in terms of both grammatical and semantic complexity. In other words, the adult's vocabulary and linguistic structures should not greatly exceed the child's language capacity, nor should they be too simplistic for the child.

Self-talk can emphasize specific aspects of language that a child needs to acquire or it can be used as a more general language stimulation approach. The idea is for the child to hear the target language behaviors frequently. However, the purpose of self-talk is not to have the child repeat the targets. Therefore, the child is not overtly directed to talk. The following three examples illustrate how self-talk might be utilized during interactions with a child. In the first two examples, a specific language goal is emphasized. The targets are repeated many times, although in slightly different ways. The last example represents a more general self-talk activity. The language level in the last example is aimed at using two- and occasional three-word combinations.

Example 1

Target: "am" + verb + "ing"

Situation: Adult and child are looking at a book.

Oh, I am looking at the book ... I am opening the book ... am opening the book ... I am looking at the picture ... I am pointing to the dog ... I am turning the page ... Oh, there is a new picture ... I am pointing to the ball ... I am looking at the cat ... I am pointing to the cat ... I am closing the book now ... Now, I am putting the book away ... am putting the book away ... I am putting the book away.

Example 2

Target: The color red

Situation: Adult and child are playing with toys of various colors, many of which are red.

I see the red car ... I have the red car ... the red car ... My car is red ... red ... Oh, here is a red ball ... The red ball ... My ball is red ... Like the apple ... The apple is red, too ... I want the red apple ... Oh, here is a red block ... I'll put my red block with my red apple ... and my red car ... These are all red ... Red toys ... The toys are red.

Example 3

Target: Two- and three-word combinations

Situation: Adult and child are cleaning up a room.

Clean the room ... Put toys away ... Put the toys away... Ball away ... Find the book ... Where's the book? ... Where's the book? ... Oh ... book's over there ... There's the book ... Put book away ... Now, where's glue? ... Put the glue away ... There, glue's away ... All gone... What now? ... I see paper ... I'll get the paper ... Paper away ... Where's the block? ... Oh ... I see blocks ... Blocks on the table ... On the

table ... There's the block ... Blocks on table ... Get the blocks ... Put blocks away.

Parallel Talk

In contrast to self-talk, in which adults describe what they are doing, **parallel talk** emphasizes what the child is doing or what is about to happen to the child or in the child's environment. Again, the purpose is not to have the child repeat the utterances used by the adults but to put the language, at the appropriate complexity level, in the child's auditory environment as the child is acting on the environment. Like self-talk, parallel talk activities can be used to emphasize specific language skills or to encourage language learning more generally. The following two examples illustrate parallel talk.

Example 1

Target: Use of elliptical responses to maintain conversation

Situation: Adult and child are playing with dolls, a dollhouse, and its furnishings.

Who has the chair? ... Oh, she does ... Here it is ... Where is the table? ... Oh yes, over there ... You get it ... Who wants it? ... You do? ... Me, too ... We'll both get it ... Where was it? ... Oh, over there. (In this example, we also see the adult using deictic terms— "here" and "there"—and presuppositions in the form of the pronoun "it.")

Example 2

Target: Three- and four-word phrases

Situation: Child is putting an animal puzzle together.

What do you have? ... You have horse ... Putting horse there ... Putting horse there ... Good, horse goes there ... What goes there? ... Oh, you have dog ... A little dog ... Oh, oh, dog fell down ... Picking up the dog ... Putting the dog in ... Dog is in ... Looking for duck ... Where's the duck? ... Can't find duck ... Oh, there's the duck ... Putting duck in ... All done now

... The puzzle is done ... All done now ... Puzzle is done.

Self-talk and parallel talk can be used together during adult–child intersecting and cooperative interactions (Van Riper, 1978). The next example incorporates both language facilitation techniques.

Example

Target: Performative intents encoded with "going to"
Situation: Adult and child are playing with various toys.

Oh, I'm going to get the toy ... You're going to get the car ... Going to get car ... You're going to get the car ... You're going to go ... I'm going to color ... You're going to color ... You're coloring ... I'm going to cut ... You're going to cut ... You are going to fall... Oops, you fell ... You are going to get up.

Imitation and Modeling

A number of terms have been used to refer to these language stimulation techniques, and as a result, there is some confusion about their meanings (Rees, 1975). *Imitation* and *mimicry* can be used synonymously. These terms refer to responses that are basically similar, if not identical, to a previously presented stimulus and that occur soon after the stimulus. The use of mimicry or imitation implies a "one-to-one process of literal matching" (Courtright & Courtright, 1976, p. 655). An interchange such as the following involves imitation by a child:

ADULT: Say "The girl is running."
CHILD: The girl is running.

In the early stages of language intervention for a specific language behavior, imitation may be a valuable technique (Gottsleben, Tyack, & Buschini, 1974; Hegde, 1980; Hegde et al., 1979; Mulac & Tomlinson, 1977; Zwitman & Sonderman, 1979). However, as "training proceeds, the child's dependence upon the imitative model is reduced" (Leonard, 1981, p. 91).

In contrast, modeling is a technique in which an adult provides several examples of slightly different utterances, each of which contains the same critical language skill to be acquired by a child. It involves a child's induction of the similar elements from a variety of previously presented stimuli. The expected response to these stimuli may not match the stimuli exactly, but it does contain the common critical element(s) of the stimuli. The following interchange represents modeling:

ADULT: This dog is big. That cat is big. The pig is big. That lion is big. Tell me about the elephant.
CHILD: Elephant is big.

A response from the child is not requested until several examples of the target language behavior are given. We can see from the child's response that common elements of the adult's utterances have been induced to produce a similar but inexact response. Modeling is frequently employed to increase children's use of specific aspects of language (Carroll, Rosenthal, & Brysh, 1973; Connell, 1987; Connell & Stone, 1992; Courtright & Courtright, 1976, 1979; Harris & Hassemer, 1972; Leonard, 1975; Rosenthal & Carroll, 1972; Wilcox & Leonard, 1978). Often, at least one other person may be included in intervention when a modeling approach is used. The third person models the target behaviors in response to the adult's stimuli. Positive reinforcements may be provided for the third person's appropriate responses as the child observes both the responses and the reinforcements. Such an approach is consistent with Bandura's (1971, 1977) social learning theory.

If we examine the examples of self-talk and parallel talk, we can see how much modeling of target language behaviors occurs. However, modeling as a language teaching technique typically asks the child for a response at some point following presentations of stimuli. In contrast, self-talk and parallel talk require no responses from the child. The following examples illustrate how modeling can be used. When it is used in language intervention, the target language behavior may receive a little extra stress as the examples are modeled in order to increase the salience of the target.

Example 1

Target: "a" + noun
Situation: Adult and child are looking at picture cards.

ADULT: Oh, look, *a* dog! This is *a* dog. *A* dog. *A* cat. This is *a* cat. *A* cat. *A* ball. Here is *a* ball. Oh, *a* top! *A* top. This is *a* cup. Oh, *a* new picture. What is this?

CHILD: A coat.

Example 2

Target: Meaning and use of "in"

Situation: Adult and child are playing with a number of small toys and a paper bag, a box, and an old purse.

ADULT: Here's a block. Let's put the block *in* the purse. *In* the purse. Put the block *in* the purse. Where's the block?—Oh, *in* the purse. (Both adult and child look.) *In* the purse. Look, here's a ball. We'll put the ball *in* the bag. *In* the bag. The ball's *in* the bag. Where's the ball?—*in* the bag. *In* the bag. Now, let's put the car *in* the box. Good, you put it *in* the box. *In* the box. Here's a spoon. Here it goes. *In* the box. Where's the spoon?—*in* the box. Oh, here's a horse. I'll put the horse *in* the box. Where's the horse?

CHILD: In box.

Reauditorization

Reauditorization is a language stimulation technique in which an adult repeats what a child says. In contrast to the previous language facilitating techniques, which are employed before a child responds, reauditorization occurs in response to the child's statements. The purpose of this approach is, again, to keep the auditory models of target language behaviors in a child's auditory environment. Although this technique can be used in isolation, this is rarely done. Instead, it is typically combined with other techniques, such as modeling. Following is an example of modeling combined with reauditorization. In this example, positive verbal reinforcement is incorporated with the two language stimulation techniques.

Example

Target: "are" + verb + "ing"

Situation: Adult and child are on a playground.

ADULT: You *are swinging*. We *are swinging*. I like swinging. Oh, now you *are running*. You *are running*. We *are running*. *Are running*. We *are jump-ing* now. You *are jumping*. We *are jumping*. Now, you *are hopping*. Me, too. What are we doing?

CHILD: We are hopping.

ADULT: We *are hopping* (reauditorization). Good, We *are hopping* up and down. You *are hopping*. We *are hopping* (reauditorization).

Expansion

Expansion is one of several language facilitation approaches suggested by Muma (1971). Some authors refer to it as a recast. In reference to language teaching, expansion is the process of taking a child's utterance and repeating it using a higher-level language skill. That is, an adult models for the child a slightly more complex way of saying what the child has said. In some instances, the structure of the expansion may be a subsequent focus of intervention for the child. Because the content and/or structure of an expansion is aimed at exceeding the child's present language capacity, the child is not expected or asked to repeat the expansion. Furthermore, the form in which the expansion occurs should not be so complex as to confuse the child. Although we can rarely accomplish this perfectly in interchanges with children, the optimal expansion is one that is at the next immediate language developmental level. Like reauditorization, expansion is typically used in combination with other language stimulation techniques. The following example combines modeling, reauditorization, and expansion, as well as positive verbal reinforcement.

Example

Target: Attributive "big" + noun

Situation: Adult and child are putting toys away.

ADULT: We need to clean up. We need to put our toys away. Clean up now. Put the *big ball* away. No, not the little ball—the *big ball*. The *big ball*. I'll take the little ball. Good, you put the *big ball* away. Now, you have the *big truck*. I'll take the little truck. You put the *big truck* away. Good. Now, what do you have?

CHILD: Big car.

ADULT: *Big car* (reauditorization). That's right. That is a *big car* (expansion). The *big car* (expansion). I want the *big car* (expansion). *Big car* (reauditorization). The *big car* (expansion).

Expatiation

Expatiation is closely related to expansion in that an adult elaborates upon what a child has said. Like expansion, expatiation is also sometimes referred to as a *recast*. Although the adult's elaboration typically incorporates somewhat more advanced language skills, the aim of **expatiation** is to demonstrate to the child how the language behavior can be used in a slightly different context with slightly different content by adding information (Muma, 1971). Example 1 demonstrates how the adult shifts the child's utterance to a somewhat new situation. It is not uncommon for both expansion and expatiation to occur in an adult's response to a child, as in this example. In fact, analysis of an adult–child interaction often shows the adult alternating among reauditorization, modeling, expansion, and expatiation, as shown in Example 2.

Example 1

Target: Irregular past tense verbs

Situation: Child and adult are looking at a story book entitled *Jack and Jill*.

CHILD: He falled down.

ADULT: He *fell* down (model). He *fell* down the hill (expansion). Oh … she *fell* down, too (expatiation). They both *fell* down (expatiation). Oh … the dog *fell* down, too (expatiation).

Example 2

Target: "will" + verb

Situation: Adult and child are decorating a bulletin board for Valentine's Day.

ADULT: I *will put* a heart here (model). *Will put* here (model). I *will put* it here (model and expansion). Where will you put your heart? (Notice that the adult's question contains a varied form of the target and is also phrased so that the child's response could include the target.)

CHILD: I put it here.

ADULT: *Will put* it here? (model) You *will put* it here? (expansion) That's a good place. I *will put* my arrow there, too (model and expatiation). I *will glue* it on (model and expatiation). Where will you glue yours?

CHILD: Will glue there.

ADULT: *Will glue* there (reauditorization). Good, *Will glue* (reauditorization). You *will glue* your arrow there (expansion). I *will get* the glue and the other arrow (model and expatiation). And I *will get* another arrow (model and expatiation). Now we *will glue* our arrows (model and expatiation). What will we do?

CHILD: We *will glue* arrows.

ADULT: We *will glue* arrows (reauditorization). Good. You *will glue* your arrow and I *will glue* mine (model, expansion, and expatiation).

Response Dialogues

When a child's language response is inadequate for the target, engaging the child in systematic interchanges may help elicit a response that more closely approximates the target. Lee, Koenigsknecht, and Mulhern (1975) have proposed seven interchange techniques: complete model, reduced model, expansion request, repetition request, repetition of error, self-correction request, and rephrased question. These interchanges, or *response dialogues,* were originally developed as part of the *Interactive Language Development Teaching* (ILDT) (Lee et al., 1975) strategy. This language teaching strategy is built around stories, usually with accompanying pictures, with different stories facilitating various language structures. The professional presents a small portion of a story and, using specific grammatical structures, questions the children about the story. Additional portions of the story are then presented and dialogue routines completed. Each question is designed to elicit a specific structure. Although the ILDT and its accompanying response dialogues were first developed to facilitate morphosyntactic development, the response dialogues are useful intervention techniques beyond their originally intended use.

Some children need more assistance than others to achieve more complete responses. Therefore, these different interchange techniques are designed to provide varying amounts of help. Some give children considerable assistance in modifying initial responses; others offer very little help. These interchange techniques will now be described. They are presented in decreasing order of assistance to children in approximating target responses.

Complete Model   In light of our previous discussion of modeling as a facilitating technique, this use of the term *model* is a misnomer. As used to describe this interchange technique, it requests an imitative or mimicked response from the child. After an inadequate response from the child, an adult provides an example of the exact target utterance that the child is expected to duplicate. Following is an example of this interchange technique.

Example

Target: Past tense verbs formed by adding the allomorph /t/ ("kicked")

ADULT: Yesterday, we read a story about a rabbit. What did the rabbit do in the story?
CHILD: He hop into a basket.
ADULT: *He hopped into a basket.*
CHILD: He hopped into a basket.
ADULT: Good. What else did the rabbit do?
CHILD: The rabbit kick the fence.
ADULT: *The rabbit kicked the fence.*
CHILD: The rabbit kicked the fence.
ADULT: Good. What else did the rabbit do?

Reduced Model   In a reduced model, the elements of a target utterance that have been omitted are included in an adult's response. The partial model cues a child as to the exact element(s) that need special focus in a reformulation. As such, a partial model is "not imitation but rather reformulation of an utterance" (Lee et al., 1975, p. 18). The following example illustrates an interchange using reduced, or partial, models.

Example

Target: Noun + "is" + verb + "ing"

ADULT: What is the boy doing?
CHILD: Boy jumping.
ADULT: *Is*
CHILD: Boy jumping.
ADULT: *Is jumping.*

CHILD: Boy is jumping.
ADULT: Good. Boy is jumping (reauditorization).

Partial models can include only the missing parts of the target or the missing elements plus closely associated grammatical units, as in the adult's second partial model in the example. The last adult utterance provides a reauditorization of the child's correct response. Such an utterance could also include an expansion.

Expansion Request   In an expansion request, the adult informs the child that the response is not adequate and that more information is needed. However, the adult does not provide the missing information. The child must decide, without the adult's identifying the missing element(s), what has been omitted and supply a complete structure on reformulation. There are a number of ways of requesting an expansion. These include "Tell me the whole thing," "Tell me more," "I didn't hear all of it," and "There's more." The following example illustrates expansion requests.

Example

Target: "Do" + subject + verb ("Do you want some glue?")

ADULT: We are going to pretend we're in a restaurant. You are the waiter. You have to ask us what we want to eat.
CHILD: You want hamburger?
ADULT: *Tell me the whole thing.*
CHILD: Do you want hamburger?
ADULT: Good. Yes, I do want hamburger.
CHILD: Want milk?
ADULT: *Say the whole thing.*
CHILD: You want milk?
ADULT: *More.*
CHILD: Do you want milk?
ADULT: Good. Yes, I do want milk. I do want milk to drink (expansion). I do want milk to drink with my hamburger (expansion). What else do you have?

Repetition Request   According to Lee et al. (1975), a repetition request does not let a child know whether the response was adequate or inadequate. As such, this interchange can be used to stabilize a correct response by having the child say it again or to reformulate adequately an incorrect response. In the latter use, a child has to reauditorize internally the first utterance, compare it to an internal standard auditory model, and restructure it. We see examples of repetition requests in the following.

Example

Target:　Use of polite requests

CHILD: Close the door.
ADULT: *What did you say? Say that again.*
CHILD: Close the door.
ADULT: *What did you say?*
CHILD: Can you close the door?
ADULT: Good. Yes, I will close the door now.

Repetition of Error　In some ways, this technique appears to provide a stimulus for a child to imitate. However, the adult is actually supplying an incorrect model. This is often accompanied by a questioning intonation or an unpleasant facial grimace. The child's task is to recognize the nonverbal cues that the response was inadequate, identify the error, and reformulate the response. Lee et al. (1975) suggest that if this interchange is used too early, the child will mistakenly interpret the adult's utterance as a correct model to be imitated. Consequently, accurate interpretation of this approach is more complex than those listed earlier. Following is an example of this interchange technique.

Example

Target:　Use of "red" to describe objects appropriately

ADULT: I have an apple. What color is the apple?
CHILD: The apple green.
ADULT: *The apple is green?*
CHILD: Apple green.
ADULT: *Green?*
CHILD: The apple red.
ADULT: You're right. The apple is red (expansion).

Self-Correction Request　As the name of this technique implies, the adult asks a child to self-evaluate an utterance. In some instances, this approach may be employed even though a child's response was correct. The purpose is to reinforce and stabilize use of the target. In other instances, the technique can be used when the child's response is inaccurate. Despite the situation in which it is utilized, the purpose is to have the child self-monitor language productions in much the same way as adult speakers monitor their own productions. Use of self-correction interchanges is illustrated in the following example.

Example

Target:　Irregular third-person present tense singular verbs

CHILD: He haves some toys.
ADULT: *Is that right?*
CHILD: He has some toys
ADULT: *Is that okay?*
CHILD: Yes.
ADULT: What else does he have?
CHILD: He has some shoes.
ADULT: *Is that right?*
CHILD: Yes.

Rephrased Question　Lee et al. indicate that this interchange may be especially effective when a number of other interchanges have occurred in order to elicit an adequate target response from a child. Rephrasing the original question may help the child stabilize use of the target language behavior. The following example shows this technique used in combination with the techniques of repetition request and repetition of an error.

Example

Target:　"is" + verb + "ing"

ADULT: What is the boy doing?
CHILD: Boy crying.
ADULT: Boy crying? (repetition of error)
CHILD: Boy is crying.
ADULT: Good. Tell me again (repetition request).
CHILD: Boy is crying.

ADULT: *Is the boy laughing?*
CHILD: No, the boy is crying.

In many instances, several of these techniques are used in combination in a set of successive utterances between child and adult, as the last example illustrates. As we indicated earlier, other language facilitating techniques, such as modeling, reauditorization, expansion, and expatiation, can also be incorporated. The following example demonstrates several interchange techniques and language facilitation approaches. An important feature in this example is that every time the child gives an inadequate response, the adult's subsequent interchange technique either provides more help or is lower in the hierarchy. It is important that a child not become frustrated as a result of giving several inaccurate responses in a row. The adult must be aware of this possibility and modify the situation so that the child will succeed.

Example

Target: Interrogative reversal of copula "is"

Situation: Adult and child are guessing the contents of a large box filled with various toys.

ADULT: What is in the box? (self-talk) Let's guess. Is it a ball? (model) I don't know (self-talk). Is it a ball? (model) Yes, it is a ball (self-talk). What else is in the box?
CHILD: It a car?
ADULT: What did you say? (repetition request)
CHILD: It a car?
ADULT: Is it? (reduced model)
CHILD: Is it a car?
ADULT: Is it a car? (reauditorization) Good. Let's look to see if you guessed right. Yes, it is a car (expatiation). It is a big red car (expatiation). Is it a big red car? (expansion) Yes, it is a big red car (self-talk). It is my turn to guess (self-talk). Let's see (self-talk). It is a . . . (model). Is it a horse? (model) No, it is not a horse (self-talk). Your turn.
CHILD: It a pig?
ADULT: It a pig (repetition of error—accompanying facial grimace).
CHILD: Is it a pig?
ADULT: Is it a pig? (reauditorization) Good. Let's see if

it is a pig. Is it a pig? (reauditorization) Yes, it is a pig (expatiation). It is a little pig (expatiation). Is it a little pig? (expansion) Yes, it is a little pig (self-talk). My turn (self-talk). Is it a . . . (model). Is it a duck? (model) No, it is not a duck (self-talk). Your turn.
CHILD: It a truck?
ADULT: Did you say that right? (self-correction request)
CHILD: It a truck?
ADULT: Tell me the whole thing (expansion request)
CHILD: Is it a truck?
ADULT: Did you say that right now? (self-correction request)
CHILD: Yes.
ADULT: What is in the box? (rephrased question)
CHILD: Is it a truck?
ADULT: Is it a truck? (reauditorization). Good question. Let's look to see.

Other Indirect Facilitating Techniques

Owens (1991) has provided examples of ways in which language can be elicited from children by relatively indirect means. These are listed in Table 15.1, and as Owens points out, there are many more that could be used and included in the list. The list is limited only by our imaginations.

PUBLISHED LANGUAGE MATERIALS

Numerous language materials are published every year. Many of them can be quite valuable in helping children discover language rules and regularities. They are, however, only as effective as the professionals who use them. Children with language disorders have differing needs. As we have emphasized throughout this book, each child is different. Therefore, "no single program can be used with all language-disordered children" (Carrow-Woolfolk & Lynch, 1982, p. 257). Likewise, no set of materials is appropriate and effective for all children. However, with careful scrutiny, sets of published materials can be used to meet the needs of some children some of the time. Furthermore, some of the materials included in these sets can be adapted to suit individual children. What is impor-

TABLE 15.1   Indirect Elicitation Techniques

There is an infinite variety of indirect elicitation techniques, although we tend to rely on two old favorites:

Tell me what you see.

Tell me in a whole sentence.

Here are a few conversational techniques that came to mind one day. The list is not exhaustive, merely illustrative.

Technique	Target	Example
The emperor's new clothes	Negative statements	CLINICIAN: Oh Shirley what beautiful yellow boots. CLIENT: I'm not wearing boots!
Pass it on	Requests for information	CLINICIAN: John, do you know where Linda's project is? CLIENT: No. CLINICIAN: Oh, see if she does? CLIENT: Linda, where's your project?
Violating routines ("Silly rabbit")	Imperatives, directives	CLINICIAN: Here's your sandwich. CLIENT: Nothing in it. CLINICIAN: Oh you must like different sandwiches than I do. What do you want? CLIENT: Peanut butter. CLINICIAN: How do I do it? (there's your opener)
Nonblabbermouth	Requests for information	CLINICIAN: (Place interesting object in front of child) Boy, is this neat. CLIENT: What is it? CLINICIAN: A flibbideejibbit. (Now *STOP*. Don't give anymore info.) CLIENT: What's it do?
What I have	Request for action	CLINICIAN: Oh I can't wait to show you what I have in this bag. It's really neat. (Wait client out)
Guess what I did	Request for information Past tense verbs	CLINICIAN: Guess what I did yesterday in the park. CLIENT: Jogged? Picked flowers? Had a picnic?
Mumble	Contingent query	At height of an interesting story or punchline of a joke, clinician should mumble so that child does not receive message. If needed, increase pressure by asking questions on what was just said.
Ask someone else	Request for information	CLINICIAN: What do you need? CLIENT: Sugar. CLINICIAN: I don't know where it is. Why don't you ask Sally where the sugar is?
Rule giving	Request for objects	CLINICIAN: I have the athletic equipment for recess. If you need some, just ask me. CLIENT: I want jump rope.
Request for assistance	Initiating conversation	CLINICIAN: John, can you ask Keith to help me?
Modeling with meaningful intent	I want _____	CLINICIAN: We have lots of colored paper for our project. Now let's see who needs some. I want a green one. (Take one and wait) CLIENT: I want blue.

TABLE 15.1,   *continued*

Technique	Target	Example
"Screw up" #1	Locatives Prepositions	CLINICIAN: Can you help me dress this doll? (Place shoe on doll's head) How's that? CLIENT: No. The shoe goes *on* the doll's foot. CLINICIAN: But now the foots all gone. CLIENT: No. It's *in* the shoe.
"Screw up" #2	Negative statements	CLINICIAN: Here's your snack. (Give child a pencil) CLIENT: That's not a snack.
Request for topic	Statements	CLINICIAN: Now let's talk about your birthday party. (Not shared information)
Expansion of child utterance into desired form	Infinitives	CLIENT: I want paste crayon. CLINICIAN: You want crayon to *sing with*? CLIENT: No, to color. CLINICIAN: What? CLIENT: I want crayon to color.

Source: From *Language Disorders: A Functional Approach to Assessment and Intervention* (pp. 373–374) by R. Owens, New York: Merrill/Macmillan, 1991. Copyright 1991 by Merrill/Macmillan. Reprinted by permission.

tant in using published language materials in intervention is to choose or adapt the materials to fit the children rather than making the children fit the materials. Materials should never be viewed as the most important factors in language intervention. They are always secondary to the objectives and principles that guide intervention and the facilitating techniques employed. Materials only support the intervention. They do not determine it.

PUTTING IT TOGETHER

We have reviewed many of the factors that go into planning and implementing language intervention. Each of these represents a decision point in the planning process, but each decision is not independent. We have seen that the factors frequently interact with each other. The decisions, therefore, interact. Figure 15.1 illustrates some of these factors and their interactions, as well as the complexity of the intervention decision-making process. There is no claim that the model includes all of the factors influencing intervention decisions. Furthermore, as we learn more about intervention and about children with language disorders, more factors will probably be added. It is also possible that some factors will combine with others. Ultimately, the factors and the decisions will combine to produce an individual child's intervention plan. Planning and implementing language intervention for individual children is a complex decision-making process.

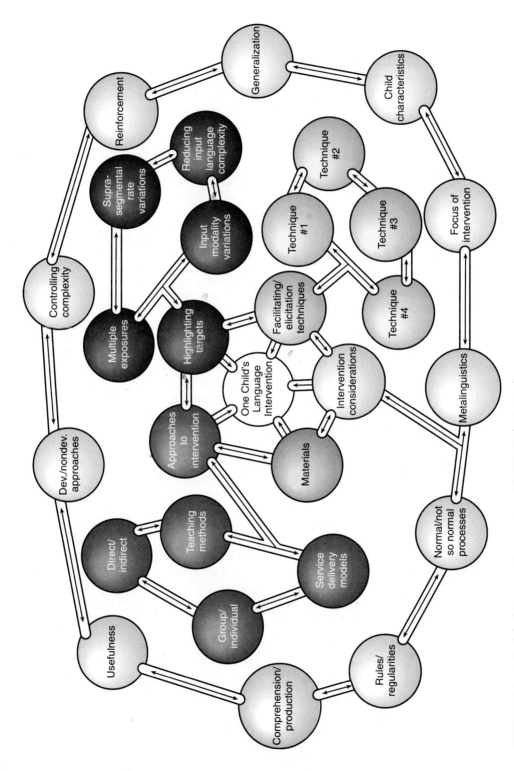

FIGURE 15.1 A Model of Language Intervention. (© 1993 Vicki A. Reed)

SUMMARY

In this chapter we have seen that:

▶ Normal language processes generally guide much of what we do in language intervention. However, there are suggestions that language-disordered children may need intervention that modifies normal processes in order to productively realize language features.

▶ Language intervention aims to help children discover rules and regularities of language.

▶ Language intervention needs to stress the usefulness of language.

▶ Developmental approaches are more frequently used to guide the sequencing of intervention objectives, although nondevelopmental approaches may sometimes be appropriate.

▶ Comprehension of a language target is sometimes taught before production; in other instances, comprehension and production are taught concomitantly. Limited data suggest that some language-disordered children need practice in producing the targeted language behavior in order to use it.

▶ The focus of intervention depends on an individual child's needs and likely changes throughout the intervention program.

▶ It is important to control all aspects of language complexity when requiring a response from a child.

▶ Reinforcement and generalization are important in planning intervention; generalization may be more successful when naturalistic reinforcers and varied contexts are incorporated in intervention.

▶ The characteristics of each child affect the intervention approaches and strategies chosen, but we still do not know how to match most efficaciously child characteristics and intervention approaches and/or strategies.

▶ Language intervention for young children does not depend heavily on metalinguistic approaches. In contrast, for older children, improvement of metalinguistic abilities may be a focus of intervention and metalinguistic approaches are sometimes employed as teaching strategies.

▶ Intervention can be direct or indirect, and can be provided via several language teaching strategies and service delivery models.

▶ In order for language-disordered children to discover the rules and regularities of language, language targets may need to be made more salient.

▶ Many direct and indirect facilitating and elicitation techniques can be employed.

▶ Published language materials can be useful, but they do not determine the intervention.

▶ Planning and implementing language intervention is a complex decision-making process in which multiple factors interact.

Each language-disordered child has unique needs that require flexibility in planning intervention. Unless intervention is viewed as an individually designed, dynamic, fluid process, the needs of language-disordered children will be met only some of the time.

REFERENCES

Bandura, A. (1971). *Psychological modeling.* Chicago: Aldine-Atherton.

Bandura, A. (1977). *Social learning theory.* Englewood Cliffs, NJ: Prentice-Hall.

Berko Gleason, J., & Weintraub, S. (1978). Input language and the acquisition of communicative competence. In K. Nelson (Ed.), *Children's language* (Vol. 1). New York: Gardner Press.

Bloom, L., Miller, P., & Hood, L. (1975). Variation and reduction as aspects of competence in language development. In A. Pick (Ed.), *Minnesota symposia on child psychology* (Vol. 9). Minneapolis: University of Minnesota Press.

Borsch, J., & Oaks, R. (1992). Effective collaboration at Central Elementary School. *Language, Speech, and Hearing Services in Schools, 23,* 367–368.

Brandel, D. (1992). Collaboration: Full steam ahead with no

prior experience! *Language, Speech, and Hearing Services in Schools, 23,* 369–370.

Broen, P. (1972). The verbal environment of the language learning child. *Monographs of the American Speech and Hearing Association, 17.*

Brown, R. (1973). *A first language: The early stages.* Cambridge, MA: Harvard University Press.

Bryen, D., & Joyce, D. (1985). Language intervention with the severely handicapped: A decade of research. *Journal of Special Education, 19,* 7–39.

Carroll, W., Rosenthal, T., & Brysh, C. (1973). Social transmission of grammatical parameters. *Journal of Educational Psychology, 63,* 589–596.

Carrow-Woolfolk, E. (1988). *Theory, assessment, and intervention in language disorders: An integrative approach.* Philadelphia: Grune & Stratton.

Carrow-Woolfolk, E., & Lynch, J. (1982). *An integrative approach to language disorders in children.* New York: Grune & Stratton.

Clark, E. (1973). Non-linguistic strategies and the acquisition of word meanings. *Cognition, 2,* 161–182.

Cole, K., & Dale, P. (1986). Direct language instruction and interactive language instruction with language delayed preschool children: A comparison study. *Journal of Speech and Hearing Research, 29,* 206–217.

Cole, P. (1982). *Language disorders in preschool children.* Englewood Cliffs, NJ: Prentice-Hall.

Committee on Language, Speech, and Hearing Services in the Schools. (1983). Recommended service delivery models and caseload sizes for speech-language pathology services in the schools. *Asha, 25,* 65–70.

Connell, P. (1982). On training language rules. *Language, Speech, and Hearing Services in Schools, 13,* 231–240.

Connell, P. (1987). An effect of modeling and imitation teaching procedures on children with and without specific language impairment. *Journal of Speech and Hearing Research, 30,* 105–113.

Connell, P. (1989). Facilitating generalization through induction teaching. In L. McReynolds & J. Spradlin (Eds.), *Generalization strategies in the treatment of communication disorders.* Philadelphia: B. C. Decker.

Connell, P., & Stone, C. A. (1992). Morpheme learning of children with specific language impairment under controlled instructional conditions. *Journal of Speech and Hearing Research, 35,* 844–852.

Courtright, J., & Courtright, I. (1976). Imitative modeling as an instructional base for instructing language-disordered children. *Journal of Speech and Hearing Research, 19,* 655–663.

Courtright, J., & Courtright, I. (1979). Imitative modeling as a language intervention strategy: Effects of two mediating variables. *Journal of Speech and Hearing Research, 22,* 389–402.

Dollaghan, C. (1987). Fast mapping in normal and language-impaired children. *Journal of Speech and Hearing Disorders, 52,* 218–222.

Dore, J. (1975). Holophrase, speech acts, and language universals. *Journal of Child Language, 2,* 21–40.

Dyer, K., Santarcangelo, S., & Luce, S. (1987). Developmental influences in teaching language forms to individuals with developmental disabilities. *Journal of Speech and Hearing Disorders, 52,* 335–347.

Ferguson, M. (1992). Implementing collaborative consultation: An introduction. *Language, Speech, and Hearing Services in Schools, 23,* 361–362.

Fey, M. (1986). *Language intervention with young children.* San Diego, CA: College-Hill Press.

Fokes, J. (1976). *Fokes sentence builder.* Hingham, MA: Teaching Resources.

Fokes, J. (1977). *Fokes sentence builder expansion.* Hingham, MA: Teaching Resources.

Friedman, P., & Friedman, K. (1980). Accounting for individual differences when comparing the effectiveness of remedial language teaching methods. *Applied Psycholinguistics, 1,* 151–170.

Gottsleben, R., Tyack, D., & Buschini, G. (1974). Three case studies in language training: Applied linguistics. *Journal of Speech and Hearing Disorders, 39,* 213–224.

Gray, B., & Fygetakis, L. (1968). The development of language as a function of programmed conditioning. *Behavior Research and Therapy, 6,* 455–460.

Hadley, P., & Rice, M. (1991). Conversational responsiveness of speech- and language-impaired preschoolers. *Journal of Speech and Hearing Research, 34,* 1308–1317.

Halliday, M. (1975). *Learning how to mean: Explorations in the development of language.* London: Edward Arnold.

Harris, M., & Hassemer, W. (1972). Some factors affecting the complexity of children's sentences: The effects of modeling, age, sex, and bilingualism. *Journal of Exceptional Child Psychology, 13,* 447–455.

Hegde, M. (1980). An experimental-clinical analysis of grammatical and behavioral distinctions between verbal auxiliary and copula. *Journal of Speech and Hearing Research, 23,* 864–877.

Hegde, M., Noll, M., & Pecora, R. (1979). A study of some factors affecting generalization of language training. *Journal of Speech and Hearing Disorders, 44,* 301–320.

Hester, P., & Hendrickson, J. (1977). Training functional expressive language: The acquisition and generalization of five-element syntactic responses. *Journal of Applied Behavior Analysis, 10,* 316.

Holland, A. (1975). Language therapy for children: Some thoughts on context. *Journal of Speech and Hearing Disorders, 40,* 514–523.

Hubbell, R. (1977). On facilitating spontaneous talking in young children. *Journal of Speech and Hearing Disorders, 42,* 216–231.

Johnson, D. (1985). Using reading and writing to improve oral language skills. *Topics in Language Disorders, 5,* 55–69.

Lahey, M. (1988). *Language disorders and language development.* New York: Merrill/Macmillan.

Lahey, M., & Bloom, L. (1977). Planning a first lexicon: Which words to teach first. *Journal of Speech and Hearing Disorders, 42,* 340–350.

Lee, L., Koenigsknecht, R., & Mulhern, S. (1975). *Interactive language development teaching.* Evanston, IL: Northwestern University Press.

Leonard, L. (1973). Teaching by the rules. *Journal of Speech and Hearing Disorders, 38,* 174–183.

Leonard, L. (1974). A preliminary view of generalization in language training. *Journal of Speech and Hearing Disorders, 39,* 429–436.

Leonard, L. (1975). Modeling as a clinical procedure in language training. *Language, Speech, and Hearing Services in Schools, 6,* 72–85.

Leonard, L. (1981). Facilitating linguistic skills in children with specific language impairment. *Applied Psycholinguistics, 2,* 89–118.

Leonard, L. (1984). Normal language acquisition: Some recent findings and clinical implications. In A. Holland (Ed.), *Language disorders in children.* San Diego, CA: College-Hill Press.

Leonard, L., Schwartz, R., Morris, B., & Chapman, K. (1981). Factors influencing early lexical acquisition: Lexical orientation and phonological composition. *Child Development, 52,* 882–887.

Lubert, N. (1981). Auditory perceptual impairments in children with specific language disorders: A review of the literature. *Journal of Speech and Hearing Disorders, 46,* 3–9.

McCormick, L., & Goldman, R. (1984). Designing an optimal learning program. In L. McCormick & R. Schiefelbusch, *Early language intervention: An introduction.* Columbus, OH: Merrill.

McLean, J., & Snyder-McLean, L. (1978). *A transactional approach to early language training.* Columbus, OH: Merrill.

Meline, T. (1980). The application of reinforcement in language intervention. *Language, Speech, and Hearing Services in Schools, 11,* 95–101.

Miller, J., & Yoder, D. (1972). A syntax teaching program. In J. McLean, D. Yoder, & R. Schiefelbusch (Eds.), *Language intervention with the retarded.* Baltimore: University Park Press.

Miller, J., & Yoder, D. (1974). An ontogenetic language teaching strategy for retarded children. In R. Schiefelbusch & L. Lloyd (Eds.), *Language perspectives—Acquisition, retardation and intervention.* Baltimore: University Park Press.

Montgomery, J. (1992). Perspectives from the field: Language, speech, and hearing services in schools. *Language, Speech, and Hearing Services in Schools, 23,* 363–364.

Mowrer, D. (1982). *Methods of modifying speech behaviors* (2nd ed.). Columbus, OH: Merrill.

Mulac, A., & Tomlinson, C. (1977). Generalization of an operant remediation program for syntax with language-delayed children. *Journal of Communication Disorders, 10,* 231–244.

Muma, J. (1971). Language intervention: Ten techniques. *Language, Speech, and Hearing Services in Schools, 2,* 7–17.

Olswang, L., & Bain, B. (1991). Intervention issues for toddlers with specific language impairments. *Topics in Language Disorders, 11,* 69–86.

Olswang, L., Kriegsmann, E., & Mastergeorge, A. (1982). Facilitating functional requesting in pragmatically impaired children. *Language, Speech, and Hearing Services in Schools, 13,* 202–222.

Owens, R. (1991). *Language disorders: A functional approach to assessment and intervention.* New York: Merrill/Macmillan.

Paul, R. (1991). Profiles of toddlers with slow expressive language development. *Topics in Language Disorders, 11,* 1–13.

Paul, R., Looney, S., & Dahm, P. (1991). Communication and socialization skills at ages 2 and 3 in "late-talking" young children. *Journal of Speech and Hearing Research, 34,* 858–865.

Rees, N. (1975). Imitation and language development: Issues and clinical implications. *Journal of Speech and Hearing Disorders, 40,* 339–350.

Rice, M., Buhr, J., & Oetting, J. (1992). Specific-language-impaired children's quick incidental learning of words:

The effect of a pause. *Journal of Speech and Hearing Research, 35,* 1040–1048.

Roller, E., Rodriquez, T., Warner, J., & Lindahl, P. (1992). Integration of self-contained children with severe speech-language needs into the regular education classroom. *Language, Speech, and Hearing Services in Schools, 23,* 365–366.

Rosenthal, T., & Carroll, W. (1972). Factors in vicarious modification of complex grammatical parameters. *Journal of Educational Psychology, 63,* 174–178.

Schwartz, R., & Leonard, L. (1982). Do children pick and choose? Phonological selection and avoidance in early lexical acquisition. *Journal of Child Language, 9,* 319–336.

Skarakis-Doyle, E., MacLellan, N., & Mullin, K. (1990). Nonverbal indicants of comprehension monitoring in language-disordered children. *Journal of Speech and Hearing Disorders, 55,* 461–467.

Slobin, D. (1973). Cognitive prerequisites for the development of grammar. In C. Ferguson & D. Slobin (Eds.), *Studies of child language development.* New York: Holt, Rinehart and Winston.

Spradlin, J., & Siegel, G. (1982). Language training in natural and clinical environments. *Journal of Speech and Hearing Disorders, 47,* 2–6.

Tallal, P., & Piercy, M. (1973). Impaired rate of non-verbal auditory processing as a function of sensory modality. *Neuropsychologia, 11,* 389–398.

Tallal, P., & Piercy, M. (1974). Developmental aphasia: Rate of auditory processing and selective impairment of consonant perception. *Neuropsychologia, 12,* 83–93.

Tallal, P., & Piercy, M. (1975). Developmental aphasia: The perception of brief vowels and extended consonants. *Neuropsychologia, 13,* 69–74.

Van Riper, C. (1978). *Speech correction: Principles and methods* (6th ed.). Englewood Cliffs, NJ: Prentice-Hall.

Wilcox, M. (1989). Delivering communication-based services to infants, toddlers, and their families: Approaches and models. *Topics in Language Disorders, 10,* 68–79.

Wilcox, M., & Leonard, L. (1978). Experimental acquisition of wh- questions in language-disordered children. *Journal of Speech and Hearing Research, 21,* 220–239.

Yoder, P., Kaiser, A., & Alpert, C. (1991). An exploratory study of the interaction between language teaching methods and child characteristics. *Journal of Speech and Hearing Research, 34,* 155–167.

Zwitman, D., & Sonderman, J. (1979). A syntax program designed to present base linguistic structures to language-disordered children. *Journal of Communication Disorders, 12,* 323–337.

APPENDIX A

International Phonetic Alphabet

CONSONANTS

Voiceless		Voiced	
Symbols	Key Words	Symbols	Key Words
p	pig	b	big
t	to	d	do
k	coat, key	g	goat
f	fine	v	vine
θ	thumb	ð	the
s	cider, sun	z	zipper
ʃ	she	ʒ	vision, azure
tʃ	chair	dʒ	jem, huge
h	hello	m	me
ʍ	when	n	new
		ŋ	ring
		l	letter
		r	run
		w	we
		j	yes

VOWELS AND DIPHTHONGS

Symbols	Key Words	Symbols	Key Words
i	feet	u	food
ɪ	hit	ʊ	foot
e	cake	o	toll
ɛ	head	ə	fog
æ	pack	ɑ	father
ʌ	dug	ɒ*	law
ə	sofa	aɪ	time
ɝ	fur	aʊ	house
ɚ	mother	ɔɪ	toil
ɜ*	bird	ju	fuse
a*	mad		

*These vowels occur in Eastern and/or Southern speech patterns.

APPENDIX B

Development of Language Comprehension

Chronological Age*	Comprehension
6 months	Responds by raising arms when mother says come here and reaches toward the child; responds appropriately to friendly or angry voices; moves or looks toward family member when named, such as where's daddy?
12 months	Up to 10 words; no, bye-bye, pat-a-cake, hot, own name; one simple direction such as sit down, or give it to me; these commands are usually accompanied by gesture.
18 months	Up to 50 words; recognizes between six and twelve objects by name such as dog, cat, show, bottle, and ball; identifies three body parts such as eyes, nose, and mouth; understands now, and simple commands unaccompanied by gesture such as give me the doll, open your mouth, and stick out your tongue.
24 months	Up to 1200 words; in, on, under; identifies dog, ball, engine, bed, doll, scissors, hair, mouth, feet, ear, nose, hand, eye, cat, button, cup, spoon, chair, box, car, key, and fork; distinguishes between one and many; formulates negative judgment—a knife is not a fork; understands soon, simple stories; follows simple directions; responds by pointing to show me questions; is beginning to make distinctions between you and me.
30 months	Up to 2400 words; identifies action in pictures and objects by use; carries out one- and two-part commands such as pick up your shoe and give it to mommy; knows what we drink out of, what goes on our feet, what we can buy candy with, what we can cut with, ride in, and what we use to iron clothes with, cook on, sleep on, sit on, and sweep the floor with; understands plurals, questions, difference between boy and girl, the concept 1, up, down, run, walk, jump, throw, fast, more and my.
36 months	Up to 3600 words; understands both, two, not today, what we do when we are thirsty, hungry, sleepy, why we have stoves, wait, later, big, new, different, strong, today, another, and taking turns at play; carries out two- and some three-item commands such as give me the ball, pick up the doll, and sit

Chronological Age*	Comprehension
	down; identifies several colors; and is aware of past and future.
42 months	Up to 4200 words; knows such words as what, where, how, see, little, funny, we, all, surprise, secret; knows first name, number concepts to 2, and how to answer questions appropriately such as do you have a doggy, which is the boy, which is the girl, where is the dress, and what toys do you have.
48 months	Up to 5600 words; carries out three-item commands consistently; knows why we have houses, books, stove, umbrella, key; knows nearly all colors, words such as somebody, anybody, even, almost, now, something, like, but, bigger, too, at least one nursery rhyme, full name, one or two songs, number concepts to 4, and understands most preschool children's stories; can complete opposite analogies such as brother is a boy, sister is a _____ ; in daytime it is light, at night it is _____ ; father is a man, mother is a _____ ; the sun shines during the day, the moon at _____ .
54 months	Up to 6500 words; knows what a house, book, window, chair, and dress are made of; what we do with our eyes and ears; understands differences in texture and composition such as hard, soft, rough, and smooth; begins to name or point to penny, nickel, and dime; inconsistently understands if, because, when, why.
60 months	Up to 9600 words; knows numbers to 5; knows and names colors; defines words in terms of use such as a horse is to ride; also defines wind, ball, hat, and stove; consistently understands words such as if, because, and when; knows what the following are for: horse, fork, and legs; begins to understand right and left.
66 months	Up to 13,500 words; knows number concepts to 7; right and left; most simple, compound, and complex sentences if not too long; knows functions of body parts—eyes, ears, etc.; understands dependent clauses such as when I open the door, put the cat out.
72 months	Up to 15,000 words; knows number concepts to 10 (this includes meaning and relationships of numbers); the meaning of morning, afternoon, night, summer, and winter; can relate differences between objects, animals, and clothing; is beginning to answer a few similarities correctly, for example, In what way are _____ and _____ alike or the same? apple and peach? piano and violin? airplane and bus?; understands differences such as how are a dog and a bird different.

Source: From *Communication Disorders* (2nd ed.) (p. 55), by C. E. Weiss and H. E. Lillywhite, 1981, St. Louis: C. V. Mosby Co. Copyright 1984 by C. E. Curtis. Reprinted by permission.

*Chronological age assumes normal or average intellectual functioning; if the child is mentally retarded or has superior intelligence, then perhaps the concept of mental age would be more appropriate.

APPENDIX C

Development of Language Usage

Chronological Age*	Expression
6 months	Repeats self-produced sounds; imitates sounds; vocalizes to persons; and uses 12 different phonemes.
12 months	Up to 3 words besides mama and dada; may say such words as bye-bye, hi, baby, kitty, and puppy; uses up to 18 different phonemes.
18 months	Up to 20 words and 21 different phonemes; jargon and echolalia are present; uses names of familiar objects, 1-word sentences such as go or eat, gestures, words such as no, mine, eat, good, bad, hot, cold, nice, here, where, more, and expressions such as oh oh, what's that, and all gone; the use of words may be quite inconsistent.
24 months	Up to 270 words and 25 different phonemes; jargon and echolalia are almost gone; averages 75 words per hour during free play; talks in words, phrases, and 2- to 3-word sentences; averages 2 words per response; first pronouns appear such as I, me, mine, it, who, and that; adjectives and adverbs are just beginning to appear; names objects and common pictures; enjoys Mother Goose; refers to self by name such as Bobby go bye-bye; and uses phrases such as I (or me) want, go bye-bye, want cookie, up daddy, nice doll, ball all gone, and where kitty.
30 months	Up to 425 words and 27 different phonemes; jargon and echolalia no longer present; averages 140 words per hour; names words such as chair, can, box, key, and door; repeats two digits from memory; average sentence length is about 2½ words; uses more adjectives and adverbs; demands repetition from others such as do it again; almost always announces intentions before acting; begins to ask questions of adults.
36 months	Up to 900 words in simple sentences averaging 3 to 4 words per sentence; averages 15,000 words per day and 170 words per hour; uses words such as when, time, today, not today, new, different, another, big, strong, surprise, and secret; can repeat three digits, name one color, say name,

Chronological Age*	Expression
	give simple account of experiences, and tell stories that can be understood; begins to use plurals; uses some prepositions and uses more pronouns, adjectives, and adverbs; describes at least one element of a picture; is aware of past and future; uses commands such as you make it, I want, you do it, and like that; also uses expressions such as I can't, I won't tell you, I don't want to, and I'm busy; verbalizes toilet needs and expresses desire to take turns; communication includes criticism, commands, requests, threats, questions, and answers.
42 months	Up to 1200 words in mostly complete sentences averaging between 4 and 5 words per sentence; has been heard to use all 50 phonemes; 7% of the sentences are compound or complex; averages 203 words per hour; rate of speech is faster; relates experiences and tells about activities in sequential order; uses words such as what, where, how, see, little, funny, they, we, she, he, some, any, several, and too; can say a nursery rhyme; and asks permission such as can I or will I.
48 months	Up to 1500 words in sentences averaging 5 to 5½ words; averages 400 words per hour; counts to 3, repeats four digits, names three objects, and repeats 9-word sentences from memory; names the primary colors, some coins, and relates fanciful tales; enjoys rhyming nonsense words and using exaggerations; demands reasons why and how; questioning is at a peak, up to 500 a day; passes judgment on own activities; can recite a poem from memory or sing a song; uses such words as even, almost, now, something, like, and but; typical expressions might include I'm so tired, you almost hit me, and now I will make something else.
54 months	Up to 1800 words in sentences averaging 5½ to 6 words; now averages only 230 words per hour—is satisfied with less verbalization; does little commanding or demanding; likes surprising; about one in ten sentences is compound or complex, and only 8% of the sentences are incomplete; can define 10 common words and count to 20; common expressions are I don't know, I said, tiny, funny, surprised, and because; asks questions for information and learns to control and manipulate persons and situations with language.
60 months	Up to 2200 words in sentences averaging 6 to 6½ words; can define ball, hat, stove, policeman, wind, horse, and fork; can count five objects and repeat four or five digits; definitions are in terms of use; can single out a word and ask its meaning; makes serious inquiries—what is this for, how does this work, who made those, and what does it

Chronological Age*	Expression
	mean; language is now essentially complete in structure and in form; uses all types of sentences, clauses, and parts of speech; reads by way of pictures and prints simple words.
66 months	Up to 2300 words; sentence length averages 6½ to 7 words; grammatical errors continue to decrease as sentences and vocabulary become more sophisticated.
72 months	Up to 2500 words in sentences averaging 7 to 7½ words; relates fanciful tales; recites numbers to 30; asks meaning of words; repeats five digits from memory; can complete analogies such as A table is made of wood, a window of _____ . A bird flies, a fish _____ . The point of a cane is blunt; the point of a knife is _____ . An inch is short; a mile is _____ .

Source: From *Communication Disorders* (2nd ed.) (pp. 57–58) by C. E. Weiss and H. E. Lillywhite, 1981, St. Louis: C. V. Mosby Co. Copyright 1984 by C. E. Curtis. Reprinted by permission.

APPENDIX D

Summaries of Stages for Language Acquisition

A. SUMMARY OF STAGES FOR ACQUISITION OF PRAGMATICS

Prelinguistic (Birth—9 Mo)	Stage I (9—18 Mo)	Stage II (18—24 Mo)	Stage III (2–3 Yr)	Stage IV (3+ Yr)	Stage V (Communicative Competence—Adult)
Perlocutionary acts gazing, crying, touching, smiling, vocalizations, grasping, sucking, laughing (Bates, 1975) Illocutionary acts nonverbal and speechlike giving, pointing, showing (Bates, 1975) Turn taking (Bruner, 1975)	Functions instrumental regulatory interactional personal heuristic imaginative informative (Halliday, 1975) Intentions label response request greeting protesting repeating description attention (Dore, 1974) Verbal turn taking procedures employed (Bloom, Rocissano, & Hood, 1976) New information coded first (Greenfield & Smith, 1976)	Functions pragmatic mathetic interpersonal textual ideational (Halliday, 1975)	Responds to contingent queries, types of revisions function of linguistic development (Gallagher, 1977) Rapid topic change (Keenan & Schieffelin, 1976)	Sustains topic (Bloom, Rocissano, & Hood, 1976) Systematic changes in speech depending on listener (Gleason, 1973; Sachs & Devin, 1976; Shatz & Gelman, 1973) Indirectives and hints (Ervin-Tripp & Mitchell-Kernan, 1977) Productive use of contingent queries to maintain the conversation (Garvey, 1975) Role-playing, ability to temporarily assume another's perspective (Anderson, 1977) Metalinguistic awareness, ability to think about language and comment on it (de Villiers & de Villiers, 1974; Gleitman, Gleitman, & Shipley, 1972)	Knowledge of who can say what, in what way, where and when, by what means, and to whom (Hymes, 1971) Behavior speakers and listeners attend to: Quality: informative but not too informative Quality: contribution should be true Relation: be relevant Manner: avoid obscurity, ambiguity, be brief and orderly (Grice, 1975)

B. SUMMARY OF STAGES FOR ACQUISITION OF SEMANTICS AND SYNTAX

Prelinguistic (Birth–9 Mo)	Stage I (9–18 Mo)	Stage II (18–24 Mo)	Stage III (2–3 Yr)	Stage IV (3+ Yr)	Stage V (Communicative Competence—Adult)
	Semantics first-words learned are general nominals, specific nominals, action words (Nelson, 1973) Overextensions regarding shape, size, function, etc. (Clark, 1973) Functions performative indicative object negative indication volition negative volition volitional object agent action/state of agent object action/state of object dative object assoc. with object or location animate assoc. with object or location location modification of event (Greenfield & Smith, 1976)	Semantics 2-word utterances agent-object agent-action action-object location nomination possessive attributive nonexistence rejection denial question recurrence acknowledgment (Bloom, 1970; Brown, 1973) Syntax 2-word utterances S-V-O-A clause level phrase level (Crystal et al., 1976)	Semantics 3–4 word utterances new structures word level (Crystal et al., 1976) Syntax 3–4 word utterances S-V-O-A new structures at clause level new structures at phrase level	Semantics word pairs—more and less, dimensional terms, before and after, verbs of expression, of causation and possession and transfer (summarized by Dale, 1976) New structures at word level (Crystal et al., 1976) Syntax new structures at clause and phrase levels, recursion, error strategies employed (Crystal et al., 1976) embeddings (Brown, 1973)	Generates and understands infinite combinations from a set of finite symbols (Chomsky, 1965)

14 morphemes in order of acquisition: present progressive, on, in, plural, past irregular, possessive, uncontractible copula, articles, past regular, third-person singular regular, third-person singular irregular, uncontractible auxiliary, contractible copula, contractible auxiliary

C. SUMMARY OF STAGES FOR ACQUISITION OF PHONOLOGY

Prelinguistic (Birth–9 Mo)	Stage I (9–18 Mo)	Stage II (18–24 Mo)	Stage III (2–3 Yr)	Stage IV (3 + Yr)	Stage V (Communicative Competence—Adult)
Discriminates phonemes during first month (Morse, 1974; Eimas, 1974)	Presented in order of acquisition	Phonological processes are employed from 18 mos. to 4 yrs. They are simplifying processes and affect classes of sounds. These are: syllable structure processes, assimilatory processes, substitution processes and multiple processes (Ingram, 1976). Hierarchically arranged constraints employed from 2 yrs–4 yrs.			Uses following rules to produce all combinations of phonemes: feature changing rules
Cooing—first 4 months vocalic velar or back consonantal sounds, denotes pleasure	first syllables CV or CVCV reduplicated				rules for deletion and insertion rules for permutation and coalescence
	first consonants labial most commonly /p/, /m/, /t/, and /k/				rules with variables (assimilation, dissimilation, multiple variables, exchange rules)
Babbling— 6 months labial consonants, sound play (Ingram, 1976)	first vowels /a/, /i/, and /u/ homorganic fricative acquired after stop (Jakobson, 1968)				Use of other aspects of phonological system such as stress contours, intonation patterns, pitch changes (Schane, 1973)

Speech perception (in order of development)
vowels
presence versus absence of consonant
sonorants versus stops
palatized versus nonpalatized consonants
Between sonorants
sonorants versus continuants
labials versus linguals
stops versus spirants
pre- versus post-linguals
voiced versus voiceless consonants
Between sibilants liquids versus /y/ (Shvachkin, 1973)

/h/ and /w/ first sounds acquired (Ferguson & Garnica, 1975)

vowel and consonant harmonization
cluster reduction
systematic simplification
grammatical simplification
(Smith, 1973)

3 yrs.—/p/, /m/, /h/, /n/, /w/

4 yrs.—/b/, /k/, /g/, /d/, /f/, /j/

6 yrs.—/t/, /ŋ/, /r/, /l/

7 yrs.—/tʃ/, /ʃ/, /z/, /dʒ/, /θ/

8 yrs.—/s/, /v/, /ð/

8½ yrs.—/ʒ/, (Sanders, 1972)

7–10 yrs. comprehension of intonation (Crutthenden, 1974)

7–12 yrs. morphophonemic development (Atkinson-King, 1973)

Note: Plus or minus six months for all age ranges reported is considered normal.

Source: From "Process: The Action of Moving Forward Progressively from One Point to Another on the Way to Completion" by C. Prutting, 1979, *Journal of Speech and Hearing Disorders, 44,* pp. 24–26. Copyright 1979 by the American Speech-Language-Hearing Association. Reprinted by permission.

APPENDIX E

Brown's Rules for Calculating MLU

A. Preferably use 100 utterances, although 50 may suffice for an estimate.

B. Determine total number of morphemes in language sample.

Count as one morpheme:

Repetitions of words used for emphasis ("yes, yes, yes")

Compound words ("birthday")

Proper names ("Jimmy Joe" or "Sally Jones")

Ritualized reduplications ("choo-choo")

Diminutives ("doggie")

Auxiliary verbs ("is" or "will")

Irregular past tense verbs ("ran" or "ate")

Catenatives ("wanna" or "gonna")

Count as two morphemes: (All grammatical inflections)

Plural nouns ("dogs")

Third-person singular present tense verbs ("runs")

Present progressive *-ing* ("running")

Possessive nouns ("baby's")

Regular past tense verbs ("jumped")

Do not count:

Stutterings or disfluencies, except for the one complete form ("I, I, I,")

Fillers ("um" or "oh"), except for "no," "yeah," "hi"

C. Divide total number of morphemes by number of utterances in language sample.

Source: Adapted from R. Brown, *A First Language: The Early Stages.* Cambridge, MA: Harvard University Press, 1973.

Glossary

Abstract unobservable associations made in thought or language; having qualities that are not directly observable through the senses; contrasts with *concrete*.

Accent differences in pronunciation that contribute to features of a dialect.

Acquired hearing loss a hearing loss that occurs sometime after birth and after an individual has had exposure to language through hearing.

Acute pertaining to the brief period following onset of a disease or injury when symptoms are most severe.

Adaptive behavior skills in areas such as social development and self-help.

Adventitious a condition occurring after birth; contrasts with *congenital*.

Aggregate occurring more than once in a family, thereby indicating a genetic pattern.

Agnosia loss of ability to interpret sensory information.

Allomorph a variation of a morpheme that does not alter the meaning signaled by the morpheme.

American Sign Language a language communicated by using a system of manually produced signs; one form of manual communication; abbreviated ASL.

Anaphoric structures that refer back to something already expressed.

Anoxia oxygen deprivation.

Apraxia of speech a neurologically based disorder that affects the ability to plan speech movements.

Asemantic without intention to communicate meaning to a conversational partner.

ASL *see* American Sign Language.

Aspiration audible breath that accompanies the production of a speech sound.

Asynchrony separation in time of two events that normally occur simultaneously.

Ataxia a type of cerebral palsy resulting from damage to the cerebellum; characterized by uncoordinated movement, reduced muscle tone, and poor balance.

Athetosis a type of cerebral palsy resulting from damage to the basal ganglia; characterized by fluctuating muscle tone and writhing movements.

Attributive descriptive.

Auditory attention the ability to focus selectively on important aspects of acoustic stimuli.

Auditory discrimination the ability to differentiate between acoustic stimuli.

Auditory memory the ability to remember acoustic stimuli.

Auditory perception the abilities involved in processing auditory stimuli; includes skills such as auditory memory and auditory discrimination.

Auditory rate the ability to process acoustic stimuli occurring at various speeds.

Auditory sensitivity the measurement of sound intensity needed to hear sound; the degree to which sound can be heard.

Auditory sequencing the ability to identify the temporal order of acoustic stimuli.

Autisticlike a clinical term for children who exhibit some behaviors characteristic of autism but who do not meet the full criteria for autistic disorder.

Auxiliary verb a verb that accompanies a main verb in order to express grammatical distinctions.

Aversive an unpleasant stimulus that is avoided and can thereby be used to change behavior.

Babbling nonmeaningful vocalizations produced by infants prior to their first words; unintelligible speech attempts by children with language disorders.

Barrier task a procedure in which two speakers are separated by a screen, thereby preventing the use of gesture or deictic language.

Behaviorism the school of thought underlying the technique of behavior modification.

Bicultural sharing aspects of two cultures.

Bilingual sharing aspects of two languages.

Black English Vernacular a variation of Standard American English that is influenced by West African and European languages and that is spoken by some black people; also known as *Ebonics* and *Black English;* abbreviated BEV.

Blissymbolics a system of pictographs and other graphic symbols used to communicate.

Bound morpheme the smallest unit of meaning that signals meaning only when attached to a free morpheme and, therefore, cannot occur alone; similar to an affix.

Catenative a main verb that governs another main verb, such as "want to go."

Cerebral palsy a label for a group of motor disorders resulting from damage to the immature brain.

Child-oriented intervention procedures in which the child provides a stimulus and the adult responds to it, such as expansion or recasting.

Circumlocution using indefinite words and/or vague descriptions rather than coming to the point or using key words; literally "talking around."

Clarification request any behavior that serves as a request for repetition or rephrasing of an utterance, such as a quizzical look, "huh?", or "excuse me?".

Class a set of words that share the same linguistic properties, such as adjectives, household vocabulary, or words that begin with /p/.

Clause a multiword unit of grammar that may or may not function as a sentence and is often defined as requiring both a subject and a verb, thereby generally differentiating it from a phrase.

Cleft lip a congenital defect in which the lip is incompletely fused.

Cleft palate a congenital defect in which the hard and/or soft palates are incompletely fused.

Closed head injury a diffuse rather than focal injury to the brain as a result of a blow to the head.

Cluster a string of adjacent consonants, such as /pl/, /fr/, /skw/, or /str/.

Code switching alternating between different types of language use (e.g., formal/informal registers, different dialects, different languages), depending on the communicative context.

Cognates two words that are derived from a common source language; for example, many English and Spanish words come from Latin.

Cohesion linkage between structures in a narrative or other discourse; for example, "then" links a sentence with preceding portions of a story.

Complex sentence a sentence containing an independent clause and at least one dependent clause; sometimes defined less specifically as a sentence containing more than one clause.

Compound sentence a sentence containing more than one independent clause.

Comprehension understanding or interpretation of a message encoded by a speaker.

Concrete observable associations made in thought or language; having qualities that are directly observable through the senses; contrasts with *abstract.*

Concreteness the tendency of a child to be limited to the "here-and-now" of objects and actions that can be directly perceived with the senses.

Conductive hearing loss an impairment of hearing caused by damage to the external or middle ear, resulting in failure of sound energy to reach the inner ear.

Confrontation naming retrieving and producing a name or label when presented with a sensory stimulus such as a picture or sound.

Congenital a condition present at the time of birth.

Connective a word or phrase that links linguistic units.

Constituent a component of a larger linguistic construction; for example, words are constituents of phrases.

Conversational repair correction of errors or misunderstandings during conversation.

Copula a form of the verb "to be" occurring as a main verb; a linking verb.

Creole a language that was learned from birth by a group of people and was formerly a pidgin; *see* pidgin.

Cued speech a system sometimes employed with hearing-impaired individuals that consists of hand signals used around the mouth to supplement information that is available through hearing and lipreading.

Decibel a measurement of sound intensity or pressure.

Decode to interpret an incoming linguistic signal.

Deep structure the meaningful base that underlies a string of words.

Deictic words words that use a speaker's perspective as a point of reference and the referents of which change as the roles of speaker and listener change.

Demonstrative a form that distinguishes between members of the same class, for example, "this," "that," "these," or "those."

Dental a consonant produced with contact between the tongue and teeth.

Devoicing production of speech sounds with reduced vocal fold vibration.

Dialect a variation of a language that may include sound, grammar, word order, and semantic differences.

Dichotic tasks in which auditory stimuli are selectively presented to the left or right ear; used to investigate hemispheric processing.

Diplegia motor impairment of all limbs but with less involvement of the arms.

Discourse connected flow of language.

Disinhibition lack of self-monitoring and control observed in individuals with brain injury.

Dissociation separation of neurological systems that normally work in unity.

Distractibility inability to attend to a specific stimulus in the presence of other stimuli; poor sensory figure/ground skills.

Dyadic communication communication between two people.

Dysarthria a term for a group of motor-based speech disorders resulting from damage to the central and/or peripheral nervous systems.

Dyslexia difficulty in learning to read in the absence of obvious causes.

Dysnomia difficulty in retrieving names or words.

Dyspraxia *see* apraxia of speech.

Echolalia repetition of speech, which is sometimes judged to be without communicative intent; parroting of the speech of others.

Egocentric unconcerned with the needs of others.

Elective language intervention language intervention provided to enhance social and academic success in the absence of a language disorder.

Elliptical response a response in which redundant or obviously shared information between conversational partners is omitted.

Embedding inserting one grammatical element within another; adding elements to the middle of an utterance so that the other elements of the utterance surround the new ones.

Emotional lability decreased control of emotions, often resulting in laughing or crying inappropriately.

Encode to produce an outgoing linguistic signal.

Ethnic dialect a variation of a language form that is related to a person's racial and/or cultural group.

Expansion an adult's repetition of a child's utterance in a longer and slightly more complex form; a language facilitation technique in which an adult repeats a child's utterance but incorporates a more advanced language form.

Expatiation a language facilitation technique in which an adult repeats a child's utterance but adds information to it.

Extralinguistic pertinent to language but not part of language.

Facilitated communication a therapeutic approach that combines elements of physical support and positive expectations to allow individuals with autism to communicate by typing messages.

Fast mapping rapid gleaning of information about a word's meaning as a result of only few exposures to it in context.

Figurative language nonliteral use of language, such as metaphors, similes, idioms.

Flap consonant produced by very rapid articulatory contact.

Focused stimulation a procedure for teaching language in which a child is exposed to frequent models of a target form but is not required to produce the form.

Formulaic language utterances produced as a unit, with little or no grammatical variation, such as "Pleased to meet you."

Free morpheme the smallest unit of meaning that can occur alone; similar to a root word.

Frequency number of cycles in 1 second of a sound wave; synonymous with Hertz (abbreviated Hz); related to the psychological phenomenon of pitch.

Genetic relating to inherited characteristics; transmitted through genes.

Glottals sounds produced by closing or narrowing the glottis, the space between the vocal folds.

Graphomotor pertaining to handwriting.

Hemiparesis motor weakness on one side of the body.

Hemiplegia motor impairment on one side of the body.

Heterogeneous a group of individuals different in behavior and general characteristics.

Homogeneous a group of individuals alike in behavior and general characteristics.

Homophones words that sound alike but have different meanings.

Hybrid intervention intervention that combines child-oriented and adult-oriented procedures.

Hyperactivity abnormally increased activity in a child; may be characterized by continuous movement and/or distractibility.

Hypernasality excessive nasal resonance.

Hypoxia *see* anoxia.

Idiolect the special or unique way each person speaks.

Idiom a saying the meaning of which is based on an abstract concept that goes beyond the literal interpretation of the words.

Idiosyncratic language forms or uses that are unique to an individual.

Idiot savant an individual whose measured general intelligence is in the range of mental retardation but who evidences a specific talent, such as sculpture, music, or feats of recall.

Illocutionary acts behaviors that reflect intents to communicate.

Impulsivity acting without thinking or considering the consequences.

Inferential reasoning from known information to reach a conclusion that was not previously stated.

Inferential meaning meaning derived from the logical relationships of statements rather than from what may be explicitly stated.

Inflection a form added to a word that signals a grammatical relationship, such as plural, possessive, or past tense word endings.

Intelligence quotient the score obtained from administration of a standardized test of intelligence; abbreviated IQ.

Intensity amount of acoustic energy producing a sound wave; related to the psychological phenomenon of loudness.

Interrogative expression of questions.

Intervocalic a consonant occurring between two vowels.

Irony language in which the meaning is the opposite of that literally conveyed.

Jargon the production of a meaningless sequence of syllables.

Kernel sentence the basic subject-verb-object sentence, often described as a simple, active, declarative, affirmative sentence.

Kernicterus a condition associated with brain damage and sensorineural hearing loss that is brought about by an excessive amount of certain blood degradation products (notably bilirubin) in the blood; may be present in an infant when there is an Rh blood factor incompatibility between the baby and the mother.

Kinesics the parameter of nonverbal communication that refers to body movement.

Language an arbitrary but agreed-on code or conventional system of symbols used to represent concepts or ideas.

Lateralization the development of neurological control by one side of the brain.

Lexicon the vocabulary of a language.

Linguistic borrowing incorporating aspects of one language into another.

Linguistic variation differences that are noted in comparing two or more languages.

Localization control of a specific behavior by a specific region of the brain.

Locutionary refers to spoken, meaningful behaviors that have communicative intents.

Mainstream as a verb, to educate children with disabilities along with children who are developing typically, as in the same classroom; as a noun, nonminority.

Mazes confused vocal behaviors in utterances and/or verbal tangles of words, such as false starts, revisions, hesitations, and fillers.

Mean length of utterance average number of morphemes per utterance; abbreviated MLU.

Meningitis inflammation of the membranes covering the brain and/or spinal cord.

Mental age the age level at which a child is functioning in a particular skill area; abbreviated MA.

Metacognition deliberate thought and/or control over one's own actions to achieve a goal; includes awareness of what the task entails and self-monitoring of one's thoughts or performance.

Metalinguistic pertaining to the ability to analyze and/or judge the acceptability of language; pertaining to the ability to think and talk about language as an action and a subject of study.

Metaphor a figurative use of language in which an attribute is employed to describe an entity or to compare entities not literally or typically associated with the attribute or each other; an expression that describes something in unreal terms so as to suggest a likeness or comparison, such as "She's a rock in a difficult situation."

Metapragmatic pertaining to the ability to talk about or analyze the appropriateness of certain language forms or behaviors in particular contexts.

Metarepresentation the ability to understand or relate to the thought processes of other people.

Microcephaly a condition in which the brain is abnormally small and poorly developed at birth.

Mixed hearing loss a hearing loss resulting from a combination of a conductive and a sensorineural component.

Modalities types of sensory input (e.g., auditory, visual, tacile) or output (e.g., motor, oral).

Modeling a language facilitation technique in which the adult provides several examples of slightly different utterances, each of which contains the same critical language skill to be acquired by the child.

Monolingual having only one language.

Monologue speech produced by one person, often differing in its characteristics from speech produced in a conversation.

Monoplegia motor impairment of one limb.

Morpheme the smallest unit of meaning in a language.

Morphology the aspect of language that concerns derivations of word forms and use of grammatical markers or inflections.

Motor impairment decreased or abnormal muscle movement or control.

Multiculturalism more than one culture; linguistic, racial, and ethnic variations in a society.

Muscular dystrophy a term used to refer to a group of progressive, degenerative muscular disorders.

Mutism inability or refusal to speak.

Mutual gaze simultaneous maintenance of reciprocal eye contact.

Narrative a story or other monologue form that requires the speaker to organize language at a level higher than a sentence.

Nasalization production of a sound with nasal resonance.

Neologism a made-up word.

Neonatal pertaining to a newborn infant.

Neuroassisted refers to alternative/augmentative communication modes that use functions such as brain waves or eye blinks to activate some type of instrument that encodes a message.

Nominals words that are nouns or are used like nouns.

Object complement a phrase or clause that functions as a direct object in a sentence.

Object permanence the concept, acquired by a child during Piaget's sensorimotor period of cognitive development, that objects continue to exist even when they are not visible.

Obligatory form language items that must be used in a particular context to form a grammatical structure.

Operant conditioning a teaching approach that emphasizes increasing the frequency of desired behaviors by differentially reinforcing them.

Otitis media a broad term referring to inflammation or infection of the middle ear; in common usage, an infection in the middle ear.

Ototoxic poisonous to the ear.

Overextension the use of a word with a wider than normal range of meaning, for example, "car" to refer to any moving vehicle with wheels.

Paralinguistic behavior vocal behavior that is superimposed on or accompanies verbal behavior and that can reinforce meaning or signal additional meaning.

Parallel talk a language facilitation technique in which an adult talks about what the child is doing at the moment.

Paraphasia fluent misnamings or sound substitutions; a characteristic sometimes seen in the language of individuals with aphasia.

Paraplegia motor impairment of both legs.

Perception recognition, interpretation, and organization of information received from the senses.

Perinatal pertaining to the time of birth.

Peripheral hearing mechanism the outer, middle, and inner ears; excludes the acoustic (auditory) nerve (cranial nerve VIII) and the central nervous system.

Perlocutionary acts behaviors that do not reflect intents to communicate but that are interpreted by others as having communicative intents.

Perseveration repetition of a particular response when it is no longer appropriate or correct.

Phoneme a speech sound that conveys differences in word meanings.

Phonology the aspect of language that concerns the speech sounds comprising a language and the rules governing their sequencing and distribution.

Phrase a group of words that form a grammatical unit, such as a noun phrase (e.g., "the big dog"); a multiword unit of grammar that does not function as a sentence and is often defined as lacking a subject and verb, thereby generally differentiating it from a clause.

Pidgin a language derived as a result of adapting one language to another.

Plasticity the ability of the brain to reorganize how functions are controlled.

Positive reinforcer an event that increases the frequency with which a behavior occurs.

Postmodifying elements of a phrase that follow the head word.

Postnatal following birth or occurring after birth.

Postonset time that has elapsed since the beginning of a disease or injury.

Postvocalic occurring after a vowel.

Pragmatics the aspect of language that concerns its use in context and the purposes for using language.

Precocious showing an advanced rate of development.

Prelinguistic prior to the beginning of meaningful language.

Prenatal prior to birth.

Presupposition the process of gauging what information a listener already knows and what may not be known in order to decide what to encode in a message.

Prevalence the number of cases of a disease or other condition that exist in a population at a given time.

Preverbal prior to the beginning of meaningful speech.

Prevocalic occurring before a vowel.

Production the encoding or expression of a message.

Propositional meaning the composite meaning derived from words used together in multiword utterances.

Prosodic features   the melodic or rhythmic aspects of a language, such as stress and intonation.

Prosthesis   an artificial device that replaces a damaged or missing body part.

Protocol   a standard set of instructions, such as those used in giving a test.

Protoword   a spoken form produced by young children during the transition from babbling to meaningful speech.

Proverb   a figurative language expression that advises, cautions, comments, or encourages, such as "A penny saved is a penny earned."

Proxemics   the parameter of nonverbal communication that refers to the use of space and distance.

Quadriplegia   motor impairment of all four extremities.

Quantifier   an item that expresses amount, such as "four," "lots," or "much."

Reauditorization   a language facilitation technique in which an adult repeats a desired utterance that has been produced by a child.

Recast   an adult's response to a child's utterance in which the same meaning is expressed in a different and usually more adequate syntactic form; related to expansion.

Reciprocal   actions that involve the taking of turns; give-and-take interactions.

Recruitment   abnormal sensitivity to loud sounds.

Reduction   the omission of linguistic elements normally found in a structure.

Reduplicated babbling   a form of babbling in which the same syllable is repeated, such as /ninini/.

Referent   item or items to which a word refers.

Referential meaning   the dictionary or lexical meaning of words.

Reflex   an involuntary motor response resulting from sensory stimulation.

Register   a variety of language used in particular social contexts.

Relational meaning   meaning conveyed by words as they are used with other words.

Relational words   words that refer to or describe relationships among objects or events.

Relative clause   a dependent or subordinate clause that modifies a noun and is often introduced by a relative pronoun such as "who," "that," or "which."

Rigidity   a type of cerebral palsy resulting from damage to the basal ganglia; characterized by limited movement.

Rubella   German measles; the contraction of this disease by a woman in the first trimester of pregnancy may cause a variety of abnormalities in the developing embryo.

SEE   *see* Seeing Essential English and Signing Exact English.

Seeing Essential English   one form of manual communication in which the English language is communicated through manually produced signs; abbreviated SEE.

Segmental   pertaining to consonants and vowels; contrasts with *suprasegmental*.

Seizure   a sudden attack in which electrical activity spreads through the body; often classified as petit mal and grand mal.

Self-talk   a language facilitation technique in which an adult talks about events that are occurring in the environment at the moment or about the activities in which the adult is engaging at the moment.

Semantic processing   the use of word meanings and relationships between word meanings to enhance comprehension and prediction.

Semantics   the aspect of language that concerns meanings of words or word sequences.

Sensorineural hearing loss   an impairment of hearing due to damage to the inner ear or the acoustic (auditory) nerve (cranial nerve VIII).

Signing Exact English   one form of manual communication in which the English language is communicated through manually produced signs; abbreviated SEE.

Simile   a figurative language expression that explicitly describes or makes a comparison, similar to a metaphor, by using the words "like" or "as," for example, "She's like a rock in a difficult situation"; *see* metaphor.

Social words   early words in a child's lexicon, such as "Hi" and "Bye," used to establish and maintain human relationships.

Spasticity   a type of cerebral palsy resulting from damage to the motor cortex or the pyramidal system; characterized by hyperactive reflexes and spastic paralysis.

Spatial   pertaining to location in space.

Speech   the sensorimotor process of producing orally the sounds and sound sequences that comprise a linguistic code.

Speech community   the environment in which people share common linguistic features.

Spina bifida   a defect in the development of the vertebral column that often results in serious disabling conditions.

Standard American English   the broadly accepted dialect of American English; abbreviated SAE.

Stereotype   behavior that is frequently produced with little variation.

Substantive words   words that refer to classes of objects or to specific, one-of-a-kind objects.

Suprasegmental   sound effects in speech that extend beyond individual consonants and vowels, such as rate or intonation.

Surface structure   the string of words used to represent a deep structure or underlying meaning.

Symbolic play   a normal play behavior of young children in which an object or toy is made to represent some other real object.

Syntax   the aspect of language that concerns the rules for combining and sequencing words in multiword utterances.

Telegraphic   omission of grammatical morphemes and other words that can be predicted from content.

Temporal   pertaining to time.

Total communication   a communication philosophy that incorporates a combination of the manual alphabet, some type of sign language, and speech; abbreviated TC.

Trainer-oriented intervention   procedures in which the adult provides a stimulus and the child responds to it, such as operant conditioning.

Traumatic brain injury   an injury to the brain as a result of an external force such as a blow to the head.

Trill   a consonant produced by rapid oscillation of an articulator, such as the "rolled" /r/ of Spanish.

Underextension   the use of a word with a narrower than normal range of meaning, often used for specific objects or events, for example "car" to refer only to the family car.

Unilateral hearing loss   an impairment of hearing restricted to one ear; contrasts with bilateral hearing loss.

Variegated babbling   a form of babbling in which successive syllables of different consonant-vowel (CV) combinations are produced.

Verbalization   production of a meaningful word or sequence of words.

Visuospatial perception   interpretation of the relative distance, direction, and position of objects or marks in space.

Vocalization   a sound that is not necessarily speechlike produced by a person's vocal mechanism.

Author Index

McLeavey, B. C., 168
McLoone, B., 221
McManus, M. D., 164
McNaughton, D., 368, 371, 372, 374, 377
McReynolds, L., 46, 47
McWilliams, B. J., 405, 406
Meadow, K., 275
Mehler, J., 42
Meier, J., 406
Meitus, I., 417
Meline, T., 211, 449
Mellits, D., 43, 123
Melnyk, T., 201, 270
Meltzer, L., 325
Meltzoff, A., 42
Membrino, I., 142, 429
Mengurt, I., 85
Menig-Peterson, C., 81
Menyuk, P., 20, 21, 44, 71, 72, 73, 102, 120, 128, 134, 236
Mercer, A. R., 200
Mercer, C. D., 200
Merkin, S., 70
Merrell, K. W., 197
Merrill, E. C., 166
Merrill, M., 154, 307, 436
Mervis, C. A., 71, 172
Mervis, C. B., 172, 179
Metraux, R., 85
Michael, A., 425
Miles, M. C., 325, 342
Milgram, N., 161, 177
Miller, D., 340
Miller, G. A., 332
Miller, J., 20, 71, 119, 140, 163, 166, 169, 170, 176, 177, 181, 218, 367, 368, 370, 371, 372, 377, 416, 425, 426, 428, 429, 445
Miller, L., 25, 26
Miller, M., 81
Miller, P., 67, 448
Miller, S. D., 237
Miller, S. R., 221
Milliken, C. H., 367
Mills, B., 53
Mills, C. J., 388
Mills, P., 427
Mindell, P., 392
Minner, S., 392
Mitchell, J., 355

Mitchell, P., 388
Mitchell-Kernan, C., 80
Mobbs, F., 353, 354
Moeller, M. P., 268, 269, 282, 283
Moerk, E., 53, 54, 55
Moffitt, A., 43
Mohay, H., 276
Molfese, D. L., 369
Molitor, C. B., 372
Moller, K., 405
Monahan, M., 232
Moneka, W., 102
Monroe, N., 19
Monsen, R. B., 272
Montague, J., 159
Montague, M., 209, 221
Montgomery, A., 344, 345, 424
Montgomery, G., 275
Montgomery, J., 457
Moog, J., 275, 281
Moores, D., 23, 259, 275, 283
Moran, M., 77, 209
Mordecai, D., 429
Morehead, D., 76, 119, 120
Morford, J. A., 282
Morgan, D., 343
Morisset, C., 73, 140
Morris, B., 74, 449
Morris, H. L., 405
Morris, R., 195
Morris, S. E., 403
Morrison, D., 122
Morrison, J. A., 171
Morse, P., 43
Morton, J., 236, 239
Mouer, D., 40
Mougey, K., 142, 429
Mowrer, D., 449
Muia, J. A., 388, 393
Mulac, A., 450, 462
Mulhern, S., 183, 464
Mullin, K., 136, 443
Mullins, J., 404
Muma, J., 35, 424, 427, 463, 464
Mundy, P., 239, 245
Murphy, V., 193, 198
Murray-Branch, J., 120
Musiek, F., 47
Musselman, C. R., 275
Myrianthopoulos, N., 405

Nair, R., 198
Nakamura, M., 145
Namy, E., 391
Naremore, R., 72
Natalicio, D., 297
Nation, J., 43, 47, 127, 319, 416, 417
Neils, J., 102
Neimark, E., 340
Nelson, D., 42
Nelson, D. S., 235, 237
Nelson, K., 20, 275
Nelson, L., 121
Nelson, N., 310
Nelson Barlow, N. L., 279
Nemeth, M., 119
Nerbonne, M. A., 283
Neuman, G., 313
Newby, H., 157
Newcomer, P., 307
Newfield, M., 76, 77, 78, 167
Newman, D., 17
Newman, L. R., 259
Newman, P. W., 175
Newsome, L., 168
Nicholls, G., 276
Nichols, R., 340
Nicholson, C. B., 335
Nickerson, N., 80
Nicolosi, L., 307
Nicolson, R. I., 221, 222
Nienhuys, T., 265
Nietupski, J., 166
Niizawa, J., 353
Nippold, M., 80, 98, 124, 132, 208, 221, 319, 331, 332, 333, 334, 335
Nober, E. H., 400
Noel, M., 211
Noffsinger, D., 47
Nolan, M., 159
Noll, M., 450
Norris, J., 29
Norris, R., 329
Northern, J., 40, 159, 259, 260, 264, 265, 272, 279, 281
Nye, C., 214

Oaks, R., 457
Ochs, E., 428
Ockwood, L., 166
O'Connor, L., 342
O'Dell, M. C., 249

Subject Index